Commissioning Editor: Michael Parkinson
Project Development Manager: Janice Urquhart
Project Manager: Nancy Arnott
Designers: Erik Bigland, Jim Farley

NEUROLOGY AND NEUROSURGERY ILLUSTRATED

Kenneth W. Lindsay PhD FRCS

Consultant Neurosurgeon, Institute of Neurological Sciences, Southern General Hospital, Glasgow;
Honorary Clinical Lecturer, University of Glasgow, Glasgow, UK
Formerly Consultant Neurosurgeon, Royal Free Hospital, London;
Honorary Senior Lecturer, Royal Free Hospital School of Medicine, University of London, UK

Ian Bone FRCP FACP

Consultant Neurologist, Institute of Neurological Sciences, Southern General Hospital, Glasgow;
Honorary Clinical Professor, University of Glasgow, Glasgow, UK

Illustrated by

Robin Callander FFPh FMAA AIMBI

Medical Illustrator, Formerly Director of Medical Illustration, University of Glasgow, Glasgow, UK

Foreword by

J. van Gijn MD FRCPE

Professor and Chairman,
University Department of Neurology,
Utrecht,
The Netherlands

FOURTH EDITION

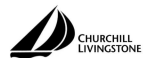

CHURCHILL
LIVINGSTONE

EDINBURGH LONDON NEW YORK OXFORD PHILADELPHIA ST LOUIS SYDNEY TORONTO 2004

CHURCHILL LIVINGSTONE
An imprint of Elsevier Limited

First edition 1986
Second edition 1991
Third edition 1997
Fourth edition 2004

ISBN 0 443 07056 3
International Edition 0 443 07057 1

British Library Cataloguing in Publication Data
A catalogue record for this book is available from the British Library

Library of Congress Cataloging in Publication Data
A catalog record for this book is available from the Library of
Congress

Notice
Medical knowledge is constantly changing. Standard safety
precautions must be followed, but as new research and clinical
experience broaden our knowledge, changes in treatment and drug
therapy may become necessary or appropriate. Readers are advised to
check the most current product information provided by the
manufacturer of each drug to be administered to verify the
recommended dose, the method and duration of administration, and
contraindications. It is the responsibility of the practitioner, relying on
experience and knowledge of the patient, to determine dosages and
the best treatment for each individual patient. Neither the Publisher
nor the authors assume any liability for any injury and/or damage to
persons or property arising from this publication.
The Publisher

**ELSEVIER
SCIENCE**
your source for books,
journals and multimedia
in the health sciences
www.elsevierhealth.com

The
publisher's
policy is to use
**paper manufactured
from sustainable forests**

Printed in China

FOREWORD

In medicine, an ideal textbook is like a good travel guide. Comprehensive but not verbose, lavishly illustrated but not confusing, it navigates the reader to foreign places and it cautions against dangers and disappointments. As the traveller continues to explore the new territory, mental images of towns and countryside gradually replace the maps and descriptions on paper. In the past, neurology has remained terra incognita for many a student because textbooks used to be crammed with long lists of forbidding terms and ancient names, while illustrations often served only to rekindle old apprehensions about the complexity of the nervous system. Only lectures by inspired clinical teachers could overcome these disadvantages – they have been and will always be the backbone of medical education, even though lecturing has for a while gone out of fashion.

The authors of this textbook have chosen a refreshing approach. A neurologist, a neurosurgeon and a medical illustrator have closely collaborated to produce the best possible substitute for real patients. The book has been so successful that three new editions have followed the initial text of 1986. This fourth edition again incorporates new advances in medical and surgical treatment for disorders of the nervous system, from endovascular occlusion of ruptured intracranial aneurysms to dexamethasone as adjunctive medication in bacterial meningitis.

The first pages of the book are rightly devoted to symptoms. The history is by far the most important part of the encounter between patient and physician. Students should not be put off by a list of questions that should be asked. Just think of someone who listens to a travel adventure, told by a friend. In that situation there is no need for a questionnaire – only a few enquiries are necessary to fill in the missing details. When obtaining a medical history, one should act in the same way: make clear that the purpose is to get the patient's own story (and not what previous doctors have said about it) and the questions will come naturally, until the symptoms are clear in the mind's eye.

In brief, this book is an invaluable guide to details of the history, to the neurological examination, to the interpretation of symptoms and signs in terms of the site and the nature of the lesion, and to the management of the most common neurological disorders. I trust this new edition will again pilot thousands of medical students through the enchanting realm of neurology.

2003   J. van Gijn

PREFACE

On writing each new edition, we are always surprised at the number of changes required, despite the relatively short time period. As before, all sections have been updated. In particular the chapter on muscle has been completely revised; the section on investigations incorporates new imaging techniques and new genetic data on disease are included throughout.

With the increasing trend to sub-specialise within clinical neuroscience, we have become increasingly dependent on colleagues for advice. The following have provided many valuable suggestions – Jennifer Brown, Graham Teasdale and Thelekat Varma (neurosurgery), Richard Petty, Keith Muir and Hugh Willison (neurology), David Graham (neuropathology) and Roy Rampling (oncology). We would like to offer sincere thanks to all. Finally we are indebted to Janice Urquhart of Elsevier for her patience and gentle encouragement.

2003

K. W. Lindsay
I. Bone

CONTENTS

CONTENTS

CONTENTS

CONTENTS

GENERAL APPROACH TO HISTORY AND EXAMINATION

NERVOUS SYSTEM – HISTORY

An accurate description of the patient's neurological symptoms is an important aid in establishing the diagnosis; but this must be taken in conjunction with information from other systems, previous medical history, family and social history and current medication. Often the patient's history requires confirmation from a relative or friend.

The following outline indicates the relevant information to obtain for each symptom, although some may require further clarification.

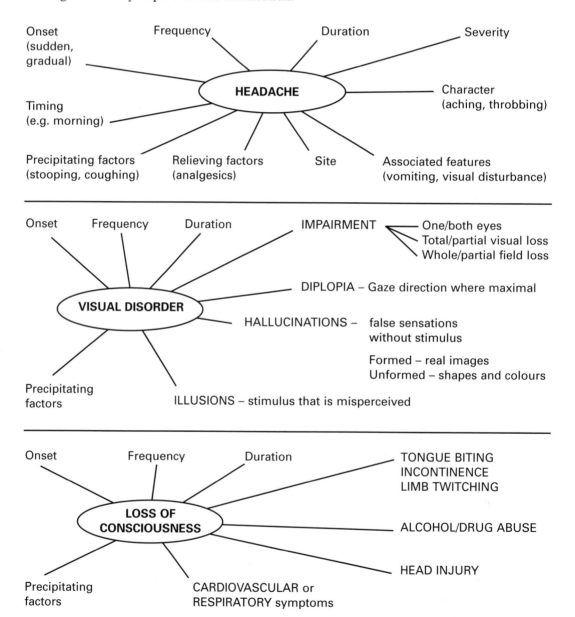

NERVOUS SYSTEM – HISTORY

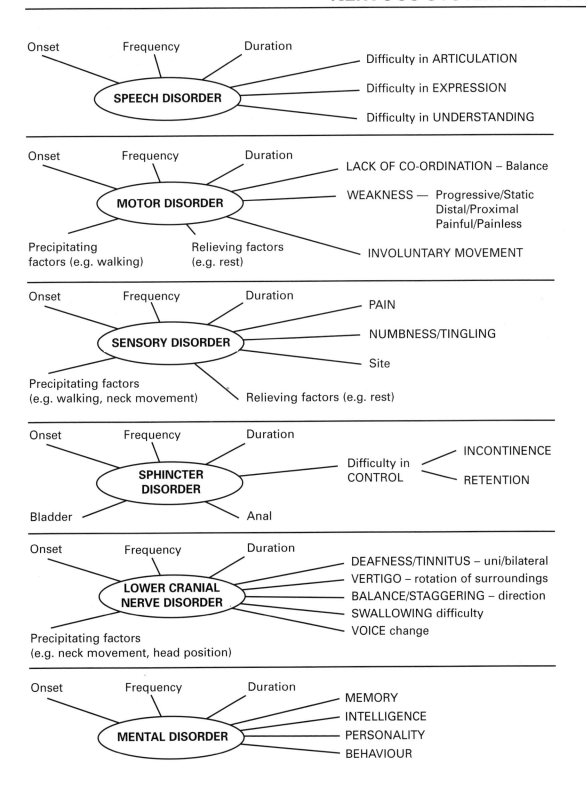

SPEECH DISORDER
- Onset
- Frequency
- Duration
- Difficulty in ARTICULATION
- Difficulty in EXPRESSION
- Difficulty in UNDERSTANDING

MOTOR DISORDER
- Onset
- Frequency
- Duration
- Precipitating factors (e.g. walking)
- Relieving factors (e.g. rest)
- LACK OF CO-ORDINATION – Balance
- WEAKNESS — Progressive/Static Distal/Proximal Painful/Painless
- INVOLUNTARY MOVEMENT

SENSORY DISORDER
- Onset
- Frequency
- Duration
- Precipitating factors (e.g. walking, neck movement)
- Relieving factors (e.g. rest)
- PAIN
- NUMBNESS/TINGLING
- Site

SPHINCTER DISORDER
- Onset
- Frequency
- Duration
- Bladder
- Anal
- Difficulty in CONTROL — INCONTINENCE / RETENTION

LOWER CRANIAL NERVE DISORDER
- Onset
- Frequency
- Duration
- Precipitating factors (e.g. neck movement, head position)
- DEAFNESS/TINNITUS – uni/bilateral
- VERTIGO – rotation of surroundings
- BALANCE/STAGGERING – direction
- SWALLOWING difficulty
- VOICE change

MENTAL DISORDER
- Onset
- Frequency
- Duration
- MEMORY
- INTELLIGENCE
- PERSONALITY
- BEHAVIOUR

3

NERVOUS SYSTEM – EXAMINATION

Neurological disease may produce systemic signs and systemic disease may affect the nervous system. A complete general examination must therefore accompany that of the central nervous system. In particular, note the following

Temperature
Blood pressure
Neck stiffness
Pulse irregularity
Carotid bruit
Cardiac murmurs
Cyanosis/respiratory insufficiency

Evidence of weight loss
Breast lumps
Lymphadenopathy
Hepatic and splenic
enlargement
Prostatic irregularity

Septic source, e.g. teeth, ears,
Skin marks, e.g. rashes
  café-au-lait spots
  angiomata
Anterior fontanelle ⎫
Head circumference ⎭ in baby

CNS examination is described systematically from the head downwards and includes:

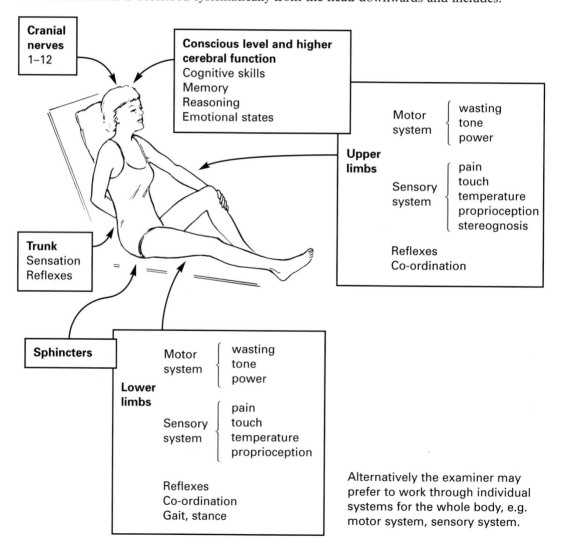

Cranial nerves 1–12

Conscious level and higher cerebral function
Cognitive skills
Memory
Reasoning
Emotional states

Upper limbs

Motor system ⎰ wasting / tone / power

Sensory system ⎰ pain / touch / temperature / proprioception / stereognosis

Reflexes
Co-ordination

Trunk
Sensation
Reflexes

Sphincters

Lower limbs

Motor system ⎰ wasting / tone / power

Sensory system ⎰ pain / touch / temperature / proprioception

Reflexes
Co-ordination
Gait, stance

Alternatively the examiner may prefer to work through individual systems for the whole body, e.g. motor system, sensory system.

EXAMINATION – CONSCIOUS LEVEL ASSESSMENT

A wide variety of systemic and intracranial problems produce depression of conscious level. Accurate assessment and recording are essential to determine deterioration or improvement in a patient's condition. In 1974 Teasdale and Jennett, in Glasgow, developed a system for conscious level assessment. They discarded vague terms such as stupor, semicoma and deep coma, and described conscious level in terms of EYE opening,
VERBAL response and
MOTOR response.

The Glasgow coma scale is now used widely throughout the world. Results are reproducible irrespective of the status of the observer and can be carried out just as reliably by paramedics as by clinicians

EYE OPENING – 4 categories

Spontaneous

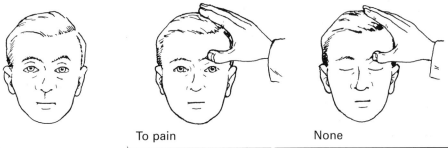

To speech

To pain   None

Supraorbital nerve or
finger nail pressure

VERBAL RESPONSE – 5 categories

Orientated   – Knows place, e.g. Southern General Hospital
                and time, e.g. day, month and year
Confused   – Talking in sentences but disorientated in time and place
Words   – Utters occasional words rather than sentences
Sounds   – Groans or grunts, but no words
None

EXAMINATION – CONSCIOUS LEVEL ASSESSMENT

MOTOR RESPONSE – 5 categories

Obeys commands

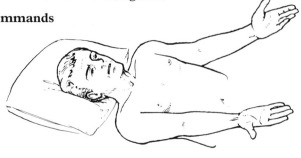

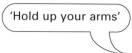

'Hold up your arms'

Pain (Supraorbital pressure)

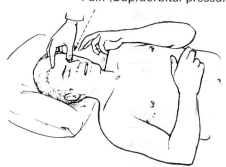

Localising to pain

Apply a painful stimulus to the supraorbital nerve, e.g. rub thumb nail in the supraorbital groove, increasing pressure until a response is obtained. If the patient responds by bringing the hand up beyond the chin = 'localising to pain'. (Pressure to nail beds or sternum at this stage may not differentiate 'localising' from 'flexing'.)

Flexing to pain

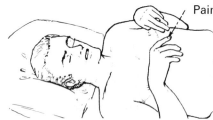

Pain (Nailbed pressure)

If the patient does not localise to supraorbital pressure, apply pressure with a pen or hard object to the nail bed. Record elbow flexion as 'flexing to pain'. Spastic wrist flexion may or may not accompany this response.

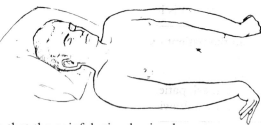

Extending to pain

If in response to the same stimulus elbow extension occurs, record as 'extending to pain'. This is always accompanied by spastic flexion of the wrist.

None

Before recording a patient at this level, ensure that the painful stimulus is adequate.

During examination the motor response may vary. Supraorbital pain may produce an extension response, whereas fingernail pressure produces flexion. Alternatively one arm may localise to pain; the other may flex. When this occurs record the best response during the period of examination (this correlates best with final outcome). For the purpose of conscious level assessment use only the arm response. Leg response to pain gives less consistent results, often producing movements arising from spinal rather than cerebral origin.

EXAMINATION – HIGHER CEREBRAL FUNCTION

COGNITIVE SKILL

	Dominant hemisphere disorders
Listen to language pattern – hesitant – fluent	Expressive dysphasia Receptive dysphasia

Does the patient understand simple/complex
    spoken commands?
    e.g. 'Hold up both arms, touch the right ear
    with the left fifth finger.'
	Receptive dysphasia

Ask the patient to name objects.	Nominal dysphasia
Does the patient read correctly?	Dyslexia
Does the patient write correctly?	Dysgraphia

Ask the patient to perform a numerical calculation,
    e.g. serial 7 test, where 7 is subtracted serially
    from 100.
	Dyscalculia

Can the patient recognise objects? e.g. ask patient to select an object from a group.	Agnosia

	Non-dominant hemisphere disorders
Note patient's ability to find his way around the ward or his home.	Geographical agnosia
Can the patient dress himself?	Dressing apraxia

Note the patient's ability to copy a geometric pattern,
    e.g. ask patient to form a star with matches or
    copy a drawing of a cube.
	Constructional apraxia

Mini Mental Status Examination (MMSE) is used
in the assessment of DEMENTIA (page 125).

EXAMINATION – HIGHER CEREBRAL FUNCTION

MEMORY TEST
Testing requires alertness and is not possible in a confused or dysphasic patient.

IMMEDIATE memory – Digit span – ask patient to repeat a sequence of 5, 6, or 7 random numbers.

RECENT memory – Ask patient to describe present illness, duration of hospital stay or recent events in the news.

REMOTE memory – Ask about events and circumstances occurring more than 5 years previously.

VERBAL memory – Ask patient to remember a sentence or a short story and test after 15 minutes.

VISUAL memory – Ask patient to remember objects on a tray and test after 15 minutes.

Note: **Retrograde amnesia** – loss of memory of events leading up to a brain injury or insult.

Post-traumatic amnesia – permanent loss of memory of events for a period following a brain injury.

REASONING AND PROBLEM SOLVING
Test patient with two-step calculations, e.g. 'I wish to buy 12 articles at 7 pence each. How much change will I receive from £1?'

Ask patient to reverse 3 or 4 random numbers.

Ask patient to explain proverbs.

Ask patient to sort playing cards into suits.

The examiner must compare patient's present reasoning ability with expected abilities based on job history and/or school work.

EMOTIONAL STATE
Note: Anxiety or excitement
Depression or apathy
Emotional behaviour
Uninhibited behaviour
Slowness of movement or responses
Personality type or change.

CRANIAL NERVE EXAMINATION

OLFACTORY NERVE (I)

Test both perception and identification using aromatic non-irritant materials that avoid stimulation of trigeminal nerve fibres in the nasal mucosa, e.g. soap, tobacco.

One nostril is closed while the patient sniffs with the other.

OPTIC NERVE (II)

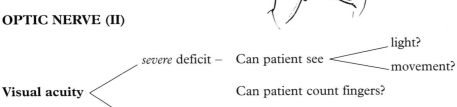

Visual acuity

severe deficit – Can patient see light? movement?

Can patient count fingers?

mild deficit – Record reading acuity with wall or hand chart.

N.B. *Refractive error* (i.e. inadequate focussing on the retina, e.g. hypermetropia, myopia) can be overcome by testing reading acuity through a pinhole. This concentrates a thin beam of vision on the macula.

Jaeger type card for near vision, labelled according to size [Normal acuity is between J1–J4].

Visual acuity is expressed as:

$$\frac{d}{D}$$

e.g. $\frac{6}{12}$

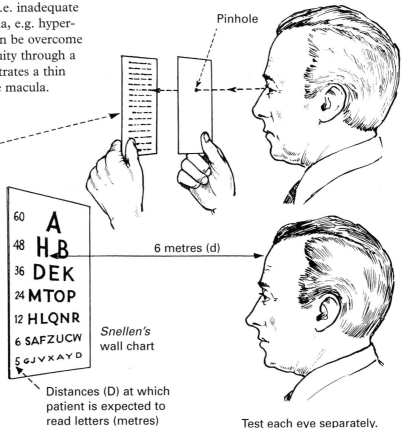

Pinhole

6 metres (d)

60	A
48	H B
36	DEK
24	MTOP
12	HLQNR
6	SAFZUCW
5	GJVXAYD

Snellen's wall chart

Distances (D) at which patient is expected to read letters (metres)

Test each eye separately.

CRANIAL NERVE EXAMINATION

Visual fields

Gross testing by CONFRONTATION. Compare the patient's fields of vision by advancing a moving finger or, more accurately, a red 5 mm pin from the extreme periphery towards the fixation point. This maps out 'cone' vision. A 2 mm pin will define central field defects which may only manifest as a loss of colour perception.

In the temporal portion of the visual field the physiological blind spot may be detected. A 2 mm object should disappear here.

The patient must fixate on the examiner's pupil.

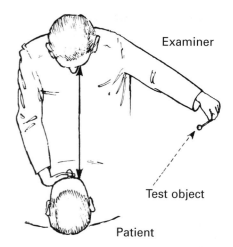

Peripheral visual fields are more sensitive to a moving target and are tested with a GOLDMANN PERIMETER.

The patient fixes on a central point. A point of light is moved centrally from the extreme periphery. The position at which the patient observes the target is marked on a chart. Repeated testing from multiple directions provides an accurate record of visual fields.

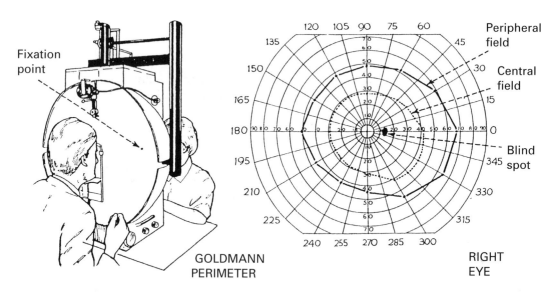

Central fields are charted with either a Goldmann perimeter using a small light source of lesser intensity or a TANGENT (BJERRUM) SCREEN. The HUMPHREY FIELD ANALYSER provides an alternative and particularly sensitive method of testing central fields. This records the *threshold* at which the patient observes a static light source of increasing intensity.

CRANIAL NERVE EXAMINATION

Optic fundus (*Ophthalmoscopy*)

Ask the patient to fixate on a distant object away from any bright light. Use the right eye to examine the patient's right eye and the left eye to examine the patient's left eye.

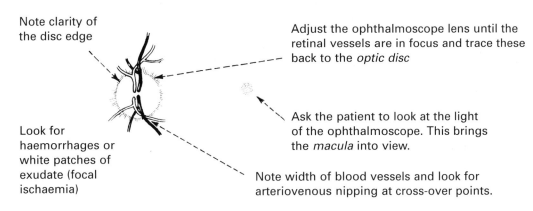

Note clarity of the disc edge

Adjust the ophthalmoscope lens until the retinal vessels are in focus and trace these back to the *optic disc*

Look for haemorrhages or white patches of exudate (focal ischaemia)

Ask the patient to look at the light of the ophthalmoscope. This brings the *macula* into view.

Note width of blood vessels and look for arteriovenous nipping at cross-over points.

If small pupil size prevents fundal examination, then dilate pupil with a quick acting mydriatic (homatropine). This is contraindicated if either an acute expanding lesion or glaucoma is suspected.

Pupils

Note: Size (small = miosis / large = mydriasis)

Shape

Equality

Reaction to light: both pupils constrict when light is shone in either eye

Reaction to accommodation and convergence: pupil constriction occurs when gaze is transferred to a near point object.

A lesion of the *optic nerve* will abolish pupillary response to light on the same side as well as in the contralateral eye.

When light is shone in the *normal* eye, it and the contralateral pupil will constrict.

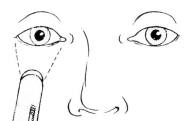

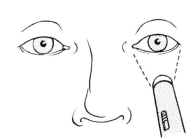

CRANIAL NERVE EXAMINATION

OCULOMOTOR (III), TROCHLEAR (IV) AND ABDUCENS (VI) NERVES

A lesion of the III nerve produces impairment of eye and lid movement as well as disturbance of pupillary response.

Pupil: The pupil dilates and becomes 'fixed' to light.

Shine torch in *affected* eye – contralateral pupil constricts (its III nerve intact). Absent or impaired response in illuminated eye.

When light is shone into the *normal* eye, only the pupil on that side constricts.

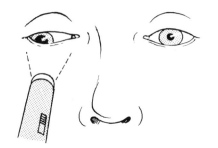

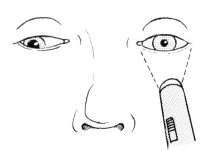

Ptosis: Ptosis is present if the eyelid droops over the pupil when the eyes are fully open. Since the levator palpebrae muscle contains both skeletal and smooth muscle, ptosis signifies either a III nerve palsy or a sympathetic lesion and is more prominent with the former.

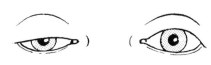

Ocular movement

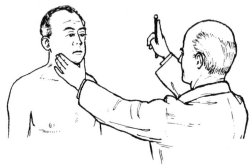

Steady the patient's head and ask him to follow an object held at arm's length. Observe the full range of horizontal and vertical eye movements.

Note any *malalignment or limitation of range.*

Examine eye movements in the six different directions of gaze representing maximal individual muscle strength.

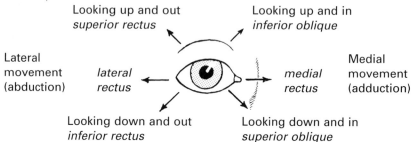

Looking up and out
superior rectus

Looking up and in
inferior oblique

Lateral movement (abduction)

lateral rectus

medial rectus

Medial movement (adduction)

Looking down and out
inferior rectus

Looking down and in
superior oblique

CRANIAL NERVE EXAMINATION

Question patient about *diplopia*; the patient is more likely to notice this before the examiner can detect impairment of eye movement. If present:
- note the *direction of maximum displacement* of the images and determine the pair of muscles involved
- identify the source of the *outer image* (from the defective eye) using a transparent coloured lens.

e.g.

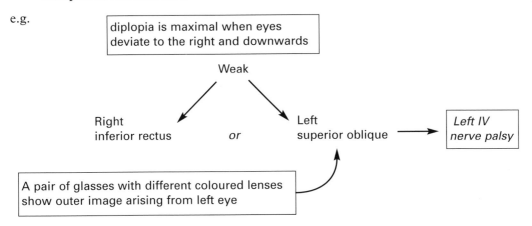

Conjugate movement: Note the ability of the eyes to move together (conjugately) in horizontal or vertical direction or tendency for gaze to fix in one particular direction.

Nystagmus: This is an upset in the normal balance of eye control. A slow drift in one direction is followed by a fast corrective movement. Nystagmus is maximal when the eyes are turned in the direction of the fast phase. Nystagmus 'direction' is usually described in terms of the fast phase and may be horizontal or vertical. Test as for other eye movements, but remember that 'physiological' nystagmus can occur when the eyes deviate to the endpoint of gaze.

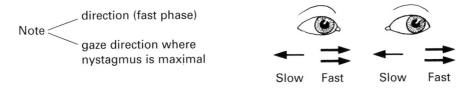

e.g. Nystagmus to the left maximal on left lateral gaze.

CRANIAL NERVE EXAMINATION

TRIGEMINAL NERVE (V)

Test *pain* (pin prick) sensation } over
temperature (cold object or } whole
hot/cold tubes) } face
light touch

Compare each side.
Map out the sensory deficit,
testing from the abnormal
to the normal region.

Does distribution involve
– a *root/division* pattern?
– or a *brain stem* 'onion skin' pattern?

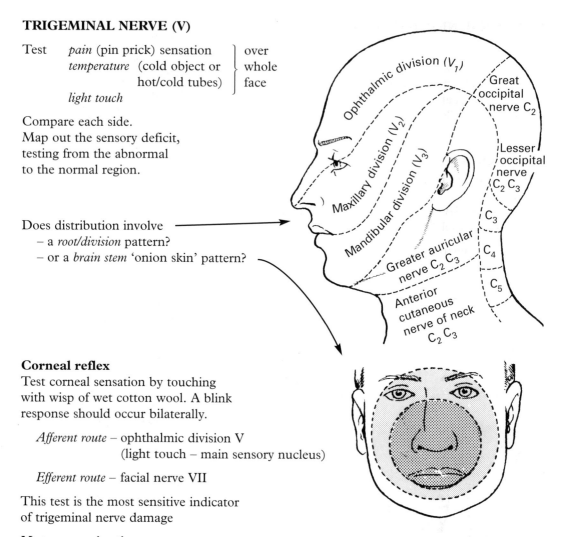

Corneal reflex
Test corneal sensation by touching
with wisp of wet cotton wool. A blink
response should occur bilaterally.

Afferent route – ophthalmic division V
(light touch – main sensory nucleus)

Efferent route – facial nerve VII

This test is the most sensitive indicator
of trigeminal nerve damage

Motor examination
Observe for wasting and thinning of temporalis muscle – 'hollowing out' the temporalis fossa.

Ask the patient to clamp jaws together. Feel temporalis and masseter muscles. Attempt to open patient's jaws by applying pressure to chin. Ask patient to open mouth. If pterygoid muscles are weak the jaw will deviate to the weak side, being pushed over by the unopposed pterygoid muscles of the good side.

CRANIAL NERVE EXAMINATION

TRIGEMINAL NERVE (V) *(cont'd)*

Jaw jerk

Ask patient to relax jaw. Place finger
on the chin and tap with hammer:
Slight jerk – normal
Increased jerk – bilateral upper neuron lesion.

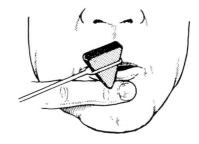

FACIAL NERVE (VII)

Observe patient as he talks and smiles, watching for:
– eye closure
– asymmetrical elevation of one corner of mouth
– flattening of nasolabial fold.

Patient is then instructed to:

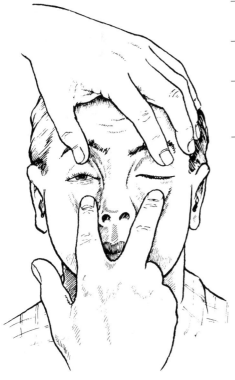

– wrinkle forehead (frontalis)
  (by looking upwards)

– close eyes while examiner attempts
  to open them (orbicularis oculi)

– purse lips while examiner
  presses cheeks
  (buccinator)

– show teeth
  (orbicularis oris)

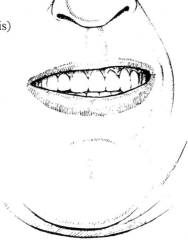

Taste may be tested by using sugar, tartaric acid or sodium chloride. A small quantity of each
substance is placed anteriorly on the appropriate side of the protruded tongue.

15

CRANIAL NERVE EXAMINATION

AUDITORY NERVE (VIII)

Cochlear component

Test by whispering numbers into one ear while masking hearing in the other ear by occluding and rubbing the external meatus. If hearing is impaired, examine external meatus and the tympanic membrane with auroscope to exclude wax or infection.

Differentiate conductive (middle ear) deafness from perceptive (nerve) deafness by:

1. **Weber's test:** Hold base of tuning fork (256 or 512 Hz) against the vertex. Ask patient if sound is heard more loudly in one ear.

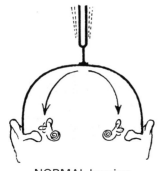 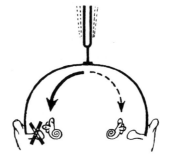 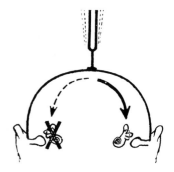

NORMAL hearing

CONDUCTIVE DEAFNESS
Sound is louder in affected ear
since distraction from external
sounds is reduced in that ear

NERVE DEAFNESS
Sound is louder in
the normal ear

2. **Rinne's test:** Hold the base of a vibrating tuning fork against the mastoid bone. Ask the patient if note is heard. When note disappears – hold tuning fork near the external meatus. Patient should hear sound again since air conduction via the ossicles is better than bone conduction.

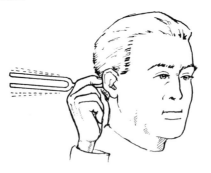

In *conductive deafness*, bone conduction is better than air conduction.
In *nerve deafness*, both bone and air conduction are impaired.

Further auditory testing and examination of the **vestibular component** requires specialised investigation (see pages 62–63).

CRANIAL NERVE EXAMINATION

GLOSSOPHARYNGEAL NERVE (IX): VAGUS NERVE (X)

These nerves are considered jointly since they are examined together and their actions are seldom individually impaired.

Note patient's *voice* – if there is vocal cord paresis (X nerve palsy), voice may be high pitched. (Vocal cord examination is best left to an ENT specialist.)

Note any *swallowing* difficulty or nasal regurgitation of fluids.

Ask patient to open mouth and say *'Ah'*. Note any asymmetry of palatal movements (X nerve palsy).

Gag reflex
Depress patient's tongue and touch palate, pharynx or tonsil on one side until the patient 'gags'. Compare sensitivity on each side (*afferent* route – IX nerve) and observe symmetry of palatal contraction (*efferent route* – X nerve).

Absent gag reflex = loss of sensation and/or loss of motor power. (Taste in the posterior third of the tongue (IX) is impractical to test).

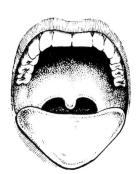

'Ah'

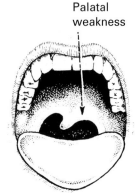

Palatal weakness

Uvula swings due to unopposed muscle action on one side

ACCESSORY NERVE (XI)

Sternomastoid
Ask patient to rotate head against resistance. Compare power and muscle bulk on each side. Also compare each side with the patient pulling head forward against resistance.

N.B. The left sternomastoid turns the head to the right and *vice versa*.

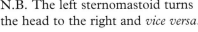

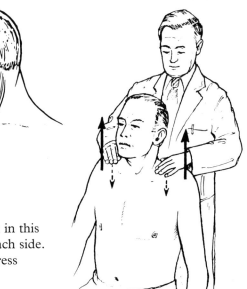

Trapezius
Ask patient to 'shrug' shoulders and to hold them in this position against resistance. Compare power on each side. Patient should manage to resist any effort to depress shoulders.

17

CRANIAL NERVE EXAMINATION

HYPOGLOSSAL NERVE (XII)

Ask patient to open mouth; inspect tongue.

Look for – evidence of atrophy (increased folds, wasting)
         – fibrillation (small wriggling movements).

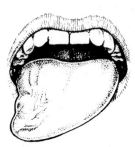

Ask patient to protrude tongue. Note any difficulty or deviation. (N.B. apparent deviation may occur with facial weakness – if present, assess tongue in relation to teeth.)
Protruded tongue deviates towards side of weakness.
Non protruded tongue cannot move to the opposite side.
Dysarthria and dysphagia are minimal.

EXAMINATION – UPPER LIMBS

MOTOR SYSTEM

Appearance

Note: – any *asymmetry* or *deformity*

– muscle *wasting*
– muscle *hypertrophy* } If in doubt, measure circumference at fixed distance above/below joint. Note muscle group involved.

– muscle *fasciculation*   irregular, non-rhythmical contraction of muscle fascicules, increased after exercise and on tapping muscle surface.

– muscle *myokimia*   a rapid rippling of muscle fibres, particularly in orbicularis oculi but occasionally in large muscles, after exercise or with fatigue – 'Benign Fasciculation'.

Tone

Ensure that the patient is relaxed, and assess tone by alternately flexing and extending the elbow or wrist.

Note: – decrease in tone

– increase in tone {
'Clasp-knife': the initial resistance to the movement is suddenly overcome (upper motor neuron lesion).
'Lead-pipe': a steady increase in resistance throughout the movement (extrapyramidal lesion).
'Cog-wheel': ratchet-like increase in resistance (extrapyramidal lesion).

Power

If a pyramidal weakness is suspect (i.e. a weakness arising from damage to the motor cortex or descending motor tracts (see pages 191–195) the following test is simple, quick, yet sensitive.

Ask the patient to hold arms outstretched with the hands supinated for up to one minute. The eyes are closed (otherwise visual compensation occurs). The weak arm gradually pronates and drifts downwards.

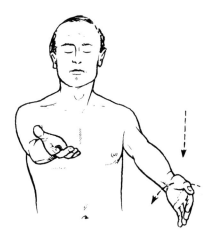

With possible involvement at the spinal root or nerve level (lower motor neuron), it is essential to test individual muscle groups to help localise the lesion.

When testing muscle groups, think of *root* and *nerve* supply.

EXAMINATION – UPPER LIMBS

Test for *Serratus anterior:*

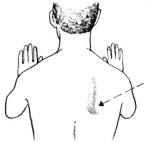

C5, C6, C7 roots
Long thoracic nerve

Patient presses
arms against wall

Look for winging of
scapula i.e. rises
from chest wall

Shoulder abduction

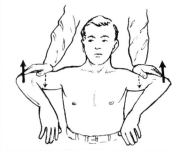

Deltoid:
C5, C6 roots
Axillary nerve

Arm (at more
than 15° from
the vertical)
abducts against
resistance

Elbow flexion

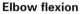

Biceps: **C5, C6** roots
Musculocutaneous
nerve

Arm flexed
against resistance
with the hand
fully supinated

Elbow extension

Triceps: C6, **C7**, C8 roots
Radial nerve

Patient
extends
arm against
resistance

Brachioradialis: C5, **C6** roots.
Radial nerve

Arm flexed against
resistance with hand
in mid-position
between pronation
and supination

Finger extension

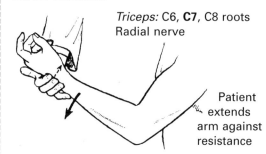

Extensor digitorum:
C7, C8 roots
Posterior
interosseous nerve

Patient extends
fingers against
resistance

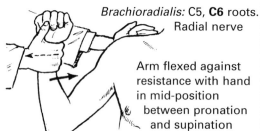

Thumb extension – terminal phalanx
Extensor pollicis longus and brevis: **C7**, C8 roots
Posterior interosseous nerve
Thumb is extended against resistance

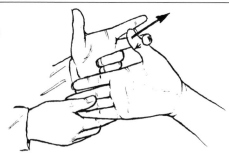

**Finger flexion –
terminal phalanx**

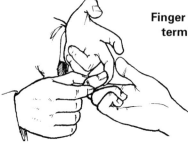

Flexor digitorum profundus I and II: C7, **C8** roots
Median nerve
Flexor digitorum profundus III and IV: C7, **C8** roots
Ulnar nerve

Examiner tries to extend patient's flexed terminal phalanges

EXAMINATION – UPPER LIMBS

Thumb opposition

Opponens pollicis: CB, **T1** roots. Median nerve

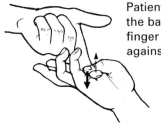

Patient tries to touch the base of the 5th finger with thumb against resistance

Finger abduction

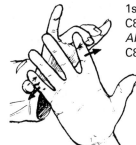

1st *dorsal interosseus:* C8, **T1** roots. Ulnar nerve
Abductor digiti minimi: C8, **T1** roots. Ulnar nerve

Fingers abducted against resistance

[Note: not all muscle groups are included in the foregoing, but only those required to identify and differentiate nerve and root lesions.]

SENSATION

Pain

Pin prick with a sterile pin provides a simple method of testing this important modality. Firstly, check that the patient detects the pin as 'sharp', i.e. painful, then rapidly test each dermatome in turn.

Memorising the dermatome distribution is simplified by noting that 'C7' extends down the middle finger.

If pin prick is impaired, then more carefully map out the extent of the abnormality, moving from the abnormal to the normal areas.

Light touch

This is tested in a similar manner, using a wisp of cotton wool.

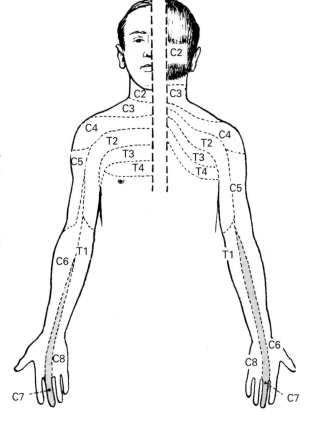

Temperature

Temperature testing seldom provides any additional information. If required, use a cold object or hot and cold test tubes.

21

EXAMINATION – UPPER LIMBS

Joint position sense

Hold the sides of the patient's finger or thumb and demonstrate 'up and down' movements.

Repeat with the patient's eyes closed. Ask patient to specify the direction of movement.

Ask the patient, with eyes closed, to touch his nose with his forefinger or to bring forefingers together with the arms outstretched.

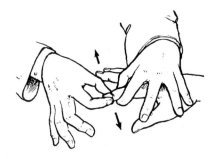

Vibration

Place a vibrating tuning fork (usually 128 c/s) on a bony prominence, e.g. radius. Ask the patient to indicate when the vibration, if felt, ceases. If impaired, move more proximally and repeat. Vibration testing is of value in the early detection of demyelinating disease and peripheral neuropathy, but otherwise is of limited benefit.

If the above sensory functions are normal and a cortical lesion is suspected, it is useful to test for the following:

Two point discrimination: the ability to discriminate two blunt points when simultaneously applied to the finger, 5 mm apart (cf, 4 cm in the legs).

Blunt ends

5 mm

Sensory inattention (perceptual rivalry): the ability to detect stimuli (pin prick or touch) in both limbs, when applied to both limbs simultaneously.

Stereognosis: the ability to recognise objects placed in the hand.

Graphaesthesia: the ability to recognise numbers or letters traced out on the palm.

REFLEXES

Biceps jerk C5, C6 roots. Musculocutaneous nerve

Supinator jerk C6, C7 roots. Radial nerve

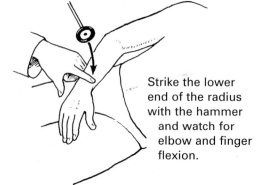

Ensure patient's arm is relaxed and slightly flexed. Palpate the biceps tendon with the thumb and strike with tendon hammer. Look for elbow flexion and biceps contraction.

Strike the lower end of the radius with the hammer and watch for elbow and finger flexion.

EXAMINATION – UPPER LIMBS

Triceps jerk

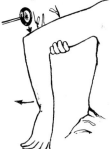

C6, **C7,** C8 roots.
Radial nerve.

Strike the patient's
elbow a few inches
above the olecranon
process. Look for
elbow extension and
triceps contraction.

Hoffman reflex C7, C8

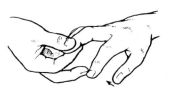

Flick the patient's
terminal phalanx,
suddenly stretching
the flexor tendon
on release. Thumb
flexion indicates
hyperreflexia. (May be present
in normal subjects with brisk
tendon reflexes.)

Reflex enhancement
When reflexes are difficult to elicit, enhancement occurs if the patient is asked to 'clench the teeth'.

CO-ORDINATION
Inco-ordination (ataxia) is often a prominent feature of cerebellar disease (see page 180).
Prior to testing, ensure that power and proprioception are normal.

Inco-ordination
Finger – nose testing

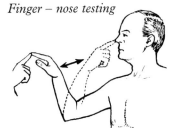

Ask patient to touch his nose with finger (eyes open).

Look for jerky movements – DYSMETRIA
or an INTENTION TREMOR (tremor
only occurring on voluntary movement).

Ask patient to alternately touch
his own nose then the examiner's
finger as fast as he can. This may
exaggerate the intention tremor
and may demonstrate
DYSDIADOCHOKINESIA –
an inability to perform rapidly alternating movements.

This may also be shown by asking the patient to rapidly supinate and pronate the forearms
or to perform rapid and repeated tapping movements.

Arm bounce

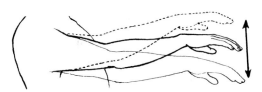

Downward pressure and sudden release
of the patient's outstretched arm causes
excessive swinging.

Rebound phenomenon

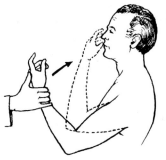

Ask the patient to
flex elbow against
resistance.
Sudden release
may cause the
hand to strike the
face due to delay
in triceps
contraction.

23

EXAMINATION – TRUNK

SENSATION

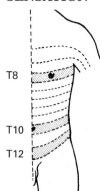

Test pin prick and light touch in dermatome distribution as for the upper limbs.

Levels to remember: T5 – at *nipple*
T10 – at *umbilicus*
T12 – at *inguinal ligament*.

Abdominal reflexes: T7 – T12 roots. Stroke or lightly scratch the skin towards the umbilicus in each quadrant in turn. Look for abdominal muscle contraction and note if absent or impaired.
(N.B. Reflexes may normally be absent in obesity, after pregnancy, or after abdominal operations.)

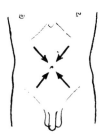

Cremasteric reflex: L1, L2 root. Scratch inner thigh. Observe contraction of cremasteric muscle causing testicular elevation.

SPHINCTERS
Examine abdomen for distended bladder.
Note evidence of urinary or faecal incontinence.
Note tone of anal sphincter during rectal examination.
Anal reflex: S4, S5 roots. A scratch on the skin beside the anus causes a reflex contraction of the anal sphincter.

EXAMINATION – LOWER LIMBS

MOTOR SYSTEM

Appearance: Note: – *asymmetry* or *deformity*
– muscle *wasting*
– muscle *hypertrophy* } as in the upper limbs
– muscle *fasciculation*
– muscle *myokimia*

Tone
Try to relax the patient and alternately flex and extend the knee joint. Note the resistance.
Roll the patient's legs from side to side. Suddenly lift the thigh and note the response in the lower leg. With increased tone the leg kicks upwards.

Clonus
Ensure that the patient is relaxed. Apply sudden and sustained flexion to the ankle. A few oscillatory beats may occur in the normal subject, but when this persists it indicates increased tone.

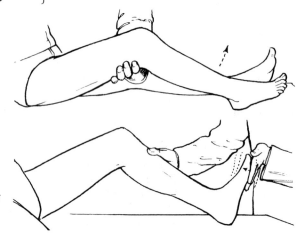

24

EXAMINATION – LOWER LIMBS

Power

When testing each muscle group, think of *root* and *nerve* supply.

Hip flexion

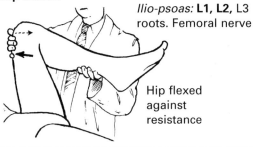

Ilio-psoas: **L1, L2,** L3 roots. Femoral nerve

Hip flexed against resistance

Hip extension

Gluteus maximus: **L5, S1,** S2 roots. Inferior gluteal nerve

Patient attempts to keep heel on bed against resistance

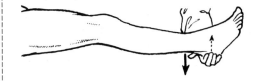

Hip abduction

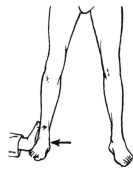

Gluteus medius and minimus and tensor fasciae latae: **L4, L5,** S1 roots. Superior gluteal nerve

Patient lying on back tries to abduct the leg against resistance

Hip adduction

Adductors: **L2, L3,** L4 roots. Obturator nerve

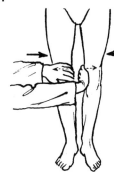

Patient lying on back tries to pull knees together against resistance

Knee flexion

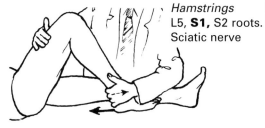

Hamstrings L5, **S1,** S2 roots. Sciatic nerve

Patient pulls heel towards the buttock and tries to maintain this position against resistance

Knee extension

Quadriceps: L2, **L3, L4** roots. Femoral nerve

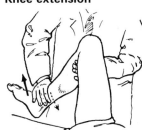

Patient tries to extend knee against resistance

Dorsiflexion

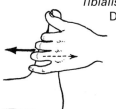

Tibialis anterior: **L4,** L5 roots. Deep peroneal nerve

Patient dorsiflexes the ankle against resistance. May have difficulty in walking on heels

Plantarflexion

Gastrocnemius, soleus: **S1, S2,** roots. Tibial nerve.

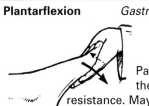

Patient plantarflexes the ankle against resistance. May have difficulty in walking on toes before weakness can be directly detected

25

EXAMINATION – LOWER LIMBS

Toe extension

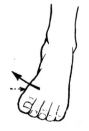

Extensor hallucis longus, extensor digitorum longus: **L5**, S1 roots.
Deep peroneal nerve

Patient dorsiflexes the toes against resistance

Inversion

Tibialis posterior: **L4, L5** root.
Tibial nerve

Patient inverts foot
against resistance

Eversion

Peroneus longus and brevis: **L5, S1** roots.
Superficial peroneal nerve

Patient everts foot
against resistance

SENSATION

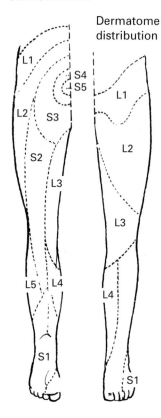

Dermatome
distribution

Test:
Pain   } follow the dermatome
Light touch } distribution as in
(Temperature) } the upper limb.

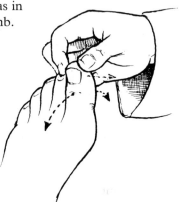

Joint position sense
Firstly, demonstrate flexion
and extension movements of
the big toe. Then ask patient
to specify the direction with
the eyes closed.

If deficient, test ankle joint
sense in the same way.

Vibration
Test vibration perception by placing a tuning fork
on the malleolus. If deficient, move up to the head
of the fibula or to the anterior superior iliac spine.

EXAMINATION – LOWER LIMBS

REFLEXES

Knee jerk: L2, L3, **L4** roots.

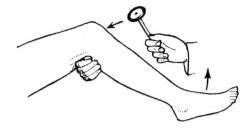

Ensure that the patient's leg is relaxed by resting it over examiner's arm or by hanging it over the edge of the bed. Tap the patellar tendon with the hammer and observe quadriceps contraction. Note impairment or exaggeration.

Ankle jerk: S1, S2 roots.

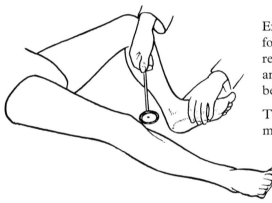

Externally rotate the patient's leg. Hold the foot in slight dorsiflexion. Ensure the foot is relaxed by palpating the tendon of tibialis anterior. If this is taut, then no ankle jerk will be elicited.

Tap the Achilles tendon and watch for calf muscle contraction and plantarflexion.

Reflex enhancement
When reflexes are difficult to elicit, they may be enhanced by asking the patient to clench the teeth or to try to pull clasped hands apart (Jendressik's manoeuvre).

Plantar response
Check that the big toe is relaxed. Stroke the lateral aspect of the sole and across the ball of the foot. Note the first movement of the big toe. Flexion should occur. Extension due to contraction of extensor hallucis longus (a 'Babinski' reflex) indicates an upper motor neuron lesion. This is usually accompanied by synchronous contraction of the knee flexors and tensor fasciae latae.

Elicit Chaddock's sign by stimulating the lateral border of the foot. The big toe extends with upper motor neuron lesions.

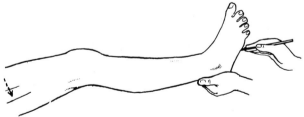

To avoid ambiguity do not touch the innermost aspect of the sole or the toes themselves.

EXAMINATION – POSTURE AND GAIT

CO-ORDINATION

Ask patient to repeatedly run the heel from the opposite knee down the shin to the big toe. Look for ATAXIA (inco-ordination). Ask patient to repeatedly tap the floor with the foot. Note any DYSDIADOCHOKINESIA (difficulty with rapidly alternating movement)

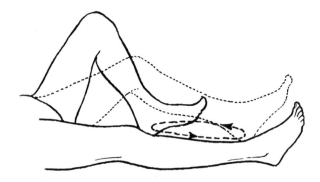

Romberg's test

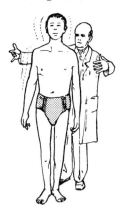

Ask patient to stand with the heels together, first with the eyes open, then with the eyes closed.

Note any excessive postural swaying or loss of balance

Present when eyes open or closed = cerebellar deficit (cerebellar ataxia)

Present only when eyes are closed ('positive' Romberg's) = proprioceptive deficit (sensory ataxia)

GAIT

Note:
  – Length of step and width of base
  – Abnormal leg movements (e.g. excessively high step)
  – Instability (gait ataxia)
  – Associated postural movements (e.g. pelvic swinging)

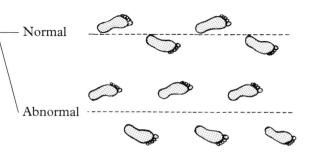

Normal

Abnormal

If normal, repeat with *tandem* walking, i.e. heel to toe. This will exaggerate any instability.

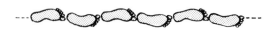

EXAMINATION OF THE UNCONSCIOUS PATIENT

HISTORY

Questioning relatives, friends or the ambulance team is an essential part of the assessment of the unconscious or the unco-operative patient.

Has the patient sustained a head injury – leading to admission, or in the preceding weeks?
Did the patient collapse suddenly?
Did limb twitching occur?
Have symptoms occurred in the preceding weeks?
Has the patient suffered a previous illness?
Does the patient take medication?

GENERAL EXAMINATION

Lack of patient co-operation does not limit general examination and this may reveal important diagnostic signs. In addition to those features described on page 4, also look for signs of head injury, needle marks on the arm and evidence of tongue biting. Also note the smell of alcohol, but beware of attributing the patient's clinical state solely to alcohol excess.

NEUROLOGICAL EXAMINATION

Conscious level: This assessment is of major importance. It not only serves as an immediate prognostic guide, but also provides a baseline with which future examinations may be compared. Assess conscious level as described previously (page 5) in terms of eye opening, verbal response and motor response.

For research purposes, a score was applied for each response, with 'flexion' subdivided into 'normal' and 'spastic flexion', giving a total coma score of '15 points'. Although of value in research, this has led to some confusion since most coma observation charts (page 5) use a '14 point scale' with 5 points on the motor score

Eye opening		Verbal response		Motor response	
Spontaneous	4	Orientated	5	Obeying commands	6
To speech	3	Confused	4	Localising	5
To pain	2	Words	3	Normal flexion	4
None	1	Sounds	2	Spastic flexion	3
		None	1	Extension	2
				None	1

For clinical purposes, the '14 point scale' provides more consistent recording. It is also important to avoid the tendency to simply quote the patient's total score. This can be misleading. Always describe the conscious level in terms of the actual responses i.e. 'no eye opening, no verbal response and extending'.

Pupil response
Fundi
Corneal reflex
    – tone
Limb – reflexes
    – plantar response

Lack of patient co-operation does not prevent objective assessment of these features described before, but elucidation of other relevant neurological signs requires a different approach.

EXAMINATION OF THE UNCONSCIOUS PATIENT

Eye movements

Observe any **spontaneous** eye movements.   (Eyes held open by examiner)

Note whether the movements, if present, are *conjugate* (i.e. the eyes move in parallel) or *dysconjugate* (i.e. the eyes do not move in parallel). These ocular movements assess midbrain and pontine function.

Elicit the **oculocephalic (doll's eye) reflex.**

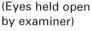 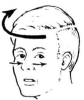

Rotation or flexion/extension of the head in a comatose patient produces transient eye movements in a direction opposite to that of the movement.

Elicit the **oculovestibular reflex** (caloric testing, see page 63).

Visual fields

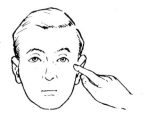

In the unco-operative patient, the examiner may detect a hemianopic field defect when 'menacing' from one side fails to produce a 'blink'.

Facial weakness

Failure to 'grimace' on one side in response to bilateral supraorbital pain indicates a facial weakness.

Supraorbital pain

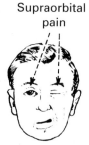

Limb weakness

Detect by comparing the response in the limbs to painful stimuli. If pain produces an *asymmetric* response, then limb weakness is present. (If the patient 'localises' with one arm, hold this down and retest to ensure that a similar response cannot be elicited from the other limb.)

Supraorbital pain

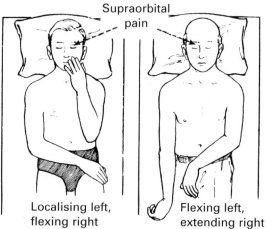

e.g.

Localising left, flexing right

Flexing left, extending right

Both patients are in coma; both have an asymmetric response to pain indicating a right arm weakness and focal brain damage.

Pain stimulus applied to the toe nails or Achilles tendon similarly tests power in the lower limbs. Variation in tone, reflexes or plantar responses between each side also indicates a focal deficit. In practice, if the examiner fails to detect a difference in response to painful stimuli, these additional features seldom provide convincing evidence.

THE NEUROLOGICAL OBSERVATION CHART

Despite major advances in intracranial investigative techniques, none has replaced clinical assessment for monitoring the patient's neurological state. The neurological observation chart produced by Jennett and Teasdale incorporates the most relevant clinical features, i.e. *coma scale (eye opening, verbal and motor response)*, *pupil size* and *reaction to light, limb responses* and *vital signs*. The frequency of observation (normally 2-hourly) depends on the individual patient's needs. The chart enables immediate evaluation of the trend in the patient's clinical state.

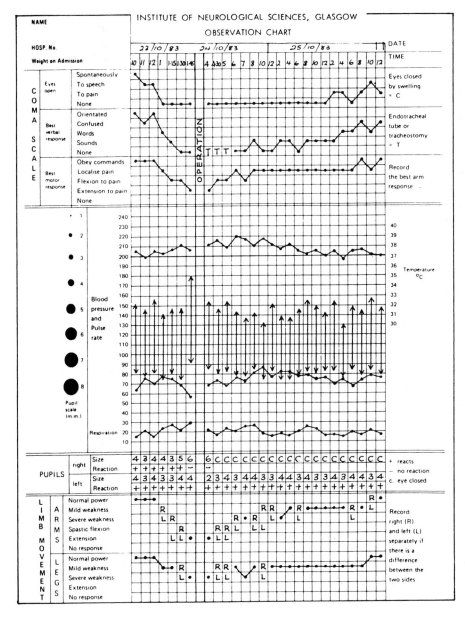

By permission of the Nursing Times

31

INVESTIGATIONS OF THE CENTRAL AND PERIPHERAL NERVOUS SYSTEMS

SKULL X-RAY

With the development of more advanced imaging techniques, skull X-ray is now less often used, but may still provide useful information.

Standard views:
Lateral
Postero-anterior
Towne's (fronto-occipital)

Learn to distinguish normal skull markings and sites of calcification (pineal and choroid plexus).

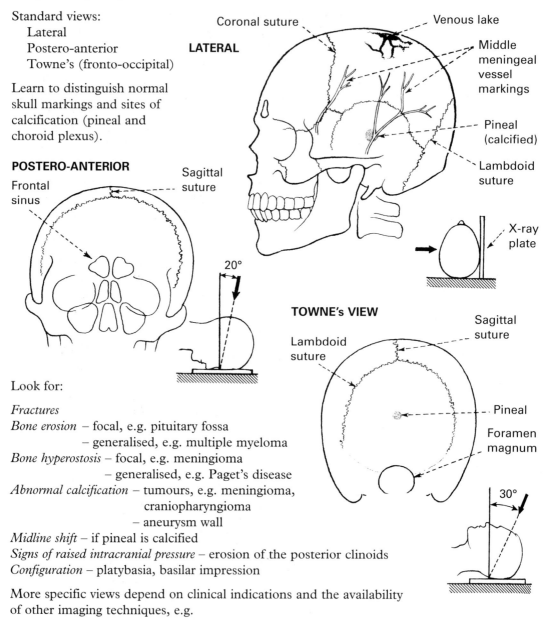

Look for:

Fractures
Bone erosion – focal, e.g. pituitary fossa
           – generalised, e.g. multiple myeloma
Bone hyperostosis – focal, e.g. meningioma
           – generalised, e.g. Paget's disease
Abnormal calcification – tumours, e.g. meningioma,
           craniopharyngioma
           – aneurysm wall
Midline shift – if pineal is calcified
Signs of raised intracranial pressure – erosion of the posterior clinoids
Configuration – platybasia, basilar impression

More specific views depend on clinical indications and the availability of other imaging techniques, e.g.

Base of skull (submentovertical) – cranial nerve palsies
Optic foramina – progressive blindness
Sella turcica – visual field defects
Petrous/internal auditory meatus – sensorineural deafness.

COMPUTERISED TOMOGRAPHY (CT) SCANNING

The development of this non-invasive technique in the 1970s revolutionised the investigative approach to intracranial pathology and it is now used routinely for 'body' and spine.

A pencil beam of X-ray traverses the patient's head and a diametrically opposed detector measures the extent of its absorption. Computer processing, multiple rotating beams and detectors arranged in a complete circle around the patient's head enable determination of absorption values for multiple small blocks of tissue (voxels). Reconstruction of these areas on a two-dimensional display (pixels) provides the characteristic CT scan appearance. For routine scanning, slices are 3–5 mm wide. With the latest 'spiral' or 'helical' CT scanners the patient moves through the field during scanning so that the X-ray beams describe a helical path. This considerably reduces scanning time and is of particular value when slices of 1–2 mm thickness provide greater detail. These 'high definition' views are usually reserved for coronal and sagittal reconstructions and examinations of the orbit and pituitary fossa.

Selecting different window levels displays tissues of different X-ray density more clearly. Some centres routinely provide two images for each scanned level of the lumbar spine, one to demonstrate bone structures, the other to show soft tissue within and outwith the spinal canal.

An intravenous iodinated water-soluble contrast medium is administered when the plain scan reveals an abnormality or if specific clinical indications exist, e.g. suspected arteriovenous malformation, acoustic neuroma or intracerebral abscess. Intravenous contrast shows areas with increased vascularity or with impairment of the blood–brain barrier.

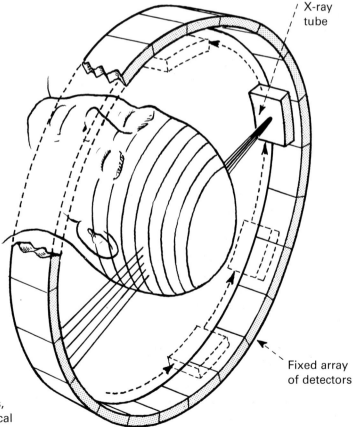

Rotating X-ray tube

Fixed array of detectors

Note: diagram illustrates individual slices. In the latest generation scanners, the beam describes a helical pathway around the head.

35

COMPUTERISED TOMOGRAPHY (CT) SCANNING

NORMAL SCAN

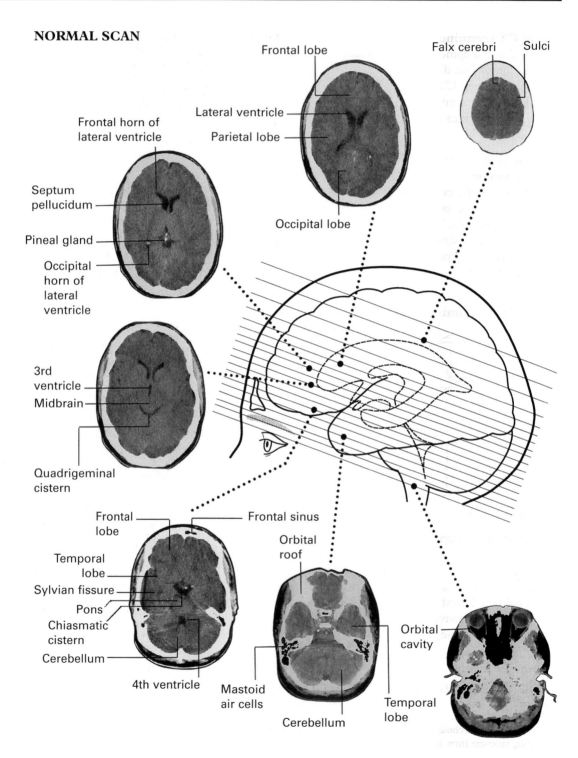

Frontal lobe

Falx cerebri

Sulci

Lateral ventricle

Parietal lobe

Frontal horn of lateral ventricle

Occipital lobe

Septum pellucidum

Pineal gland

Occipital horn of lateral ventricle

3rd ventricle

Midbrain

Quadrigeminal cistern

Frontal lobe

Frontal sinus

Orbital roof

Temporal lobe

Sylvian fissure

Pons

Chiasmatic cistern

Cerebellum

4th ventricle

Mastoid air cells

Cerebellum

Orbital cavity

Temporal lobe

COMPUTERISED TOMOGRAPHY (CT) SCANNING

Spinal CT scanning

Plain CT of the spine provides useful information of disc disease, particularly at the lumbosacral level. CT scanning after instilling a small amount of intrathecal contrast more clearly demonstrates lesions compressing the spinal cord or the cervico-medullary junction.

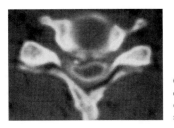

Cervical disc compressing one side of the spinal cord.

Coronal and sagittal reconstruction

CT imaging in the coronal plane is difficult and in the sagittal plane, virtually impossible. Two dimensional reconstruction of a selected plane may provide more information, but requires CT slices of narrow width e.g. 1–2 mm.

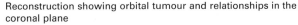

Reconstruction showing orbital tumour and relationships in the coronal plane

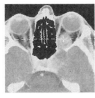
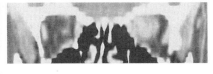

Coronal CT scanning

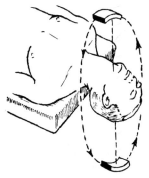

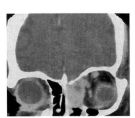

Coronal scan showing a tumour of the ethmoidal sinus

Full neck extension combined with maximal angulation of the CT gantry permits direct coronal scanning and may give greater definition than reconstructed views.

3-D CT angiogram showing an anterior communicating artery aneurysm

CT angiography

Helical scanning during infusion of intravenous contrast provides a non-invasive method of demonstrating intracranial vessels in 2 and 3-D format. The ability to rotate the image through 360° more clearly demonstrates vessels and any abnormalities. Latest reports claim that 3-D CT angiography is as accurate as conventional angiography in detecting small aneurysms, but these claims await further validation.

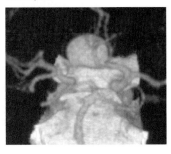

CT perfusion imaging

Following the infusion of contrast it is possible to construct brain perfusion maps. Ischaemic regions receive less contrast and appear as low density areas. This technique is of value in predicting outcome from acute stroke.

Xenon-enhanced computed tomography (XE-CT)

Inhaled stable xenon mixed with O_2 crosses the intact blood–brain barrier. CT scanning detects changes in tissue density as xenon accumulates producing quantitative maps of regional blood flow. This technique determines the degree and extent of cerebral ischaemia.

COMPUTERISED TOMOGRAPHY (CT) SCANNING

Interpretation of the cranial CT scan
Before contrast enhancement note:

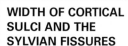

VENTRICULAR SYSTEM

Size
Position
Compression of
one or more horns,
i.e. frontal, temporal
or occipital

WIDTH OF CORTICAL SULCI AND THE SYLVIAN FISSURES

SKULL BASE AND VAULT

Hyperostosis
Osteolytic lesion
Remodelling
Depressed fracture

MULTIPLE LESIONS

may result from:

Tumour – metastases
        – lymphoma
Abscesses
Granuloma
Infarction
Trauma

ABNORMAL TISSUE DENSITY

Identify the site, and whether the lesion lies
within or without the brain substance.
Note the 'MASS EFFECT':
– midline shift
– ventricular compression
– obliteration of the basal cisterns, sulci

High density
    Blood
    Calcification – tumour
    – arteriovenous malformation/aneurysm
    – hamartoma
(Calcification of the pineal gland, choroid
plexus, basal ganglia and falx may occur
in normal scans.)

Low density
Infarction (arterial/venous)
Tumour
Abscess
Oedema
Encephalitis
Resolving haematoma

Mixed density
Tumour
Abscess
Arteriovenous malformation
Contusion
Haemorrhagic infarct

After contrast enhancement:

Vessels in the circle of Willis appear in the basal slices. Look at the extent and pattern of contrast uptake in any abnormal region. Some lesions may only appear after contrast enhancement.

MAGNETIC RESONANCE IMAGING (MRI)

For many years, magnetic resonance techniques aided chemical analysis in the food and petrochemical industries. The development of large-bore homogeneous magnets and computer assisted imaging (as in CT scanning) extended its use to the mapping of hydrogen nuclei (i.e. water) densities and their effect on surrounding molecules in vivo. Since these vary from tissue to tissue, MRI can provide a detailed image of both head and body structures. The latest echo-planer MR imaging permits rapid image acquisition.

Physical basis

When a substance is placed in a magnetic field, spinning protons within the nuclei act like small magnets and align themselves within the field.

A superimposed electromagnetic pulse (radiowave) at a specific frequency displaces the hydrogen protons.

The transverse component of the magnetisation vector generates the MRI signal.

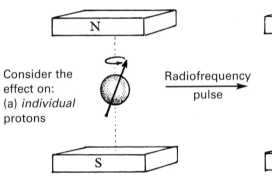

Consider the effect on:
(a) *individual* protons

Radiofrequency pulse

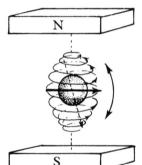

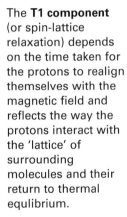

The **T1 component** (or spin-lattice relaxation) depends on the time taken for the protons to realign themselves with the magnetic field and reflects the way the protons interact with the 'lattice' of surrounding molecules and their return to thermal equlibrium.

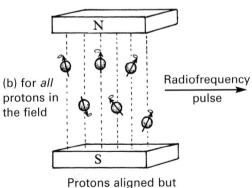

(b) for *all* protons in the field

Radiofrequency pulse

Protons aligned but spinning out of phase

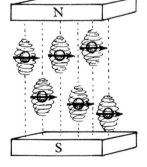

Protons spin in phase (i.e. 'resonate')

The **T2 component** (spin-spin relaxation) is the time taken for the protons to return to their original 'out of phase' state and depends on the locally 'energised' protons and their return to electro-magnetic equilibrium.

A variety of different radiofrequency pulse sequences (saturation recovery (SR), inversion recovery (IR) and spin echo (SE)) combined with computerised imaging produce an image of either proton density or of T1 or T2 weighting depending on the sequence employed.

MAGNETIC RESONANCE IMAGING (MRI)

Normal MRI images (T1/T2 weighting in relation to normal grey/white matter)

axial views – head

Sagittal view – head

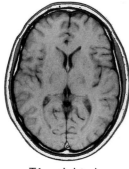 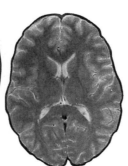 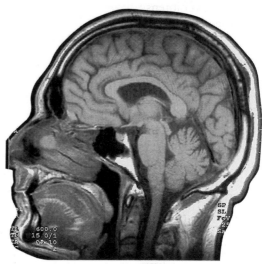

T1 weighted

T2 weighted

T1 weighted

Cervicodorsal spine (sagittal view)

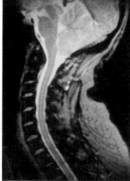

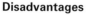T2 weighted

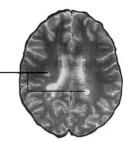

T2 weighted

Advantages (compared to CT scanning)
Can select any plane, e.g. coronal,
    sagittal, oblique.
No ionising radiation.
More sensitive to tissue change, e.g. demyelination plaques
(but not specific for each pathology,
    i.e. does not distinguish demyelination
    from ischaemia).
No bone artifacts, e.g. intracanalicular acoustic neuroma.

Disadvantages
Limited slice thickness – 3 mm (cf. CT – 1 mm).
Bone imaging limited to display of marrow.
Claustrophobia.
Cannot use with pacemaker or ferromagnetic implant.

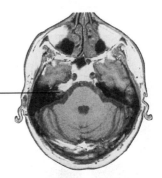

T1 weighted

MAGNETIC RESONANCE IMAGING (MRI)

Interpretation of abnormal MRI image

Look for structural abnormalities and abnormal intensities indicating a change in tissue T1 or T2 weighting *in relation to normal grey and white matter*. (A prolonged T1 relaxation time gives hypointensity, i.e. more black; a prolonged T2 relaxation time gives hyperintensity, i.e. more white).

Tissue/lesion			T1 weighting Intensity –	T2 weighting Intensity –
CSF, cyst, hygroma, cerebromalacia			↓↓	↑
Ischaemia, oedema, demyelination, most malignant tumours			↓	↑
Fat e.g. dermoid tumour, lipoma, some metastasis, atheroma			↑	↑
Meningioma (usually identified from structural change or surrounding oedema)			=	=
Evolution of haemorrhage				
Hyperacute	0–2 hours	Intracellular Oxy-Hb	=, slight ↓	↑
Acute	2 hours – 5 days	Intracellular Deoxy-Hb	=, slight ↓	↓↓
Early subacute	5 – 10 days	Intracellular Met-Hb	↑↑	↓↓
Late subacute	10 days – weeks	Free Met-Hb	↑↑	↑↑
Chronic	Months – years	Haemosiderin, Ferritin	=, ↓	↓↓

Paramagnetic enhancement

Some substances e.g. gadolinium, induce strong local magnetic fields – particularly shortening the T1 component. After intravenous administration, leakage of gadolinium through regions of damaged blood–brain barrier produces marked enhancement of the MRI signal, e.g. in ischaemia, infection, tumours and demyelination. Gadolinium may also help differentiate tumour tissue from surrounding oedema.

MR Angiography (MRA)

Rapidly flowing protons can create different intensities from stationary protons and the resultant signals obtained by special sequences can demonstrate vessels, aneurysms and arteriovenous malformations. Vessels

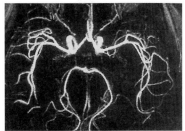

Cerebral arteries from below

displayed simultaneously, may make interpretation difficult, but selection of a specific MR section can demonstrate a single vessel or bifurcation. By selecting a specific flow velocity, MRA will show either arteries or veins. The resolution does not match other techniques. MRA will only detect 85–95% of those aneurysms seen on intra-arterial DSA (see page 44).

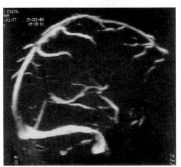

Cerebral veins – oblique view showing sagittal sinus

MAGNETIC RESONANCE IMAGING (MRI)

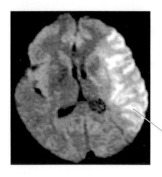

Diffusion-weighted MRI (DWI)

Images are based on an assessment of thermally driven translational movement of water and other small molecules within the brain. In acute ischaemia, cytotoxic oedema restrains diffusion. The degree of restricted diffusion is quantified with a parameter termed the apparent diffusion coefficient (ADC). ADC values fall initially, then normalise and prolong as ischaemic tissues become necrotic and are replaced by extracellular fluid. DWI shows size, site and age of ischaemic change. Whilst the volume normally increases within the first few days, the initial lesion size correlates best with the final outcome. This image shows restricted diffusion in a left middle cerebral artery infarct 3 hours from the onset.

Perfusion-weighted MRI (PWI)

Images are obtained by 'bolus tracking' after rapid contrast injection. A delay in contrast arrival and reduced concentration signifies hypoperfusion of that brain region. Soon after onset, ischaemic changes on PWI appear larger than on DWI. *The difference between PWI and DWI reflects dysfunctional salvagable tissue* (ischaemic penumbra see page 242). Early resolution of the PWI abnormality indicates recanalisation of an occluded vessel, whereas in those who do not recanalise the DWI volume expands to fill a large part of the original PWI lesion.

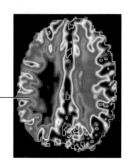

Hypoperfusion following a right middle cerebral infarction

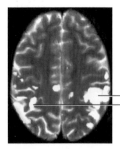

Areas of brain activation caused by bilateral finger movements

Functional MRI (fMRI)

The oxygenated state of haemoglobin influences the T2 relaxation time of perfused brain. A mismatch between the supply of oxygenated blood and oxygen utilisation in activated areas, produces an increase in venous oxygen content within post capillary venules causing signal change due to blood oxygenation level dependent (BOLD) contrast. Improved spatial and temporal resolution has increased the scope of functional imaging, leading to greater understanding of normal and abnormal brain function. A demonstration of the exact proximity of eloquent regions to areas of proposed resection, help minimise damage.

Magnetic resonance spectroscopy (MRS)

Spectroscopic techniques generate information on in vivo biochemical changes in response to disease. Concentrations of chemicals of biological interest are minute but measurement can be undertaken in single or multiple regions of interest of around $1.5\,cm^3$. N-acetylaspartate (a neuronal marker) and lactate are studied by ^{1}H-MRS, whilst adenosine triphosphate phosphocreatine and inorganic phosphate are measured by ^{31}P-MRS. MRS is gradually emerging from being a research tool to play a role in tumour characterisation, the confirmation of metabolic brain lesions and the study of degenerative disease.

^{1}H-MRS from both regions of normal brain and from a grade II astrocytoma. The tumour trace shows a high choline peak, due to high membrane turnover, a grossly reduced peak of N-acetylaspartate and the presence of lactate, confirming anaerobic metabolism.

Cho – Choline, Cr/PCr – Creatine/phosphocreatine, NAA – N-acetylaspartate.

NAA

Cho
Cr/PCr

MRS: normal

Cho

Cr/PCr NAA

MRS: tumour

Lactate

4   3   2   1   0 ppm

ULTRASOUND

Extracranial

When the probe (i.e. a transducer) – frequency 5–10 MHz, is applied to the skin surface, a proportion of the ultrasonic waves emitted are reflected back from structures of varying acoustic impedance and are detected by the same probe. These reflected waves are reconverted into electrical energy and displayed as a two-dimensional image (β-mode).

When the probe is directed at moving structures, such as red blood cells within a blood vessel lumen, frequency shift of the reflected waves occurs (the Doppler effect) proportional to the velocity of flowing blood. Doppler ultrasound uses *continuous wave* (CW) or *pulsed wave* (PW). The former measures frequency shift anywhere along the path of the probe. Pulsed ultrasound records frequency shift at a specific depth.

Duplex scanning combines β-mode with doppler, simultaneously providing images from the vessels from which the velocity is recorded.

Colour Coded Duplex (CCD) uses colour coding to superimpose flow velocities on a two dimensional ultrasound image.

Normal vessels exhibit laminar flow and the probe detects a constant velocity.

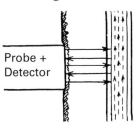

With stenosis the probe detects a wide spectrum of velocity

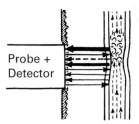

β-mode (real time) scanning images the arterial wall rather than the passage of red blood cells – producing a 'map' of the lumen.

Applications: assessment of extracranial carotid and vertebral arteries.

Intracranial – transcranial Doppler ultrasound

By selecting lower frequencies (2 MHz), ultrasound is able to penetrate the thinner parts of the skull bone. Combining this with a pulsed system gives reliable measurements and flow velocity in the anterior, middle and posterior cerebral arteries and in the basilar artery.

Applications:

Assessment of intracranial haemodynamics in extracranial occlusive/stenotic vascular disease. Detection of vasospasm in subarachnoid haemorrhage.

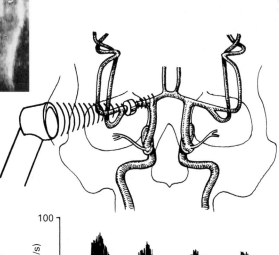

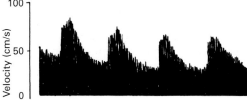

43

ANGIOGRAPHY

Many neurological and neurosurgical conditions require accurate delineation of both intra- and extracranial vessels. Intra-arterial injection of contrast remains the standard angiographic technique, imaged by digital subtraction (DSA).

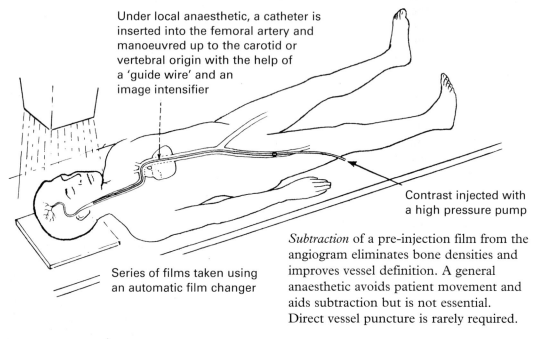

Under local anaesthetic, a catheter is inserted into the femoral artery and manoeuvred up to the carotid or vertebral origin with the help of a 'guide wire' and an image intensifier

Contrast injected with a high pressure pump

Series of films taken using an automatic film changer

Subtraction of a pre-injection film from the angiogram eliminates bone densities and improves vessel definition. A general anaesthetic avoids patient movement and aids subtraction but is not essential. Direct vessel puncture is rarely required.

Phase – arterial
– capillary
– venous

Most information is now derived from the arterial phase. Prior to the availability of CT scanning, the position of the cerebral vessels helped localise intracranial structures.

Digital subtraction angiography (DSA) depends upon high-speed digital computing. Exposures taken before and after the administration of contrast agents are instantly subtracted 'pixel by pixel'. Data manipulation allows enhancement of small differences of shading as well as magnification of specific areas of study.

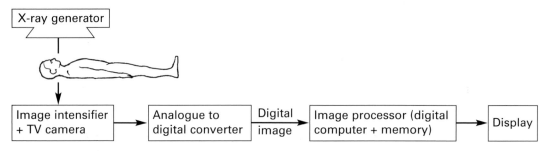

X-ray generator

Image intensifier + TV camera → Analogue to digital converter → Digital image → Image processor (digital computer + memory) → Display

DSA results in improved contrast sensitivity, permitting the use of much lower concentrations of contrast material compared to the older method of imaging directly on to X-ray film.

ANGIOGRAPHY

CAROTID ANGIOGRAPHY

Lateral view

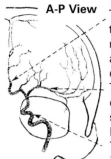

A-P View

The *anterior cerebral arteries* run over the corpus callosum, supplying the medial aspects of the frontal lobes. Both anterior cerebral arteries may fill from each carotid injection.

The *middle cerebral artery* runs in the depth of the Sylvian fissure. Branches supply the frontal and temporal lobes.

The *internal carotid artery* bifurcates into the anterior and middle cerebral arteries.

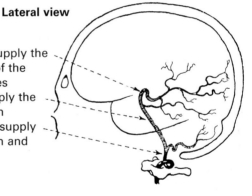

Oblique views may aid identification of some lesions, e.g. aneurysms.

VERTEBRAL ANGIOGRAPHY

Towne's view

Lateral view

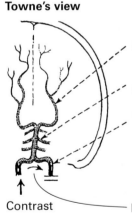

Posterior cerebral arteries supply the occipital lobes and parts of the parietal and temporal lobes

Basilar artery: branches supply the brain stem and cerebellum

Vertebral arteries: branches supply the spinal cord, brain stem and cerebellum

Contrast medium

Retrograde flow may demonstrate both vessels with one injection

In *carotid* and *vertebral* angiography look for:
Vessel *occlusion, stenosis* or *plaque formation*
Aneurysms
Arterio-venous malformations
Abnormal *tumour circulation*
Vessel *displacement* or *compression.*

Although superseded by the CT scan in tumour detection, angiography may give useful information about feeding vessels and the extent of vessel involvement with the tumour.

45

ANGIOGRAPHY

Complications

The development of non-ionic contrast mediums, e.g. iohexol, iopamidol, has considerably reduced the risk of complications during or following angiography.

Cerebral ischaemia: caused by emboli from an arteriosclerotic plaque broken off by the catheter tip, hypotension or vessel spasm following contrast injection. The reduced amount of contrast used for intra-arterial DSA carries less risk. In the hands of experienced radiologists, permanent neurological deficit occurs in only one in every 1000 investigations (one in 100 in arteriopaths)

Contrast sensitivity: mild sensitivity to the contrast occasionally develops, but this rarely causes severe problems.

Magnetic Resonance Angiography (MRA) (see page 41)

INTERVENTIONAL ANGIOGRAPHY

With recent advances, endovascular techniques now play an important role in neurosurgical management.

Embolisation: *Particles* (e.g. Ivalon sponge) injected through the arterial catheter will occlude small vessels; e.g. those feeding meningioma or glomus jugulare tumours, thus minimising operative haemorrhage.

'Glue' (isobutyl-2-cyanocrylate) can be injected into both high and low flow arteriovenous malformations. Operative excision is greatly facilitated; if the lesion is completely obliterated, this may even serve as a definitive treatment.

Balloons inflated, then detached from the catheter tip will occlude high flow systems involving large vessels, e.g. carotico-cavernous fistula, high flow arteriovenous malformations.

Platinum coils inserted into the aneurysm fundus through a special catheter can produce complete or partial obliteration. This technique is now often used as a first line treatment for aneurysms at certain sites e.g. basilar bifurcation and for certain anterior circulation aneurysms (see page 287). Temporary inflation of a balloon within the parent vessel during coiling can help prevent occlusion of the parent vessel in wide necked aneurysms (see page 286).

Stents may become routinely available for use in intracranial vessels in the future, but at present are only used on a trial basis in a few centres.

All techniques carry some risk of cerebral (or spinal) infarction from inadvertent distal embolisation when used in the internal carotid or spinal systems.

Angioplasty: Inflation of an intravascular balloon within a vasospastic segment of a major vessel may reverse cerebral ischaemia, but the technique is not without risk. No large trials exist and experience in individual centres tends to be limited.

RADIONUCLIDE IMAGING

Single photon emission computed tomography (SPECT)

There are two components to imaging with radioactive tracers – the detecting system and the labelled chemical. Each has become increasingly sophisticated in recent years. SPECT uses compounds labelled with gamma-emitting tracers (ligands), but unlike conventional scanning, acquires data from multiple sites around the head. Similar computing to CT scanning provides a two-dimensional image depicting the radioactivity emitted from each 'pixel'. This gives improved definition and localisation. Various ligands have been developed but a $^{99}Tc^m$ labelled derivative of propylamine oxime (HMPAO) is the most frequently used. This tracer represents *cerebral blood flow* since it rapidly diffuses across the blood–brain barrier, becomes trapped within the cells, and remains long enough to allow time for scanning. Of the total injected dose, 5% is taken up by the brain and 86% of this activity remains in the brain at least 24 hours.

Ligands for SPECT scanning	Purpose
HMPAO	Cerebral blood flow
^{123}I–FP–CIT	Dopamine presynaptic receptors
^{123}I–IBZM	Dopamine postsynaptic receptors
^{123}I–Iomazenil	Benzodiazepine receptors
^{123}I–CNB	Cholinergic receptors
^{123}I–MK801	Glutamate receptors
$^{201}Thallium$–chloride	High grade tumour/breakdown blood–brain barrier
^{123}I–tyrosine	Low grade tumour component

A rotating gamma camera is often used for detection, although fixed multidetector systems will produce higher quality images. Data are normally reconstructed to give axial images but coronal and sagittal can also be produced.

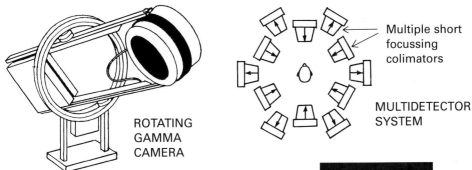

ROTATING GAMMA CAMERA

Multiple short focussing colimators

MULTIDETECTOR SYSTEM

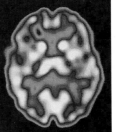

The normal scan – HMPAO (10 mm resolution)

The tomogram is examined in conjunction with structural imaging (CT or MRI) to aid interpretation.

RADIONUCLIDE IMAGING

Single photon emission computed tomography (SPECT) *(contd)*

Clinical applications

– Detection of early ischaemia in
OCCLUSIVE and HAEMORRHAGIC CEREBROVASCULAR DISEASE

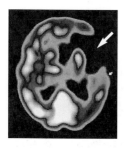

Absence of blood flow corresponds with area of infarction and tissue loss seen on structural imaging.

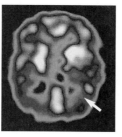

– Assessment of blood flow changes in DEMENTIA

Blood flow is generally reduced, especially in temporal and parietal lobes

– Evaluation of patients with intractable EPILEPSY of temporal lobe origin

Normal subject

Scan of temporal lobe showing symmetrical pattern of blood flow more prominent in grey matter

Patient with temporal lobe epilepsy

An *interictal* scan shows reduced flow throughout the temporal lobe

An *ictal* scan (i.e. HMPAO injected during the seizure) shows a marked hyperperfusion of the temporal lobe

The plane of scan lies in the same axis as the temporal lobe

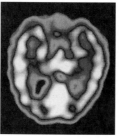

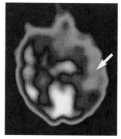

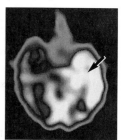

Such findings aid localisation of the epileptic focus and selection of patients for surgical treatment.

Thallium SPECT: a high uptake of thallium indicates rapidly dividing cells and can help differentiate low and high grade TUMOURS.

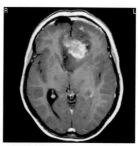

MRI showing apparent high grade tumour

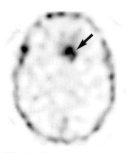

^{201}Thallium scan showing high uptake

RADIONUCLIDE IMAGING

Positron emission tomography (PET)

This technique utilises positron-emitting isotopes (radionuclides) bound to compounds of biological interest to study specific physiological processes quantitatively. Positron-emitting isotopes depend on a cyclotron for production and their half-life is short, thus PET scanners only exist on adjacent sites. This limits availability for routine clinical use but PET scanners provide valuable research information.

Each decaying positron results in the release of two photons in diametric opposition; these activate two coincidental detectors. Multiple pairs of detectors and computer processing techniques enable quantitative determination of local radioactivity (and density of the labelled compound) for each 'voxel' (a cube of tissue) within the imaged field. Reconstruction using similar imaging techniques to CT scanning produces the positron emission scan.

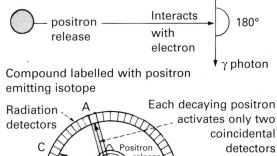

few millimetres — γ photon

positron release — Interacts with electron — 180°

γ photon

Compound labelled with positron emitting isotope

Radiation detectors

Each decaying positron activates only two coincidental detectors e.g. A and B

Positron release

Rejected by AB but coincident for CD

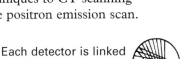

Each detector is linked to several others in a fan shaped distribution

Isotope	Binding compound		Measurement under study
^{15}Oxygen	Carbon monoxide	– inhalation	*Cerebral blood volume (CBV)*
^{15}Oxygen	Water	– i.v. bolus	*Cerebral blood flow (CBF)*
^{18}Fluorine	Fluorodeoxyglucose	– i.v. bolus	*Cerebral glucose metabolism (CMRgl)*
^{15}Oxygen	Oxygen	– inhalation	*Cerebral oxygen utilisation (CMRO$_2$)*
			Oxygen extraction factor (OEF)
^{11}Carbon	Drug, e.g. phenytoin	– i.v. bolus	*Drug receptor site*
^{11}Carbon	Methyl spiperone	– i.v. bolus	*Dopamine binding site*

Clinical and research uses

PET scanning is of particular value in elucidating the relationships between cerebral blood flow, oxygen utilisation and extraction in focal areas of ischaemia or infarction (page 242) and has been used to study patients with dementia, epilepsy and brain tumours. Identification of neurotransmitter and drug receptor sites has aided the understanding and management of psychiatric (schizophrenia) and movement disorders.

PET scan several days after a left middle cerebral infarct showing a reduction in blood flow

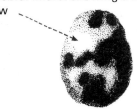

Oxygen utilisation is also reduced with a slight increase in oxygen extraction

ELECTROENCEPHALOGRAPHY (EEG)

Electroencephalography examines by means of scalp electrodes the spontaneous electrical activity of the brain. Tiny electrical potentials, which measure millionths of volts, are recorded, amplified and displayed on either 8 or 16 channels of a pen recorder. Low and high frequency filters remove unwanted signals such as muscle artefact and mains interference.

The system of electrode placement is referred to as the 10/20 system because the distance between bony points, i.e. inion to nasion, is divided into lengths of either 10% or 20% of the total, and the electrodes placed at each distance.

A switch changes recording from A (parasagittal) to B (transverse). Other electrode arrangements are also 'preset'. The numbering indicates the write out from top to bottom of an 8-channel record.

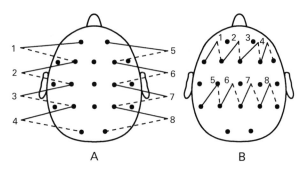

A   B

Normal rhythms

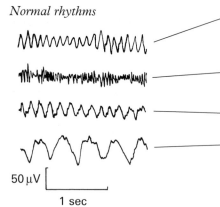

50 µV

1 sec

Alpha rhythm (8–13 Hz – cycles/second). Symmetrical and present posteriorly with the eyes closed – will disappear or 'block' with eye opening

Beta rhythm (> 13 Hz). Symmetrical and present frontally. Not affected by eye opening

Theta rhythm (4–8 Hz) ⎱ Seen in children and young
adults with frontal and
Delta rhythm (< 4 Hz) ⎰ temporal predominance

These 'immature' features should disappear in adult life as the EEG shows 'maturation'

As well as recording a resting EEG using various 'preset' electrode arrangements, stressing the patient by hyperventilation and photic stimulation (a flashing strobe light) may result in an electrical discharge supporting a diagnosis of epilepsy.

More advanced methods of telemetry and foramen ovale recording may be necessary
- to establish the diagnosis of 'epilepsy' if doubt remains
- to determine the exact frequency and site of origin of the attacks
- to aid classification of seizure type.

Telemetry: utilises a continuous 24–48 hour recording of EEG, often combined with a videotape recording of the patient. Increasing availability of this and ambulatory recording has greatly improved diagnostic accuracy and reliability of seizure classification.

Foramen ovale recording: a needle electrode is passed percutaneously through the foramen ovale to record activity from the adjacent temporal lobe.

INTRACRANIAL PRESSURE MONITORING

Although CSF pressure may be measured during lumbar puncture, this method is of limited value in intracranial pressure measurement:

An isolated pressure reading does not indicate the trend or detect pressure waves.

Lumbar puncture is contraindicated in the presence of an intracranial mass.

Pressure gradients exist between different intracranial and spinal compartments, especially in the presence of brain shift.

Many techniques are now available to measure intracranial pressure. In most instances a transducer either lying on the brain surface or inserted a few millimetres into the brain substance suffices, but a catheter inserted into the lateral ventricle remains the 'gold' standard by which other methods are compared.

Ventricular catheter insertion

A ventricular catheter is inserted into the frontal horn of the lateral ventricle through a frontal burr hole or small drill hole situated two finger breadths from the midline, behind the hairline and anterior to the coronal suture.

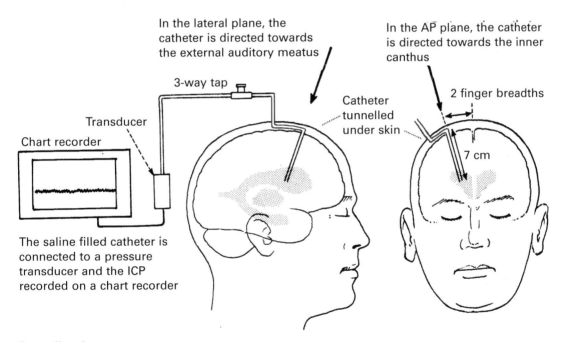

In the lateral plane, the catheter is directed towards the external auditory meatus

In the AP plane, the catheter is directed towards the inner canthus

3-way tap

Transducer

Chart recorder

Catheter tunnelled under skin

2 finger breadths

7 cm

The saline filled catheter is connected to a pressure transducer and the ICP recorded on a chart recorder

Complications

Intracerebral haemorrhage following catheter insertion rarely occurs.

Ventriculitis occurs in from 10 – 17%. Minimise this risk by tunnelling catheter under the skin and removing as soon as is practicable.

INTRACRANIAL PRESSURE MONITORING

NORMAL PRESSURE TRACE

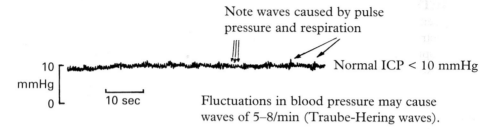

Note waves caused by pulse pressure and respiration

Normal ICP < 10 mmHg

Fluctuations in blood pressure may cause waves of 5–8/min (Traube-Hering waves).

ABNORMAL PRESSURE TRACE

Look for: *Increase in the mean pressure* – > 20 mmHg – moderate elevation
> 40 mmHg – severe increase in pressure

N.B. As ICP increases, the amplitude of the pulse pressure wave increases.

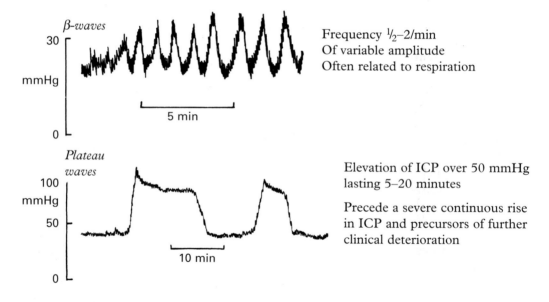

Frequency ½–2/min
Of variable amplitude
Often related to respiration

Elevation of ICP over 50 mmHg lasting 5–20 minutes

Precede a severe continuous rise in ICP and precursors of further clinical deterioration

CLINICAL USES OF ICP MONITORING
– Investigation of normal pressure hydrocephalus – the presence of β waves for > 5% of a 24-hour period suggests impaired CSF absorption and the need for a drainage operation.
– Postoperative monitoring – a rise in ICP may precede clinical evidence of haematoma formation or cerebral swelling.
– Small traumatic haematomas – ICP monitoring may guide management and indicate the need for operative removal.
– ICP monitoring is required during treatment aimed at reducing a raised ICP and maintaining cerebral perfusion pressure.

EVOKED POTENTIALS – VISUAL, AUDITORY AND SOMATOSENSORY

RECORDING METHODS

Stimulation of any sensory receptor evokes a minute electrical signal (i.e. microvolts) in the appropriate region of the cerebral cortex. Averaging techniques permit recording and analysis of this signal normally lost within the background electrical activity. When sensitive apparatus is triggered to record cortical activity at a specific time after the stimulus, the background electrical 'noise' averages out, i.e. random positive activity subtracts from random negative activity, leaving the signal evoked from the specific stimulus.

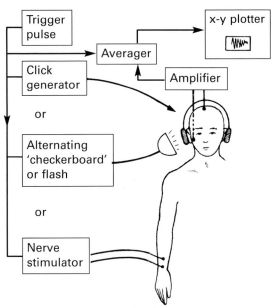

Visual evoked potential (VEP)

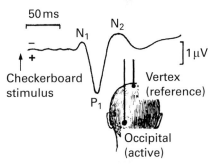

A stroboscopic flash diffusely stimulates the retina; alternatively an alternating checkerboard pattern stimulates the macula and produces more consistent results. The evoked visual signal is recorded over the occipital cortex. The first large positive wave (P_1) provides a useful point for measuring conduction through the visual pathways.

Uses: *Multiple sclerosis detection* – 30% with normal ophthalmological examination have abnormal VEP.
Peroperative monitoring – pituitary surgery.

Brain stem auditory evoked potential (BAEP)

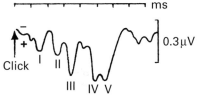

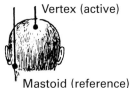

Electrical activity evoked in the first 10 milliseconds after a 'click' stimulus provides a wave pattern related to conduction through the auditory pathways in the VIII nerve and nucleus (waves I and II) and in the pons and midbrain (waves III–V). Longer latency potentials (up to 500 ms), recorded from the auditory cortex in response to a 'tone' stimulus, are of less clinical value.

Uses: *Hearing assessment* – especially in children.
Detection of intrinsic and extrinsic brain stem and cerebellopontine angle lesions, e.g. acoustic tumours.
Peroperative recording during acoustic tumour operations.
Assessment of brain stem function in coma.

EVOKED POTENTIALS – SOMATOSENSORY

Somatosensory evoked potentials (SEP)

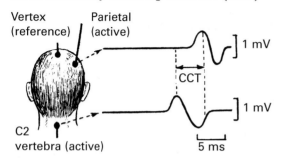

The sensory evoked potential is recorded over the parietal cortex in response to stimulation of a peripheral nerve (e.g. median nerve). Other electrodes sited at different points along the sensory pathway record the ascending activity. Subtraction of the latencies between peaks provides conduction time between these sites.

Central conduction time (CCT): sensory conduction time from the dorsal columns (or nuclei) to the parietal cortex.

Uses: *Detection of lesions in the sensory pathways* – brachial plexus injury

– spinal cord and brainstem tumours or demyelination.

Peroperative recording – straightening of scoliosis
– removal of spinal tumours/AVM } spinal conduction
– aneurysm operation with temporary vessel occlusion – CCT.

Motor Evoked Potential (MEP)

Subtraction of the latencies between motor evoked potentials elicited by applying a brief magnetic stimulus to either the motor cortex, the spinal cord or the peripheral nerves gives *peripheral* and *central motor conduction velocities*. The use of MEP in clinical practice awaits further evaluation.

MYELOGRAPHY

Now rarely used due to availability of MRI and CT scanning. Injection of water-soluble contrast into the lumbar theca and imaging flow up to the cervicomedullary junction provides a rapid (although invasive) method of screening the whole spinal cord and cauda equina for compressive lesions (e.g. disc disease or spondylosis, tumours, abscesses or cysts). For suspected lumbosacral disc disease, contrast is screened up to the level of the conus i.e. RADICULOGRAPHY (but a normal study does not exclude the possibility of a laterally situated disc). CT scanning and MRI have gradually replaced the need for myelography, but the introduction of a low dose of water-soluble contrast considerably enhances axial CT scan images of the spinal cord and nerve roots.

Problems

Headache occurs in 30%, *nausea* and *vomiting* in 20% and *seizures* in 0.5%.
Arachnoiditis – previously a major complication with oil based contrast MYODIL, but rarely occurs with water soluble contrast.
Subdural injection (accidental) – prevents correct interpretation.
Haematoma – occurs rarely at the injection site.
Impaction of spinal tumour – may follow CSF escape and aggravate the effects of cord compression, leading to clinical deterioration.

LUMBAR PUNCTURE

Lumbar puncture permits: – acquisition of cerebrospinal fluid for analysis.
– CSF drainage and pressure reduction, e.g. in communicating hydrocephalus/CSF fistula.

TECHNIQUE

Both 'traumatic' and 'atraumatic' needles are available; use the smallest gauge possible.

1. *Correct positioning of the patient is essential.* Open the vertebral laminae by drawing the knees up to the chest and flexing the neck. Ensure the back is parallel to the bed to avoid rotation of the spinal column.

2. Identify the site. The L3/4 space lies level with the iliac crests and this is most often used, but since the spinal cord ends at L1 any space from L2/L3 to L5/S1 provides a safe approach.

3. Clean the area and insert a few millilitres of local anaesthetic.

4. Ensure the stylet of a 20G lumbar puncture needle is fully home (22G for children) and insert at a slight angle towards the head, so that it parallels the spinous processes. Some resistance is felt as the needle passes through the ligamentum flavum, the dura and arachnoid layers.

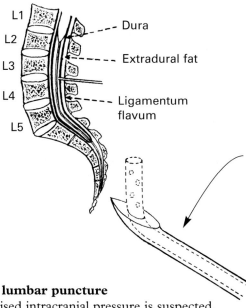

L1
L2
L3
L4
L5

- - - Dura

- - - Extradural fat

- - - Ligamentum flavum

5. Withdraw the stylet and collect the CSF. If bone is encountered, withdraw the needle and reinsert at a different angle. If the position appears correct yet no CSF appears, rotate the needle to free obstructive nerve roots.

A similar technique employing a TUOHY needle allows insertion of intra- or epidural cannula (for CSF drainage or drug instillation) or stimulating electrodes (for pain management).

Avoid lumbar puncture

- if raised intracranial pressure is suspected.
  Even a fine needle leaves a hole through which CSF will leak. In the presence of a space-occupying lesion, especially in the posterior fossa, CSF withdrawal creates a pressure gradient which may precipitate tentorial herniation.
- if platelet count is less than 40 000 and prothrombin time is less than 50% of control.

55

CEREBROSPINAL FLUID

CSF COLLECTION

Subarachnoid haemorrhage (SAH), or puncture of a blood vessel by the needle, may account for blood-stained CSF. To differentiate, collect CSF in three bottles.

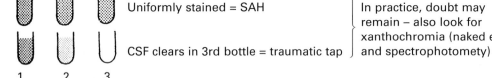

Uniformly stained = SAH

CSF clears in 3rd bottle = traumatic tap

In practice, doubt may remain – also look for xanthochromia (naked eye and spectrophotomety)

1   2   3

CSF PRESSURE MEASUREMENT

Check that the patient's head (foramen of Munro) is level with the lumbar puncture. Connect a manometer via a 3-way tap to the needle and allow CSF to run up the column. Read off the height. Normal value: 100–150 mm CSF.

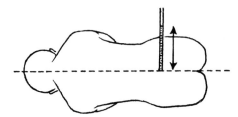

CSF ANALYSIS

Standard tests

1. Bacteriological – RBC and differential WBC (normal = < 5 WBCs per mm^3)
   - Gram stain and culture
   - appearance of supernatant. Xanthochromia (yellow staining) results from subarachnoid haemorrhage with RBC breakdown, high CSF protein or jaundice.

2. Biochemical – protein (normal = 0.15–0.45 g/l)
   - glucose (normal = 0.45–0.70 g/l) 40–60% of blood glucose simultaneously sampled.

Special tests

Suspected:

Subarachnoid haemorrhage –	spectrophotometry for blood breakdown products
Malignant tumour	– cytology
Tubercle	– Ziehl-Neelson stain, Lowenstein-Jensen culture, polymerase chain reaction (PCR)
Non-bacterial infection	– virology, fungal and parasitic studies
Demyelinating disease	– oligodonal bands
Neurosyphilis	– VDRL (Venereal Disease Research Laboratory) test
	– FTA-ABS (Fluorescent treponemal antibody absorption) test
	– *Treponema pallidum* immobilisation test (TPI)
Cryptococcus	– culture and antigen detection
HIV	– culture, antigen detection and antiviral antibodies (anti-HIV-IgG).

Complications

- tonsillar herniation (see page 81)
- transient headache (10%), radicular pain (10%), or ocular palsy (1%)
- epidural haemorrhage very rare.

ELECTROMYOGRAPHY/NERVE CONDUCTION STUDIES

Needle electromyography records the electrical activity occurring within a particular muscle.

Nerve conduction studies measure conduction in nerves in response to an electrical stimulus.

Both are essential in the investigation of diseases of nerve (neuropathy) and muscle (myopathy).

Repetitive nerve stimulation tests are important in the evaluation of disorders of neuromuscular transmission, e.g. myasthenia gravis.

ELECTROMYOGRAPHY

A concentric needle electrode is inserted into muscle. The central wire is the active electrode and the outer casing the reference electrode. This records from an area of $300\,\mu$ radius.

The potential difference between the two electrodes is amplified and displayed on an oscilloscope. An audio monitor enables the investigator to 'hear' the pattern of electrical activity.

Normal muscle at rest is electrically 'silent' with a resting potential of 90 mV; as the muscle gradually contracts, *motor unit potentials* appear … followed by the development of an *interference pattern*

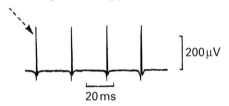

200 µV

20 ms

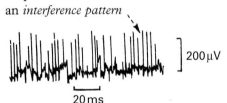

200 µV

20 ms

Abnormalities take the form of:
Spontaneous activity in muscle when at rest.
Abnormalities of the motor unit potential.
Abnormalities of the interference pattern.
Special phenomena, e.g. myotonia.

The recruitment of more and more motor units prevents identification of individual potentials

Spontaneous activity at rest

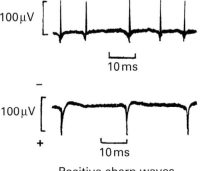

100 µV

10 ms

100 µV

10 ms

Positive sharp waves

Fibrillation potentials are due to single muscle fibre contraction and indicate active denervation. They usually occur in neurogenic disorders, e.g. neuropathy.

Slow negative waves preceded by sharp positive spikes. Seen in chronically denervated muscle, e.g. motor neuron disease, but also in acute myopathy, e.g. polymyositis. These waves probably represent injury potentials.

57

ELECTROMYOGRAPHY/NERVE CONDUCTION STUDIES

Abnormalities (contd)

Motor unit potential

In myopathies and muscular dystrophies, potentials are polyphasic and of small amplitude and short duration.

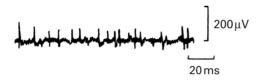

200 μV

20 ms

In neuropathy, the surviving motor unit potentials are also polyphasic but of large amplitude and long duration.

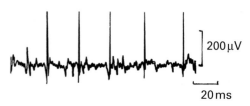

200 μV

20 ms

The enlarged potentials result from collateral reinnervation.

Interference pattern

In myopathy, recruitment of motor units and the interference pattern remain normal. The interference pattern may even appear to increase due to fragmentation of motor units.

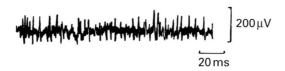

200 μV

20 ms

In neuropathy, there is a reduction in interference due to a loss of motor units under voluntary control.

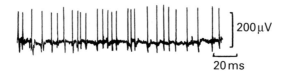

200 μV

20 ms

Myotonia

High frequency repetitive discharge may occur after voluntary movement. The amplitude and frequency of the potentials wax and wane giving rise to the typical 'dive bomber' sound on the audio monitor.

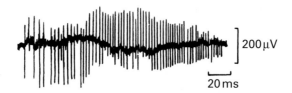

200 μV

20 ms

An abnormal myotonic discharge provoked by moving the needle electrode.

ELECTROMYOGRAPHY/NERVE CONDUCTION STUDIES

NERVE CONDUCTION STUDIES

Distal latency (latency from stimulus to recording electrodes), *amplitude* of the evoked response and *conduction velocity* all provide information on motor and sensory nerve function.

Conduction velocity: measurement made by stimulating or recording from two different sites along the course of a peripheral nerve.

$$\frac{\text{Distance between two sites}}{\text{Difference in conduction times between two sites}} = \text{Conduction velocity}$$

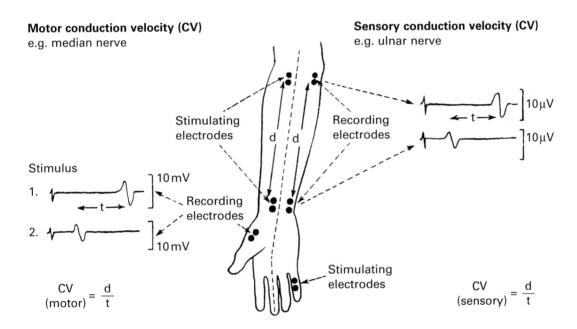

Motor conduction velocity (CV)
e.g. median nerve

Sensory conduction velocity (CV)
e.g. ulnar nerve

$$\underset{\text{(motor)}}{\text{CV}} = \frac{d}{t}$$

$$\underset{\text{(sensory)}}{\text{CV}} = \frac{d}{t}$$

Normal values (motor)

Ulnar and median nerves – 50–60 m/s
Common peroneal nerve – 45–55 m/s

Normal values (sensory)

Ulnar and median nerves – 60–70 m/s
Common peroneal nerve – 50–70 m/s

Motor conduction velocities slow with age.

Body temperature is important; a fall of 1°C slows conduction in motor nerves by approximately 2 metres per second.

Pathological delay occurs with nerve entrapments, demyelinating neuropathies (Guillain–Barré syndrome) and multifocal motor neuropathy.

ELECTROMYOGRAPHY/NERVE CONDUCTION STUDIES

REPETITIVE STIMULATION

In the normal subject, repetitive stimulation of a motor nerve at a frequency of <30/second produces a muscle potential of constant form and amplitude. Increasing the stimulus frequency to >30/second results in fatigue manifest by a decline or 'decrement' in the amplitude. In patients with disorders of neuromuscular transmission, repetitive stimulation aids diagnosis:

Myasthenia gravis
A decrementing response occurs
with a stimulus rate of 3–5/second.

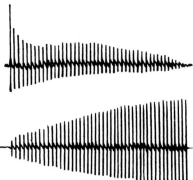

Myasthenic (Eaton Lambert) syndrome
With a stimulation rate of 20–50/second
(i.e. rapid) a small amplitude response
increases to normal amplitude –
incrementing response.

SINGLE FIBRE ELECTROMYOGRAPHY

A standard concentric needle within muscle will record electrical activity 0.5–1 mm from its tip – sampling from up to 20 motor units. A 'single fibre' electromyography needle with a smaller recording surface detects electrical activity within 300 μm of its tip – sampling 1–3 muscle fibres from a single motor unit.

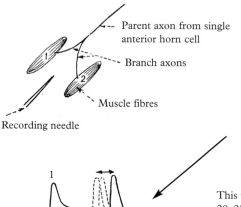

Parent axon from single
anterior horn cell

Branch axons

Muscle fibres

Recording needle

Record:

1   2

Action potentials recorded from two muscle fibres are not synchronous. The gap between each is variable and can be measured if the first recorded potential is 'locked' on the oscilloscope.

This variability is referred to as JITTER – normally 20–25 μs (2–5 μs due to transmission in the branch axon – 15–20 μs to variation in neuromuscular transmission).

Single fibre electromyography is occasionally helpful in the investigation of disorders of neuromuscular transmission. In ocular myasthenia, the affected muscles are not accessible and frontalis is sampled instead.

NEURO-OTOLOGICAL TESTS

AUDITORY SYSTEM

Neuro-otological tests help differentiate conductive, cochlear and retrocochlear causes of impaired hearing. They supplement Weber's and Rinne's test (page 16).

PURE TONE AUDIOMETRY   Thresholds for air and bone conduction are measured at different frequencies from 250 Hz to 8 kHz.

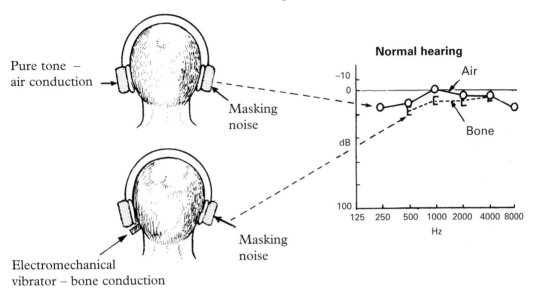

Sound conducted through air requires an intact ossicular system as well as a functioning cochlea and VIII nerve. Sound applied directly to the bone bypasses the ossicles.

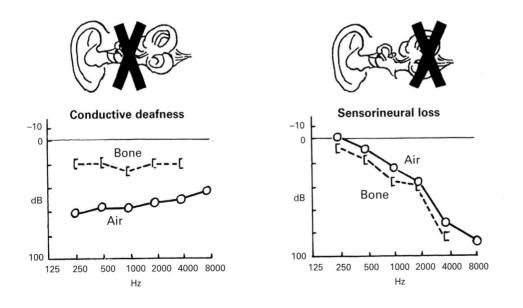

NEURO-OTOLOGICAL TESTS

SPEECH AUDIOMETRY

This test measures the percentage of words correctly interpreted as a function of the intensity of presentation and indicates the usefulness of hearing. The graph shows how different types of hearing loss can be differentiated.

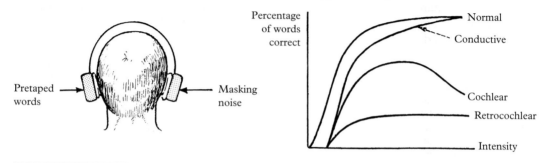

STAPEDIAL REFLEX DECAY

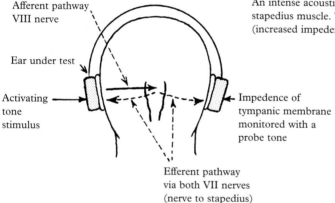

An intense acoustic stimulus causes reflex contraction of the stapedius muscle. This in turn causes reduced compliance (increased impedence) of the tympanic membrane.

Impedence of tympanic membrane monitored with a probe tone

Rapid decay of the reflex response suggests a lesion of the auditory nerve

AUDITORY BRAINSTEM EVOKED POTENTIAL

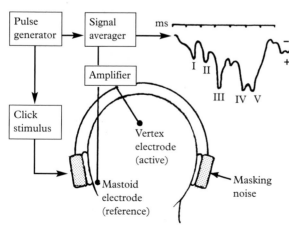

Averaging techniques (page 53) permit the recording and analysis of small electrical potentials evoked in response to auditory stimuli. Activity in the first 10 ms provides information about the VIII nerve and nucleus (waves I and II) and the pons and midbrain (waves III – V). Lesions of the VIII nerve diminish the amplitude and/or increase the latency of wave I or II and increase the wave I to V interpeak latency. In comparison, cochlear lesions seldom affect either wave pattern or latency.

NEURO-OTOLOGICAL TESTS

VESTIBULAR SYSTEM

Caloric testing (vestibulo-ocular reflex)

Compensatory mechanisms may mask clinical evidence of vestibular damage – spontaneous and positional nystagmus. Caloric testing provides useful supplementary information and may reveal undetected vestibular dysfunction.

Method: Water at 30°C irrigated into the external auditory meatus. Nystagmus usually develops after a 20 second delay and lasts for more than a minute. The test is repeated after 5 minutes with water at 44°C.

Cold water effectively reduces the vestibular output from one side, creating an imbalance and producing eye drift towards the irrigated ear. Rapid corrective movements result in 'nystagmus' to the opposite ear. Hot water (44°) reverses the convection current, increases the vestibular output and changes the direction of nystagmus.

N.B. Ice water ensures a maximal stimulus when caloric testing for brain death or head injury prognostication.

Time from onset of irrigation to the cessation of nystagmus is plotted for each ear, at each temperature.

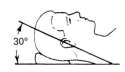

Stimulus is maximal with the head supported 30° from the horizontal (with the lateral semicircular canal in a vertical plane).

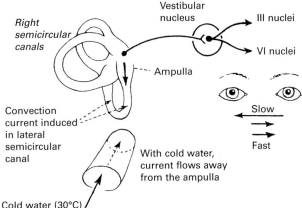

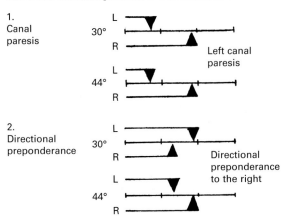

Damage to the labyrinth, vestibular nerve or nucleus results in one of two abnormal patterns, or a combination of both.

Electronystagmography: The potential difference across the eye (the corneoretinal potential) permits recording of eye movements with laterally placed electrodes and enables detection of spontaneous or reflex induced nystagmus in darkness or with eyes closed.

This eliminates optical fixation which may reduce or even abolish nystagmus.

Canal paresis implies reduced duration of nystagmus on one side. It may result from either a peripheral or central (brain stem or cerebellum) lesion on that side.

Directional preponderance implies a more prolonged duration of nystagmus in one direction than the other. It may result from a central lesion on the side of the preponderance or from a peripheral lesion on the other side.

These tests combined with audiometry should differentiate a peripheral from a central lesion.

CLINICAL PRESENTATION, ANATOMICAL CONCEPTS AND DIAGNOSTIC APPROACH

HEADACHE – GENERAL PRINCIPLES

Headache is a common symptom arising from psychological, otological, ophthalmological, neurological or systemic disease. In clinical practice tension-type headache is encountered most frequently.

Definition: Pain or discomfort between the orbits and occiput, arising from pain-sensitive structures.

Intracranial pain-sensitive structures are:
venous sinuses, cortical veins, basal arteries, dura of anterior, middle and posterior fossae.

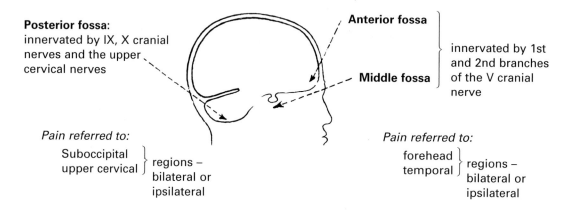

Posterior fossa:
innervated by IX, X cranial nerves and the upper cervical nerves

Anterior fossa
Middle fossa
innervated by 1st and 2nd branches of the V cranial nerve

Pain referred to:
Suboccipital upper cervical } regions – bilateral or ipsilateral

Pain referred to:
forehead temporal } regions – bilateral or ipsilateral

Extracranial pain-sensitive structures are:
Scalp vessels and muscles, orbital contents, mucous membranes of nasal and paranasal spaces, external and middle ear, teeth and gums.

International classification of headache type (1988)
% Frequency in General Practice

Type	Percentage
Tension type headache	45
Migraine	30
With disease of the eye/sinuses	< 8
With systemic infection	7
With head trauma	3
With drugs	2
With cerebrovascular disease	< 1
With other intracranial disease	< 1
With metabolic disease	< 1
Cluster headache	< 1
Neuralgias	< 1

Examination
Full general examination, including:
  Ocular – acuity, tenderness, strabismus
  Teeth and scalp
  Percussion over frontal and maxillary
    sinuses
Full neurological examination.

HEADACHE – DIAGNOSTIC APPROACH

History: most information is derived from determining:
– the first attack or previous attacks
– whether onset is acute or gradual (days or weeks)
– whether attacks have recurred for many years (chronic)
– site of headache
– accompanying symptoms
– precipitating factors

The following table classifies causes in these categories:

Cause	Associated features which (if present) aid diagnosis	RECURRENT ATTACKS	Further investigations (if required)
ACUTE			
Sinusitis	Preceding 'cold' nasal discharge	*	X-ray nasal sinuses
Migraine	Visual/neurological aura, nausea, vomiting	*	
Cluster headache	Lacrimation, rhinorrhoea	*	
Glaucoma	'misting' of vision 'haloes' around objects	*	Ophthalmological referral
Retrobulbar neuritis	Loss of vision (unilateral)		Visual evoked response
Post-traumatic	Following head injury		Skull X-ray, CT scan
Drugs/toxins	On vasodilator drugs		
Haemorrhage	Instantaneous onset vomiting, neck stiffness impaired conscious level		CT scan, lumbar puncture (see page 55)
Infection (meningitis, encephalitis)	As above but more gradual onset with pyrexia	* (if CSF fistula)	
Hydrocephalus	Impaired conscious levels, leg weakness impaired upward gaze	*	CT scan
SUBACUTE			
Infection (subacute, chronic meningitis, e.g. TB cerebral abscess)	Impaired conscious level, pyrexia, neck stiffness, focal neurological signs		CT scan lumbar puncture
Intracranial tumour Chronic subdural haematoma Hydrocephalus	Vomiting, papilloedema, impaired conscious level ± focal neurological signs	*	CT scan CT scan
Benign intracranial hypertension	Vomiting, papilloedema	*	CSF pressure monitoring
Temporal arteritis	Thickened, tender, scalp arteries		ESR, temporal artery biopsy
CHRONIC			
Tension-type headache	Anxiety, depression	*	
Ocular 'eye strain'	Impaired visual acuity	*	Refractive errors
Drugs/toxins	On vasodilator drugs		
Cervical spondylosis	Neck, shoulder, arm pain	*	X-ray cervical spine

HEADACHE – DIAGNOSTIC APPROACH

Headache in children

All causes of adult headache (except in retrobulbar neuritis, glaucoma, temporal arteritis and cervical spondylosis) may cause headache in children. In this age group, the commonest type of headache is that accompanying any *febrile illness* or *infection of the nasal passages or sinuses*.

The clinician must not take a complaint of headache lightly; the younger the child, the more likely the presence of an underlying organic disease. Pyrexia may not only represent a mild 'constitutional' upset, but may result from *meningitis, encephalitis* or *cerebral abscess*. The presence of neck stiffness and/or impaired conscious level indicates the need for urgent investigation.

Although *intracranial tumours* are uncommon in childhood, when they occur they tend to lie in the *midline* (e.g. medulloblastoma, pineal region tumours). As a result, obstructive hydrocephalus often develops acutely with headache as a prominent initial symptom.

In a child with 'unexplained' headache, *CT scan* should be performed:
- if the presentation is acute
- if the severity progressively increases
- if school performance declines, or other symptoms, e.g. personality change, develop
- if the head circumference increases
- if the child is under 5 years.

HEADACHE – SPECIFIC CAUSES

TENSION TYPE HEADACHE

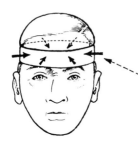

This is the commonest form of headache experienced by 70% of males and 90% of females at some time in their lives.

Characteristics: Diffuse, dull, aching, 'band-like' headache, worse on touching the scalp and aggravated by noise; associated with 'tension' but not with other physical symptoms. Attacks may be chronic or episodic. Depression commonly co-exists.

Duration: Many hours – days.

Frequency: Infrequent or daily; worse towards the end of the day. May persist over many years.

Mechanism: 'Muscular' due to persistent contraction, e.g. clenching teeth, head posture, furrowing of brow.

Treatment: Reassurance
Attempt to reduce psychological stress and analgesic over-use.
Antidepressants or β-blockers.

HEADACHE – SPECIFIC CAUSES

MIGRAINE

Migraine is a common, often familial disorder characterised by *unilateral throbbing headache*.

Onset: Childhood or early adult life.
Incidence: Affects 5–10% of the population.
Female:male ratio: 2 :1
Family history: Obtained in 70% of all sufferers.

Two recognisable forms exist:
Specific diagnostic criteria are required for migraine with and without aura.

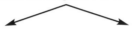

MIGRAINE WITH AURA

An *aura* or warning of visual, sensory or motor type followed by headache – throbbing, unilateral, worsened by bright light, relieved by sleep, associated with nausea and, occasionally, vomiting.

MIGRAINE WITHOUT AURA (COMMON MIGRAINE)

The *aura* is absent. The headache has similar features, but it is often poorly localised and its description may merge with that of 'tension' headache.

The aura of migraine may take many forms. The visual forms comprise: flashing lights, zig-zags (fortifications), scintillating scotoma (central vision) and may precede visual field defects. Such auras are of visual (occipital) cortex origin.

The headache is recurrent, lasting from 2 to 48 hours and rarely occurring more frequently than twice weekly. In *migraine equivalents* the aura occurs without ensuing headache.

Mechanism

Mutations in mitochondrial DNA and Ca^{2+} channel genes may explain familial cases. Vascular and neuronal processes probably co-exist with changes in serotonin activity initiating attacks.

Specific types of migraine with aura

Basilar: Characterised by bilateral visual symptoms, unsteadiness, dysarthria, vertigo, limb paraesthesia, even tetraparesis. Loss of consciousness may ensue and precede the onset of headache. This form of migraine affects young women.

Hemiplegic: Characterised by an aura of unilateral paralysis (hemiplegia) which unusually persist for some days after the headache has settled. Often misdiagnosed as a 'stroke'. When familial, mendelian dominant inheritance is noted. Recovery is the rule.

Ophthalmoplegic: Characterised by extraocular nerve palsies, usually the IIIrd, rarely the VIth. These may result from dilatation of the internal carotid artery with stretching of the III or VI cranial nerve within the cavernous sinus.

Rarely migraine can present as episodic coma – **MIGRAINE COMA.**

Retinal

Unilateral (monocular) visual loss which is reversible and followed by headache. Ophthalmological examination between episodes is normal.

HEADACHE – SPECIFIC CAUSES

Precipitating factors in migraine
- Dietary: alcohol, chocolate and cheese (contain tyramine).
- Hormonal: often premenstrual or related to oral contraceptive (fluctuations in oestrogen).
- Stress, physical fatigue, exercise, sleep deprivation and minor head trauma.

Diagnosis
Clinical history with   – occasional positive family history
                         – travel sickness or migraine variants (abdominal pains) in childhood
                         – onset in childhood, adolescence, early adult life or menopause
Distinguish – partial (focal) epilepsy (in hemiplegic or hemisensory migraine)
                 – aneurysm compressing III cranial nerve (in ophthalmoplegic migraine)
                 – transient ischaemic attack (in hemiplegic or hemisensory migraine)
                 – arteriovenous malformation – gives well localised but chronic headache)
                 – hypoglycaemia

Management
(i)   Identification and avoidance of precipitating factors
(ii) Prophylaxis: use only for frequent and severe attacks
    Pizotifen (5HT$_2$ receptor blocker)
    Propranolol (beta adrenergic receptor blocker)
    Methysergide (5HT$_2$ receptor blocker) – use with caution in view of side effects,
       e.g. retroperitoneal fibrosis.
    In resistant cases, use *calcium antagonists, antidepressants* and *anticonvulsants,*
       e.g.Topiramate.
(iii) Treatment of an acute attack:
    Simple *analgesics* (e.g. aspirin) with *metoclopramide* to enhance reduced absorption
       during an attack.
    Sumatriptan (a selective 5HT$_1$ agonist) and other triptans e.g. Naratriptan, Rizatriptan
       and Zolmitriptan – effectively reverse dilatation in extracranial vessels. Given orally
       or subcutaneously.
    Ergotamine – widespread action on 5HT receptors reversing dilatation. Give orally or
       by inhalation, injection or by suppository.
    Methylprednisolone i.m. or i.v. will halt the attack when prolonged (status migrainosus).

CLUSTER HEADACHES (Histamine cephalgia or migrainous neuralgia)
Cluster headaches occur less frequently than migraine, and more often in men than women, with onset in middle age.

Characteristics: Severe unilateral pain around one eye, associated with conjunctival injection, lacrimation, rhinorrhea and occasionally a transient Horner's syndrome.

Duration: 10 minutes to 2 hours.

Frequency: Once to many times per day, often wakening from sleep at night. 'Clusters' of attacks separated by weeks or even many months. Alcohol may precipitate the attacks.

Mechanism: Serum histamine levels rise during the attacks, hence 'histamine cephalgia'.

Treatment: Antihistamines give disappointing results. *Ergotamine* and *sumatriptan* may give relief. Use *prednisolone* 30 mg daily in refractory cases. For prevention, use *methysergide, calcium channel blockers* or *lithium carbonate.*

HEADACHE – SPECIFIC CAUSES

POST-TRAUMATIC HEADACHE

A 'common migraine' or 'tension-like' headache may arise after head injury and accompany other symptoms including light-headedness, irritability, difficulty in concentration and in coping with work. Although once thought to have a purely 'psychological' origin, especially with impending litigation, it is now recognised that injuries severe enough to cause loss of consciousness or a period of post-traumatic amnesia result in some neuronal damage and abnormalities of evoked responses. A headache similar to migraine can occur after neck injury and responds to propranolol.

Treatment: As for tension headache.

GIANT CELL (TEMPORAL) ARTERITIS

Giant cell arteritis, an autoimmune disease of unknown cause, presents with headache in the elderly. This is severe and throbbing in nature and overlies the involved vessel – usually the superficial temporal artery, although the condition may affect any extra- or intracranial vessel.

Palpation reveals a thickened, tender, but nonpulsatile artery.
Neurological symptoms: strokes, hearing loss, myelopathy and neuropathy may result.
Jaw claudication: pain when chewing or talking due to ischaemia of the masseter muscles is pathognomonic and occurs in a high proportion of patients.
Visual symptoms are common with blindness (transient or permanent) or diplopia.
Associated systemic symptoms – weight loss, lassitude and generalised muscle aches – polymyalgia rheumatica in one-fifth of cases.
Duration: the headache is intractable, lasting until treatment commences.

Mechanism:

Large and medium-sized arteries undergo intense 'giant cell' infiltration, with fragmentation of the lamina and narrowing of the lumen, resulting in distal ischaemia as well as stimulating pain sensitive fibres. Occlusion of important end arteries, e.g. the ophthalmic artery, may result in blindness; occlusion of the basilar artery may cause brain stem or bilateral occipital infarction.

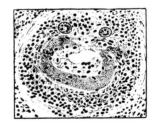

Thickened wall with giant cell infiltrate

Diagnosis: ESR usually high. Blood film shows anaemia or thrombocytosis. C-reactive protein and hepatic alkaline phosphatase elevated. Biopsy of 1 cm length of temporal artery is often diagnostic.

Treatment: Urgent treatment, prednisolone 60 mg daily, prevents visual loss or brain-stem stroke, as well as relieving the headache. If complications have already occurred e.g. blindness, give parenteral high dose steroids. Monitoring the ESR allows gradual reduction in steroid dosage over several weeks to a maintenance level, e.g. 5 mg daily. Most patients eventually come off steroids; 25% require long-term treatment and if so, complications commonly occur.

HEADACHE – SPECIFIC CAUSES

HEADACHE FROM RAISED INTRACRANIAL PRESSURE

Characteristics:
– generalised.
– aggravated by bending or coughing.
– worse in the morning on awakening; may awaken patient from sleep.
– the severity of the headache gradually progresses.

Associated features:
– vomiting in later stages.
– transient loss of vision (obscuration) with sudden change in posture.
– eventual impairment of conscious level

Management:
    further investigations are essential – CT or MRI

Low Pressure headache
(Spontaneous intracranial hypotension/post lumbar puncture headache) Due to obvious or occult CSF leak. Headache is posturally dependent (worse when erect and eased by lying flat). MRI shows downward displacement of midline structures e.g. cerebellar tonsils, meningeal enhancement with contrast (Gd) and an elevated CSF protein. Spontaneous improvement is usual, occasionally a dural 'blood patch' at the site of CSF leak (post LP or epidural anaesthesia) is necessary.

HEADACHE DUE TO INTRACRANIAL HAEMORRHAGE

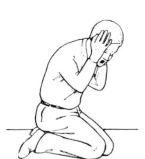

Characteristics:
– instantaneous onset.
– severe pain, spreading over the vertex to the occiput, or described as a 'sudden blow to the back of the head'.
– patient may drop to knees or lose consciousness.

Associated features:
– usually accompanied by vomiting.
– focal neurological signs suggest a haematoma.

Management: further investigation – CT scan/lumbar puncture (see Meningism, page 73).

NON-NEUROLOGICAL CAUSES OF HEADACHE

Local causes:

Sinuses: Well localised. Worse in morning. Affected by posture, e.g. bending.
    X-ray – sinus opacified. Treatment – decongestants or drainage.

Ocular: Refraction errors may result in 'muscle contraction' headaches
    – resolves when corrected with glasses.
    Glaucoma does not produce headache without other symptoms,
    e.g. misting of vision, 'haloes'. Cupping seen on fundoscopy.

Dental disease: Discomfort localised to teeth. Check for malocclusion.
        Check temporomandibular joints.

Systemic causes:

Headache may accompany any febrile illness or may be the presenting feature of accelerated hypertension or metabolic disease, e.g. hypoglycaemia, hypercalcaemia.

Many drugs produce headache
    – through vasodilatation e.g. bronchodilators, antihistamines
    – on withdrawal e.g. amphetamines, benzodiazepines, caffeine.

MENINGISM

Evidence of meningeal irritation caused by infection or subarachnoid haemorrhage results in characteristic clinical features:

SYMPTOMS
1. Headache
2. Vomiting
3. Photophobia

SIGNS

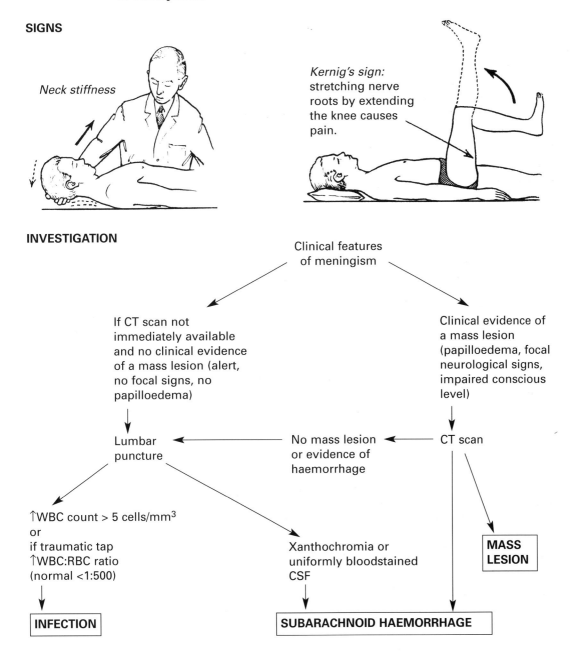

Neck stiffness

Kernig's sign: stretching nerve roots by extending the knee causes pain.

INVESTIGATION

Clinical features of meningism

If CT scan not immediately available and no clinical evidence of a mass lesion (alert, no focal signs, no papilloedema)

Clinical evidence of a mass lesion (papilloedema, focal neurological signs, impaired conscious level)

Lumbar puncture ←— No mass lesion or evidence of haemorrhage ←— CT scan

↑WBC count > 5 cells/mm³
or
if traumatic tap
↑WBC:RBC ratio
(normal <1:500)

Xanthochromia or uniformly bloodstained CSF

MASS LESION

INFECTION

SUBARACHNOID HAEMORRHAGE

73

RAISED INTRACRANIAL PRESSURE

The skull is basically a rigid structure. Since its contents – brain, blood and cerebrospinal fluid (CSF) – are incompressible, an increase in one constituent or an expanding mass within the skull results in an increase in intracranial pressure (ICP) – the 'Monro-Kellie doctrine'.

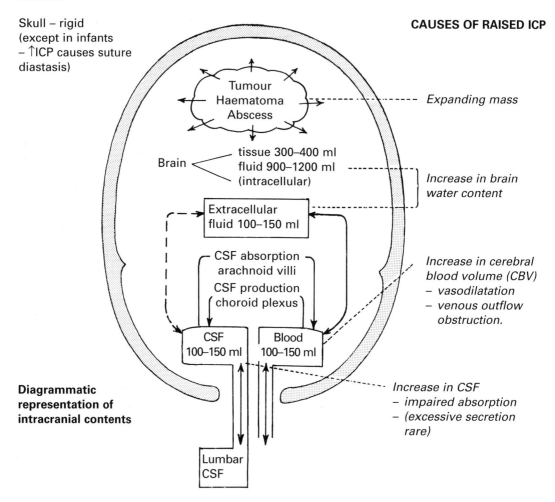

Skull – rigid
(except in infants
– ↑ICP causes suture
diastasis)

CAUSES OF RAISED ICP

Tumour
Haematoma
Abscess

Expanding mass

Brain

tissue 300–400 ml
fluid 900–1200 ml
(intracellular)

Increase in brain
water content

Extracellular
fluid 100–150 ml

CSF absorption
arachnoid villi
CSF production
choroid plexus

Increase in cerebral
blood volume (CBV)
– vasodilatation
– venous outflow
obstruction.

CSF
100–150 ml

Blood
100–150 ml

**Diagrammatic
representation of
intracranial contents**

Increase in CSF
– impaired absorption
– (excessive secretion
rare)

Lumbar
CSF

Compensatory mechanisms for an expanding intracranial mass lesion:

– Immediate $\begin{cases} 1. \downarrow \text{CSF volume – CSF outflow to the lumbar theca} \\ 2. \downarrow \text{Cerebral blood volume} \end{cases}$

– Delayed –   3. ↓ Extracellular fluid

RAISED INTRACRANIAL PRESSURE

CEREBROSPINAL FLUID (CSF)

Secreted at a rate of 500 ml per day from the choroid plexus, CSF flows through the ventricular system and enters the subarachnoid space via the 4th ventricular foramina of Magendie and Luschka.

Under normal conditions, CSF flows freely through the subarachnoid space and is absorbed into the venous system through the arachnoid villi. If flow is obstructed at any point in the pathway, *hydrocephalus* with an associated rise in intracranial pressure develops, as a result of continued CSF production. With an expanding intracranial mass lesion, normal pressure is initially maintained by CSF expulsion to the expandable lumbar theca. Further expansion and subsequent brain shift may obstruct the free flow of CSF not only to the lumbar theca but also to the arachnoid villi, causing an acute rise in intracranial pressure.

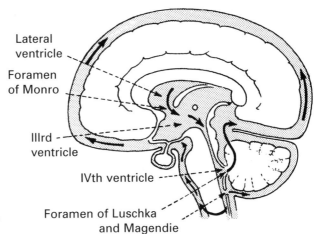

Lateral ventricle

Foramen of Monro

IIIrd ventricle

IVth ventricle

Foramen of Luschka and Magendie

BRAIN WATER/OEDEMA

Cerebral oedema – an excess of brain water – may develop around an intrinsic lesion within the brain tissue, e.g. tumour or abscess or in relation to traumatic or ischaemic brain damage, and contribute to the space-occupying effect.

Different forms of cerebral oedema exist:

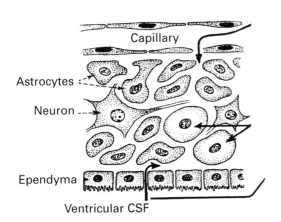

Capillary

Astrocytes

Neuron

Ependyma

Ventricular CSF

Vasogenic: excess fluid (protein rich) passes through damaged vessel walls to the extracellular space – especially in the white matter. The extracellular fluid gradually infiltrates throughout normal brain tissue towards the ventricular CSF and this drainage route may aid clearance. E.g. adjacent to tumour.

Cytotoxic: fluid accumulates within cells – neurons and glia i.e. intracellular. E.g. toxic or metabolic states.

Interstitial: when obstructive hydrocephalus develops, CSF is forced through to the extracellular space especially in the periventricular white matter.

With *ischaemic* damage, as cell metabolism fails, intracellular Na^+ and Ca^{2+} increase and the cells swell i.e. cytotoxic oedema. Capillary damage follows and vasogenic oedema supervenes.

75

RAISED INTRACRANIAL PRESSURE

CEREBRAL BLOOD FLOW (CBF)/CEREBRAL BLOOD VOLUME (CBV)

Blood flow is dependent on blood pressure and the vascular resistance:

$$\text{Flow} = \frac{\text{Pressure}}{\text{Resistance}}$$

Inside the skull, intracranial pressure must be taken into account:

$$\text{Cerebral blood flow (CBF)} = \frac{\text{Cerebral perfusion pressure (CPP)}}{\text{(i.e. systemic BP – intracranial pressure)}}{\text{Cerebral vascular resistance (CVR)}}$$

Under normal conditions the cerebral blood flow is coupled to the energy requirements of brain tissue. Various regulatory mechanisms acting on the arterioles maintain a cerebral blood flow sufficient to meet the metabolic demands.

FACTORS AFFECTING THE CEREBRAL VASCULATURE

Chemoregulation

- Change in extracellular pH or an accumulation of metabolic by-products directly affects the vessel calibre.

- Any change in arteriolar P_{CO_2} has a direct effect on cerebral vessels, but only a reduction of P_{O_2} to < 50 mmHg has a significant effect.

Autoregulation

- A change in the cerebral perfusion pressure results in a compensatory change in vessel calibre.

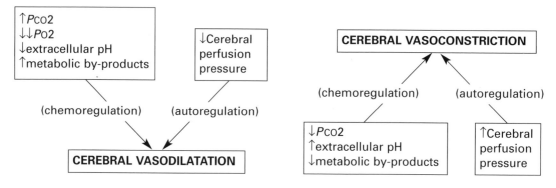

Any change in blood vessel diameter results in considerable variation in cerebral blood volume and this, in turn, directly affects intracranial pressure.

Energy requirements differ in different parts of the brain. To meet such needs in the white matter, flow is 20 ml/100 g/min, whereas in the grey matter flow is as high as 100 ml/100 g/min.

RAISED INTRACRANIAL PRESSURE

CEREBRAL BLOOD FLOW *(cont'd)*

Autoregulation is a compensatory mechanism which permits fluctuation in the cerebral perfusion pressure within certain limits without significantly altering cerebral blood flow.

A drop in cerebral perfusion pressure produces vasodilation (probably due to a direct 'myogenic' effect on the vascular smooth muscle) thereby maintaining flow; a rise in the cerebral perfusion pressure causes vasoconstriction.

Neurogenic influences appear to have little direct effect on the cerebral vessels but they may alter the range of pressure changes over which autoregulation acts.

Autoregulation fails when the cerebral perfusion pressure falls below 60 mmHg or rises above 160 mmHg. At these extremes, cerebral blood flow is more directly related to the perfusion pressure.

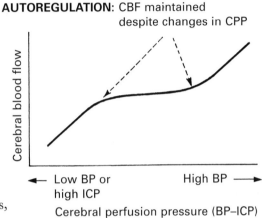

In damaged brain (e.g. after head injury or subarachnoid haemorrhage), autoregulation is impaired; a drop in cerebral perfusion pressure is more likely to reduce cerebral blood flow and cause ischaemia. Conversely, a high cerebral perfusion may increase the cerebral blood flow, break down the blood–brain barrier and produce cerebral oedema as in hypertensive encephalopathy.

INTRACRANIAL PRESSURE (ICP)

Intracranial pressure, measured relative to the foramen of Monro, under normal conditions ranges from 0–135 mm CSF (0–10 mmHg) although very high pressure, e.g., 1000 mm CSF may occur transiently during coughing or straining.

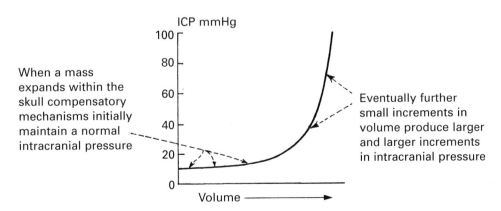

RAISED INTRACRANIAL PRESSURE

ICP *(cont'd)*

When intracranial pressure is monitored with a ventricular catheter, regular waves due to pulse and respiratory effects are recorded (page 52). As an intracranial mass expands and as the compensatory reserves diminish, transient pressure elevations (pressure waves) are superimposed. These become more frequent and more prominent as the mean pressure rises.

Eventually the rise in intracranial pressure and resultant fall in cerebral perfusion pressure reach a critical level and a significant reduction in cerebral blood flow occurs. Electrical activity in the cortex fails at flow rates about 20 ml/100 g/min. If autoregulation is already impaired these effects develop even earlier. When intracranial pressure reaches the mean arterial blood pressure, cerebral blood flow ceases.

INTERRELATIONSHIPS

Many factors affect intracranial pressure and these should not be considered in isolation. Inter-relationships are complex and feedback pathways may merely serve to compound the brain damage.

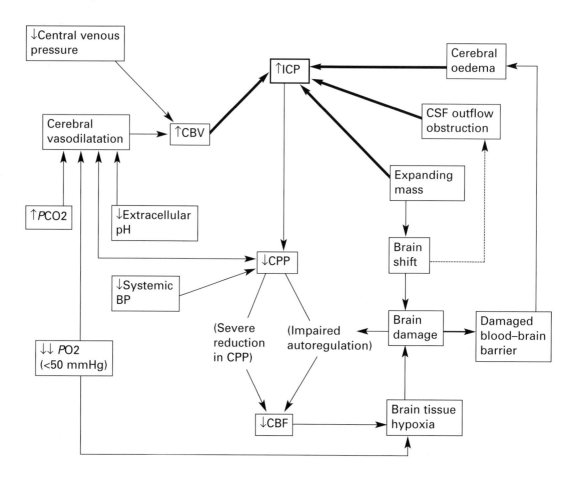

RAISED INTRACRANIAL PRESSURE

CLINICAL EFFECTS OF RAISED INTRACRANIAL PRESSURE

A raised ICP will produce symptoms and signs but does not cause neuronal damage provided cerebral blood flow is maintained. Damage does, however, result from brain shift – tentorial or tonsillar herniation.

Clinical features due to ↑ICP:

1. *Headache* – worse in the mornings, aggravated by stooping and bending.
2. *Vomiting* – occurs with an acute rise in ICP.
3. *Papilloedema* – occurs in a proportion of patients with ↑ICP. It is related to CSF obstruction and does not necessarily occur with brain shift alone. Increased CSF pressure in the optic nerve sheath impedes venous drainage and axoplasmic flow in optic neurons. Swelling of the optic disc and retinal and disc haemorrhages result. Vision is only at risk when papilloedema is both severe and prolonged.

BRAIN SHIFT – TYPES

TENTORIAL HERNIATION (lateral):
a unilateral expanding mass causes tentorial (uncal) herniation as the medial edge of the temporal lobe herniates through the tentorial hiatus. As the intracranial pressure continues to rise, 'central' herniation follows.

SUBFALCINE 'MIDLINE' SHIFT: occurs early with unilateral space-occupying lesions. Seldom produces any clinical effect, although ipsilateral anterior cerebral artery occlusion has been recorded.

TONSILLAR HERNIATION:
a subtentorial expanding mass causes herniation of the cerebellar tonsils through the foramen magnum. A degree of *upward* herniation through the tentorial hiatus may also occur. Clinical effects are difficult to distinguish from effects of direct brainstem/midbrain compression.

TENTORIAL HERNIATION (central):
a midline lesion or diffuse swelling of the cerebral hemispheres results in a vertical displacement of the midbrain and diencephalon through the tentorial hiatus. Damage to these structures occurs either from mechanical distortion or from ischaemia secondary to stretching of the perforating vessels.

Unchecked lateral tentorial herniation leads to central tentorial and tonsillar herniation, associated with progressive brain stem dysfunction from midbrain to medulla.

RAISED INTRACRANIAL PRESSURE

CLINICAL EFFECTS OF BRAIN SHIFT

The rate of symptom progression is related to the rate of lesion expansion.

TENTORIAL HERNIATION – Lateral

The posterior cerebral artery is sometimes occluded but the resultant *homonymous hemianopia* is rarely detected in the acute stage

Pressure against the reticular formation in the midbrain causes *deterioration of conscious level*

Pressure from the edge of the tentorium cerebelli on the opposite cerebral peduncle (Kernohan's notch) may produce *limb weakness on the same side* as the lesion i.e. 'false localising sign'

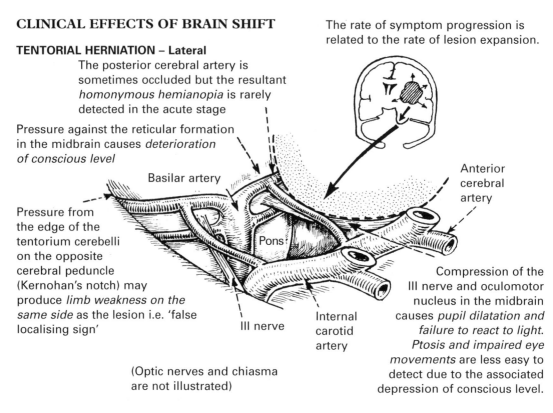

Basilar artery

Pons

III nerve

Internal carotid artery

Anterior cerebral artery

Compression of the III nerve and oculomotor nucleus in the midbrain causes *pupil dilatation and failure to react to light. Ptosis and impaired eye movements* are less easy to detect due to the associated depression of conscious level.

(Optic nerves and chiasma are not illustrated)

TENTORIAL HERNIATION – Central

Pressure on dorsal aspect (pretectum and superior colliculi) *impairs eye movements* – upward gaze is initially lost

Diencephalon and midbrain damage from buckling and distortion and stretching of perforating vessels causes: *deterioration of conscious level. Pupils initially small, become moderately dilated and fixed to light*

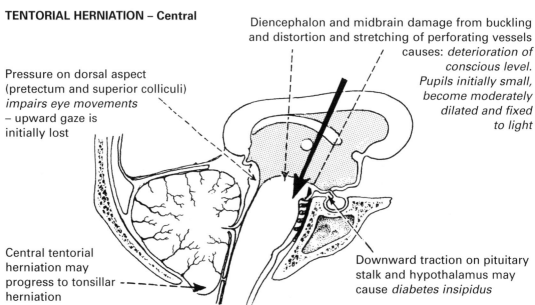

Central tentorial herniation may progress to tonsillar herniation

Downward traction on pituitary stalk and hypothalamus may cause *diabetes insipidus*

RAISED INTRACRANIAL PRESSURE

CLINICAL EFFECTS OF BRAIN SHIFT *(cont'd)*

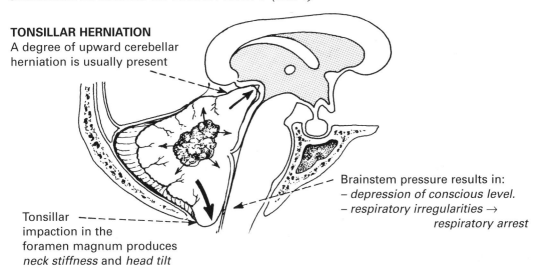

TONSILLAR HERNIATION
A degree of upward cerebellar herniation is usually present

Tonsillar impaction in the foramen magnum produces *neck stiffness* and *head tilt*

Brainstem pressure results in:
– *depression of conscious level.*
– *respiratory irregularities* → *respiratory arrest*

An injudicious lumbar puncture in the presence of a subtentorial mass may create a pressure gradient sufficient to induce tonsillar herniation.

N.B. Harvey Cushing described cardiovascular changes – an increase in blood pressure and a fall in pulse rate, associated with an expanding intracranial mass, and probably resulting from direct medullary compression. The clinical value of these observations is often overemphasised. They are often absent; when present they are invariably preceded by a deterioration in conscious level.

INVESTIGATIONS
Patients with suspected raised intracranial pressure require an urgent CT/MRI scan. Intracranial pressure monitoring where appropriate (see page 52).

TREATMENT OF RAISED INTRACRANIAL PRESSURE
When a rising intracranial pressure is caused by an expanding mass, or is compounded by respiratory problems, treatment is clear-cut; the mass must be removed and blood gases restored to normal levels – by ventilation if necessary.

In some patients, despite the above measures, cerebral swelling may produce a marked increase in intracranial pressure. This may follow removal of a tumour or haematoma or may complicate a diffuse head injury. Artificial methods of lowering intracranial pressure may prevent brain damage and death from brain shift, but some methods lead to reduced cerebral blood flow, which in itself may cause brain damage (see page 82).

Intracranial pressure is monitored with a ventricular catheter or surface pressure recording device (see page 51).

Treatment may be instituted when the mean ICP is > 25 mmHg.

RAISED INTRACRANIAL PRESSURE

TREATMENT *(cont'd)*

Methods of reducing intracranial pressure

Mannitol infusion: An i.v. bolus of 100 ml of 20% mannitol infused over 15 minutes reduces intracranial pressure by establishing an osmotic gradient between the plasma and brain tissue. *This method 'buys' time prior to craniotomy in a patient deteriorating from a mass lesion.* Mannitol is also used 6 hourly for a 24–48 hour period in an attempt to reduce raised ICP. Repeated infusions, however, lead to equilibration and a high intracellular osmotic pressure, thus counteracting further treatment. In addition, repeated doses may precipitate lethal rises in arterial blood pressure and acute tubular necrosis. Its use is therefore best reserved for emergency situations.

CSF withdrawal: Removal of a few ml of CSF from the ventricle immediately reduces the intracranial pressure. Within minutes, however, the pressure will rise and further CSF withdrawal will be required. In practice, this method is of limited value, since CSF outflow to the lumbar theca results in a diminished intracranial CSF volume and the lateral ventricles are often collapsed. Continuous CSF drainage may make most advantage of this method.

Sedatives: If intracranial pressure fails to respond to standard measures then sedation may help under carefully controlled conditions.

Propofol, a short acting anaesthetic agent, reduces intracranial pressure but causes systemic vasodilatation. If this occurs pressor agents may be required to prevent a fall in blood pressure and a reduction in cerebral perfusion.

Barbiturates (thiopentone) reduce neuronal activity and depress cerebral metabolism; a fall in energy requirements theoretically protects ischaemic areas. Associated vasoconstriction can reduce cerebral blood volume and intracranial pressure but systemic hypotension and myocardial depression also occur. *Clinical trials of barbiturate therapy have not demonstrated any improvement in outcome.*

Etomidate also provides cerebral protection by reducing cerebral metabolism and intracranial pressure without producing cardiodepression. It inhibits endogenous steroid synthesis, and therefore requires steroid cover.

Controlled hyperventilation: Bringing the PCO_2 down to 3.5 kPa by hyperventilating the sedated or paralysed patient causes vasoconstriction. Although this reduces intracranial pressure, the resultant reduction in cerebral blood flow may aggravate ischaemic brain damage and do more harm than good (see page 229). Maintaining the blood pressure and the *cerebral perfusion pressure* (CPP) (>70 mmHg) appears to be as important as lowering intracranial pressure.

Decompressive craniectomy: This technique is gaining renewed interest in treating raised ICP unresponsive to other methods. The principal concern is that although reducing mortality, unacceptable levels of morbidity may result.

Hypothermia: Cooling to 34°C lowers ICP, but trials in head injured patients have failed to demonstrate significant benefit.

Steroids: By stabilising cell membranes, steroids play an important role in treating patients with oedema surrounding intracranial tumours. As yet there is no evidence of benefit after traumatic or ischaemic damage, but a further trial is underway assessing their use in serious head injury.

COMA AND IMPAIRED CONSCIOUS LEVEL

Consciousness is regarded as a state of awareness of self and surroundings. Impaired consciousness is due to disturbed arousal or content of mental function.

Many pathological processes may impair conscious level and numerous terms have been employed to describe the various clinical states which result, including obtundation, stupor, semicoma and deep-coma. These terms result in ambiguity and inconsistency when used by different observers. Recording conscious level with the *Glasgow coma scale* (page 5) avoids these difficulties and clearly describes the level of arousal. With this scale:

CoMA = NO SPEECH, NO EYE OPENING, NO MOTOR RESPONSE

In this section we describe conditions which may present with, or lead to, coma. Patients experiencing 'transient disturbance of conscious level' require a different approach.

Pathophysiology of coma

A 'conscious' state depends on intact cerebral hemispheres, interacting with the ascending reticular activating system in the brain stem, midbrain, hypothalamus and thalamus. Lesions diffusely affecting the cerebral hemispheres, or directly affecting the reticular activating system cause impairment of conscious level:

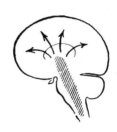

Diffuse hemisphere damage
e.g.   – trauma
       – ischaemia
       – hypoglycaemia
       – hepatic or renal
         failure

[Note: focal damage
   to part of the
   cortex does *not*
   affect conscious
   level]

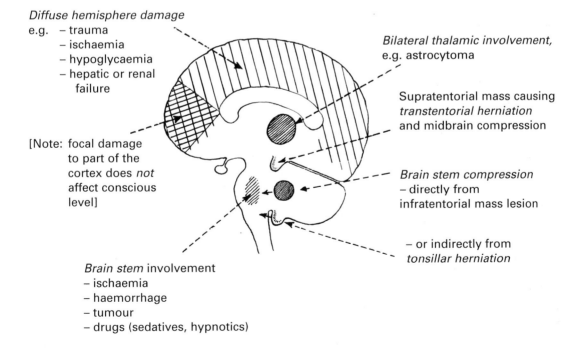

Bilateral thalamic involvement,
e.g. astrocytoma

Supratentorial mass causing
transtentorial herniation
and midbrain compression

Brain stem compression
– directly from
infratentorial mass lesion

– or indirectly from
tonsillar herniation

Brain stem involvement
 – ischaemia
 – haemorrhage
 – tumour
 – drugs (sedatives, hypnotics)

COMA AND IMPAIRED CONSCIOUS LEVEL

CAUSES

INTRACRANIAL

Trauma
Diffuse white matter injury
Haematoma   – extradural
              – subdural
              – 'burst' lobe

Neoplastic
Tumour with oedema

Other
Epilepsy
Hydrocephalus

Vascular
Subarachnoid haemorrhage
'Spontaneous' intracerebral haematoma
Cerebral infarct with oedema and 'shift'
Brain stem infarction or haemorrhage

Infective
Meningitis
Abscess
Encephalitis

EXTRACRANIAL

Metabolic
Hypo/hypernatraemia
Hypo/hyperkalaemia
Hypo/hypercalcaemia
Hypo/hyperglycaemia
Diabetic ketoacidosis
Lactic acidosis
Hypo/hyperthermia
Uraemia
Hepatic failure
Porphyria
Hypercapnia
Hypoxia

Endocrine
Diabetes
Hypopituitarism
Adrenal crisis (Addison's disease)
Hypo/hyperparathyroidism
Hypothyroidism

Respiratory insufficiency
Hypoventilation
Diffusion deficiency
Perfusion deficiency
Anaemia

Arterial occlusion
Vertebral artery disease
Bilateral carotid disease

Reduced cerebral blood flow

Decreased cardiac output
Vasovagal attack
Blood loss
Valvular disease
Myocardial infarction
Cardiac arrhythmias
Hypotensive drugs

Drugs
Sedatives
Opiates
Antidepressants
Anticonvulsants
Anaesthetic agents

Psychiatric disorders
Hysteria
Catatonia (mutism with decreased motor activity)
Fugue states

Toxins
Alcohol
Carbon monoxide
Heavy metals

COMA AND IMPAIRED CONSCIOUS LEVEL

Examination of the unconscious patient *(see pages 29, 30)*

DIAGNOSTIC APPROACH

Questioning friends, relatives or the ambulance team, followed by general and neurological examination all provide important diagnostic information.

History	**Possible cause of coma/impaired conscious level**
Head injury leading to admission ⟶	*Diffuse shearing injury and/or intracranial haematoma*
Previous head injury (e.g. 6 weeks) ⟶	*Chronic subdural haematoma*
Sudden collapse ⟶	*Intracerebral haemorrhage* *Subarachnoid haemorrhage*
Limb twitching, incontinence ⟶	*Epilepsy/postictal state*
Gradual development of symptoms ⟶	*Mass lesion, metabolic or infective cause*
Previous illness – diabetes ⟶	*Hypo- or (less likely) hyperglycaemia*
– epilepsy ⟶	*Postictal state*
– psychiatric illness ⟶	*Drug overdose*
– alcoholism or drug abuse ⟶	*Drug toxicity*
– viral infection ⟶	*Encephalitis*
– malignancy ⟶	*Intracranial metastasis*

General examination

Note the presence of:

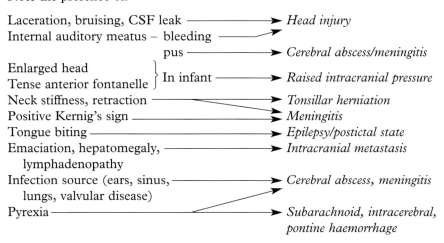

Laceration, bruising, CSF leak ⟶	*Head injury*
Internal auditory meatus – bleeding ⟶	
pus ⟶	*Cerebral abscess/meningitis*
Enlarged head ⎫ In infant ⟶ Tense anterior fontanelle ⎭	*Raised intracranial pressure*
Neck stiffness, retraction ⟶	*Tonsillar herniation*
Positive Kernig's sign ⟶	*Meningitis*
Tongue biting ⟶	*Epilepsy/postictal state*
Emaciation, hepatomegaly, lymphadenopathy ⟶	*Intracranial metastasis*
Infection source (ears, sinus, lungs, valvular disease) ⟶	*Cerebral abscess, meningitis*
Pyrexia ⟶	*Subarachnoid, intracerebral, pontine haemorrhage*

85

COMA AND IMPAIRED CONSCIOUS LEVEL

DIAGNOSTIC APPROACH *(cont'd)*

General examination *(cont'd)*

Possible cause of coma/impaired conscious level

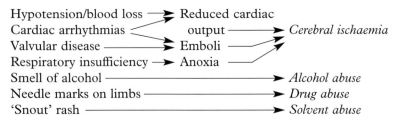

Hypotension/blood loss → Reduced cardiac
Cardiac arrhythmias ⟨ output → *Cerebral ischaemia*
Valvular disease → Emboli →
Respiratory insufficiency → Anoxia

Smell of alcohol ⟶ *Alcohol abuse*
Needle marks on limbs ⟶ *Drug abuse*
'Snout' rash ⟶ *Solvent abuse*

Neurological examination

Signs of raised intracranial pressure (ICP)
  – papilloedema
  – tense anterior fontanelle ⟶ *Intracranial mass lesion*
    (in infants) *Hydrocephalus*
Neurological signs
  – unilateral, dilated, fixed pupil ⟶ *Diffuse cerebral swelling, e.g. anoxia*
  – bilateral dilated, fixed pupils ⟨ *Drugs – anticholinergics* ⟩
      sympathomimetics ⟩ *overdose*

  – pinpoint pupils ⟶ *Drugs – opiates*
      parasympathomimetics
    ⟶ *Pontine haemorrhage*

  – eye movements absent   pupils fixed ⟶ *Severe – trauma*
    (spontaneous or reflex) ⟨   *– ischaemia*
      pupils   *– haemorrhage*
      usually   *Drugs (transient effect)*
      reacting ⟶ *Hypoxic/hepatic encephalopathy*
  – asymmetric limb response ⟶ *Focal brain damage, e.g.*
    (i.e. hemi/monoparesis)   *– tumour*
         – trauma
         – haematoma
         – encephalitis

    ⎡ N.B. – *hepatic encephalopathy* ⎤
    ⎢   – *hypoglycaemia* ⟩ ⟶ occasionally produce ⎥
    ⎣   – *uraemia*   asymmetrical responses ⎦

– Symmetrical limb responses ⎫
– Reacting pupils   ⟩ ⟶ suggest a *metabolic encephalopathy*
– Full eye movements   ⎭   *or drug toxicity*
– Subhyaloid/vitreous haemorrhage (on fundoscopy) ⟶ *Subarachnoid haemorrhage*

COMA AND IMPAIRED CONSCIOUS LEVEL

Investigations

The sequence of investigations depends on clinical suspicion:

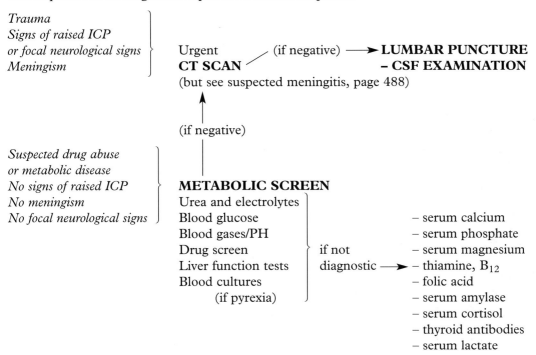

Trauma
Signs of raised ICP
or focal neurological signs } Urgent   (if negative) ⟶ **LUMBAR PUNCTURE**
Meningism   **CT SCAN**   **– CSF EXAMINATION**
(but see suspected meningitis, page 488)

(if negative)

Suspected drug abuse
or metabolic disease
No signs of raised ICP } **METABOLIC SCREEN**
No meningism   Urea and electrolytes
No focal neurological signs Blood glucose   – serum calcium
                       Blood gases/PH   – serum phosphate
                       Drug screen   } if not   – serum magnesium
                       Liver function tests   diagnostic ⟶ – thiamine, B_{12}
                       Blood cultures   – folic acid
                            (if pyrexia)   – serum amylase
                                                – serum cortisol
                                                – thyroid antibodies
                                                – serum lactate

In addition

SKULL X-RAY – may reveal an unsuspected fracture, pineal shift, calcification
                       or an osteolytic lesion.
CHEST X-RAY – may reveal a bronchial carcinoma.
ELECTROENCEPHALOGRAPHY – may provide evidence of – subclinical epilepsy
                                              – herpes simplex encephalitis
                                              – metabolic encephalopathy.

MRI – has a limited role in the investigation of coma. More sensitive than CT scan in demonstrating small ischaemic changes and early encephalitis.

Prognosis

Although *conscious level examination* does not aid diagnosis, it plays an essential role in patient management and along with the *duration of coma, pupil response* and *eye movements* provides valuable prognostic information. Non-traumatic coma tends to carry a better prognosis (see page 212).

TRANSIENT LOSS OF CONSCIOUSNESS

Many conditions causing coma may also transiently affect a patient's conscious level. This results from:

Reduction in cerebral
arterial oxygen supply
 – *cardiac arrhythmias*
 – *cardiac outflow obstruction*
 – *vasovagal attack*
 – *vertebrobasilar ischaemia*
} *reduced cardiac output*

Neuronal suppression
 – *basilar migraine*
 – *hypoglycaemia*

Neuronal excitation
 – *epilepsy*

} Clinical details – *see page 97*

Drug abuse – *alcohol, solvents or barbiturates* – may cause transient, intermittent confusion.

DIAGNOSTIC APPROACH

History
The patient's own description of the attack or that of an eyewitness may establish the diagnosis. Prodromal features of pallor, nausea and sweating accompany *vasovagal attacks*. Clonic/tonic movements occur shortly after the onset of an *epileptic 'grand mal' attack* (but either movement can occur with a prolonged vasovagal attack or cardiac arrhythmia).

Palpitations, sweating, behavioural disturbances and seizures may precede loss of consciousness from *hypoglycaemia*. Vertigo and scintillating teichopsia often precede *basilar migraine*.

Electroencephalography (EEG) may reveal a focal disturbance – *epilepsy*.

Electrocardiography (ECG) may reveal a *cardiac arrythmia*.

Echocardiography may reveal *cardiomyopathy*.

Blood glucose may indicated *hypoglycaemia*.

If an eyewitness account and the above tests provide no evidence of the cause, proceed to:

1. **Telemetric EEG and ECG monitoring** over a 24-hour period.
2. **24–36-hour fast** – if symptoms appear, check **blood glucose** and **insulin (insulinoma)** levels.

Often attacks of unconsciousness remain unexplained and possibly have a psychological or attention-seeking basis. The circumstances of the attack (e.g. during an argument), the non-stereotyped nature of the episode and the lack of personal trauma with repeated falls all suggest a *non-organic* explanation.

CONFUSIONAL STATES AND DELIRIUM

Of all acute medical admissions, 5–10% present with a **confused verbal response**, i.e. disorientation in time and/or place. Most patients are easily distracted, have slowed thought processes and a limited concentration span. Some may lose interest in the examination to the point of drifting off to sleep.

Perceptual disorders (illusions and hallucinations) may accompany the confused state – **delirium**. This is often associated with withdrawal and lack of awareness or with restlessness and hyperactivity.

Primary neurological disorders contribute to only 10% of those patients presenting with an acute confusional state. In the elderly, postoperative disorientation is particularly common and multiple factors probably apply; in these patients the prognosis is good.

The Confusion Assessment Method (CAM) is used to confirm delirium.
        Feature 1 – Acute onset and fluctuating course.
        Feature 2 – Inattention.
        Feature 3 – Disorganised thinking.
        Feature 4 – Altered level of consciousness.
The presence of features 1 and 2 and either 3 or 4 are diagnostic.

DIAGNOSTIC APPROACH

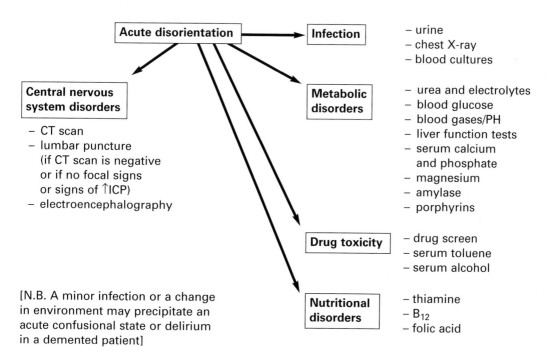

Acute disorientation → **Infection**
 – urine
 – chest X-ray
 – blood cultures

Central nervous system disorders
 – CT scan
 – lumbar puncture
 (if CT scan is negative
 or if no focal signs
 or signs of ↑ICP)
 – electroencephalography

Metabolic disorders
 – urea and electrolytes
 – blood glucose
 – blood gases/PH
 – liver function tests
 – serum calcium
 and phosphate
 – magnesium
 – amylase
 – porphyrins

Drug toxicity
 – drug screen
 – serum toluene
 – serum alcohol

[N.B. A minor infection or a change in environment may precipitate an acute confusional state or delirium in a demented patient]

Nutritional disorders
 – thiamine
 – B$_{12}$
 – folic acid

EPILEPSY

Definitions

A seizure or epileptic attack is the consequence of a paroxysmal uncontrolled discharge of neurons within the central nervous system. The clinical manifestations range from a major motor convulsion to a brief period of lack of awareness.

The *prodrome* refers to mood or behavioural changes which may precede the attack by some hours.
The *aura* refers to the symptom immediately before a seizure and will localise the attack to its point of origin within the nervous system.
The *ictus* refers to the attack or seizure itself.
The *postictal period* refers to the time immediately after the ictus during which the patient may be confused, disorientated and demonstrate automatic behaviours.
The stereotyped and uncontrollable nature of the attack is characteristic of epilepsy.

Pathogenesis

Epilepsy has been described since ancient times. The 19th century neurologist Hughlings-Jackson suggested 'a sudden excessive disorderly discharge of cerebral neurons' as the causation of the attack. Berger (1929) recorded the first electroencephalogram (EEG) and not long after, it was appreciated that certain seizures were characterised by particular EEG abnormalities.

Recent studies in animal models of *focal epilepsy* suggest a central role for the excitatory neurotransmitter glutamate. This produces a depolarisation shift by activating receptors which in turn facilitate cellular influx of Na^+, K^+ and Ca^{2+}. Gamma amino butyric acid (GABA) has an important inhibitory influence in containing abnormal cortical discharges and preventing the development of generalised seizures.

Epilepsies have complex inheritance; molecular genetics studies in rarer syndromes with autosomal dominant features have identified genes that code for ion channel subunits, either ligand or voltage gated (Channelopathies).

Incidence and course

Epilepsy usually presents in childhood or adolescence but may occur for the first time at any age.

5% of the population suffer a single seizure at some time.

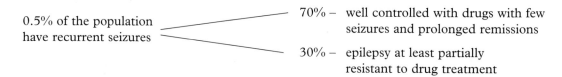

0.5% of the population have recurrent seizures

70% – well controlled with drugs with few seizures and prolonged remissions

30% – epilepsy at least partially resistant to drug treatment

Though there is considerable variability depending on seizure type, 6 years after diagnosis 40% of patients have had a substantial remission; after 20 years – 75%.

EPILEPSY IS A SYMPTOM OF NUMEROUS DISORDERS, BUT IN THE MAJORITY OF SUFFERERS THE CAUSE REMAINS UNCLEAR DESPITE CAREFUL HISTORY TAKING, EXAMINATION AND INVESTIGATION.

EPILEPSY – CLASSIFICATION

The modern classification of the epilepsies is based upon the *nature* of the attack rather than the presence or absence of an underlying cause. The use of the electroencephalogram (EEG) has greatly increased our understanding of the source of 'point of origin' of any particular type of epileptic attack.

Attacks which begin **focally** from a single location within one hemisphere are thus distinguished from those of a **generalised** nature which probably commence in deeper midline structures and project to both hemispheres simultaneously.

CLASSIFICATION OF EPILEPSIES
(Revised classification of International League Against Epilepsy [ILAE] 1989)

1. PARTIAL (focal, local) SEIZURE

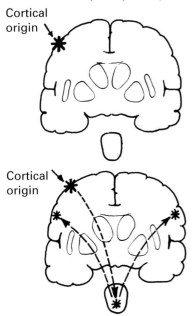

Cortical origin

Cortical origin

A. Simple partial seizures
   – motor
   – sensory

B. Complex partial seizures (when partial seizure is accompanied by any degree of impaired conscious level)

C. Partial seizures evolving to tonic/clonic convulsion

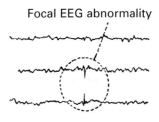

Focal EEG abnormality

Focal → generalised EEG abnormality

2. GENERALISED SEIZURES (convulsive or non-convulsive)

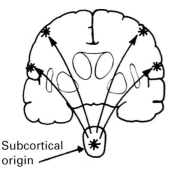

Subcortical origin

A. Absences
B. Myoclonic seizures
C. Clonic seizures
D. Tonic seizures
E. Tonic/clonic seizures
F. Atonic seizures

Generalised EEG abnormality

3. UNCLASSIFIED SEIZURES, e.g. Some neonatal seizures
Rhythmic eye movement disorders

THE PARTIAL SEIZURES

Partial seizures account for 80% of adult epilepsies.

SIMPLE MOTOR SEIZURES

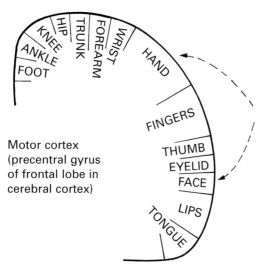

Motor cortex
(precentral gyrus
of frontal lobe in
cerebral cortex)

These arise in the frontal motor cortex with movements occurring in contralateral face, trunk or limbs.

The **Jacksonian** motor seizure consists of a 'march' of involuntary movement from one muscle group to the next.

Movement is clonic (shaking) and usually begins in hand or face – these having the largest representative cortical area.

Motor seizures with the above 'march' are quite rare, usually they are less localised, involving many muscle groups simultaneously and are tonic (rigid) or clonic.

After a motor seizure the affected limb(s) may remain weak for some hours before return of function occurs – **Todd's paralysis.**

Adversive seizures

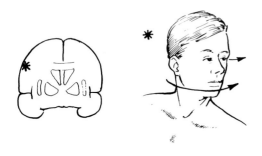

The patient is aware of movement of the head. Attacks often progress to loss of consciousness and tonic/clonic epilepsy.

The patient's eyes and head turn away from the site of the focal origin usually in the supplementary motor cortex of the frontal lobe with involvement of the frontal 'gaze centre'. Some doubt the localising value of such an attack.

SIMPLE SENSORY SEIZURES

These arise in the sensory cortex, the patient describing paraesthesia or tingling in an extremity or on the face sometimes associated with a sensation of distortion of body image. A 'march' similar to the Jacksonian motor seizure may occur. Motor symptoms occur concurrently – the limb appears weak without involuntary movement.

The representation of limbs, trunk, etc. in the post-Rolandic sensory cortex is similar to that of the motor cortex.

VISUAL, AUDITORY and AUTONOMIC simple partial seizures occur, but are rare.

Motor and sensory seizures indicate structural brain disease, the focal onset localising the lesion. Full investigation is mandatory.

THE PARTIAL SEIZURES

COMPLEX PARTIAL SEIZURES

These attacks usually originate within the temporal lobe and are characterised by a complex aura (initial symptom) and some impairment of consciousness.

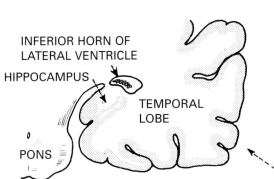

INFERIOR HORN OF
LATERAL VENTRICLE

HIPPOCAMPUS

TEMPORAL
LOBE

PONS

Complex partial seizures are generally synonymous with **psychomotor epilepsy** and **temporal lobe epilepsy** (though motor, sensory and other partial seizures can be associated with impaired consciousness when propagated through the temporal lobe – extratemporal complex partial seizures).

The seizure origin lies in the medial part of the temporal lobe, hippocampus or lateral surface of the lobe.

Coronal section through the pons showing medial aspect of the temporal lobe and hippocampus

The nature of the attack

The content of attacks may vary in an individual patient. Commonly encountered symptoms include:

Visceral disturbance: Gustatory (taste) and olfactory (smell) hallucinations, lip smacking, epigastric fullness, choking sensation, nausea, pallor, pupillary changes (dilatation), tachycardia.

Memory disturbance: Déjà vu ('something has happened before'), jamais vu ('feeling of unfamiliarity'), depersonalisation, derealisation, flashbacks, formed visual or auditory hallucinations.

Motor disturbance: Fumbling movement, rubbing, chewing, semi-purposeful limb movements.

Affective disturbance: Displeasure, pleasure, depression, elation, fear.

A constellation of these symptoms associated with subtle clouding of consciousness characterises a complex partial seizure.

AUTOMATISM occurs during the state of clouding of consciousness either during or after the attack (postictal) and takes the form of involuntary, often complicated, motor activity. In ambulatory automatism, subjects may 'wander off'.

Confusion and headache after an attack are common. The whole episode may last for seconds but occasionally may be prolonged and a rapid succession or cluster of attacks may occur. Attacks show an increased incidence in adolescence and early adult life. A history of birth trauma or febrile convulsions in infancy may be obtained. Lesions in the hippocampus occur as a result of anoxia or from the convulsion itself and act as a source of further epilepsy. When surgery is carried out, hippocampal sclerosis is often found. Occasionally other pathologies are identified, such as hamartomas, vascular malformations and low-grade malignant astrocytomas.

PARTIAL SEIZURES EVOLVING TO TONIC/CLONIC CONVULSION

Seizure discharges have the capacity to spread from their point of origin and excite other structures. When spread occurs to the subcortical structures (thalamus and upper reticular formation) their excitation releases a discharge which spreads back to the cerebral cortex of both hemispheres, resulting in a tonic/clonic seizure. This chain of events is reflected in the electroencephalogram (EEG).

The symptoms before the tonic/clonic convulsion give a clue to the site of the initial discharge (simple partial or complex partial).

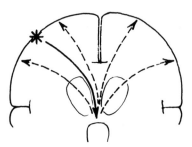
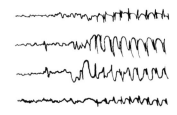

An eyewitness account is important because retrograde amnesia may prevent recall of the onset.

TONIC/CLONIC ATTACKS
Loss of consciousness; falls to the ground.

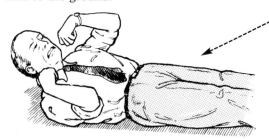

1. **Tonic phase (10 seconds)**
   Eyes open. Elbows flexed.
   Arms pronated. Legs extended.
   Teeth clenched. Pupils dilated.
   Breath held – cyanosis.
   Bowel/bladder control may be
   lost at the end of this phase.

2. **Clonic phase (1–2 minutes)**
   Tremor gives way to violent
     generalised shaking.
   Eyes roll backwards and forwards.
   Tongue may be bitten.
   Tachycardia develops.
   Breathing recommences at end of phase.

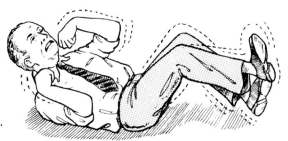

The patient then sleeps with stertorous respiration and cannot be roused. On regaining consciousness, confusion and headache are present. He may feel exhausted for hours or even days afterwards. Muscles may ache as a result of violent movement and muscle damage occurs with elevation of the muscle enzyme creatinine phosphokinase (CPK). Trauma occurs frequently, either as a result of the fall, or as a result of the movements, e.g. posterior dislocation of the shoulder. Very rarely sudden death may occur from inhalation or an associated cardiac arrhythmia.

The differentiation of these attacks from pseudoseizures will be discussed later.

GENERALISED SEIZURES

Generalised seizure attacks arise from subcortical structures and involve both hemispheres. Consciousness may be impaired and motor manifestations are bilateral.

ABSENCES (*SYN*: **Petit mal**)

Onset usually in childhood (between 4 and 12 years of age). Family history in 40% of patients.

The absence may occur many times a day with a duration of 5–15 seconds.

The patient stares vacantly, eyes may blink and myoclonic jerks occur.

Attacks may be induced by hyperventilation.

Frequent episodes lead to falling off in scholastic performance.

Attacks rarely present beyond adolescence.

In 30% of children, adolescence may bring tonic/clonic seizures (**Grand mal**).

Distinction of absences from complex partial seizures is easy; the latter are longer – 30 seconds or more – and followed by headache, lethargy, confusion and automatism.

The *ELECTROENCEPHALOGRAM (EEG)* is diagnostic.

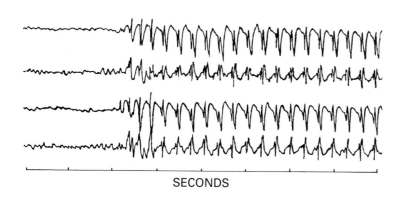

SECONDS

3 per second spike and wave activity occurs in all leads, persisting as long as the seizure. Hyperventilation evokes this appearance during recording.

Similarly, photic stimulation – flashing a light in both eyes – may produce spike and wave discharge.

PETIT MAL STATUS

Long periods of clouding of consciousness with continuing 'spike and wave' activity on the EEG.

MYOCLONIC SEIZURES

Sudden, brief, generalised muscle contractions. They often occur in the morning and are occasionally associated with tonic/clonic seizures. The commonest disorder is benign juvenile myoclonic epilepsy (JME) with onset after puberty. Myoclonus also occurs in degenerative and metabolic disease (see page 188).

TONIC SEIZURES

Sudden sustained muscular contraction associated with immediate loss of consciousness.

Tonic episodes occur as frequently as tonic/clonic episodes in children and should alert the physician to a possible anoxic aetiology.

In adults, tonic attacks are rare.

GENERALISED SEIZURES

TONIC/CLONIC SEIZURES (*SYN:* **Grand mal**)

It is the absence of a focal onset which may distinguish this primary generalised seizure from that evolving from a partial seizure.

The *epileptic cry* must not be confused with a seizure of focal onset. This results from tonic contraction of respiratory muscles with partial closure of vocal cords. The tonic phase is associated with rapid neuronal discharge. The clonic phase begins as neuronal discharge slows.

The *EEG* during an attack is, not surprisingly, marred by movement artefact. 10–14 Hz spike activity may be seen. When the seizure ends, the record may be 'silent' and then gradually picks up. Slow rhythm may persist for some hours – postictal changes.

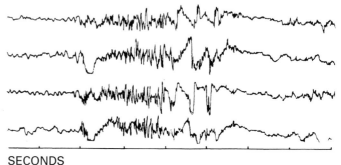

SECONDS

The record between attacks may be normal or slow with occasional clinically silent bursts of seizure activity. ---------➤

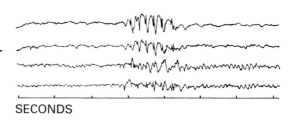

SECONDS

Again, hyperventilation or photic stimulation may bring out abnormalities.

ATONIC SEIZURES

These are characterised by a loss of muscle tone and a sudden fall. Consciousness may only be lost briefly. The EEG shows polyspike activity or low voltage fast activity.

SYNDROMES AND UNCLASSIFIED SEIZURES

West Syndrome

Infants present with diffusely abnormal EEGs, tonic clonic convulsions, myoclonic jerks and mental retardation following perinatal trauma or asphyxia. The seizures are sometimes called infantile spasms and the abnormal EEG pattern between events – hypsarrhythmia. Mortality or severe disability is high.

Lennox-Gastaut Syndrome

This similar syndrome presents later between 1–7 years of age. The response to anticonvulsant treatment and the degree of retardation is variable. The condition is associated with a large number of disorders including hypoxia, intracranial haemorrhage, toxoplasmosis, cytomegalovirus infection and tuberous sclerosis.

The **REFLEX EPILEPSIES** are a rare group of seizure disorders in which tonic/clonic or complex partial seizures are evoked by sensory stimuli. A primary generalised seizure induced by photic stimulation may be regarded as a reflex epilepsy, but the term is usually reserved for:

1. **Musicogenic epilepsy** in which certain musical themes or tones 'trigger' seizures.
2. **Reading epilepsy** in which reading a passage will evoke involuntary jaw movements followed by a seizure.
3. **Arithmetical epilepsy** in which performing calculations will 'trigger' seizures.

EPILEPSY – DIFFERENTIAL DIAGNOSIS

The following should be considered in the differential diagnosis of epilepsy –

SYNCOPE (VASOVAGAL) ATTACKS

These attacks occur usually when the patient is standing and result from a global reduction of cerebral blood flow.

Prodromal pallor, nausea and sweating occur; if the patient sits down, the attack may pass off or proceed to a brief loss of consciousness.

Tonic and clonic movements may develop if impaired cerebral blood flow is prolonged ('anoxic' seizures).

Mechanism: Peripheral vasodilatation with drop in blood pressure followed by vagal over-activity with fall in heart rate.

Syncopal attacks occur in hot, crowded rooms (e.g. classroom) or in response to pain or emotional disturbance.

'Reflex' syncope from cardiac slowing may occur with carotid sinus compression. Similarly, cough syncope may result from vigorous coughing.

CARDIAC ARRHYTHMIAS

Seen in situations such as complete heart block (Adams-Stokes attacks).

Prolonged arrest of cardiac rate or critical reduction will progressively lead to loss of consciousness – tonic jerks – cyanosis/stertorous respiration – fixed pupils and extensor plantar responses.

On recovery of normal cardiac rhythm, the degree of persisting neurological damage depends upon the duration of the episode and the presence of pre-existing cerebrovascular disease. In suspected patients, electrocardiography is mandatory. Continuous (24 hours) ECG monitoring may be necessary.

MIGRAINE

The slow evolution of focal hemisensory or hemimotor symptoms in complicated migraine contrasts with the more rapid 'spread' of such manifestations in simple partial seizures. Basilar migraine may produce a transient loss of consciousness.

HYPOGLYCAEMIA

Amongst other neuroglycopenic manifestations, seizures or intermittent behavioural disturbances may occur. A rapid fall of blood sugar is associated with symptoms of catecholamine release, e.g. palpitations, sweating, etc. In 'atypical' seizures exclude a metabolic cause by blood sugar estimation when symptomatic.

EPISODIC CONFUSION

Intermittent confusional episodes caused by drugs (e.g. barbiturates) or toxins (e.g. solvents).

PANIC ATTACKS Hyperventilation can induce focal motor and sensory symptoms.

NARCOLEPSY

Inappropriate sudden sleep episodes may easily be confused with epilepsy (see page 105).

PSEUDOSEIZURES (non-epileptic attack disorder, NEAD)

A difficult distinction lies between genuine epilepsy and attention seeking, hysterical or malingering episodes in which violent shaking and feigned loss of consciousness occurs. Often true epileptics will also manifest such attacks. Patients are usually suggestible, manipulative and with personality disorder. Many affected women have histories of sexual exploitation. EEG studies, serum prolactin and muscle enzyme studies may help discriminate.

EPILEPSY – CAUSATION

Epilepsy is often a symptom of disease rather than a disease itself. The approach to investigation depends on knowledge of potential causes:

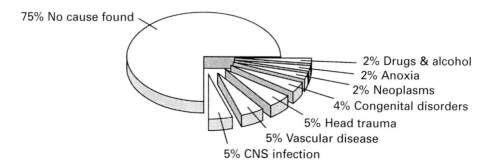

75% No cause found

2% Drugs & alcohol
2% Anoxia
2% Neoplasms
4% Congenital disorders
5% Head trauma
5% Vascular disease
5% CNS infection

Where no obvious cause is found there is often an increase in 'risk factors' – family history, febrile convulsion or difficult delivery.

Partial seizures with or without secondary generalisation
Age of onset gives a clue to causation. Each list is in order of frequency.

Newborn
Asphyxia
Intracranial haemorrhage
Hypocalcaemia
Hypoglycaemia
Hyperbilirubinaemia
Water intoxication
Inborn errors of metabolism
Trauma

Infancy
Febrile convulsions
CNS infection
Trauma
Congenital defects
Inborn errors of metabolism

Childhood
Trauma
CNS infection
Arteriovenous malformations
Congenital defects
Tumours

Adolescence and early adulthood
Trauma
CNS infection
Tumours
Arteriovenous malformation
Drugs and alcohol

Late adult
Drugs and alcohol
Trauma
Neoplasms
Vascular disease
Degenerative disease
CNS infection

Other general or systemic disorders may be associated with seizures e.g. metabolic disease and collagen vascular disorder. Seizures may rarely occur in multiple sclerosis. Some drugs may cause seizures. Antidepressants, antipsychotics, sympathomimetics, antineoplastics and certain general anaesthetic agents have all been incriminated.

Generalised epilepsies
There appears to be no clearly definable cause. Genetic factors play a role; concordance in monozygote twins is 75% for petit mal. An autosomal dominant gene would appear responsible for spike and wave abnormalities seen in the EEGs of parents and siblings of patients with generalised epilepsy. Some generalised epilepsies appear to be channelopathies and are associated with similar overlapping disorders (e.g.: hemiplegic migraine).

EPILEPSY – INVESTIGATION

With an incidence of 0.5% in the population, selectivity in investigation is often necessary. CT scanning is not always routinely available.

The concern of the clinician is that epilepsy may be symptomatic of a treatable cerebral lesion. Investigations serve to define a cause and to aid diagnosis in difficult cases.

Routine investigations
    Haematology
    Biochemistry (electrolytes, urea and calcium)
    Chest X-ray
    Electroencephalogram (EEG)

Neuroimaging (CT/MRI) should be performed in all persons aged 25 or more presenting with first seizure as well as in those with focal epilepsy irrespective of age.

MRI is more sensitive and will detect subtle lesions (see below). More sophisticated techniques e.g. Magnetisation Transfer and Spectroscopy remain research tools.

In doubtful cases the diagnosis should be deferred rather than labelling the patient 'epileptic'.

Specialised neurophysiological investigations
Indicated if attacks of unconsciousness are frequent or persistent and the diagnosis remains unclear.

        Sleep deprived electroencephalography (EEG).
        'Activated' EEG recording with procyclidine or other drugs.
        Telemetric EEG recording over 24–48 hours often combined with
        video recording of the patients (split screen display).

These investigations may reveal 'diagnostic' epileptic discharges or confirm non-epileptiform seizures.

Advanced investigations
These are reserved for cases of intractable epilepsy where surgery is considered.

    Telemetric, sphenoidal, foramen ovale and intraoperative EEG recording.
    Magnetic resonance imaging may display low grade gliomas, hamartomas, neuronal migration disorders or mesial temporal sclerosis, lesions often missed on CT scanning.
    Positron emission tomography (PET) or single photon emission computed tomography (SPECT) localise functional changes in cerebral blood flow and metabolism.

EPILEPSY – TREATMENT

The majority of patients respond to drug therapy (anticonvulsants). In intractable cases surgery may be necessary. Drug treatment should be simple, preferably using one anticonvulsant (monotherapy). Polytherapy is to be avoided especially as drug interactions occur between major anticonvulsants.

Treatment is aimed at rendering the patient 'fit free', though not always achieved. If the patient goes three years without an attack, withdrawal of therapy should be considered. Withdrawal should be carried out only if the patient is satisfied that a further fit would not ruin employment etc. (e.g. car driver). The risk of teratogenicity is well known (6%) especially with phenytoin, but withdrawing drug therapy in pregnancy is perhaps more risky than continuation. All anticonvulsants probably have some risk of producing fetal abnormalities, though these are usually mild. Sodium valproate has been incriminated in neural tube defects – spinal bifida.

The introduction of blood level monitoring, from early promise, is now regarded as being of limited value. Compliance can be confirmed but clinical responses balanced against symptomatic side effects are a much better guide to dosing. Some drugs do require monitoring of blood film and liver enzymes though rarely do abnormal results necessitate their withdrawal.

The commonest drugs used in clinical practice are
    Carbamazepine; Sodium valproate; Phenytoin; Phenobarbitone; Lamotrigine;
    Gabapentin; Topiramate; Tiagabine; Zonisamide; Oxcarbazepine; Levetiracetam
The first few drugs being licensed for monotherapy others as 'add-on' therapy when control sub-optimal. Fosphenytoin is a safer intravenous alternative to phenytoin.

	Sodium valproate	Phenobarbitone	Phenytoin	Carbamazepine
Mode of action	Inhibitor of GABA transaminase and glutamate decarboxylase	Opens postsynaptic Cl⁻ ion channels decreasing Na⁺ & Ca²⁺ influx	Blocks voltage dependent Na⁺ channels in neuronal cell membrane	Blocks voltage dependent Na⁺ channels in neuronal cell membrane
Metabolised	Liver Protein bound Short variable half-life	Liver or excreted in urine unchanged Long half-life (60 hours)	Liver Can saturate enzyme systems Long half-life	Liver Enzyme inducer Short half-life (10 hours)
Dose (ADULT)	2–3 × daily 600 mg to 3 g total daily dose	Can be given as single dose, e.g. 90 mg at night	Can be given as single dose e.g. 150–400 mg at night	2–3 × daily 600 mg to 1.2 g total daily dose
Side effects	Gastrointestinal upset Thrombocytopenia Drug-induced hepatitis Hair loss Tremor/chorea	Sedation. Depression Behavioural disturbance in children Skin rashes Withdrawal seizures	Gum hypertrophy Acne. Coarsening of facial characteristics At toxic levels – nystagmus – ataxia, diplopia – neuropathy	Gastrointestinal upset Ataxia Skin rash Agranulocytosis Antidiuretic effect

New (novel) anti-epilepsy drugs have specific modes of action and may have a synergistic effect. Topiramate and Tiagabine are GABA-ergic compounds. Lamotrigine inhibits glutamate release. Levetiracetam selectively binds to glial membranes.

EPILEPSY – SURGICAL TREATMENT

In some patients, particularly those with complex partial epilepsy, seizures remain intractable despite adequate drug administration and prevent a normal lifestyle; of those, a proportion will benefit from surgery.

Operation is contraindicated in patients with severe mental retardation or with an underlying psychiatric problem.

Investigations: *Videotelemetry* (24–48 hr EEG) and imaging with *MRI, SPECT* or *PET* scanning help identify the primary focus. Coronal MRI may show a small, sclerotic (high T2 signal) hippocampus on one side indicating 'mesial temporal sclosis' or a structural abnormality (e.g. tumour, AVM, hamartoma or a neuronal migration disorder). The presence of such a lesion improves the chance of a good result with resective surgery.

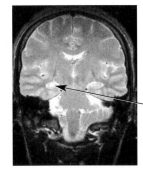

T2 weighted MRI showing right mesial temporal sclerosis

Operative techniques

Extra-temporal cortical resection: incorporates a frontal, parietal or occipital epileptogenic focus. Results are less satisfactory than for temporal resection.

Anterior temporal lobectomy: incorporating the usual epileptogenic focus (hippocampus and amygdala), the usual epileptogenic focus. The most commonly employed technique; over half become seizure free, a further 30% gain significant improvement in seizure control.

Selective amygdalo-hippocampectomy: less extensive resection than with temporal lobectomy, but no evidence that this improves seizure control or reduces the mild cognitive changes occasionally seen.

Hemispherectomy/ hemispherotomy: used in children with irreversible damage to a hemisphere. Good results with >80% becoming seizure free. Hemispherotomy involves disconnection of all cortical grey matter on one side without tissue resection. Despite the extent of these procedures, crude limb movements in the opposite limbs and walking are often preserved.

Corpus callosal section: prevents spread and reverberation of seizure activity between hemispheres. Most useful with generalized atonic seizures, but only about two-thirds obtain some benefit. Few become seizure free. In future may be replaced by vagal nerve stimulation.

Vagal nerve stimulation (VNS): involves periodic stimulation of the left vagus nerve by an implanted stimulator. Considered in patients with intractable epilepsy not suited to the resective procedures. VNS appears to reduce neuronal excitability, but the exact mechanism remains obscure. From 30–40% of patients show a 50% seizure reduction within two years.

STATUS EPILEPTICUS

A succession of tonic/clonic convulsions, one after the other with a gap between each, is referred to as **serial epilepsy**.

When consciousness does not return between attacks the condition is then termed **status epilepticus**. This state may be life-threatening with the development of pyrexia, deepening coma and circulatory collapse.

Status epilepticus may occur with frontal lobe lesions, following head injury, on reducing drug therapy (especially phenobarbitone), with alcohol or other sedation withdrawal, drug intoxications (tricyclic antidepressants), infections, metabolic disturbances (hyponatraemia) or pregnancy.

TREATMENT
There is no completely satisfactory approach.
Death occurs in 5–10%

> NOTE: ALL DOSE REGIMES APPLY TO ADULTS AND NOT TO CHILDREN

General
Establish an airway.
    O_2 inhalation 10 litres/minute.
    I.V. infusion: 500 ml 5% dextrose/0.9N saline.
    Vital signs recorded regularly – especially temperature.
        Prevent hyperthermia (sponging, etc.).

Specific
Diazepam 5 mg i.v. followed, after 2 minutes gap, by further 5 mg i.v.
    Effective for 10–20 minutes then seizures may return.
    Beware respiratory depression with repeated injections.
    When the effect of bolus injection wears off, a continuous diazepam infusion can be used
        (50–100 mg of diazepam in 500 ml dextrose/saline).

If not controlled then proceed to longer acting drug.

Fosphenytoin
This pro-drug is converted to phenytoin in the plasma (75 mg of fosphenytoin is equivalent to 50 mg phenytoin). Because it is water-soluble it causes less thrombophlebitis when given intravenously. It is also infused more rapidly than phenytoin with less risk of cardiac arrhythmias, hypotension or respiratory depression. Fosphenytoin is measured in phenytoin equivalents (PE) and infused at 100–150 mg PE/min.

At this point status should be controlled and oral maintenance therapy re-established.

If control has not been achieved, the stage of **refractory status** is reached and general anaesthesia with Propofol should be commenced immediately (2 mg/kg i.v. bolus followed by continuous infusion of 5–10 mg/kg/h). Alternatively Thiopentone can be used (100–250 mg i.v. bolus over 20 sec with further 50 mg boluses every 2–3 min until control is achieved. This is then followed by continuous infusion.) These treatments where possible should be used under EEG control to induce and maintain a 'burst suppression' pattern.

EPILEPSY – GENERAL

PROGNOSIS ON WITHDRAWAL OF DRUG TREATMENT

Several factors increase the likelihood of relapse of epilepsy after drug withdrawal:
- epilepsy associated with known cerebral disease   – seizure type
- response to starting treatment   – early childhood onset

Drug withdrawal should be performed slowly. Within 2 years of withdrawing treatment, 20% of persons will suffer a further attack. EEG appearance does not predict outcome after withdrawing therapy. Withdrawal should only be considered after 3–5 years of continuing freedom from seizures.

EPILEPSY AND PREGNANCY

Best practice guidelines are available for managing women with epilepsy (Seizure 1999:8:201–17). The frequency of seizures may decrease in pregnancy. The patient may present with the first seizure during pregnancy (when investigation is limited) or during the puerperium. Tumours and arteriovenous malformations can enlarge in pregnancy and produce such seizures; however, these causes are rare and most attacks are idiopathic. Cortical venous thrombosis and systemic lupus erythematosus should be considered as alternative explanations. Care must be taken when prescribing treatment in pregnancy although a change or withdrawal of medication is rarely necessary. The role of drugs in teratogenesis is complex; genetic mechanisms in epilepsy account for an increased incidence of birth defects. Over 90% of pregnant women with epilepsy will deliver a normal child.

THE FEBRILE CONVULSION

Febrile convulsions occur in the immature brain as a response to high fever, probably as a result of water and electrolyte disturbance.

Usually occurs between 6 months and 3 years of age.

Long-term follow up suggests a liability to develop seizures in later life (unassociated with fever) especially in males, when seizures are prolonged and have focal features.

Treatment is aimed at preventing a prolonged seizure by sponging the patient and using rectal diazepam. The role of prophylaxis after one seizures is debatable.

SUDDEN UNEXPLAINED DEATH IN EPILEPSY (SUDEP)

The Standardised Mortality Ratio (SMR) compares mortality in a group with a specific illness to age and sex matched controls. The SMR is increased 2–3 times in epilepsy. When accidental death and suicide are excluded it appears that some persons with epilepsy die abruptly of no clear cause. Such deaths could be seizure related (cardiac arrhythmias/suffocation); autopsy is usually uninformative. A community-based study suggests 1 SUDEP/year/370 persons with epilepsy. Patients and carers should be compassionately informed of this small risk.

DRIVING AND EPILEPSY (DVLA UK REGULATIONS)

Off treatment   Isolated (single) seizure: 1 year off driving
Withdrawal of treatment: 6 months off driving (excluding period of drug withdrawal)

On treatment   Patients must be free of attacks (whilst awake) for 1 year
Patients must be free of attacks whilst asleep for 1 year unless they have a 3 year history of sleep related attacks alone.

DISORDERS OF SLEEP

PHYSIOLOGY

Sleep results from activity in certain sleep producing areas of
the brain rather than from reduced sensory input to the
cerebral cortex. Stimulation of these areas produces sleep;
damage results in states of persistent wakefulness.

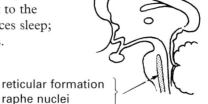

Pontine ⎫
Medullary ⎭ → { reticular formation }
{ raphe nuclei }

Two states of sleep are recognized:

1. **Rapid eye movement (REM) sleep**	2. **Non-rapid eye movement (non-REM) sleep**
Characterised by: – Rapid conjugate eye movement – Fluctuation of temperature, BP, heart rate and respiration – Muscle twitching – Presence of dreams	– Absence of eye movement – Stability of temperature, BP, heart rate and respiration – Absence of muscle twitching – Absence of dreams
Originates in: – Pontine reticular formation	– Midline pontine and medullary nuclei (raphe nuclei)
Mediated by: – Noradrenaline (norepinephrine)	– Serotonin

The **electroencephalogram** shows characteristic patterns which correspond to the type and
death of sleep.

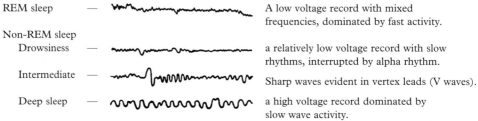

REM sleep — A low voltage record with mixed frequencies, dominated by fast activity.

Non-REM sleep
Drowsiness — a relatively low voltage record with slow rhythms, interrupted by alpha rhythm.

Intermediate — Sharp waves evident in vertex leads (V waves).

Deep sleep — a high voltage record dominated by slow wave activity.

The sleep pattern

In adults non-REM and REM sleep
alternate throughout the night.

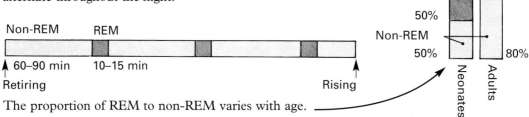

Non-REM   REM

↑ 60–90 min   10–15 min
Retiring   Rising

REM
50%
Non-REM
50%

20%
80%

Neonates   Adults

The proportion of REM to non-REM varies with age.

In view of the important role of serotonin and noradrenaline (norepinephrine)
in sleep, it is understandable that drugs may affect the duration and/or content of sleep.

DISORDERS OF SLEEP

NARCOLEPSY AND CATAPLEXY

> **Narcolepsy:** an irresistible desire to sleep in inappropriate circumstances and places. Attacks occur suddenly and are of brief duration unless patient remains undisturbed.

> **Cataplexy:** sudden loss of postural tone. The patient crumples to the ground. Consciousness is preserved. Emotion – laughter or crying – can bring on an attack.

The narcolepsy/cataplexy tetrad
Only 10% of patients manifest the complex tetrad

> **Sleep paralysis:** on awakening, the patient is unable to move. This may last for 2–3 minutes.

> **Hypnagogic hallucinations:** vivid dreams or hallucinations occur as the patient falls asleep or occasionally when apparently awake.

Males are affected more than females. Prevalence 1:2000.

Onset is in adolescence/early adult life. The disorder is life long, but becomes less troublesome with age. It may have a familial incidence, or may occur after head injury, with multiple sclerosis, or with hypothalamic tumours. The cause remains unknown, though the increased incidence of certain histocompatiblity antigens (DR2) in sufferers does suggest an immunological basis.

Diagnosis
The suggestive history is supported by EEG studies. The multiple sleep latency test (MSLT) is diagnostic in showing onset of REM within 15 min of sleep onset in 2 of 4 naps (short sleeps).

Treatment
The non-amphetamine stimulant Modafinal, a wake promoting agent, reduces daytime sleepiness. Amphetamines are more potent but carry the risk of habituation. Selegilene, metabolised in part to amphetamine, has a stimulant effect and also reduces cataplexy. Other drugs, Maxindol, Pemoline and Clomipramine can be helpful. Occasionally modifying life-style alone by 'cat-napping' is sufficient.

OTHER SLEEP DISORDERS (PARASOMNIAS)

NIGHT TERRORS (pavor nocturnus)
These occur in children, shortly after falling asleep and during deep to intermediate non-REM sleep. The child awakes in a state of fright with a marked tachycardia, yet in the morning cannot recollect the attack. Such attacks are not associated with psychological disturbance, are self limiting and if necessary will respond to diazepam.

NIGHTMARES
These occur during REM sleep. Drug or alcohol withdrawal promotes REM sleep and is often associated with vivid dreams.

SOMNAMBULISM (sleep walking)
Sleep walking varies from just sitting up in bed to walking around the house with the eyes open, performing complex major tasks. Episodes occur during intermediate or deep non-REM sleep. In childhood, somnambulism is associated with night terrors and bed wetting, but not with psychological disturbance. In adults, there is an increased incidence of psychoneurosis. Prevention of injury is important.

Cerebral degenerative disorders such as dementia and Parkinson's disease can present with REM sleep disturbance and associated behavioural abnormality (nocturnal confusion)

DISORDERS OF SLEEP

SLEEP STARTS (HYPNIC JERKS)

On entering sleep, sudden jerks of the arms or legs commonly occur and are especially frequent when a conscious effort is made to remain awake, e.g. during a lecture. This is a physiological form of myoclonus.

Other movement disorders in sleep: Restless legs, Dystonia, Bruxism (teeth grinding) and head banging.

HYPERSOMNIA

Lesions which affect the structures in the floor of the third ventricle may produce excessive sleepiness, e.g. tumours or encephalitis, and are often associated with diabetes insipidus.

Systemic disease such as myxoedema may result in hypersomnia, as may conditions which produce hypercapnia – chronic bronchitis, or primary muscle disease, e.g. dystrophia myotonica.

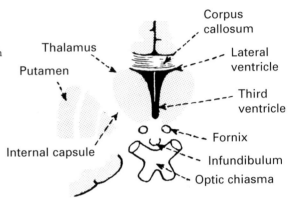

SLEEP APNOEA SYNDROMES

Respiratory rate fluctuates during REM sleep with occasional short episodes of apnoea. These are normal physiological events and are brief and infrequent.

Prolonged sleep apnoea results from central reduction of respiratory drive, a mechanical obstruction of the airway or a mixture of both.

Central causes:
Brain stem medullary infarction or following cervical/foramen magnum surgery.

Mechanical causes:
Obesity. Tonsillar enlargement.
Myxoedema. Acromegaly.

When breathing ceases, the resultant hypercapnia and hypoxia eventually stimulate respiration.

Patients may present with daytime sleepiness, nocturnal insomnia and early morning headache. Snoring and restless movements are characteristic. In severe cases of sleep apnoea, hypertension may develop with right heart failure secondary to pulmonary arterial hypertension. Polycythaemia and left heart failure may ensue.

Evaluation requires sleep oximetry and video recording with low level illumination. Fall in oxygen saturation may be as much as 50%.

Treatment depends on aetiology. Mechanical airway obstruction should be relieved; drugs such as theophylline are occasionally helpful. Continuous positive airway pressure (CPAP) applied to the nose may help. Surgical reconstruction of palate and oropharynx is offered in extreme cases.

The *Pickwickian syndrome*: sleep apnoea associated with obesity, named after the Dickens' fat boy who repeatedly fell asleep.

INSOMNIA

The most common sleep disorder, difficult to evaluate and of multiple causation including psychiatric, alcohol, drug related or due to systemic illness. Treatment depends on cause e.g. antidepressant.

HIGHER CORTICAL DYSFUNCTION

Specific parts of the cerebral hemispheres are responsible for a certain aspect of function. In normal circumstances these functions are integrated and the patient operates as a whole. Damage to part of the cortex will result in a characteristic disturbance of function. Interruption by disease of 'connections' between one part of the cortex and another will 'disconnect' function.

GENERAL ANATOMY

Brodmann, on the basis of histological differences, divided the cortex into 47 areas. Knowledge of these areas is not practical, though they are referred to often in some texts.

Six layers can be recognized in the cerebral cortex superficial to the junction with the underlying white matter.

The relative preponderance of each layer varies in different regions of the cortex and appears to be related to function.

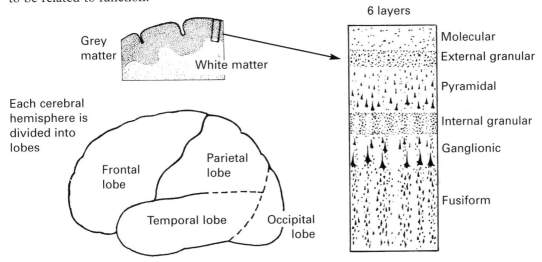

The frontal motor cortex, dominated by pyramidal rather than granular layers, is termed the AGRANULAR CORTEX.

The parietal sensory cortex, dominated by granular layers, is termed the GRANULAR CORTEX.

The largest cells of the granular cortex are the giant cells of Betz. These give rise to some of the motor fibres of the corticospinal tract.

RIGHT AND LEFT HEMISPHERE FUNCTION

Unilateral brain damage reveals a difference in function between hemispheres. The left hemisphere is 'dominant' in right-handed people. In left-handed subjects the left hemisphere is dominant in the majority (up to 75%).

Hand preference may be hereditary, but in some cases disease of the left hemisphere in early life determines left-handedness.

107

HIGHER CORTICAL DYSFUNCTION

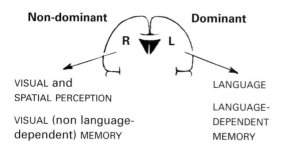

Non-dominant | Dominant

R | L

VISUAL and SPATIAL PERCEPTION

VISUAL (non language-dependent) MEMORY

LANGUAGE

LANGUAGE-DEPENDENT MEMORY

Hemisphere dominance may be demonstrated by the injection of sodium amytal into the internal carotid artery. On the dominant side this will produce an arrest of speech for up to 30 seconds – the WADA TEST. Such a test may be important before temporal lobectomy for epilepsy when handedness/hemisphere dominance is in doubt.

FRONTAL LOBES

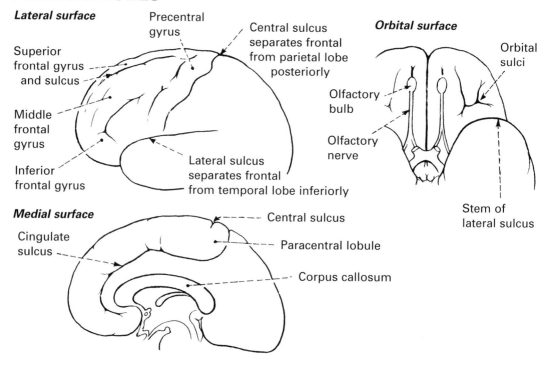

Lateral surface

Precentral gyrus

Central sulcus separates frontal from parietal lobe posteriorly

Superior frontal gyrus and sulcus

Middle frontal gyrus

Inferior frontal gyrus

Lateral sulcus separates frontal from temporal lobe inferiorly

Orbital surface

Orbital sulci

Olfactory bulb

Olfactory nerve

Stem of lateral sulcus

Medial surface

Cingulate sulcus

Central sulcus

Paracentral lobule

Corpus callosum

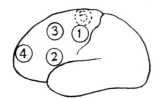

FRONTAL LOBE FUNCTION

1 Precentral gyrus – motor cortex contralateral movement – face, arm, leg, trunk.
2. Broca's area – dominant hemisphere – expressive centre for speech.
3. Supplementary motor area – contralateral head and eye turning.
4. Prefrontal areas – 'personality', initiative.
5. Paracentral lobule – cortical inhibition of bladder and bowel voiding.

FRONTAL LOBES

IMPAIRMENT OF FRONTAL LOBE FUNCTION

1. Precentral gyrus
Monoplegia or hemiplegia depending on extent of damage.

2. Broca's area (inferior part of dominant frontal lobe)
Results in Broca's dysphasia (see page 122) (motor or expressive).

3. Supplementary motor area
Paralysis of head and eye movement to opposite side. Head turns 'towards' diseased hemisphere and eyes look in the same direction.

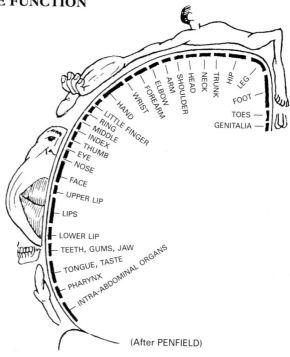

(After PENFIELD)

4. Prefrontal areas (the vast part of the frontal lobes anterior to the motor cortex as well as undersurface – orbital – of frontal lobes)
Damage is often bilateral, e.g. infarction, following haemorrhage from anterior communicating artery aneurysm, neoplasm, trauma or anterior dementia, resulting in a change of personality with antisocial behaviour/loss of inhibitions.
Three pre-frontal syndromes are recognised

Orbitofrontal syndrome	Frontal convexity syndrome	Medial frontal syndrome
Disinhibition	Apathy	Akinetic
Poor judgement	Indifference	Incontinent
Emotional lability	Poor abstract thought	Sparse verbal output

Pre-frontal lesions are also associated with:
1. Primitive reflexes – grasp, pout, etc. (see page 125).
2. Disturbance of gait – 'gait apraxia'.
3. Resistance to passive movements of the limbs – paratonia.

Unilateral lesions may show minor degrees of such change.

5. Paracentral lobule

Damage to the posterior part of the superior frontal gyrus results in incontinence of urine and faeces – 'loss of cortical inhibition'. This is particularly likely with ventricular dilatation and is an important symptom of normal pressure hydrocephalus.

PARIETAL LOBES

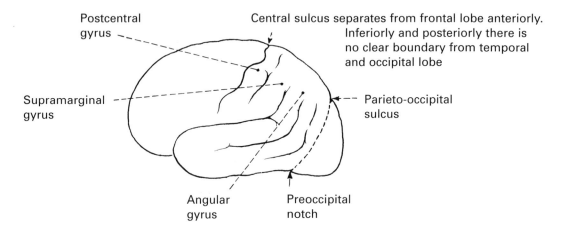

Postcentral gyrus

Central sulcus separates from frontal lobe anteriorly. Inferiorly and posteriorly there is no clear boundary from temporal and occipital lobe

Supramarginal gyrus

Parieto-occipital sulcus

Angular gyrus

Preoccipital notch

PARIETAL LOBE FUNCTION

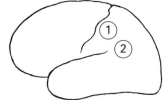

1. **Postcentral gyrus** (*granular cortex*)
The sensory cortex (representation similar to the motor cortex) receives afferent pathways for appreciation of posture, touch and passive movement.
2. **Supramarginal and angular gyri** (*dominant hemisphere*) make up part of Wernicke's language area.
This is the receptive area where auditory and visual aspects of comprehension are integrated.
The **non-dominant** parietal lobe is important in the concept of body image and the awareness of the external environment. The ability to construct shapes, etc. results from such visual/proprioceptive skills.
The **dominant** parietal lobe is implicated in the skills of handling numbers/calculation.
The **visual pathways** – the fibres of the optic radiation (lower visual field) – pass deep through the parietal lobe.

IMPAIRMENT OF PARIETAL LOBE FUNCTION

Disease of **either dominant or non-dominant** sensory cortex (postcentral gyrus) will result in contralateral disturbance of cortical sensation:
Postural sensation disturbed.
Sensation of passive movement disturbed.
Accurate localization of light touch may be disturbed.
Discrimination between one and two points (normally 4 mm on finger tips) is lost.
Appreciation of size, shape, texture and weight may be affected, with difficulty in distinguishing coins placed in hand, etc. (astereognosis).
Perceptual rivalry (sensory inattention) is characteristic of parietal lobe disease. Presented with two stimuli, one applied to each side (e.g. light touch to the palm of the hand) simultaneously, the patient is only aware of that one contralateral to the normal parietal lobe. As the gap between application of stimuli is increased (approaching 2–4 seconds) the patient becomes aware of both.

2. **Supramarginal and angular gyri** – Wernicke's dysphasia (see page 122).

PARIETAL LOBES

3. Non-dominant   **4. Dominant**

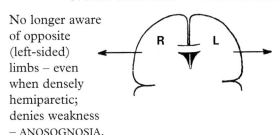

No longer aware of opposite (left-sided) limbs – even when densely hemiparetic; denies weakness – ANOSOGNOSIA.

Difficulty in dressing, e.g. getting arm into pyjamas – DRESSING APRAXIA.

Disturbance of geographical memory – GEOGRAPHICAL AGNOSIA (e.g. patient cannot find his bed in ward).

Cannot copy geometrical pattern – CONSTRUCTIONAL APRAXIA.

Confusion of right and left limbs. Difficulty in distinguishing fingers on hand – FINGER AGNOSIA.

Disturbance of calculation – ACALCULIA.

Disturbance of writing – AGRAPHIA.

These comprise GERSTMANN'S SYNDROME

5. Damage to the **optic radiation** deep in the parietal lobe will produce a lower homonymous quadrantanopia

TEMPORAL LOBES

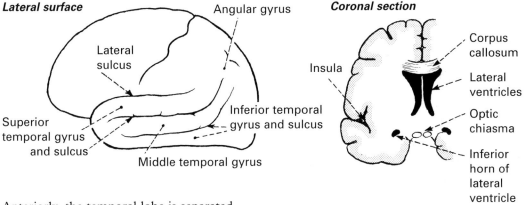

Lateral surface

Angular gyrus

Lateral sulcus

Superior temporal gyrus and sulcus

Middle temporal gyrus

Inferior temporal gyrus and sulcus

Coronal section

Insula

Corpus callosum

Lateral ventricles

Optic chiasma

Inferior horn of lateral ventricle

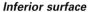

Anteriorly, the temporal lobe is separated from the frontal lobe by the lateral sulcus. Posteriorly and superiorly, separation from occipital and parietal lobes is less clearly defined.

The lateral sulcus is deep and contains 'buried' temporal lobe. The buried island of cortex is referred to as the INSULA.

The temporal lobe also has a considerable inferior and medial surface in contact with the middle fossa.

Inferior surface

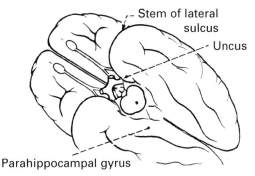

Stem of lateral sulcus

Uncus

Parahippocampal gyrus

111

TEMPORAL LOBES

TEMPORAL LOBE FUNCTION

1. The **auditory cortex** lies on the upper surface of the superior temporal gyrus, buried in the lateral sulcus (Heschl's gyrus).
The **dominant** hemisphere is important in the hearing of language.
The **non-dominant** hemisphere is important in the hearing of sounds, rhythm and music.
Close to the auditory cortex labyrinthine function is represented.

2. The **middle and inferior temporal gyri** are concerned with learning and memory (see later).

3. The **limbic lobe**: the inferior and medial portions of the temporal lobe, including the hippocampus and parahippocampal gyrus.
The sensation of olfaction is mediated through this structure as well as emotional/affective behaviour.
Olfactory fibres terminate in the uncus.
The limbic lobe or system also incorporates inferior frontal and medial parietal structures and will be discussed later.

4. The **visual pathways** pass deep in the temporal lobe around the posterior horn of the lateral ventricle.

IMPAIRMENT OF TEMPORAL LOBE FUNCTION

1. Auditory cortex

Cortical deafness: Bilateral lesions are rare but may result in complete deafness of which the patient may be unaware.
Lesions which involve surrounding association areas may result in difficulty in hearing spoken words (dominant) or difficulty in appreciating rhythm/music (non-dominant) – *AMUSIA*. Auditory hallucinations may occur in temporal lobe disease.

2. Middle and inferior temporal gyri

Disturbance or memory/learning will be discussed later.
Disordered memory may occur in complex partial seizures either after the event – postictal amnesia – or in the event – déjà vu, jamais vu.

3. Limbic lobe damage may result in:

Olfactory hallucination with complex partial seizures.
Aggressive or antisocial behaviour.
Inability to establish new memories (see later).

4. Damage to **optic radiation** will produce an upper homonymous quadrantanopia.
Dominant hemisphere lesions are associated with Wernicke's dysphasia.

OCCIPITAL LOBE

The occipital lobe merges anteriorly with the parietal and temporal lobes.

On the medial surface the calcarine sulcus extends forwards and the parieto-occipital sulcus separates occipital and parietal lobes.

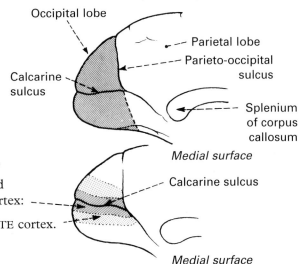

OCCIPITAL LOBE FUNCTION

The occipital lobe is concerned with the perception of vision (the visual cortex).

The visual cortex lies along the banks of the calcarine sulcus – this area is referred to as the STRIATE cortex:

above and below this lies the PARASTRIATE cortex.

The *striate* cortex is the primary visual cortex and when stimulated by visual input relays information to the *parastriate* – association visual cortex. This, in turn, connects with the parietal, temporal and frontal lobes both on the same side and on the opposite side (through the posterior part of the corpus callosum) so that the meaning of a visual image may be interpreted, remembered, etc.

The visual field is represented upon the cortex in a specific manner (page 138).

IMPAIRMENT OF OCCIPITAL LOBE FUNCTION

A cortical lesion will result in a homonymous hemianopia with or without involvement of the macula, depending on the posterior extent of the lesion.

When only the occipital pole is affected, a central hemianopia field defect involving the macula occurs with a normal peripheral field of vision.

Cortical blindness

Extensive bilateral cortical lesions of the striate cortex will result in cortical BLINDNESS. In this, the pupillary light reflex is normal despite the absence of conscious perception of the presence of illumination (light reflex fibres terminate in the midbrain).

Anton's syndrome

Involvement of both the striate and the parastriate cortices affects the interpretation of vision. The patient is unaware of his visual loss and denies its presence. This denial in the presence of obvious blindness characterizes Anton's syndrome.

Cortical blindness occurs mainly in vascular disease (posterior cerebral artery), but also following hypoxia and hypertensive encephalopathy or after surviving tentorial herniation.

Balint's syndrome

Inability to direct voluntary gaze, associated with visual agnosia (loss of visual recognition) due to bilateral parieto-occipital lesions.

113

OCCIPITAL LOBE

Visual hallucinations are common in migraine when the occipital lobe is involved; also in epilepsy when the seizure source lies here.

Hallucinations of occipital origin are elementary – unformed – appearing as patterns (zig-zags, flashes) and fill the hemianopic field, whereas hallucinations of temporal lobe origin are formed, complex and fill the whole of the visual field.

Visual illusions also may occur as a consequence of occipital lobe disease. Objects appear smaller (MICROPSIA) or larger (MACROPSIA) than reality. Distortion of a shape may occur or disappearance of colour from vision.

These illusions are more common with non-dominant occipital lobe disease.

Prosopagnosia: the patient, though able to see a familiar face, e.g. a member of the family, cannot name it. This is usually associated with other disturbances of 'interpretation' and naming with intact vision such as colour agnosia (recognition of colours and matching of pairs of colours). Bilateral lesions at occipito-temporal junction are responsible.

APRAXIA

A loss of ability to carry out skilled movement despite adequate understanding of the task and normal motor power.

Constructional and dressing apraxia: See page 111, non-dominant parietal disease.

Gait apraxia: Difficulty in initiating walking – frontal lobe/anterior corpus callosum disease.

Oculomotor apraxia: Impaired voluntary eye movement – parieto-occipital disease.

Ideamotor apraxia: Separation of idea of movement from execution – cannot carry out motor command but can perform the required movement under different circumstances – dominant hemisphere (see later).

Ideational apraxia: Inability to carry out a sequence of movements each of which can be performed separately – frontal lobe disease.

HIGHER CORTICAL DYSFUNCTION – DISCONNECTION SYNDROMES

Cortical function is described, on the previous pages, 'lobe by lobe'. These functions integrate by means of connections between hemispheres and lobes. Lesions of these connecting pathways disorganise normal function, resulting in recognizable syndromes – the disconnection syndromes. APRAXIA is a feature of some of these disorders.

The connecting pathways may be divided into:

*Intra*hemispheric: lying in the subcortical white matter and linking parts of the same hemisphere.

*Inter*hemispheric: traversing the corpus callosum and linking related parts of the two hemispheres.

THE INTRAHEMISPHERIC DISCONNECTION SYNDROMES

1. Conduction aphasia

Lesion of the arcuate fasciculus linking Wernicke's and Broca's speech areas.

Characterised by:
Fluent dysphasic speech. Good comprehension of written/spoken material. Poor repetition.

2. Pure word deafness

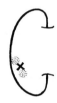

Lesion of the connection between the primary auditory cortex (Heschl's gyrus) and auditory association cortex.

Characterised by:
Impaired comprehension of spoken word. Self-initiated language is normal. The patient seems deaf, but audiometry is normal.

3. Buccal lingual and 'sympathetic' apraxia

Involves the links between left and right association motor cortices in the subcortical region.

Premotor motor cortex Broca's area

Characterised by:
Right brachiofacial weakness and apraxia of tongue, lip and left limb movements.

THE INTERHEMISPHERIC DISCONNECTION SYNDROMES

1. Left side apraxia

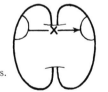

Lesion of the anterior corpus callosum with interruption of the connections between the left and right association motor cortices.

Characterised by:
Apraxia of left sided limb movements.

2. Pure word blindness or alexia without agraphia

Lesion of the posterior corpus callosum and dominant occipital lobe with interruption of connections between the visual cortex and the angular gyrus/Wernicke's area.

Characterised by:
Inability to read, to name colours, to copy writing, but with normal spontaneous writing and the ability to identify colours.

3. Agenesis of the corpus callosum

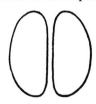

This is a developmental disorder with no connection between the two hemispheres.

Characterised by:
A failure to name an object presented visually or by touch to the non-dominant hemisphere. (The right and left visual fields cannot match presented objects.)

115

HIGHER CORTICAL FUNCTION – MEMORY

Normal memory involves the recognition, registering and cataloguing of a stimulus – *acquisition*, as well as the skill of appropriate recall – *retrieval*.

Verbal memory: refers to material presented in the verbal form.
Visual memory: denotes material presented without words or verbal mediation.
Short term memory: immediate recall of a short message.
Long term memory: retrieval of recent or remote events.
Semantic memory: refers to long established factual knowledge.

Disordered memory may be confused with disturbances of attention, motivation and concentration and requires detailed neuropsychological examination to properly assess.

THE ANATOMICAL BASIS OF MEMORY

The structures of the limbic system involved in the memory process are inferred from the pathological examination of diseases that disorder function. The *hippocampus*, a deep structure in the temporal lobe, ridges the floor of the lateral ventricle. Fimbriae of the hippocampus connect this structure to the *fornix*. There appears to be a loop from hippocampus → fornix → mamillary body → thalamus → cingulate gyrus → back to hippocampus.

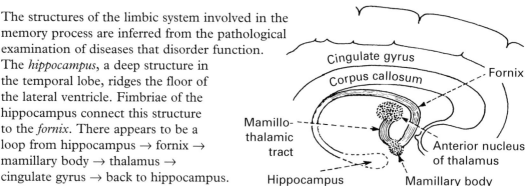

	Mamillary bodies	Thalamus	Orbito-frontal cortex	Medial temporal cortex/ hippocampus	Fornix
Korsakoff's	+	+			
Head trauma		+	+	+	+
Stroke		+		+	+
Encephalitis				+	+
Anoxia				+	+
Metabolic				+	+
Temporal lobectomy				+	
3rd ventricular operations					+

TESTS OF MEMORY (see examination, page 8)

These aim to distinguish loss of immediate, recent or remote memory.
Disorders may be further classified into those which affect memories established before the injury or damage – RETROGRADE AMNESIA – and those which affect memory of events following the injury or damage – ANTEROGRADE or POST-TRAUMATIC AMNESIA.

DISORDERS OF MEMORY

THE AMNESIC SYNDROME is characterised by –

Retrograde amnesia – impairment of memory for events that antedate illness or injury
Anterograde amnesia – inability to learn new verbal or non verbal information from onset of the illness or injury
Intact retrieval of old information
Intact intellectual function
Intact personality
Tendency to confabulate

CAUSES

Korsakoff's syndrome: results from – alcoholism
– encephalitis
– head injury

Lesions occur within the thalamus and the mamillary bodies. Commonly associated with confabulation – a false rationalization of events and circumstances.

Post-traumatic amnesia: after trauma, retrograde amnesia may span several years, but with recovery, this gradually diminishes. The duration of post-traumatic amnesia on the other hand remains fixed and relates directly to the severity of the injury.

Amnesic stroke: bilateral medial temporal lobe infarction from a posterior circulation stroke is usually associated with hemiplegia and visual disturbance or loss e.g. Anton's or Balint's syndrome (page 113).

Amnesia with tumours: tumours that compress thalamic structures or the fornix may produce amnesia – e.g. colloid cyst of the 3rd ventricle.

Temporal lobectomy: amnesia will only occur if function in the unoperated temporal lobe is abnormal. Pre-operative assessment during a unilateral carotid injection of sodium amytal minimises this risk.

Transient global amnesia: memory loss of less than 36 hours during which time patients will often carry out complex cognitive tasks e.g. drive to the office and do a day's work. There is usually nothing objectively wrong. Episodes are sometimes precipitated by exercise. The disorder is benign but requires investigation to exclude temporal lobe disease.

Psychogenic amnesia: affects overlearned and personally relevant aspects of memory e.g. 'What is my name?', while less well learned memory remains unaffected.
Clinically evident acute mental stress may precipitate this. This inadequate defence mechanism suggests a serious underlying psychiatric or personality disorder.

DISORDERS OF MEMORY RETRIEVAL

Senescence – as part of normal aging, rapid retrieval of stored memory becomes defective.

Depression – impaired memory is a common complaint in depressive illness. The disorder is one of motivation and concentration.

Subcortical dementia – This will be described later (page 124). The major abnormality is that of a slowed (but correct) response rate to questions of memory function.

NB DEMENTIA, TUMOURS and CEREBROVASCULAR DISEASE are all often associated with memory loss but this is usually combined with evidence of more widespread disordered cognitive function.

DISORDERS OF SPEECH AND LANGUAGE

Introduction

Disturbed speech and language are important symptoms of neurological disease. The two are not synonymous. Language is a function of the dominant cerebral hemisphere and may be divided into (a) *emotional* – the instinctive expression of feelings representing the earliest forms of language acquired in infancy and (b) *symbolic or prepositional* – conveying thoughts, opinion and concepts. This language is acquired over a 20-year period and is dependent upon culture, education and normal cerebral development.

An understanding of disorders of speech and language is essential, not just to the clinical diagnosis but also to improve communication between patient and doctor. All too often patients with language disorders are labelled 'confused' as a consequence of superficial evaluation.

DYSARTHRIA

Dysarthria is a *disturbance of articulation* in which the content of speech – language – is unaffected.

Mechanism of articulation

① Speech initiated

② Descending corticobulbar pathway from left hemisphere to nuclei X and XII

③ Connection through corpus callosum to motor cortex of right hemisphere

④ Descending corticobulbar pathway from right hemisphere to nuclei X and XII

Nuclei X and XII receive corticobulbar pathway from both ipsilateral and contralateral hemispheres (bilateral innervation). This 'safety factor' means that a lesion of one corticobulbar pathway does not produce symptoms.

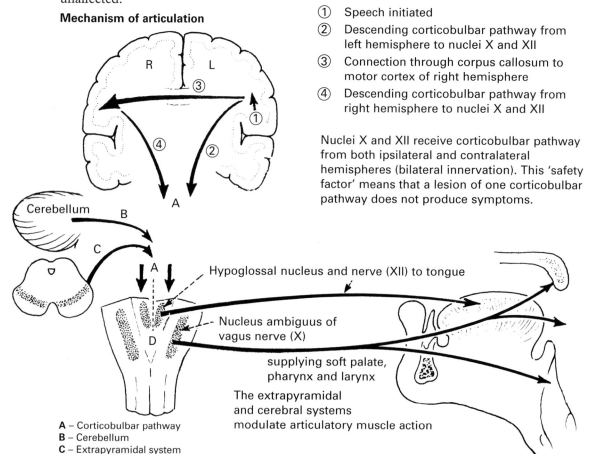

Hypoglossal nucleus and nerve (XII) to tongue

Nucleus ambiguus of vagus nerve (X)

supplying soft palate, pharynx and larynx

The extrapyramidal and cerebral systems modulate articulatory muscle action

A – Corticobulbar pathway
B – Cerebellum
C – Extrapyramidal system
D – Nuclei of lower motor neurons of X, XII cranial nerves

Muscles of expression, innervated by the facial nerve, play an additional role in articulation and weakness also results in dysarthria.

DISORDERS OF SPEECH – DYSARTHRIA

DIAGNOSTIC APPROACH

Listen to spontaneous speech and ask the patient to read aloud.

Observe: lingual consonants – 'ta ta ta' (made with the tongue), labial consonants – 'mm mm mm' (made with the lips), guttural consonants – 'ga ga ga' (laryngeal and pharyngeal/palatal). Difficulty with articulation = **DYSARTHRIA**

N.B. Beware misinterpretation of dialect or poorly fitting teeth.

Speech hoarse and strained; labial consonants especially affected.

Speech slow and monotonous with abnormal separation of syllables – 'scanning speech'; at times may sound explosive – **Associated signs of cerebellar disease**

Soft and monotonous with poor volume and little inflection – and short rushes of speech **Associated signs of extrapyramidal disease**

Labial consonants first affected, later gutturals. *Nasal speech* and progression to total loss of articulation (*anarthria*). **Associated signs of l.m.n. weakness of X and XII**

Associated contralateral hemiparesis or dysphasia ——▶ SPASTIC DYSARTHRIA (Cortical origin)

Other signs of pseudobulbar palsy (impaired chewing, swallowing) ——▶ SPASTIC DYSARTHRIA (Corticobulbar origin)

——▶ ATAXIC DYSARTHYRIA

(Lesion in cerebellar vermis and paravermis)

HYPOKINETIC (slow) HYPER-KINETIC (fast) DYSARTHYRIA (Lesion of the extrapyramidal system)

——▶ FLACCID DYSARTHYRIA

(Involvement of X and XII nuclei or emergent nerves to muscles of articulation)

Causative diseases e.g. Middle cerebral artery occlusion.

Neoplasm.

e.g. Bilateral small vessel occlusion.

Motor neuron disease.

e.g. Multiple sclerosis. Hereditary ataxias.

Parkinson's disease.

Huntington's chorea.

e.g. Motor neuron disease.

Bulbar poliomyelitis.

Cranial polyneuritis.

Many diseases affect multiple sites and a 'mixed' dysarthria occurs.

For example, multiple sclerosis with corticobulbar and cerebellar involvement will result in a mixed spastic/ataxic dysarthria.

DISORDERS OF SPEECH – DYSPHONIA

Sound is produced by the passage of air over the vocal cords.

Respiratory disease or vocal cord paralysis results in a disturbance of this facility – **dysphonia**. A complete inability to produce sound is referred to as aphonia. Dysarthria often co-exists.

DIAGNOSTIC APPROACH
If, despite attempts, there is deficient sound production then examine the vocal cords by indirect laryngoscopy.

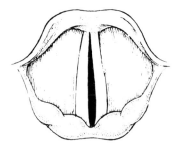

Causative diseases
e.g. Medullary damage:
– infarction
– syringobulbia

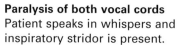

Paralysis of both vocal cords
Patient speaks in whispers and inspiratory stridor is present.

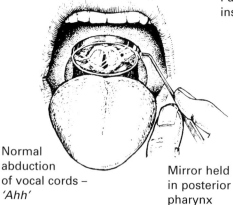

Normal abduction of vocal cords – *'Ahh'*

Mirror held in posterior pharynx

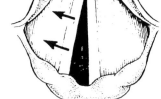

e.g. Recurrent laryngeal nerve palsy:
– following thyroid surgery
– bronchial neoplasm
– aortic aneurysm

Spastic dysphonia
Sounds as though speaking while being strangled! May be a functional disorder, form of 'focal' dystonia, occurs with essential tremor or hypothyroidism.

Paralysis of left vocal cord
which does not move with *'Ahh'* while right abducts. When patient says *'E'* normal cord will move towards paralysed cord. The voice is weak and 'breathy' and the cough 'bovine'.

OTHER DISORDERS OF SPEECH
Mutism: An absence of any attempt at oral communication. It may be associated with bilateral frontal lobe or third ventricular pathology (see Akinetic mutism).

Echolalia: Constant repetition of words or sentences heard in dementing illnesses.

Palilalia: Repetition of last word or words of patient's speech. Heard in extrapyramidal disease.

Logorrhoea: Prolonged speech monologues; associated with Wernicke's dysphasia.

DISORDERS OF SPEECH – DYSPHASIA

Dysphasia is an acquired loss of production or comprehension of spoken and/or written language secondary to brain damage.

Hand preference is associated with 'hemisphere dominance' for language. In right-handed people the left hemisphere is dominant; in left-handed people the left hemisphere is dominant in most, though 25% have a dominant right hemisphere.

The cortical centres for language reside in the dominant hemisphere.

1. Broca's area

Executive or motor area for the production of language – lies in the inferior part of the frontal lobe on the lateral surface of the cerebral hemisphere abutting the mouth of the Sylvian fissure.

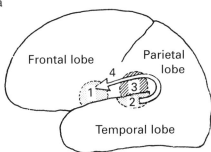

2 and 3. Receptive areas

Here the spoken word is understood and the appropriatae reply or action initiated. These areas lie at the posterior end of the Sylvian fissure on the lateral surface of the hemisphere.

The temporal lobe receptive area (**2**) lies close to the auditory cortex of the transverse gyrus of the temporal lobe. The parietal lobe receptive area (**3**) lies within the angular gyrus.

Receptive and expressive areas must be linked in order to integrate function. The link is provided by (**4**), the **arcuate fasciculus,** a fibre tract which runs forward in the subcortical white matter.

Dysphasia may develop as a result of vascular, neoplastic, traumatic, infective or degenerative disease of the cerebrum when language areas are involved.

DISORDERS OF SPEECH – DYSPHASIA

DIAGNOSTIC APPROACH

Listen to content and fluency of speech. Test comprehension, i.e. simple then complex commands

Assess
– Spontaneous speech
– Naming objects
– Repetition
– Reading
– Writing

Non-fluent, hesitant speech; may be confined to a few repeated utterances or, in less severe cases, is of a 'telegraphic' nature with articles and conjunctions omitted. Good comprehension. Handwriting poor. Look for coexisting right arm and face weakness.

BROCA'S DYSPHASIA (Motor or expressive dysphasia)

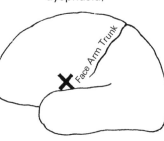

Causative diseases

Vascular disease
Neoplasm
Trauma
Infective disease
Degenerative disease

Comprehension impaired. ⟶ WERNICKE'S DYSPHASIA
Speech nonsensical but fluent. (Sensory or receptive dysphasia)
   neologisms –
     nonexistent words.
   paraphrasia –
     half right words.
Patient unaware
   of language problem.
Handwriting poor.

Vascular disease
Neoplasm
Trauma
Infective disease
Degenerative disease

Differentiate from confused patient – construction of words and sentences are normal.

Non-fluent speech and ⟶ GLOBAL DYSPHASIA
impaired comprehension. Damage involving a
Often associated with large area of the
hemiplegia/hemianaesthesia dominant hemisphere.
and visual field deficit.

Vascular disease
Neoplasm
Trauma
Infective disease
Degenerative disease

Speech nonsensical but ⟶ CONDUCTION
fluent (neologisms and DYSPHASIA
paraphrasia) yet comprehension is normal. Repetition is poor.

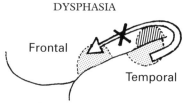

Vascular disease
Neoplasm
Trauma
Infective disease
Degenerative disease

DEMENTIAS

Definition

Progressive deterioration of intellect, behaviour and personality as a consequence of diffuse disease of the cerebral hemispheres, maximally affecting the cerebral cortex and hippocampus.

Distinguish from *delirium* which is an acute disturbance of cerebral function with impaired conscious level, hallucinations and autonomic overactivity as a consequence of toxic, metabolic or infective conditions.

Dementia may occur at any age but is more common in the elderly, accounting for 40% of long-term psychiatric in-patients over the age of 65 years. A recent study shows an annual incidence rate of 187/100 000 persons. Dementia is a symptom of disease rather than a single disease entity. When occurring under the age of 65 years it is labelled 'presenile' dementia. This term is artificial and does not suggest a specific aetiology.

Clinical course:

The rate of progression depends upon the underlying cause.

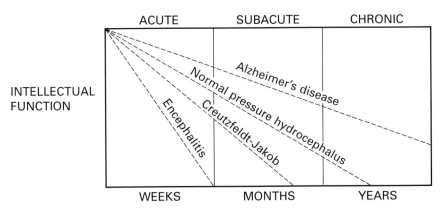

The duration of history helps establish the cause of dementia; Alzheimer's disease is slowly progressive over years, whereas encephalitis may be rapid over weeks. Dementia due to cerebrovascular disease appears to occur 'stroke by stroke'.

All dementias show a tendency to be accelerated by change of environment, intercurrent infection or surgical procedures.

Development of symptoms

Introspective. Unsure of self. → Difficulty in coping with work and ordinary routine (retained insight). → Loss of insight, behavioural changes, Loss of inhibition.
↓
Mutism, incontinence and DEATH ← Long-term care. Cannot be left unattended.

This initial phase of dementia may be inseparable from the *pseudodementia* of *depressive illness*.   123

DEMENTIAS – CLASSIFICATION

Based on cause

Alzheimer's
Cerebrovascular
   Multi-infarct state
   Subcortical small vessel
   Amyloid angiopathy
   CADASIL (see later)
Neurodegenerative
   Pick's disease
   Huntington's chorea
   Parkinson's disease
Infectious
   Sporadic and variant
      Creutzfeld–Jakob disease.
   HIV infection
   Progressive multifocal
      leucoencephalopathy
Normal pressure hydrocephalus

Nutritional
   Wernicke Korsakoff
      (thiamine deficiency)
   B_{12} deficiency
   Folate deficiency
Metabolic
   Hepatic disease
   Thyroid disease
   Parathyroid disease
   Cushing's syndrome
Chronic inflammatory
   Collagen vascular
   Primary and secondary vasculitis
   Multiple sclerosis
Trauma
   Head injury
   'Punch drunk' syndrome
Tumour
   e.g. Subfrontal meningioma

Alzheimer's disease accounts for 60% of all dementias; cerebrovascular disease 20%.

It is important to investigate all patients with dementia as many causes are treatable; in practice 10–15% can be reversed.

Based on site

Subdividing dementia depending upon the site of predominant clinical involvement is of questionable diagnostic value. However, many clinicians use this classification:

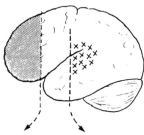 or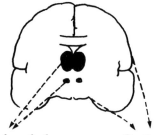

Anterior	**Posterior**	**Subcortical**	**Cortical**
(Frontal premotor cortex)	(Parietal and temporal lobes)	Apathetic	Higher cortical abnormalities
↓	↓	Forgetful and slow, poor ability to use knowledge	– dysphasia
Behavioural changes/loss of inhibition, antisocial behaviour, facile and irresponsible	Disturbance of cognitive function (memory and language) without marked changes in behaviour	Associated with other neurological signs and movement disorders	– agnosia – apraxia
↓	↓	↓	↓
e.g. Normal pressure Hydrocephalus Huntington's chorea Metabolic disease	ALZHEIMER'S DISEASE	e.g. PARKINSON'S DISEASE AIDS DEMENTIA COMPLEX	e.g. ALZHEIMER'S DISEASE

DEMENTIAS — HISTORY AND CLINICAL EXAMINATION

When obtaining a history from a demented person and relative, establish:

- Rate of intellectual decline
- Impairment of social function
- General health and relevant disorders, e.g. stroke, head injury
- Nutrition status
- Drug history
- Family history of dementia.

Tests to assess intellectual function are designed to check

- memory
- abstract thought
- judgement
- specific focal cortical functions

The Mini Mental Status Examination (MMSE)

Date orientation	Serial sevens
Place orientation	Naming
Register 3 objects	Repeating
Obeying verbal command	
Obeying written command	
Writing/drawing	

This is the standard tool of evaluation. Top Score = 30; score >24 normal; <24 suggests dementia
Folstein at el J. Psych Res 12:196–198 1975

On neurological examination note:

- Focal signs
- Involuntary movements
- Pseudobulbar signs
- Primitive reflexes:

Pout reflex

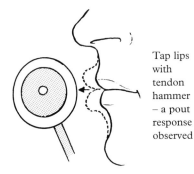

Tap lips with tendon hammer – a pout response is observed

Glabellar reflex

Patient cannot inhibit blinking in response to stimulation (tapping between the eyes)

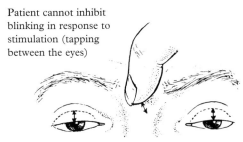

Grasp reflex

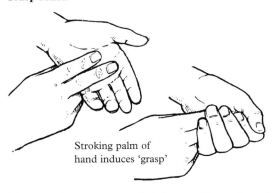

Stroking palm of hand induces 'grasp'

Palmomental reflex

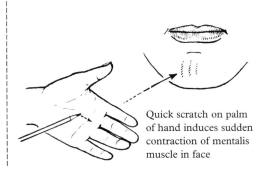

Quick scratch on palm of hand induces sudden contraction of mentalis muscle in face

Primitive reflexes are present in infancy and in aged people, as well as in dementia.

DEMENTIAS — SPECIFIC DISEASES

ALZHEIMER'S DISEASE

This is the commonest cause of dementia with an estimated half million sufferers in the UK. The disorder rarely occurs under the age of 45 years. The incidence increases with age. Up to 30% of cases are familial.

Pathology

(i) **Neuritic plaque:** a complex extracellular lesion of 15–100 μm. Aggregates of filaments with a central core of *amyloid*. Found in the hippocampus and parietal lobes

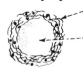

(ii) **Neurofibrillary tangle:** an intracellular lesion. Paired helical strands of protein close to nuclei of neurons. Mainly affecting pyramidal cells of cortex

These lesions are associated with neuronal loss and granulovacuolar degeneration

The brain is small with atrophy most evident in the superior and middle temporal gyri.

Subcortical origins of cholinergic projections are also involved.

Diagnosis This may be established during life by early memory failure, slow progression and exclusion of other causes. Specific clinical criteria have been established, mainly for research purposes. Whilst certain blood tests can identify populations at risk (i.e. APOE genotyping) these are of no diagnostic value in individual cases.

CT scanning: aids diagnosis by excluding multiple infarction or a mass lesion.

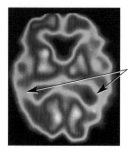

SPECT: confirms selective temporo-parietal hypoperfusion

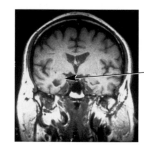

MRI: coronal views show early unilateral (as shown) or bilateral peri-hippocampal atrophy

Causation

The cause of Alzheimer's disease is not known. An association with Down's syndrome suggests a disease locus on chromosome 21 (on which amyloid precursor protein is coded), and this has been confirmed in familial cases. The role of environmental toxins, especially aluminium, is uncertain. Early research suggested selective lesions of neurotransmitter pathways occurred and a disorder of cholinergic innervation was postulated. It is now known that many neurotransmitter pathways are defective.

Treatment

Centrally acting drugs such as acetylcholinesterase inhibitors (e.g. Donepezil and Rivastigmine) have been shown in trials to enhance cognitive performance in early disease. However they do not cure.

DEMENTIAS — SPECIFIC DISEASES

MULTI-INFARCT (arteriosclerotic dementia)

This is an overdiagnosed condition which accounts for less than 10% of cases of dementia. Dementia occurs 'stroke by stroke', with progressive focal loss of function. Clinical features of stroke profile – hypertension, diabetes, etc. – are present.

Diagnosis is obtained from the history and confirmed by CT scan.

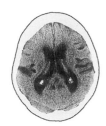

Low density areas of infarction

These areas are not space-occupying and do not enhance after intravenous contrast

Treatment: Maintain adequate blood pressure control. Anti-platelet aggregants (aspirin).

PICK'S DISEASE

This progressive condition accounts for 5% of all dementias. Usually sporadic, it more commonly affects women between 40 and 60 years. Frontal lobe dysfunction predominates with apathy, lack of initiative and personality changes. CT scan shows frontal atrophy. Blood flow studies (SPECT (HMPAO)) reveal anterior hypoperfusion. The disorder is characterised pathologically by *argyrophilic inclusion bodies* within the cytoplasm of cells of the frontotemporal cortex. There is no treatment, death occurring within 2–3 years of the onset.

Cerebral autosomal dominant arteriopathy with subcortical infarcts and leukoencephalopathy (CADASIL)

This inherited disorder presents with migraine (often hemiplegic) in early adult life, progessing through TIAs and subcortical strokes to early dementia. The advent of MRI with its characteristic appearance has led to increasing recognition of what was previously only identified at autopsy. CADASIL has been mapped to the 'Notch 3' gene on chromosome 19 in many (though not all) cases allowing diagnostic testing. The role of the gene is uncertain and specific treatments not available.

Primary progressive aphasia

This condition is one of a group of disorders characterised by asymmetrical cortical degeneration. Dominant hemisphere perisylvian atrophy is associated with loss of language, which, after many years, becomes a more widespread dementia. Pathologically non-specific cell loss, Pick's pathology or spongiform changes are described. MRI and SPECT confirm focal changes.

AIDS DEMENTIA COMPLEX (see pages 511–512)

Approximately two-thirds of persons with AIDS develop dementia, mostly due to AIDS dementia complex. In some patients HIV is found in the CNS at postmortem. In others an immune mechanism or an unidentified pathogen is blamed. Dementia is initially of a 'subcortical' type. CT shows atrophy; MRI shows increased T2 signal from white matter. Imaging excludes other infections and neoplastic causes of intellectual decline.

Treatment with Zidovudine (AZT) halts and partially reverses neuropsychological deficit.

METABOLIC DEMENTIA

General medical examination is important in suggesting underlying systemic disease. B_{12} deficiency may produce dementia rather than subacute combined degeneration of the spinal cord. In alcoholics, consider not only Wernicke Korsakoff syndrome but also *chronic subdural haematoma.*

DEMENTIAS – SPECIFIC DISEASES

NORMAL PRESSURE HYDROCEPHALUS

Normal pressure hydrocephalus (NPH) is the term applied to the triad of:

Dementia	occurring in conjunction with
Gait disturbance	*hydrocephalus* and *normal*
Urinary incontinence	CSF pressure.

Two types occur:
- NPH with a *preceding cause* – subarachnoid haemorrhage
  - meningitis
  - trauma
  - radiation-induced

(This must be distinguished from hydrocephalus with raised intracranial pressure associated with these causes.)

- NPH with no known preceding cause – *idiopathic* (50%).

Aetiology is unclear. It is presumed that at some preceding period, impedence to normal CSF flow causes raised intraventricular pressure and ventricular dilatation. Compensatory mechanisms permit a reduction in CSF pressure yet the ventricular dilatation persists and causes symptoms:

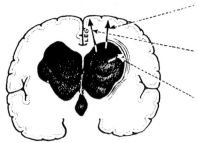

Pressure on frontal lobes ——▶ Dementia
(possibly related to decreased
cerebral blood flow).

Pressure on the cortical centre ——▶ Incontinence
for bladder and bowel control
in the paracentral lobe.

Pressure on the 'leg fibres' from ——▶ Gait disturbance
the cortex passing around the   and pyramidal
ventricle towards the internal capsule. signs in the legs.

Diagnosis is based on clinical picture plus CT scan/MRI evidence of ventricular enlargement.

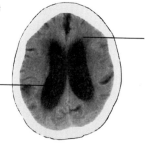

The lateral ventricles are often dilated more than the 3rd and 4th

Note the presence or absence of periventricular lucency (PVL) and width of cortical sulci

Normal pressure hydrocephalus must be differentiated from patients whose ventricular enlargement is merely the result of shrinkage of the surrounding brain, e.g. Alzheimer's disease. These patients do not respond to CSF shunting, whereas a proportion of patients with NPH (but not all) show a definitive improvement with shunting.

DEMENTIAS – SPECIFIC DISEASES

Investigations

Numerous tests have been assessed to predict those most likely to benefit from operation. The most reliable are –

(i) The presence of *beta waves* on *continuous intracranial pressure* monitoring for more than 5% of a 24 hour period.

(ii) Clinical improvement with *continuous lumbar CSF drainage* of 200 ml per day for three to five days.

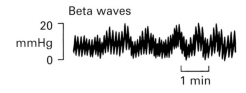

Beta waves

20 mmHg

0

1 min

Other tests include the presence of periventricular lucency or disproportionate sulcal width on CT scan, isotope cisternography and CSF infusion studies but none appear to produce a reliable guide.

Operation: Ventriculo-peritoneal shunting (see page 373).
Results: Improvement occurs in 50–70% of those patients with a known preceding cause e.g. subarachnoid haemorrhage. Only 30% of the idiopathic group respond to shunting.

TRAUMA

Reduction of intellectual function is common after severe head injury. Chronic subdural haematoma can also present as progressive dementia, especially in the elderly.
Punch-drunk encephalopathy (dementia pugilistica) is the cumulative result of repeated cerebral trauma. It occurs in both amateur and professional boxers and is manifest by dysarthria, ataxia and extrapyramidal signs associated with 'subcortical' dementia. There is no treatment for this progressive syndrome.

TUMOUR presenting as dementia

Concern is always expressed at the possibility of dementia being due to intracranial tumour. This is rare, but may happen when tumours occur in certain sites.

Mental or behavioural changes occur in 50–70% of all brain tumours as distinct from dementia which is associated with **frontal lobe tumours** (and subfrontal tumours), **III ventricle tumours** and **corpus callosum tumours**.

Suspect in recent onset dementia with focal signs, e.g. subfrontal lesions may be associated with loss of smell (I cranial nerve involvement) and optic atrophy (II cranial nerve involvement).

Cognitive impairment also occurs as a non metastatic complication of systemic malignancy.

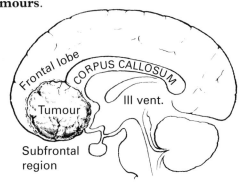

Frontal lobe

CORPUS CALLOSUM

III vent.

Tumour

Subfrontal region

N.B. Dementia can occur as a symptom of a more widespread degenerative disorder

e.g. Parkinson's disease
Diffuse Lewy body disease
Progressive supranuclear palsy

Huntington's disease
Motor neuron disease
These will be considered later

DEMENTIA – DIAGNOSTIC APPROACH

It is neither practical nor essential to perform all the screening tests in every patient with dementia. The presenting features should guide investigations.

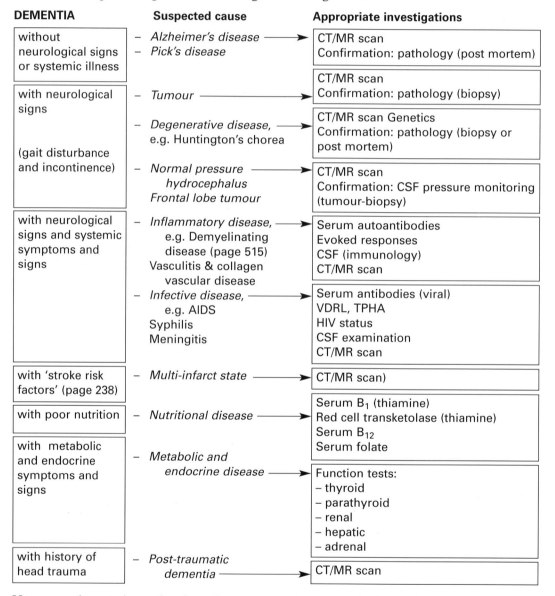

DEMENTIA	Suspected cause	Appropriate investigations
without neurological signs or systemic illness	– *Alzheimer's disease* – *Pick's disease*	CT/MR scan Confirmation: pathology (post mortem)
with neurological signs	*Tumour*	CT/MR scan Confirmation: pathology (biopsy)
(gait disturbance and incontinence)	– *Degenerative disease,* e.g. Huntington's chorea	CT/MR scan Genetics Confirmation: pathology (biopsy or post mortem)
	– *Normal pressure* *hydrocephalus* *Frontal lobe tumour*	CT/MR scan Confirmation: CSF pressure monitoring (tumour-biopsy)
with neurological signs and systemic symptoms and signs	– *Inflammatory disease,* e.g. Demyelinating disease (page 515) Vasculitis & collagen vascular disease	Serum autoantibodies Evoked responses CSF (immunology) CT/MR scan
	– *Infective disease,* e.g. AIDS Syphilis Meningitis	Serum antibodies (viral) VDRL, TPHA HIV status CSF examination CT/MR scan
with 'stroke risk factors' (page 238)	– *Multi-infarct state*	CT/MR scan)
with poor nutrition	– *Nutritional disease*	Serum B_1 (thiamine) Red cell transketolase (thiamine) Serum B_{12} Serum folate
with metabolic and endocrine symptoms and signs	– *Metabolic and* *endocrine disease*	Function tests: – thyroid – parathyroid – renal – hepatic – adrenal
with history of head trauma	– *Post-traumatic* *dementia*	CT/MR scan

Neuropsychometric testing is performed – to diagnose early dementia.
 – evaluate atypical dementia.
 – separate out depressive illness.
 – monitor therapies.

When the reason for dementia is unclear, comprehensive investigation is essential to ensure that treatable nutritional, infective, metabolic and structural causes are not overlooked.

IMPAIRMENT OF VISION

ANATOMY AND PHYSIOLOGY

Anatomically the visual system is contained in the supratentorial compartment. It is composed of peripheral receptors in the retina, central pathways and cortical centres. The control of ocular movement and pupillary responses are closely integrated.

The retina: three distinct layers of the retina are identified:

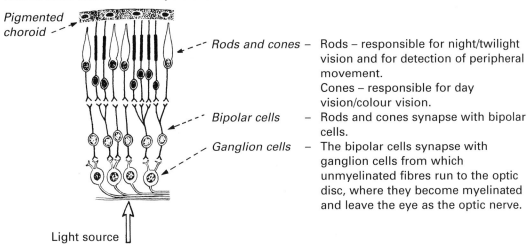

Pigmented choroid

Rods and cones – Rods – responsible for night/twilight vision and for detection of peripheral movement.
Cones – responsible for day vision/colour vision.

Bipolar cells – Rods and cones synapse with bipolar cells.

Ganglion cells – The bipolar cells synapse with ganglion cells from which unmyelinated fibres run to the optic disc, where they become myelinated and leave the eye as the optic nerve.

Light source

The *macular region* of the retina is its most important area for visual acuity. Here, cones lie in the greatest concentration whereas rods are more numerous in the surrounding retina.

The optic nerve leaves the orbit through the *optic foramen* and passes posteriorly to unite with the opposite optic nerve at the *optic chiasma*. Here, partial decussation occurs (axons from ganglion cells on the nasal side of the retina cross over to the opposite side).

The *optic tract* consisting of ipsilateral temporal and contralateral nasal fibres passes to the *lateral geniculate body*. A few fibres leave the tract before the lateral geniculate body and pass to the *superior colliculus* (fibres concerned with pupillary light reflex).

Axons of cell bodies in the lateral geniculate body make up the *optic radiation*. This enters the hemisphere in the most posterior part of the internal capsule, courses deep in parietal and temporal lobes and terminates in the *calcarine cortex* of the occipital lobe.

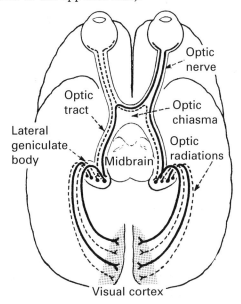

Optic nerve

Optic tract

Optic chiasma

Lateral geniculate body

Midbrain

Optic radiations

Visual cortex

IMPAIRMENT OF VISION

CLINICAL APPROACH AND DIFFERENTIAL DIAGNOSIS

Patients presenting with visual impairment require a systematic examination, not only of *vision*, but also of the *pupillary response*, *eye movements*, and, unless the cause clearly lies within the globe, *a full neurological examination.*

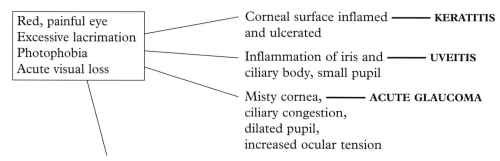

The findings aid localisation of the lesion, e.g.

Impairment of vision + impaired pupil response indicates a lesion anterior to the lateral geniculate body

A homonymous hemianopia + sensory and cognitive deficit indicates a parieto-temporal lesion

An isolated homonymous hemianopia usually indicates an occipital lesion

Refractive errors are excluded by testing visual acuity through a pinhole or by correcting a lens deformity (page 9).

Four types of refractive error exist:

PRESBYOPIA – failure of accommodation with age
HYPERMETROPIA (long sightedness) – short eyeball
MYOPIA (short sightedness) – long eyeball
ASTIGMATISM – variation in corneal curvature

If this examination is normal, then the lesion lies in the retina, visual pathways or visual cortex.

Examine the globe and anterior chamber

Red, painful eye
Excessive lacrimation
Photophobia
Acute visual loss

Corneal surface inflamed and ulcerated ——— **KERATITIS**

Inflammation of iris and ciliary body, small pupil ——— **UVEITIS**

Misty cornea, ciliary congestion, dilated pupil, increased ocular tension ——— **ACUTE GLAUCOMA**

Involvement of the vitreous, uvea and retina; pus and debris present in the anterior chamber. ——— **ENDOPHTHALMITIS**

Examine the lens with an ophthalmoscope

Opacification indicates CATARACT.

IMPAIRMENT OF VISION

CLINICAL APPROACH AND DIFFERENTIAL DIAGNOSIS (*cont'd*)

Examine the posterior segment of the eye with an ophthalmoscope. Pupil dilatation may be required.

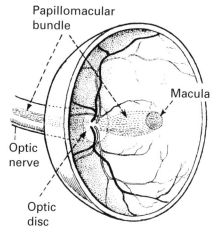

Papillomacular bundle

Macula

Optic nerve

Optic disc

In the normal fundus, the *disc* is pale with a central cup and reddish-brown surrounding retina. Arteries and veins emerge from the optic disc. The *macula* is darker than the rest of the fundus and lies on the temporal side of the disc. One-third of all retinal fibres arise from the small macular region and pass to the optic nerve head (disc) as the *papillomacular bundle*. The macula is the region of sharpest vision (cone vision), whereas peripheral vision (rod vision) serves the purpose of perception of movement and directing central/macular vision. The optic nerve head contains no rods or cones and accounts for the physiological *blind spot* in normal vision. The macular fibres being so functionally active, are the most susceptible to damage and produce a specific defect in the visual field – a **scotoma**.

Retinal abnormality with acute impairment of vision

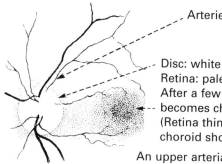

Arteries: narrow – branch occlusion, one vessel absent, embolus may be visualised → **ARTERIAL OCCLUSION**

Disc: white
Retina: pale and oedematous
After a few days the macular area becomes cherry red in appearance (Retina thinned here and the choroid shows through.)

An upper arterial branch occlusion is associated with a lower field defect in one eye.

Confirm with visual field examination.

Altitudinal field defect

Look for embolic source, e.g. carotid stenosis.

Loss of retinal colour (becomes milky white) and macular blush. → **CENTRAL RETINAL ARTERY OCCLUSION**

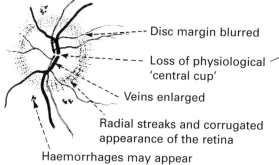

Disc margin blurred

Loss of physiological 'central cup'

Veins enlarged

Radial streaks and corrugated appearance of the retina

Haemorrhages may appear

Papillitis: *visual acuity severely affected* due to associated inflammation of the optic nerve (retrobulbar neuritis).

Papilloedema does not affect visual acuity (unless the macular area is affected by haemorrhage) although the blind spot is enlarged.

IMPAIRMENT OF VISION

CLINICAL APPROACH AND DIFFERENTIAL DIAGNOSIS (*cont'd*)

N.B. Distinguish:

HYPERMETROPIC patients who have a pale indistinct disc often difficult to differentiate from early papilloedema.

HYPERTENSIVE RETINOPATHY – superficial haemorrhages and 'cotton wool' exudates.

PSEUDOPAPILLOEDEMA – **'DRUSEN'** – hyaline bodies near the optic disc which raise the disc and blur the margin. This normal variant may be inherited.

Separation of the superficial retina from the pigment layer → **RETINAL DETACHMENT**
(traumatic or spontaneous)

Retinal abnormalities with gradual impairment of vision

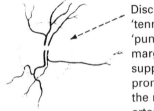

Disc white like a ——→ **OPTIC ATROPHY**
'tennis ball' with
'punched out'
margins: blood
supply is less
prominent and
the number of
arteries reduced

Primary (optic nerve disease): *compression, toxins, ischaemia, optic neuritis*
Secondary (following papilloedema):
↓
visual field charting (see later) may
help differentiate cause

N.B. Any disease of the optic nerve or anterior visual pathway causing loss of vision will eventually result in optic atrophy.

Pigmentary deposits in the ——→ **RETINITIS PIGMENTOSA**
periphery of the retina

Progressive pallor
of the optic disc

Areas of white sclera ——→ **CHOROIDITIS**
exposed along with areas
of proliferation of retinal
pigmentary epithelium –
follows atrophy of the
choroid

Occurs in *toxoplasmosis* and
in *cytomegalovirus* infection

Field examination reveals
a patchy loss.

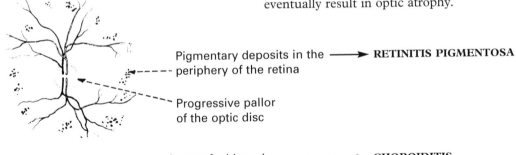

LEFT   RIGHT

Fixation point ---

Blind spot ---

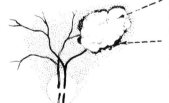

IMPAIRMENT OF VISION

CLINICAL APPROACH AND DIFFERENTIAL DIAGNOSIS (*cont'd*)

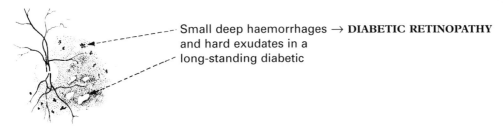

Small deep haemorrhages → **DIABETIC RETINOPATHY**
and hard exudates in a
long-standing diabetic

Dark oval mass – possibly related to — in middle aged → **MALIGNANT MELANOMA**
secondary retinal   patient
detachment

White mass behind the pupil — in infancy → **RETINOBLASTOMA**

Examine the visual fields

If ophthalmoscopic examination is normal, or if optic atrophy is evident, then visual field examination is essential. Visual confrontation is useful for detecting large defects, but smaller defects require visual field charting with a Goldmann perimeter (page 10).

In interpreting the results of examination it is important to remember that the ocular system *reverses* the image. The nasal side of the fundus picks up the temporal image and vice versa. Damage, therefore, to the nasal side of the retina will produce a temporal visual field defect.

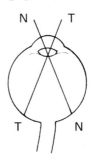

IMPAIRMENT OF VISION

CLINICAL APPROACH AND DIFFERENTIAL DIAGNOSIS (*cont'd*)

Central scotoma   Characteristic of most optic nerve lesions.

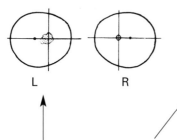

L   R

RETROBULBAR NEURITIS – associated papillitis may be evident on fundoscopy; may be first sign of *multiple sclerosis.*

OPTIC NERVE COMPRESSION
X-ray optic foramen ——— ***Orbital lesion*** (usually with proptosis)

CT/MRI scan
(orbital/intracranial)
     – *tumour*
     – *granuloma*

Lesion within optic canal
– *tumour*, e.g. meningioma
– *granuloma*
– *hyperostosis*, e.g. Paget's disease, fibrous dysplasia

Intracranial lesions
– *tumour*, e.g. meningioma (chordoma, dermoid)
– *granuloma*, e.g. tuberculoma, sarcoid (rare)
– *aneurysm*, e.g. ophthalmic → angiography confirms

Pupil response may be impaired (Marcus-Gunn pupil, see page 144)

OPTIC NERVE GLIOMA →   CT/MRI → exploration
LEBER'S OPTIC ATROPHY → large bilateral scotoma

Centro-caecal scotoma

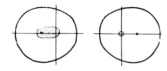

The scotoma extends to involve the blind spot. Characteristic of *toxic amblyopia* – alcohol, tobacco.

Monocular blindness

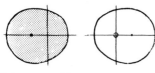

Direct pupillary response absent; consensual present.

Arcuate scotoma

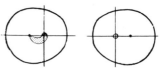

The scotoma extends from the blind spot following the course of nerve fibres.

Characteristic of *glaucoma*; seen also in small lesions close to the optic disc such as *choroiditis.*

The end result of an inflammatory, vascular or compressive optic nerve lesion.

Junctional scotoma

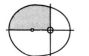

– indicates the presence of an *optic nerve lesion immediately anterior to the chiasma.*

Nasal fibres not only decussate in the chiasma, but also loop forward into the opposite optic nerve. This lesion emphasises the importance of examining the 'normal' eye in monocular impairment of vision.

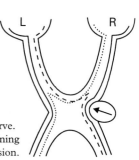

L   R

IMPAIRMENT OF VISION

CLINICAL APPROACH AND DIFFERENTIAL DIAGNOSIS (*cont'd*)

Bitemporal hemianopia/quadrantanopia

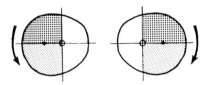 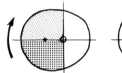 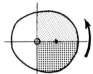

Involvement of the upper quadrants first indicates compression of the optic chiasma from below and suggests:

– **PITUITARY ADENOMA**
– **NASOPHARYNGEAL**
  CARCINOMA $\Big\} \rightarrow$ Skull X-ray/
– **SPHENOID SINUS**   CT scan/MRI
  MUCOLELE

Involvement of the lower quadrants first indicates compression of the optic chiasma from above and suggests:

– **CRANIOPHARYNGIOMA**
– **THIRD VENTRICULAR TUMOUR**
  $\downarrow$
  CT scan/MRI

The optic chiasma is closely associated with the pituitary fossa.

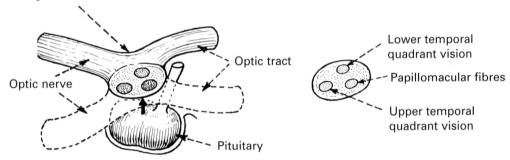

Homonymous hemianopia

An incongruous homonymous hemianopia (i.e. one eye more affected than the other) suggests a compressive lesion of the **optic tract** near the chiasma.

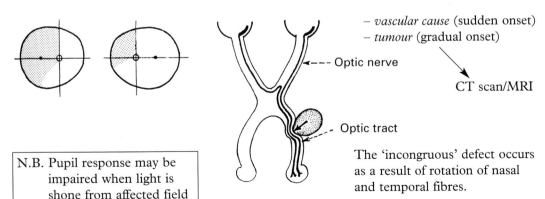

N.B. Pupil response may be impaired when light is shone from affected field

– *vascular cause* (sudden onset)
– *tumour* (gradual onset)

CT scan/MRI

The 'incongruous' defect occurs as a result of rotation of nasal and temporal fibres.

IMPAIRMENT OF VISION

CLINICAL APPROACH AND DIFFERENTIAL DIAGNOSIS (*cont'd*)

Congruous homonymous hemianopia (fields can be exactly superimposed)

Inferior quadrantanopia

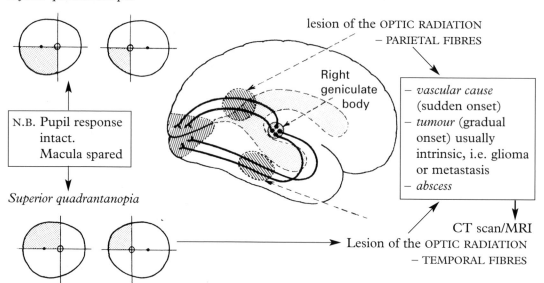

lesion of the OPTIC RADIATION
– PARIETAL FIBRES

Right
geniculate
body

N.B. Pupil response
intact.
Macula spared

– *vascular cause*
(sudden onset)
– *tumour* (gradual
onset) usually
intrinsic, i.e. glioma
or metastasis
– *abscess*

Superior quadrantanopia

CT scan/MRI

Lesion of the OPTIC RADIATION
– TEMPORAL FIBRES

At the temporo-parietal junction where fibres meet, lesions produce a complete 'homonymous hemianopia'.

Homonymous hemianopia with macular involvement

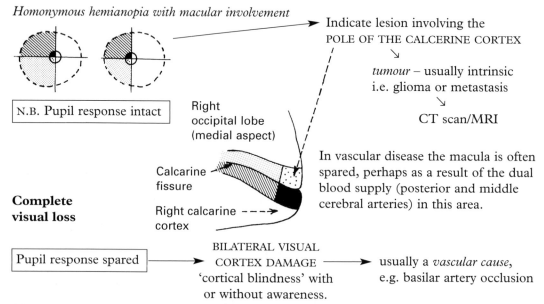

Indicate lesion involving the
POLE OF THE CALCERINE CORTEX

tumour – usually intrinsic
i.e. glioma or metastasis

CT scan/MRI

N.B. Pupil response intact

Right
occipital lobe
(medial aspect)

In vascular disease the macula is often
spared, perhaps as a result of the dual
blood supply (posterior and middle
cerebral arteries) in this area.

Calcarine
fissure

**Complete
visual loss**

Right calcarine
cortex

Pupil response spared

BILATERAL VISUAL
CORTEX DAMAGE
'cortical blindness' with
or without awareness.

usually a *vascular cause*,
e.g. basilar artery occlusion

The interpretation of the visual image and its integration with other cortical functions is
discussed under 'Higher cortical function'.

DISORDERS OF SMELL

OLFACTORY (I) cranial nerve conveys the sensation of smell.

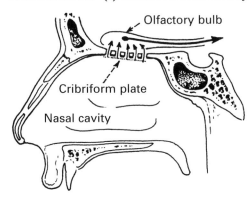

A number of fine nerves arising from receptor cells in the nasal mucosa pierce the *cribriform plate* of the ethmoid bone. These pass to the *olfactory bulb* where they synapse with neurons of the olfactory tract.

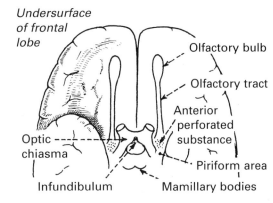

The axons partially decussate as they pass back in the olfactory tract to the *piriform area* of the temporal lobe and the *amygdaloid nucleus*.

Differential diagnosis

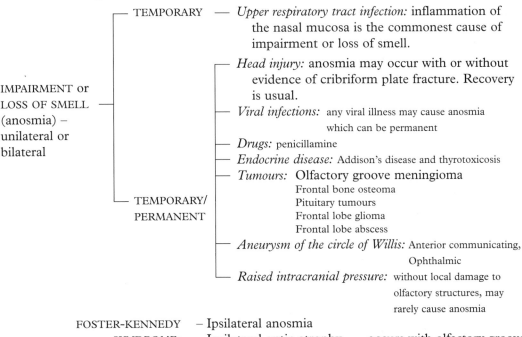

IMPAIRMENT or LOSS OF SMELL (anosmia) – unilateral or bilateral

TEMPORARY — *Upper respiratory tract infection:* inflammation of the nasal mucosa is the commonest cause of impairment or loss of smell.

TEMPORARY/ PERMANENT

Head injury: anosmia may occur with or without evidence of cribriform plate fracture. Recovery is usual.

Viral infections: any viral illness may cause anosmia which can be permanent

Drugs: penicillamine

Endocrine disease: Addison's disease and thyrotoxicosis

Tumours: Olfactory groove meningioma
Frontal bone osteoma
Pituitary tumours
Frontal lobe glioma
Frontal lobe abscess

Aneurysm of the circle of Willis: Anterior communicating, Ophthalmic

Raised intracranial pressure: without local damage to olfactory structures, may rarely cause anosmia

FOSTER-KENNEDY SYNDROME:
– Ipsilateral anosmia
– Ipsilateral optic atrophy — occurs with olfactory groove or sphenoid ridge masses
– Contralateral papilloedema

OLFACTORY HALLUCINATIONS — occur in complex partial seizures and migraine.

139

PUPILLARY DISORDERS

ANATOMY/PHYSIOLOGY

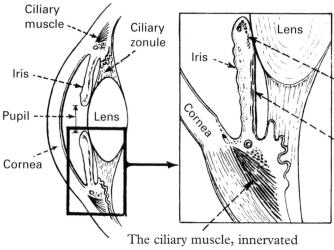

The iris controls the size of the pupil. It contains two groups of smooth muscle fibre:

1. *Sphincter pupillae*; a circular constrictor, innervated by the parasympathetic nervous system.
2. *Dilator pupillae*; a radial dilator, innervated by the sympathetic nervous system.

Pupillary size (normal 2–6 mm) depends on the balance between sympathetic and parasympathetic tone.

The ciliary muscle, innervated by the parasympathetic, controls the degree of convexity of the lens through the ciliary zonule.

Pathway of pupillary constriction and the light reflex (parasympathetic)

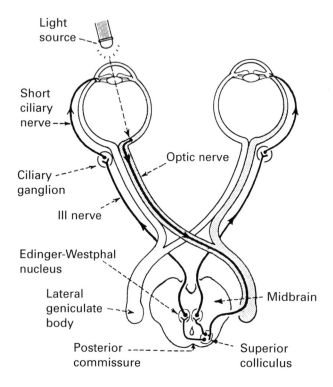

A stimulus, such as a bright light shone in the left eye, will send an afferent impulse along the **optic nerve** to the midbrain (superior colliculus); here a second order fibre passes to the *Edinger-Westphal nucleus* (part of the III nerve nucleus) on the same and opposite side (through the posterior commissure). Efferent fibres leave in the **oculomotor nerve,** pass to the ciliary ganglion and thence, in the short ciliary nerve, to the constrictor fibres of the sphincter pupillae muscle.

If all pathways are intact, shining a light in one eye will constrict *both pupils* at an equal rate and to a similar degree.

PUPILLARY DISORDERS

Pathway of pupillary dilatation (sympathetic)

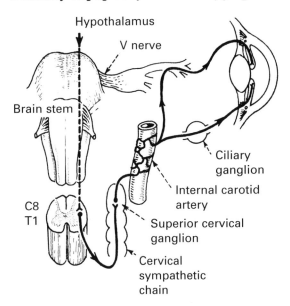

Sympathetic fibres descend from the ipsilateral hypothalamus through the lateral aspect of the brain stem into the spinal cord. The pupillary fibres pass out in the anterior roots of C8 and T1, enter the sympathetic chain and, in the superior cervical ganglion, give rise to postganglionic fibres which ascend on the wall of the internal carotid artery to enter the cranium. The fibres eventually leave the intracranial portion of the internal carotid artery and pass directly through the ciliary ganglion to the iris or join the cranial nerves III, IV, V and VI, running to the eye and iris. Sudomotor fibres (concerned with sweating) run up the external carotid artery to the dermis of the face.

Interruption of sympathetic supply affects:
1. Dilator pupillae causing a small pupil (miosis)
2. Levator palpebrae muscle (30% supplied by sympathetic) causing drooping of eyelid (ptosis)
3. Vasoconstrictor fibres to orbit, eyelid and face causing absence of sweating.

Interruption of parasympathetic supply affects:
Sphincter pupillae causing a large pupil (mydriasis)

Mechanism of accommodation
When gaze is focused on a near object the medial rectus muscles contract, producing convergence, the ciliary muscles contract enabling the lens to produce a more convex shape and the pupil constricts (accommodation for near vision).

The pathway is poorly understood but must involve the visual cortex, Edinger-Westphal nuclei and both medial rectus components of the III nerve nucleus in the midbrain.

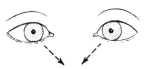

Inability of the pupil to constrict during accommodation need not always be associated with impairment of convergence, though usually this is the case.

Pupillary inequality (anisocoria)
A difference in pupil size occurs in 20% of the normal population and is distinguished from pathological states by a normal response to bright light.

PUPILLARY DISORDERS

PUPIL DILATATION – CAUSES

III nerve lesion

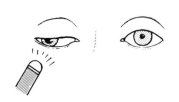

Examination of the light reflex (page 11) distinguishes lesions of the optic (II) and oculomotor (III) nerves. Failure of the pupil to constrict when light is shone into either the affected or the contralateral eye indicates a lesion of the parasympathetic component of the III nerve.

Look for – **ptosis** – 70% of levator palpebrae muscle is supplied by the oculomotor nerve

– **impaired eye movements**.

Causes of a III nerve lesion are described on page 151.

In comatose patients, pupil dilatation and failure to react to light is the simplest way of detecting a III nerve lesion; after head injury or in patients with raised intracranial pressure this is an important sign of transtentorial herniation.

The tonic pupil – Adie's pupil

This is a benign condition usually affecting young women. Onset is usually acute and unilateral in 80%.

The pupil dilates and the patient complains of mistiness in the affected eye.

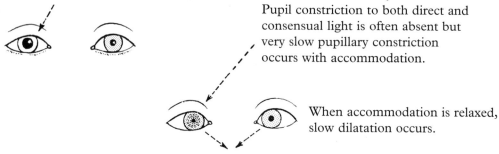

Pupil constriction to both direct and consensual light is often absent but very slow pupillary constriction occurs with accommodation.

When accommodation is relaxed, slow dilatation occurs.

Occasionally the pupil appears completely unreactive to both light and accommodation. When the pupil is associated with reduced or absent limb reflexes this is termed the *Holmes-Adie* syndrome. More widespread autonomic dysfunction – orthostatic hypotension, segmental disturbance of sweating and diarrhoea can co-exist.

Diagnosis: confirmed by pupillary response to pilocarpine (0.1% or 0.05%) – the tonic pupil will constrict (denervation hypersensitivity); the normal eye is not affected.

The cause is unknown; the lesion probably lies in the midbrain or ciliary ganglion.

Migraine: Mydriasis persisting for some hours can accompany headache.

Drugs: Mydriasis occurs with anticholinergic drugs (atropine), tricyclic antidepressants, non-steroidal anti-inflammatories, antihistamines and oral contraceptives. Mydriasis can precipitate an attack of acute angle-closure glaucoma.

PUPILLARY DISORDERS

PUPILS CONSTRICTION – CAUSES

Horner's syndrome

Lesion

 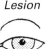

MIOSIS: the affected pupil is smaller than the opposite pupil. It does not dilate when the eye is shaded.

PTOSIS: the affected eyelid droops and may be slightly raised voluntarily. Ptosis is less marked than with a III nerve palsy.

DISTURBANCE OF SWEATING: depends on the site of the lesion. Absence of sweating occurs when the lesion is proximal to fibre separation along the internal and external carotid arteries.

Horner's syndrome may result from sympathetic damage at the following sites:

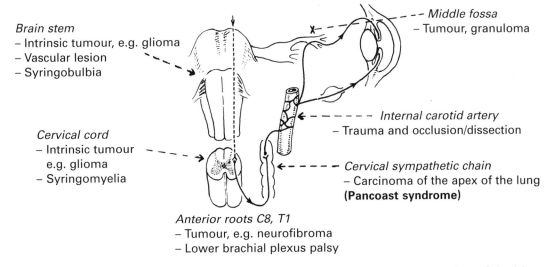

Brain stem
– Intrinsic tumour, e.g. glioma
– Vascular lesion
– Syringobulbia

Middle fossa
– Tumour, granuloma

Internal carotid artery
– Trauma and occlusion/dissection

Cervical cord
– Intrinsic tumour
 e.g. glioma
– Syringomyelia

Cervical sympathetic chain
– Carcinoma of the apex of the lung
(Pancoast syndrome)

Anterior roots C8, T1
– Tumour, e.g. neurofibroma
– Lower brachial plexus palsy

The congenital or familial form exists, often associated with lack of pigmentation of the iris. The lesion site is unknown.

Distinguish peripheral and central lesions by instilling drugs, e.g. 1% cocaine in eyes.

Preganglionic lesions

Right sided Horner's

Cocaine acts at the adrenergic nerve endings and, by preventing adrenaline uptake, causes pupil dilatation when the lesion is preganglionic.

Postganglionic lesions

Right sided Horner's

When the lesion is postganglionic, cocaine has little affect because there are no nerve endings on which the drug may act.

Investigative approach: depends on associated signs. Chest X-ray is mandatory to exclude an apical lung tumour.

PUPILLARY DISORDERS

PUPILS CONSTRICTION – CAUSES *(cont'd)*

The Argyll-Robertson pupil
Small pupils irregular in shape, which do not
react to light but react to accommodation.

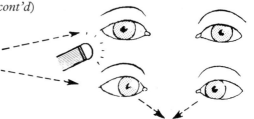

They respond inadequately to pupillary
dilator drugs.

Argyll-Robertson pupils are usually synonymous with *syphilitic infection*, but they may also result from any *midbrain lesion – neoplastic, vascular, inflammatory or demyelinative.*

The Argyll-Robertson pupil has also been described in *diabetes* and in *alcoholic neuropathy* as well as following infectious mononucleosis. The lesion could lie in the midbrain, involving fibres passing to the Edinger-Westphal nucleus, in the posterior commissure, or alternatively, in the ciliary ganglion. A central lesion seems most likely.

Investigative approach: – look for associated signs of neurosyphilis
– blood serology – VDRL, Captia G.

Drugs
Parasympathomimetic drugs – Carbachol, phenothiazines and opiates produce miosis.

N.B. Do not confuse with small pupils, normally occurring in the elderly.

OTHER PUPILLARY DISORDERS

Failure of accommodation and convergence

Impaired accommodation and convergence are of limited diagnostic value since other clinical features are usually more prominent

Causes – extrapyramidal disease, e.g. Parkinson's
– tumours of the pineal region.

The Marcus Gunn pupil (pupillary escape)

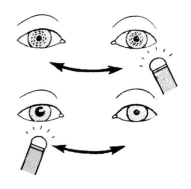

Illumination of one eye normally produces
pupillary constriction with a degree of waxing
and waning (hippus).

When afferent transmission in the optic nerve
is impaired, this 'escape' becomes more evident.

If the light source is 'swung' from eye to eye,
dwelling 2–3 seconds on each, the affected pupil
may eventually, paradoxically, dilate – a 'Marcus
Gunn' pupil.

The swinging light test is a sensitive test of optic nerve damage but is also abnormal in retinal or macular disease.

DIPLOPIA – IMPAIRED OCULAR MOVEMENT

Diplopia or double vision results from impaired ocular movement.

RELATED ANATOMY AND PHYSIOLOGY

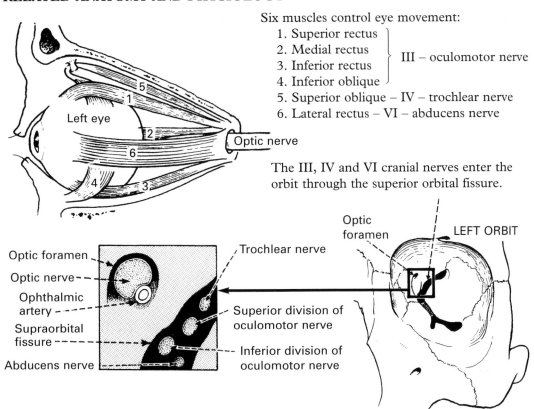

Six muscles control eye movement:
1. Superior rectus ⎫
2. Medial rectus ⎪ III – oculomotor nerve
3. Inferior rectus ⎬
4. Inferior oblique ⎭
5. Superior oblique – IV – trochlear nerve
6. Lateral rectus – VI – abducens nerve

The III, IV and VI cranial nerves enter the orbit through the superior orbital fissure.

The line of action of individual ocular muscles

Eye movements result from a continuous interplay of all the ocular muscles, but each muscle has a direction of maximal efficiency. The oblique muscles move the eye up and down when it is turned in. The superior and inferior recti move the eye up and down when it is turned out.

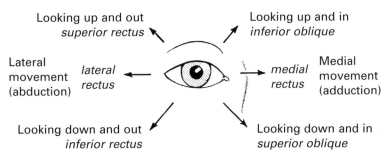

Eye movements are examined in the six different directions of gaze representing individual muscle action.

145

DIPLOPIA – IMPAIRED OCULAR MOVEMENT

The line of action of individual ocular muscles (*cont'd*)

As a result of the angle of insertion into the globe, the inferior and superior recti and the oblique muscles also have a rotatory or torsion effect.

When the eye is turned out, the oblique muscles rotate the globe; when turned in, the inferior or superior recti rotate the globe.

OCULOMOTOR (III) nerve

The oculomotor nucleus lies in the *ventral periaqueductal grey matter* at the level of the *superior colliculus*. Nerve fibres pass through the *red nucleus* and *substantia nigra* and emerge medial to the *cerebral peduncle*.

The nucleus has a complex structure:

Perlia's nuclei (parasympathetic) concerned with convergence and accommodation.
Edinger-Westphal nuclei (parasympathetic) concerned with pupil constriction

Medial rectus and inferior oblique

Inferior rectus

Superior rectus

Caudal nucleus of Perlia (levator of eyelid)

The nucleus is a paired structure which lies close to the midline, the portion representing the medial rectus abutting its neighbour.

DIPLOPIA – IMPAIRED OCULAR MOVEMENT

III nerve (*cont'd*)

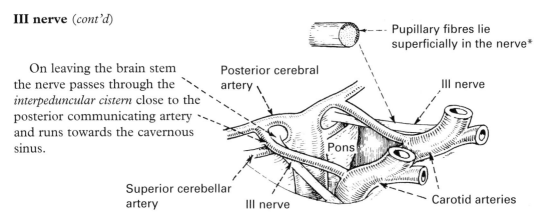

On leaving the brain stem the nerve passes through the *interpeduncular cistern* close to the posterior communicating artery and runs towards the cavernous sinus.

*This in part explains early pupillary involvement with III nerve compression and pupillary sparing with nerve infarction in hypertension and diabetes.

The nerve runs within the lateral wall of the *cavernous sinus* and then finally through the *superior orbital fissure* into the *orbit*.

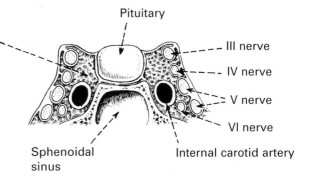

Here it divides into:
1. Superior branch to the levator of the eyelid and the superior rectus.
2. Inferior branch to the inferior oblique, medial and inferior recti.

TROCHLEAR (IV) nerve

This nerve supplies the *superior oblique muscle* of the eye.

The nucleus lies in the midbrain at the level of the *inferior colliculus*, near the ventral *periaqueductal grey matter*. The nerve passes laterally and dorsally around the central grey matter and decussates in the dorsal aspect of the brain stem in close proximity to the *anterior medullary velum* of the cerebellum.

Emerging from the brain stem the nerve passes laterally around the *cerebral peduncle* and pierces the dura to lie in the lateral wall of the *cavernous sinus*. Finally, it passes through the *superior orbital fissure* into the orbit.

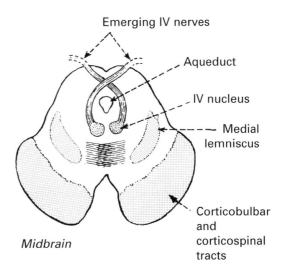

Midbrain

DIPLOPIA – IMPAIRED OCULAR MOVEMENT

ABDUCENS (VI) nerve

This nerve supplies the *lateral rectus muscle* of the eye.

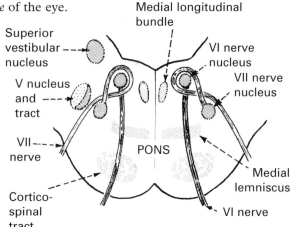

The nucleus lies in the floor of the IV ventricle within the lower portion of the *pons*. The axons pass ventrally through the pons without decussating.

Note the close association of the VI and VII nuclei.

Emerging from the brain stem the nerve runs up anterior to the pons for approximately 15 mm before piercing the dura overlying the *basilar portion* of the *occipital bone*.

Under the dura the nerve runs up the *petrous portion* of the temporal bone and from its apex passes on to the lateral wall of the *cavernous sinus* and finally through the *superior orbital fissure*.

Note the long intracranial course and the proximity of the VI to the V cranial and greater superficial petrosal nerves at the apex of the petrous temporal bone.

DIPLOPIA

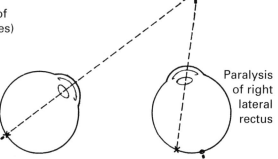

When the eyes fix on an image, impairment of movement of one eye results in projection of the image upon the macular area in the normal eye and to one side of the macula in the paretic eye; two images of the single object are thus perceived.

The image seen by the paretic eye is the false image; that seen by the normal eye is the *true image*. The false image is always outermost; this may lie in the vertical or the horizontal plane.

DIPLOPIA – IMPAIRED OCULAR MOVEMENT

CLINICAL ASSESSMENT

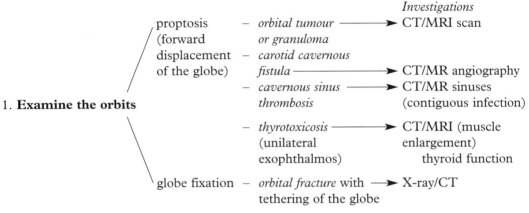

1. **Examine the orbits**

proptosis (forward displacement of the globe)
– *orbital tumour or granuloma* ——→ CT/MRI scan
– *carotid cavernous fistula* ——→ CT/MR angiography
– *cavernous sinus thrombosis* ——→ CT/MR sinuses (contiguous infection)
– *thyrotoxicosis* ——→ CT/MRI (muscle enlargement) thyroid function (unilateral exophthalmos)

Investigations

globe fixation – *orbital fracture* with ——→ X-ray/CT tethering of the globe

2. **Examine ocular movement** (page 12)
   – note the presence of a squint or *strabismus* ——→
   i.e. when the axes of the eyes are not parallel.

Differentiate

Concomitant squint (heterotropia) – an ocular disorder. The eyes adopt an abnormal position in relation to each other and the deviation is constant in all directions of gaze. Such squints develop in the first few years of life before binocular vision is established. Usually they are convergent (esotropia), occasionally divergent (exotropia). Suppression of vision from one eye (*amblyopia ex anopsia*) results in *absence of diplopia*.
Occasionally patients subconsciously alternate vision from one eye to the other, retaining equal visual function in both – *strabismus alternans*. Correction of an underlying hypermetropia with convex lenses may offset the tendency for the eyes to converge.

Paralytic squint:
– Affected eye shows limited movement.
– Angle of eye deviation and diplopia greatest when looking in the direction controlled by the weak muscle.
– Diplopia is always present.
– The patient may assume a head tilt posture to minimise the diplopia.
Paralytic squint results from disturbance of function of nerves or muscles.

III NERVE LESION
In the primary position, the affected eye deviates laterally (due to unopposed action of the lateral rectus) ——→
and **ptosis** and **pupil dilatation** are evident.

(Ptosis may be complete, unlike the partial ptosis of a Horner's syndrome which disappears on looking up.)

149

DIPLOPIA – IMPAIRED OCULAR MOVEMENT

IV NERVE LESION

The eyes appear conjugate in the primary position.

Testing eye movements reveals defective depression of the adducted eye.

Symptomatically the patient complains of double vision when looking downwards, e.g. when descending stairs or reading, and the head may tilt to the side opposite the weak superior oblique to minimise the diplopia.

A IV nerve palsy is difficult to detect when associated with a III nerve palsy. If inward rotation (intorsion) is absent on looking downwards when the eye is abducted, then a IV nerve palsy coexists with the III nerve palsy.

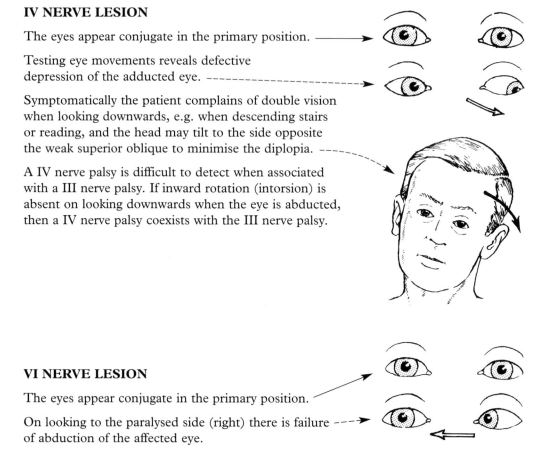

VI NERVE LESION

The eyes appear conjugate in the primary position.

On looking to the paralysed side (right) there is failure of abduction of the affected eye.

Diplopia is horizontal (true and fake image side by side), is present only when looking to the paralysed side and is maximal at the extreme of binocular lateral vision.

NOTE: In partial oculomotor palsies, the patient may be aware of diplopia, although eye movements appear normal. When this occurs:
- check diplopia is 'true' by noting its disappearance on covering one eye.
- determine the direction of maximal image displacement and the eye responsible for the outermost image (see page 13).

This information is sufficient to differentiate a III, IV and VI nerve lesion.

OCULAR MUSCLES

If the limitation of eye movement is not restricted to one muscle, or group of muscles with a common innervation, and affects both eyes, look for:

- involvement of extraocular muscles (levator palpebrae superioris, orbicularis oculi)   *myasthenia gravis*
- signs of fatigue on repeated testing   *ocular myopathy*

DIPLOPIA – IMPAIRED OCULAR MOVEMENT

CAUSES OF III NERVE LESION

Midbrain

When BILATERAL → oculomotor nucleus

When III nerve lesion is associated with

TREMOR → red nucleus
OR
CONTRALATERAL
HEMIPARESIS → cerebral
(WEBER'S SYNDROME) peduncles

Infarction, demyelination, intrinsic tumour, e.g. glioma, basilar aneurysm compression

Orbital fissure/orbit

Look for PROPTOSIS and associated involvement of the IV, VI and FIRST DIVISION of the V NERVES
– *Orbital tumour, granuloma,*
– *Periosteitis*

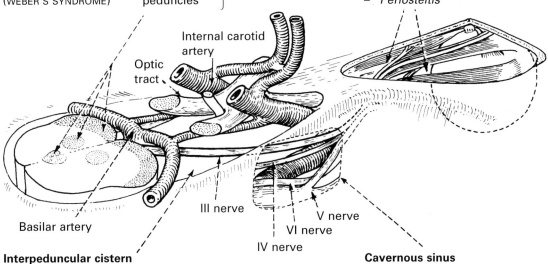

Internal carotid artery

Optic tract

III nerve

Basilar artery

V nerve

VI nerve

IV nerve

Interpeduncular cistern

WHEN III NERVE LESION IS ASSOCIATED WITH:

DETERIORATION OF → *Transtentorial*
CONSCIOUS LEVEL *herniation*

RETRO-ORBITAL PAIN → *Aneurysm compression*
± SUBARACHNOID *(posterior communicating*
HAEMORRHAGE *or basilar aneurysm)*

MENINGISM + OTHER → *Basal meningitis*
CRANIAL NERVE PALSIES *– TB, syphilitic, bacterial, fungal*
– carcinomatous

PUPIL REACTION SPARED → Nerve trunk infarction
SUDDEN ONSET *– hypertension,*
– diabetes,
– polyarteritis nodosa,
– SLE

Cavernous sinus

Look for associated involvement of IV, VI and 1st DIVISION OF V NERVE
– *Tumour e.g. pituitary adenoma, meningioma, metastasis, nasopharyngeal carcinoma*
– *Intracavernous aneurysm*
– *Cavernous sinus thrombosis*

DIPLOPIA – IMPAIRED OCULAR MOVEMENT

CAUSES OF IV AND VI NERVE LESIONS

Midbrain
When IV nerve lesion is associated with:

CONTRALATERAL
HEMIPARESIS,
CONTRALATERAL
HEMISENSORY LOSS
} Intrinsic
midbrain
lesion
} *Infarction,
demyelination,
intrinsic tumour,
e.g. glioma*

Proximity to
anterior
medullary velum
and superior
vermis
} *cerebellar
tumour, e.g.
medullo-
blastoma*

**Orbital fissure
orbit
Cavernous sinus** } *Causes as
for III nerve
lesion*

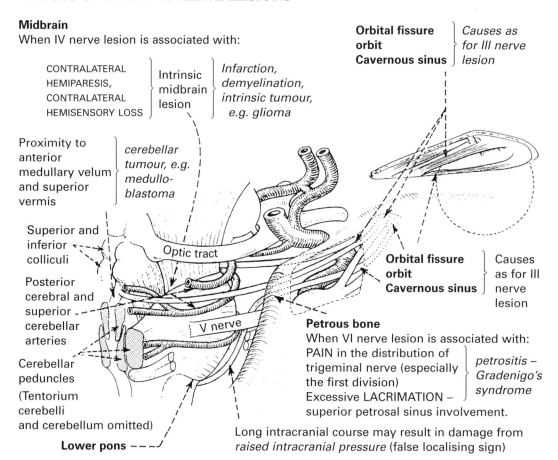

Superior and
inferior
colliculi

Optic tract

Posterior
cerebral and
superior
cerebellar
arteries

**Orbital fissure
orbit
Cavernous sinus** } Causes
as for III
nerve
lesion

Cerebellar
peduncles
(Tentorium
cerebelli
and cerebellum omitted)

V nerve

Petrous bone
When VI nerve lesion is associated with:
PAIN in the distribution of
trigeminal nerve (especially
the first division)
Excessive LACRIMATION –
superior petrosal sinus involvement.
} *petrositis –
Gradenigo's
syndrome*

Lower pons – – – –

Long intracranial course may result in damage from
raised intracranial pressure (false localising sign)

When VI nerve lesion is associated with:

CONTRALATERAL HEMIPARESIS,
CONTRALATERAL HEMISENSORY,
LOWER MOTOR NEURON VII LESION
} Nuclear or
intramedullary
lesion
} *Infarction,
demyelination,*
intrinsic tumour, e.g. glioma

NOTE: Infective or carcinomatous meningitis and nerve trunk infarction may also involve the IV and VI nerves, although less often than the III nerve.

Investigative approach
Impaired ocular movement from III, IV or VI nerve lesions requires full investigation with *CT/MR angiography* and, where appropriate, *CSF cytology, CT/MRI, CT/MR angiography*; only in elderly hypertensive or diabetic patients with pupillary sparing may angiography be omitted.

When myopathy or myasthenia gravis is suspected then appropriate investigations – acetyl choline receptor antibodies, EMG studies and occasionally muscle biopsy – may be necessary.

DISORDERS OF GAZE

ANATOMY AND PHYSIOLOGY

Two cortical centres of ocular control are recognised:
1. Middle gyrus of frontal lobe (frontal eye field).
2. Occipital cortex.

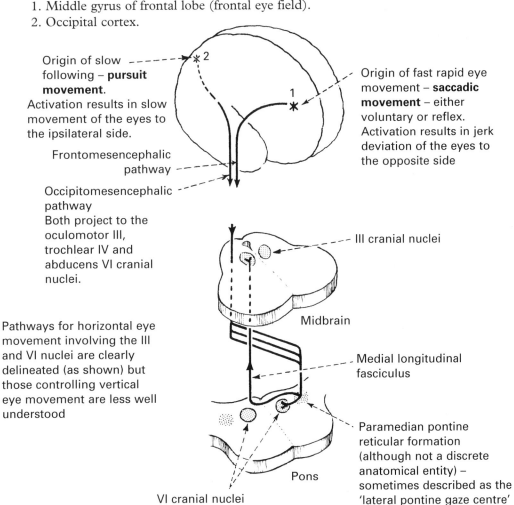

Origin of slow following – **pursuit movement**.
Activation results in slow movement of the eyes to the ipsilateral side.

Frontomesencephalic pathway

Occipitomesencephalic pathway
Both project to the oculomotor III, trochlear IV and abducens VI cranial nuclei.

Pathways for horizontal eye movement involving the III and VI nuclei are clearly delineated (as shown) but those controlling vertical eye movement are less well understood

Origin of fast rapid eye movement – **saccadic movement** – either voluntary or reflex.
Activation results in jerk deviation of the eyes to the opposite side

III cranial nuclei

Midbrain

Medial longitudinal fasciculus

Paramedian pontine reticular formation (although not a discrete anatomical entity) – sometimes described as the 'lateral pontine gaze centre'

Pons

VI cranial nuclei

Note that the cortical descending pathways from one side activate the ipsilateral III nucleus and the contralateral VI nucleus thus swinging the direction of gaze to the opposite side.

It is important to distinguish between **saccadic** and **pursuit** movement. When following an object a slow pursuit movement maintains the image on the macular area of the retina. To fixate on a new object, rapid saccadic movement aligns the new target on the macular area. When locked into the new target, pursuit movement maintains fixation.

Eye movement occurs voluntarily in a conjugate (parallel) manner in any direction. Eye movements also occur reflexly to labyrinthine stimulation.

DISORDERS OF GAZE

Gaze disorders usually follow vascular episodes (infarct or haemorrhage) but may also occur in traumatic, inflammatory or neoplastic disease. In gaze palsy eye movements are symmetrically limited in one direction.

CONJUGATE DEVIATION OF THE EYES

Occurring during a seizure

Eyes deviate towards the affected limbs in a jerking fashion.

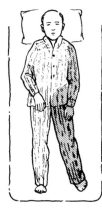

Indicates an epileptic focus in the frontal lobe contralateral to the direction of eye deviation.

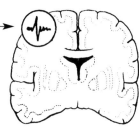

Accompanying a hemiparesis

Tonic deviation of the eyes *away* from the hemiparetic limb.

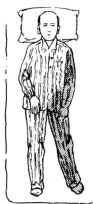

Indicates a lesion in the frontal lobe *ipsilateral* to the direction of eye deviation.

Haemorrhage deep in the cerebral hemisphere (thalamic) can cause deviation of eyes to the side of hemiparesis – *wrong-way eyes*

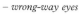
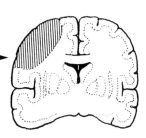

Tonic deviation of the eyes *towards* the hemiparetic limb.

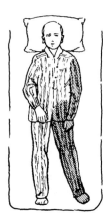

Usually indicates a lesion in the pons *contralateral* to the direction of eye deviation and results from damage to the paramedian pontine reticular formation (PPRF)

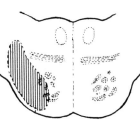

DISORDERS OF GAZE

VERTICAL GAZE PALSY

Midbrain or pontine lesions may produce failure of upward or downward gaze. Disturbed downward gaze alone occurs with periaqueductal (Sylvian aqueduct) lesions. Impaired vertical eye movement is common in extrapyramidal disease (Progressive supranuclear palsy, page 367).

PARINAUD'S SYNDROME

This syndrome is characterised by impaired upward eye movements in association with a dorsal midbrain lesion (✚).

Pineal gland
Superior colliculus
Inferior colliculus

Corpus callosum

III ventricle

– upward gaze and convergence are lost
– the pupils may dilate and the response to light and accommodation is impaired

Causes:

Third ventricular tumours   Multiple sclerosis
Pineal region tumours   Wernicke's encephalopathy
Hydrocephalus   Encephalitis

INTERNUCLEAR OPHTHALMOPLEGIA (ataxic nystagmus)

This disorder, caused by damage to the medial longitudinal bundle, is dealt with on page 184. It is an internuclear disorder of eye movement and produces a disconjugate gaze palsy.

Two unusual disconjugate gaze palsies are –

Webino syndrome (wall eyes – bilateral internuclear ophthalmoplegia): midbrain lesion characterised by bilateral exotropia and loss of convergence

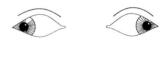

'Look right'

The 'One and a half' syndrome: Conjugate gaze palsy to one side and impaired adduction on looking to the other side. Lesion involves the PPRF or abducens nucleus and adjacent median longitudinal bundle on the side of the complete palsy.

'Look left'

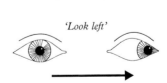

OCULAR APRAXIA

Bilateral prefrontal motor cortex damage will produce this unusual finding in which the patient does not move the eyes voluntarily to command, yet has a full range of random eye movement.

FACIAL PAIN AND SENSORY LOSS

The fifth cranial nerve subserves facial sensation and innervates the muscles of mastication.

Anatomy

The anatomical arrangement of the trigeminal central connections are complex.

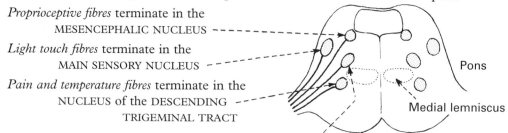

Proprioceptive fibres terminate in the
MESENCEPHALIC NUCLEUS

Light touch fibres terminate in the
MAIN SENSORY NUCLEUS

Pain and temperature fibres terminate in the
NUCLEUS of the DESCENDING
TRIGEMINAL TRACT

Pons

Medial lemniscus

Motor fibres arise from the TRIGEMINAL MOTOR NUCLEUS

The separate location of the main sensory nucleus and nucleus of the descending trigeminal tract account for
dissociated sensory loss,
i.e. a low pontine or medullary lesion will result in loss of pain and temperature sensation with pre-servation of light touch.

Longitudinal arrangement of the trigeminal nuclei (sensory paths)

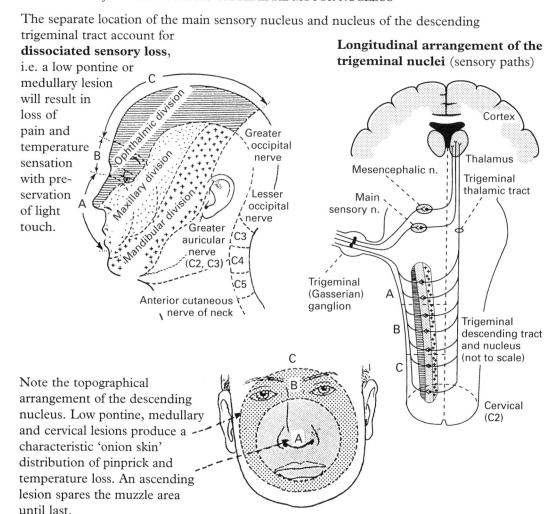

Note the topographical arrangement of the descending nucleus. Low pontine, medullary and cervical lesions produce a characteristic 'onion skin' distribution of pinprick and temperature loss. An ascending lesion spares the muzzle area until last.

FACIAL PAIN AND SENSORY LOSS

The peripheral course of the V nerve

The motor and sensory nerve roots emerge separately from the lateral aspect of the brain stem at the midpontine level. The Gasserian ganglion of the sensory root contains bipolar sensory nuclei and lies on the apex of the petrous bone in the middle fossa. Here the three divisions of the trigeminal nerve merge. Each passes through its own foramen and carries sensation from a specific area of the face.

The **ophthalmic** division passes through the superior orbital fissure, divides into branches within the orbit and emerges from the supraorbital foramen to innervate the forehead.

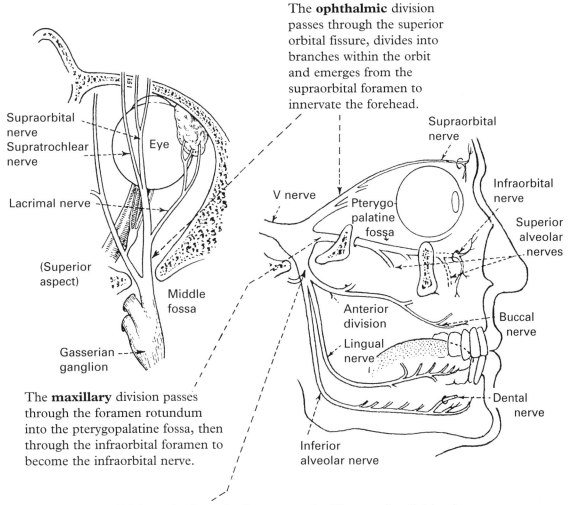

The **maxillary** division passes through the foramen rotundum into the pterygopalatine fossa, then through the infraorbital foramen to become the infraorbital nerve.

The **mandibular** division exits from the foramen ovale. The anterior division incorporates the motor branch of the V nerve, innervating the muscles of mastication – masseter, pterygoids and temporalis – as well as innervating the cheek and gums (buccal nerve).

The lingual branch of the posterior trunk innervates the anterior two-thirds of the tongue (and is joined by the chordi tympani from the facial nerve carrying salivary secretomotor fibres and taste from the anterior two-thirds of the tongue).

157

FACIAL PAIN AND SENSORY LOSS

EXAMINATION OF TRIGEMINAL NERVE FUNCTION

This should include examination of the corneal reflex and masticatory muscle function (page 14).

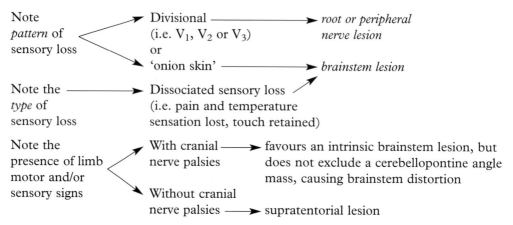

Note *pattern* of sensory loss → Divisional (i.e. V_1, V_2 or V_3) → *root or peripheral nerve lesion*

or

'onion skin' → *brainstem lesion*

Note the *type* of sensory loss → Dissociated sensory loss (i.e. pain and temperature sensation lost, touch retained)

Note the presence of limb motor and/or sensory signs → With cranial nerve palsies → favours an intrinsic brainstem lesion, but does not exclude a cerebellopontine angle mass, causing brainstem distortion

Without cranial nerve palsies → supratentorial lesion

CAUSES OF V NERVE LESIONS

Pons

When associated with other cranial nerve lesions and long tract signs:
– *vascular*
– *neoplastic*
– *demyelination*
– *syringobulbia* (especially dissociated sensory loss)

(Tentorium cerebelli omitted)

Other causes
– *diabetes*
– *SLE*

Orbital fissure
Orbit
Cavernous sinus

First division of V nerve ± III, IV and VI nerve palsies

(see III nerve lesions, page 151).

Petrous apex
associated VI nerve palsy
– *petrositis (Gradenigo's syndrome)*

Skull base
One or more V divisions involved:
– *nasopharyngeal or metastatic carcinoma*
– *trauma (e.g. infraorbital nerve – malar fracture)*

Cerebello-pontine angle
When associated with other cranial nerve lesions ± long tract signs:
– *acoustic neuroma*
– *trigeminal neuroma*
– *subacute (chronic) meningitis*

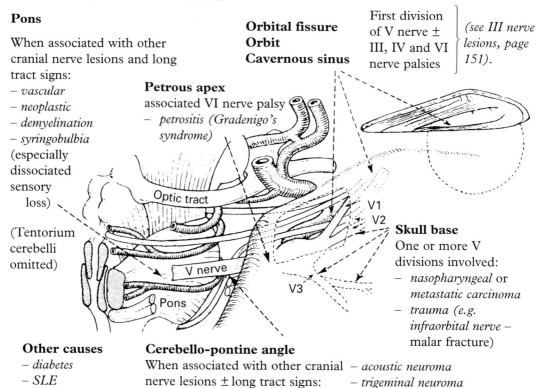

Optic tract

V nerve

Pons

V1

V2

V3

FACIAL PAIN AND SENSORY LOSS

Sensory trigeminal neuropathy:

Progressive, painless loss of trigeminal sensation. Normally unilateral and without trigeminal motor weakness, the sensory loss may affect one or all trigeminal divisions. This condition is often associated with established connective tissue disease (scleroderma, Sjögren's syndrome and mixed connective tissue disease (MCTD)). Diagnosis requires exclusion of intracranial granuloma and tumour compressing the trigeminal nerve – meningioma, schwannoma, epidermoid – by contrast enhanced MRI.

Mental neuropathy (numb chin syndrome):

Caused by a lesion of the mandibular nerve or inferior alveolar or mental branches, usually the result of metastatic compression of the nerve within the mandible. Bone scans or an enhanced CT/MRI combined with image-guided aspiration is diagnostic.

Infraorbital neuropathy (numb cheek syndrome) has similar etiology.

Gradenigo's syndrome:

Lesions located at the petrous-temporal bone apex (osteitis or meningitis associated with otitis media) irritate the ophthalmic division of the trigeminal and abducens (VI) nerve. Forehead pain is accompanied by ipsilateral lateral rectus palsy and a Horner's syndrome if sympathetic fibres are also involved. Tumours and trauma can also produce this syndrome.

Neuropathic keratitis

Corneal anaesthesia from a central or peripheral V nerve lesion may lead to a neuropathic keratitis. The corneal surface becomes hazy, ulcerated and infected and blindness may follow.

Patients with absent corneal sensation should wear a protective shield, attached to the side of spectacles, when out of doors.

FACIAL PAIN – DIAGNOSTIC APPROACH

Pain in the face may result from many different disorders and often presents as a diagnostic problem to the neurologist or neurosurgeon.

Consider:

1. Site of pain

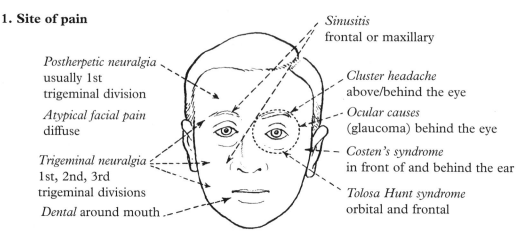

Sinusitis frontal or maxillary

Postherpetic neuralgia usually 1st trigeminal division

Atypical facial pain diffuse

Cluster headache above/behind the eye

Ocular causes (glaucoma) behind the eye

Trigeminal neuralgia 1st, 2nd, 3rd trigeminal divisions

Costen's syndrome in front of and behind the ear

Dental around mouth

Tolosa Hunt syndrome orbital and frontal

2. Quality of pain

Trigeminal neuralgia – sharp, stabbing, shooting, paroxysmal
Atypical facial pain – dull, persisting
Postherpetic neuralgia – dull, burning, persisting, occasional paroxysm
Dental – dull
Sinusitis – sharp, boring, worse in the morning
Ocular – dull, throbbing
Costen's syndrome – severe aching, aggravated by chewing
Cluster headache – sharp, intermittent

3. Associated symptoms/signs

Trigeminal neuralgia – often no neurological deficit, but occasional blunting of pinprick over involved region
Atypical facial pain – accompanying features of depressive illness
Postherpetic neuralgia – evidence of scarring associated with sensory loss
Dental – swelling of lips/face
Sinusitis – puffy appearance around eyes, tenderness to percussion over involved sinus
Ocular – glaucoma: associated visual symptoms – blurring/haloes/loss
Costen's syndrome – tenderness over temporomandibular joint
Cluster headache – associated lacrimation/rhinorrhoea

Investigations
– guided by clinical suspicion

Blood tests: ESR, FBC, biochemistry.
Imaging: CT/MRI, dental X-rays, isotope bone scan.

FACIAL PAIN – TRIGEMINAL NEURALGIA

TRIGEMINAL NEURALGIA (tic douloureux)

Trigeminal neuralgia is characterised by paroxysmal attacks of severe, short, sharp, stabbing pain affecting one or more divisions of the trigeminal nerve. The pain involves the second or third divisions more often than the first; it rarely occurs bilaterally and never simultaneously on each side, occasionally more than one division is involved. Paroxysmal attacks last for several days or weeks; they are often superimposed on a more constant ache. When the attacks settle, the patient may remain pain free for many months.

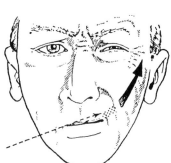

Chewing, speaking, washing the face, tooth-brushing, cold winds, or touching a specific 'trigger spot', e.g. upper lip or gum, may all precipitate an attack of pain.

Trigeminal neuralgia more commonly affects females and patients over 50 years of age.

Aetiology
Trigeminal pain may be symptomatic of disorders which affect the nerve root or its entry zone.

Root or root entry zone compression
– *arterial vessels* often abut and sometimes clearly indent the trigeminal nerve root at the entry-zone into the pons, causing ephaptic transmission (short circuiting).
– *tumours* of the cerebellopontine angle lying against the V nerve roots, e.g. meningioma, epidermoid cyst, frequently present with trigeminal pain.

Demyelination – such a lesion in the pons should be considered in a 'young' person with trigeminal neuralgia. Trigger spots are rare. Remission occurs infrequently and the response to drug treatment is poor.

In some patients the cause remains unexplained, as do the long periods of remission.

Investigation
CT or preferably MR scan to exclude a cerebello-pontine angle lesion or demyelination.

Management
Drug therapy
CARBAMAZEPINE proves effective in most patients (and helps confirm the diagnosis). Provided toxicity does not become troublesome, i.e. drowsiness, ataxia, the dosage is increased until pain relief occurs (600–1600 mg/day). When remission is established, drug treatment can be discontinued.

If pain control is limited, other drugs – BACLOFEN, LAMOTRIGINE, GABAPENTIN, PHENYTOIN – may benefit.

Persistence of pain on full drug dosage or an intolerance of the drugs, indicates the need for more radical measures.

FACIAL PAIN — TRIGEMINAL NEURALGIA

MANAGEMENT (*cont'd*)

Operative therapy

Peripheral nerve techniques: Nerve block with alcohol or phenol provides temporary relief (up to two years). *Avulsion* of the supra- or infraorbital nerves gives more prolonged pain relief.

A **radiosurgical lesion** of the trigeminal ganglion provides another alternative for high risk surgical patients.

Traumatising the trigeminal ganglion/roots within Meckel's cave by either **glycerol injection** or by Fogarty **balloon inflation** usually produces good pain relief with minimal sensory loss.

Trigeminal root section: Through either a subtemporal (extra- or intradural) or posterior fossa approach, the appropriate trigeminal root is identified and divided.

Microvascular decompression: Exploration of the cerebellopontine angle reveals blood vessels in contact with the trigeminal nerve root or root entry zone in the majority of patients. Separation of these structures and insertion of a non absorbable sponge produces pain relief in most patients, without the associated problems of nerve destruction.

Radiofrequency thermocoagulation: The site of facial 'tingling' produced by electrical stimulation of a needle inserted into the trigeminal ganglion, accurately identifies the location of the needle tip. When the site of tingling corresponds to the trigger spot or site of pain origin, radiofrequency thermocoagulation under general anaesthetic, produces a permanent lesion – usually resulting in analgesia of the appropriate area with retention of light touch.

Results and complications

Pain relief – accurate comparison of the wide variety of techniques used for trigeminal neuralgia is difficult; all but peripheral nerve avulsion appear to produce similar results. Approximately 80–85% of patients remain pain free for a 5-year period, although some may relapse in the long term, particularly after balloon compression or glycerol injection. Results of peripheral nerve avulsion are less satisfactory with pain recurring in 50% within 2 years.

Dysaesthesia/Anaesthesia dolorosa – this troublesome sensory disturbance follows any destructive technique to nerve or root in 5–30% of patients. Microvascular decompression avoids this problem and the risk of a severe deficit is low with glycerol injection.

Corneal anaesthesia – this occurs when root section or thermocoagulation involves the first division and keratitis may result.

Mortality – microvascular decompression and open root section carry a very low mortality (< 1%), but this must not be ignored when comparing results with safer methods.

Treatment selection: This largely depends on the surgeon's personal preference and experience.

In most centres, the absence of sensory complications make microvascular decompression the procedure of first choice, particularly for 1st division pain and for the younger patient.

Frail and elderly patients may tolerate glycerol injection, balloon compression and thermocoagulation more easily than other procedures.

FACIAL PAIN – OTHER CAUSES

Temporomandibular joint dysfunction (Costen's syndrome)

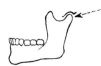

Aching pain occurring around the ear, aggravated by chewing; due to malalignment of one temporomandibular joint as a consequence of dental loss with altered 'bite' or involvement of the joint in rheumatoid arthritis. This condition requires dental treatment with realignment.

Raeder's syndrome (the paratrigeminal syndrome)

Pain and sensory loss in 1st and 2nd trigeminal divisions, maximal around the eye and associated with a sympathetic paresis (ptosis and small pupil). Sweating in the lower face is preserved. This may be associated with involvement of the other cranial nerves (IV & VI). The syndrome occurs with lesions of the middle fossa, e.g. nasopharyngeal carcinoma, granulomas and infection.

Tolosa Hunt syndrome

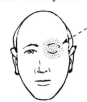

A condition in which an inflammatory process involving the cavernous sinus or superior orbital fissure presents with pain, loss of ocular movement and ophthalmic division sensory loss. The diagnosis is based on exclusion of tumour and response to steroids. Pathological examination confirms non-specific granulomatous change.

Atypical facial pain

The patient, often a young or middle-aged woman, experiences a dull, persistent pain, spreading diffusely over one or both sides of the face. These symptoms often result from an underlying depression and may respond well to antidepressant therapy.

Herpes zoster

Frequently affects the trigeminal territory, especially the ophthalmic division producing a painful 'herpetic rash' and often involving the cornea. The acute symptoms may resolve but lead to a chronic postherpetic neuralgia which slowly improves. Surgical procedures such as trigeminal root section do not help. The incidence of postherpetic neuralgia is not influenced by treatment with antiviral agents (acyclovir) in the acute phase.

Carotidynia

A form of migraine characterised by intermittent facial pain associated with vasomotor rhinitis and tenderness of the carotid artery. It may be precipitated by alcohol.

Carotid artery dissection

This presents as acute retro-orbital pain with a Horner's syndrome (page 143).

'Cluster' headaches – see page 70.

FACIAL WEAKNESS

Related anatomy

The facial (VII) nerve contains mainly motor fibres supplying the muscles of facial expression, but also visceral efferent (parasympathetic) and visceral afferent (taste) fibres.

The motor nucleus lies in the lower pons medial to the descending nucleus and tract of the Vth cranial nerve. Axons from the motor nucleus wind around the nucleus of the VIth cranial nerve. The facial nerve and its visceral root (*nervus intermedius*) exit from the lateral aspect of the brain stem and cross the cerebellopontine angle immediately adjacent to the VIII cranial nerve. They enter the internal auditory meatus and, passing through the facial canal of the temporal bone, lie in close proximity to the inner ear and tympanic membrane. The facial nerve gives off several branches before exiting from the skull through the stylomastoid foramen.

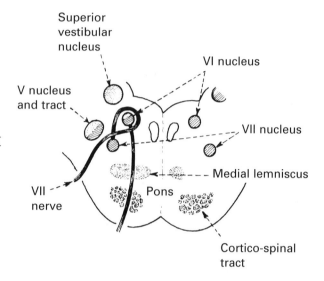

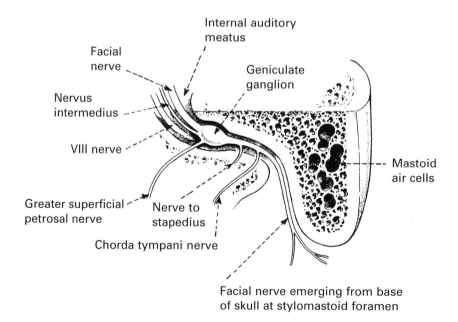

FACIAL WEAKNESS

Visceral efferent and visceral afferent fibres arise and terminate in the superior salivary nucleus and nucleus/tractus solitarius respectively.

They run together as the nervus intermedius and accompany the facial nerve to the internal auditory meatus. The parasympathetic fibres (visceral efferent) pass in the greater petrosal nerve to the sphenopalatine ganglion and thence to the lacrimal gland to produce tears and in the chorda tympani nerve to the submandibular ganglion.

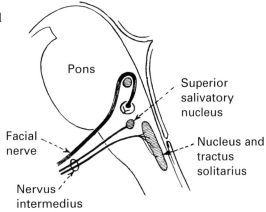

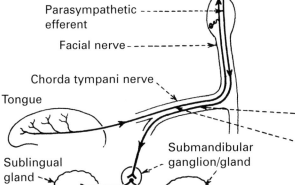

The chorda tympani nerve contains both parasympathetic efferent and visceral afferent fibres. Parasympathetic fibres are responsible for salivation. Visceral afferent fibres convey sensations of taste from the anterior two-thirds of the tongue. The geniculate ganglion contains the bipolar cell bodies of these afferent fibres.

Supranuclear control of facial muscles

The muscles in the lower face are controlled by the contralateral hemisphere, whereas those in the upper face receive control from both hemispheres (bilateral representation). Hence a lower motor neuron lesion paralyses all facial muscles on that side, but an upper motor neuron (supranuclear) lesion paralyses only the muscles in the lower half of the face on the opposite side.

Clinical examination of the facial nerve (see page 15)

In addition to examining for facial weakness and taste impairment, also note whether the patient comments on reduced lacrimation or salivation on one side, or hyperacusis (exaggeration of sounds due to loss of the stapedius reflex).

FACIAL WEAKNESS

LESION, LOCALISATION AND CAUSE

Note the *distribution:*

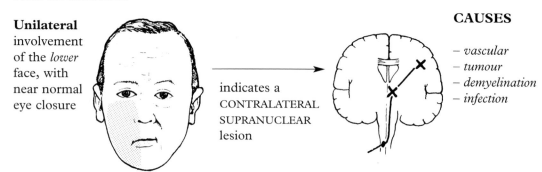

Unilateral involvement of the *lower* face, with near normal eye closure

indicates a CONTRALATERAL SUPRANUCLEAR lesion

CAUSES

– *vascular*
– *tumour*
– *demyelination*
– *infection*

(Spontaneous emotional expression may be unaffected with subcortical lesions)

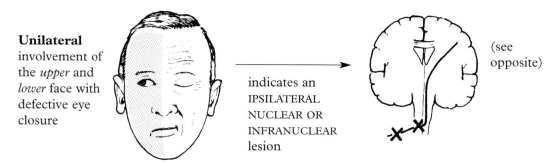

Unilateral involvement of the *upper* and *lower* face with defective eye closure

indicates an IPSILATERAL NUCLEAR OR INFRANUCLEAR lesion

(see opposite)

(Spontaneous emotional expression affected).

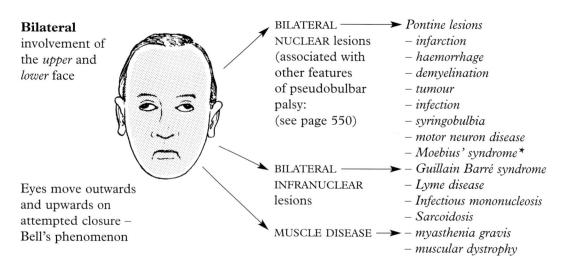

Bilateral involvement of the *upper* and *lower* face

Eyes move outwards and upwards on attempted closure – Bell's phenomenon

BILATERAL NUCLEAR lesions (associated with other features of pseudobulbar palsy: (see page 550)

Pontine lesions
– *infarction*
– *haemorrhage*
– *demyelination*
– *tumour*
– *infection*
– *syringobulbia*
– *motor neuron disease*
– *Moebius' syndrome* ★

BILATERAL INFRANUCLEAR lesions

– *Guillain Barré syndrome*
– *Lyme disease*
– *Infectious mononucleosis*
– *Sarcoidosis*

MUSCLE DISEASE → – *myasthenia gravis*
– *muscular dystrophy*

★ Moebius' syndrome: a congenital failure of the development of the facial and abducens nuclei (bilateral).

FACIAL WEAKNESS

NUCLEAR/INFRANUCLEAR LESIONS

The following features (if present) help in lesion location:

- VI nerve palsy → **Pons**
- contralateral limb weakness
  - *vascular*
  - *demyelination*
  - *tumour*
  - *encephalitis*
  - *syringobulbia*
  - *motor neuron disease*

- V, VIII, (IX, X, XI) nerve palsies
- loss of taste, salivation, and lacrimation
- hyperacusis

→ **Cerebellopontine angle or internal auditory meatus**
  - *acoustic tumours*
  - *meningioma*
  - *epidermoid*
  - *glomus jugulare tumour*

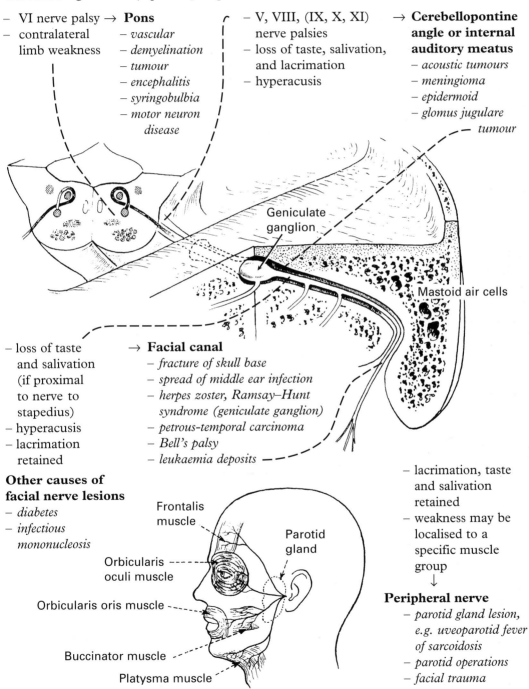

Geniculate ganglion

Mastoid air cells

- loss of taste and salivation (if proximal to nerve to stapedius)
- hyperacusis
- lacrimation retained

→ **Facial canal**
  - *fracture of skull base*
  - *spread of middle ear infection*
  - *herpes zoster, Ramsay–Hunt syndrome (geniculate ganglion)*
  - *petrous-temporal carcinoma*
  - *Bell's palsy*
  - *leukaemia deposits*

Other causes of facial nerve lesions
- *diabetes*
- *infectious mononucleosis*

Frontalis muscle

Parotid gland

Orbicularis oculi muscle

Orbicularis oris muscle

Buccinator muscle

Platysma muscle

- lacrimation, taste and salivation retained
- weakness may be localised to a specific muscle group
  ↓

Peripheral nerve
  - *parotid gland lesion, e.g. uveoparotid fever of sarcoidosis*
  - *parotid operations*
  - *facial trauma*

167

BELL'S PALSY

Bell's palsy is characterised by an acute paralysis of the face related to 'inflammation' and swelling of the facial nerve within the facial canal or at the stylomastoid foramen. It is usually unilateral, rarely bilateral, and may occur repetitively. In some, a family history of the condition is evident.

Aetiology

Uncertain, but may be associated with viral infections, e.g. herpes simplex and varicella-zoster; epidemics of Bell's palsy occur sporadically. Bell's palsy may be part of the syndrome of polyneuritis cranialis.

Symptoms

Pain of variable intensity over the ipsilateral mastoid precedes weakness, which develops over a 48-hour period.

Impairment of taste, hyperacusis and salivation depend on the extent of inflammation and will be lost in more severe cases. Lacrimation is seldom affected.

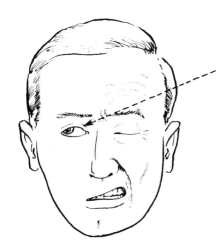

On attempting to close the eyes and show the teeth, the one eye does not close and the eyeball rotates upwards and outwards – Bell's phenomenon (normal eyeball movement on eye closure).

Diagnosis

Based on typical presentation and exclusion of middle ear disease, diabetes, sarcoidosis and Lyme disease.

Treatment

During the acute stage protect the exposed eye during sleep.

Prednisolone given in high dosage in the acute stage (40–60 mg per day for 5 days) may reduce inflammation, but there is no conclusive evidence of benefit. Antiviral therapy – similarly. Eye care (shielding) is important in preventing corneal abrasion.

Prognosis

Most patients (80%) recover in 4–8 weeks without treatment. In the remainder, residual facial asymmetry may require corrective surgery. Incomplete paralysis indicates a good prognosis. In patients with complete paralysis, electrical absence of denervation on electromyography is an optimistic sign.

Occasionally aberrant reinnervation occurs – movement of the angle of the mouth on closing the eyes (jaw winking) or lacrimation when facial muscles contract (crocodile tears).

OTHER FACIAL NERVE DISORDERS

RAMSAY HUNT SYNDROME

Herpes zoster infection of the geniculate (facial) ganglion causes sudden severe facial weakness with a typical zoster vesicular eruption within the external auditory meatus. Pain is a major feature and may precede the facial weakness. Serosanguinous fluid may discharge from the ear.

Deafness may result from VIII involvement. Occasionally, other cranial nerves from V–XII are affected.

Treatment

Antiviral agents (acyclovir) may help.

HEMIFACIAL SPASM

This condition is characterised by unilateral clonic spasms beginning in the orbicularis oculi and spreading to involve other facial muscles. The stapedius muscle can be affected producing a subjective ipsilateral clicking sound.

Contractions are irregular, intermittent and worsened by emotional stress and fatigue. Onset usually occurs in middle to old age and women are preferentially affected.

The aetiology remains unknown but 'irritation' from an adjacent blood vessel (or from a tumour) may cause demyelination and 'short-circuiting' within the nerve. Occasionally hemifacial spasm follows a Bell's palsy or traumatic facial injury.

The clinician must distinguish hemifacial spasm from milder habit spasms or tics which tend to be familial, and also from 'focal' seizures selectively affecting the face.

Investigations

CT/MR scan of the posterior fossa excludes the presence of a cerebellar pontine angle lesion and may show an ectatic basilar artery.

Treatment

Drugs – Anxiolytics and carbamazepine may produce some benefit but are of no lasting value. When spasm is confined to orbicularis oculi, local infiltration with botulinum toxin is helpful.

Surgery – Posterior fossa exploration and microvascular decompression i.e. dissecting blood vessels off the facial nerve root entry zone, gives excellent results (cure rate 80%), but carries the risk of producing deafness and rarely brainstem damage. Alternative, less successful treatments include phenol injection or partial section of the facial nerve; these methods inevitably cause some facial weakness.

TONIC FACIAL SPASM

Less common than hemifacial spasm. Occurs with cerebellar pontine angle lesions. It produces tonic elevation of the corner of the mouth with narrowing of the eye. The diagnosis is confirmed by CT/MR scanning and treatment is surgical.

FACIAL MYOKYMIA

A rare condition seen most often in multiple sclerosis. Flickering of facial muscles results from spontaneous discharge in the facial motor nucleus. Other brainstem signs are present. The facial movements respond to carbamazepine.

MYOCLONUS

Rhythmic facial movement associated with similar palatal movements and characteristic of dentate or olivary nucleus disease.

BLEPHAROSPASM

Spasmodic closing or screwing up of eyes (see page 367).

DEAFNESS, TINNITUS AND VERTIGO

Deafness, tinnitus and vertigo result from disorders affecting the auditory and vestibular apparatus or their central connections transmitted through the VIII cranial nerve.

MECHANISMS OF AUDITORY AND VESTIBULAR FUNCTION

Auditory function: the cochlea converts sound waves into action potentials in cochlear neurons. Sound waves are transmitted by the tympanic membrane and the ossicles to the oval window, setting up waves in the perilymph of the cochlea. The action of the waves on the spiral organ (of Corti) generates action potentials in the cochlear division of the VIII cranial nerve.

Vestibular function: the vestibular system responds to rotational and linear acceleration (including gravity) and along with a visual and proprioceptive input maintains equilibrium and body orientation in space. Relative inertia of the endolymph within the semicircular canals during angular acceleration displaces hair cells imbedded in the cupula, activates the hair cells and transmits action potentials to the vestibular division of the VIII cranial nerve. Linear acceleration results in displacement of the otoliths within the utricle or saccule. This distorts the hair cells and increases or decreases the frequency of action potentials in the vestibular division of the VIII cranial nerve.

CENTRAL CONNECTIONS

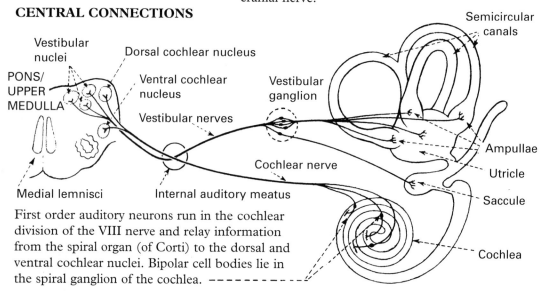

First order auditory neurons run in the cochlear division of the VIII nerve and relay information from the spiral organ (of Corti) to the dorsal and ventral cochlear nuclei. Bipolar cell bodies lie in the spiral ganglion of the cochlea.

First order vestibular neurons lie in the vestibular division of the VIII nerve and relay information from the utricle, saccule and semicircular canals to the vestibular nuclei (superior, inferior, medial and lateral). Bipolar cell bodies lie in the vestibular ganglion.

The cochlear (acoustic) and vestibular divisions travel together through the petrous bone to the internal auditory meatus where they emerge to pass through the subarachnoid space in the cerebellopontine angle, each entering the brain stem separately at the pontomedullary junction.

DEAFNESS, TINNITUS AND VERTIGO

CENTRAL CONNECTIONS (*cont'd*)

Auditory: From the cochlear nucleus, second order neurons either pass upwards in the lateral lemniscus to the ipsilateral inferior colliculus or decussate in the trapezoid body and pass up in the lateral lemniscus to the contralateral inferior colliculus.
Third order neurons from the inferior colliculus on each side run to the medial geniculate body on both sides.
Fourth order neurons pass through the internal capsule and auditory radiation to the auditory cortex.
The bilateral nature of the connections ensures that a unilateral central lesion will not result in lateralised hearing loss.

Vestibular

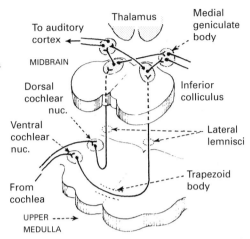

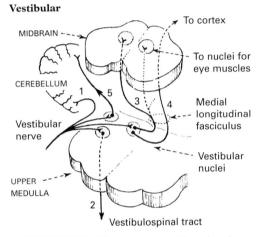

1. Directly to cerebellum.
2. Second order neurons arise in the vestibular nucleus and descend in the ipsilateral vestibulospinal tract.
3. Second order neurons project to the oculomotor nuclei (III, IV, VI) through the medial longitudinal fasciculus.
4. Second order neurons project to the cortex (temporal lobe). The pathway is unclear.
5. Second order neurons project to the cerebellum.

(There is a bilateral feedback loop to the vestibular nuclei from the cerebellum though the fastigial nucleus.)

DEAFNESS: Three types of hearing loss are recognised:

1. *Conductive deafness:* failure of sound conduction to the cochlea.
2. *Sensorineural deafness:* failure of action potential production or transmission due to disease of the cochlea, cochlear nerve or cochlear central connections.
   Further subdivision into cochlear and retrocochlear deafness helps establish the causative lesion.
3. *Pure word or cortical deafness:* a bilateral or dominant posterior temporal lobe (auditory cortex) lesion produces a failure to understand spoken language despite preserved hearing.

TINNITUS: a sensation of noise of ringing, buzzing, pulsing, hissing or singing quality. Tinnitus may be (i) continuous or intermittent, (ii) unilateral or bilateral, (iii) high or low pitch.
As a rule, when hearing loss is accompanied by tinnitus, conductive deafness is associated with low pitch tinnitus – sensorineural deafness is associated with high pitch tinnitus, except Menière's disease where tinnitus is low pitch. Pulsing tinnitus has a vascular cause.

VERTIGO: an illusion of rotatory movement due to disturbed orientation of the body in space. The sufferer may sense that the environment is moving. Vertigo may result from disease of the labyrinth, vestibular nerve or their central connections.

171

DEAFNESS, TINNITUS AND VERTIGO

Clinical examination

Examination of the external auditory meatus, tympanic membrane and eye movements (for nystagmus) and Weber's and Rinne's tests (page 16) provide valuable information, but more detailed neuro-otological tests (pages 61, 62) are usually required to determine the exact nature of the auditory or vestibular dysfunction and to locate the lesion site. The results of these tests may indicate the need for further investigation (e.g. CT/MR scan).

Causes of deafness

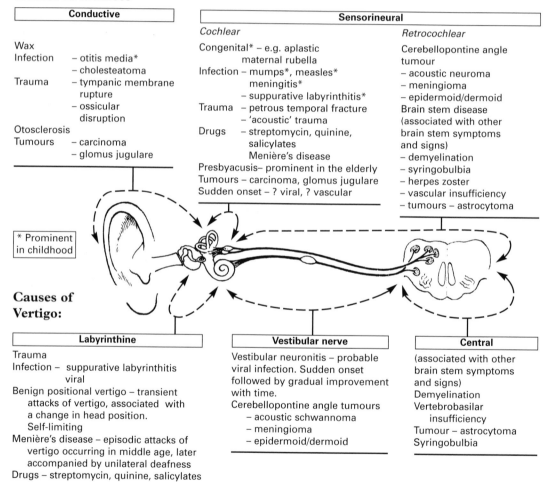

Conductive

Wax
Infection   – otitis media*
           – cholesteatoma
Trauma   – tympanic membrane
            rupture
           – ossicular
            disruption
Otosclerosis
Tumours   – carcinoma
           – glomus jugulare

Sensorineural	
Cochlear	Retrocochlear

Cochlear:
Congenital* – e.g. aplastic
      maternal rubella
Infection – mumps*, measles*
           meningitis*
          – suppurative labyrinthitis*
Trauma   – petrous temporal fracture
          – 'acoustic' trauma
Drugs   – streptomycin, quinine,
          salicylates
          Menière's disease
Presbyacusis– prominent in the elderly
Tumours – carcinoma, glomus jugulare
Sudden onset – ? viral, ? vascular

Retrocochlear:
Cerebellopontine angle tumour
   – acoustic neuroma
   – meningioma
   – epidermoid/dermoid
Brain stem disease
(associated with other brain stem symptoms and signs)
   – demyelination
   – syringobulbia
   – herpes zoster
   – vascular insufficiency
   – tumours – astrocytoma

* Prominent in childhood

Causes of Vertigo:

Labyrinthine

Trauma
Infection – suppurative labyrinthitis
          viral
Benign positional vertigo – transient
   attacks of vertigo, associated with
   a change in head position.
   Self-limiting
Menière's disease – episodic attacks of
   vertigo occurring in middle age, later
   accompanied by unilateral deafness
Drugs – streptomycin, quinine, salicylates

Vestibular nerve

Vestibular neuronitis – probable
viral infection. Sudden onset
followed by gradual improvement
with time.
Cerebellopontine angle tumours
   – acoustic schwannoma
   – meningioma
   – epidermoid/dermoid

Central

(associated with other
brain stem symptoms
and signs)
Demyelination
Vertebrobasilar
   insufficiency
Tumour – astrocytoma
Syringobulbia

Causes of tinnitus

Any lesion causing deafness may also cause tinnitus. Occasionally patients perceive a vibratory noise inside the head, transmitted from an arteriovenous malformation or carotid stenosis.

In addition, patients with non-specific disease, e.g. anaemia, fever, hypertension, occasionally complain of tinnitus.

DISORDERS OF THE LOWER CRANIAL NERVES

NINTH (GLOSSOPHARYNGEAL) CRANIAL NERVE

This is a mixed nerve with motor, sensory and parasympathetic functions.

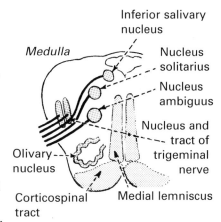

1. Motor fibres to stylopharyngeus muscle arise in the nucleus ambiguus.
2. Preganglionic parasympathetic fibres arise in the inferior salivatory nucleus and pass to the otic ganglion. From there postganglionic fibres innervate the parotid gland.
3. General somatic sensory fibres innervate the area of skin behind the ear, pass to the superior ganglion and end in the nucleus and tract of the trigeminal nerve.
4. Sensory fibres innervate the posterior third of the tongue (taste), pharynx, eustachian tube and carotid body/sinus and terminate centrally in the nucleus solitarius. The cell bodies lie in the inferior ganglion.

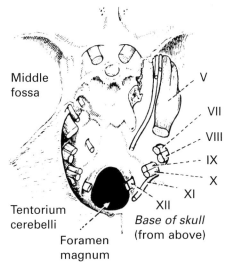

The IX nerve emerges as 5 or 6 rootlets from the medulla, dorsal to the olivary nucleus and passes with the vagus and accessory nerves through the jugular foramen in the neck.

Within the neck the nerve lies in close proximity to the internal carotid artery and internal jugular vein.

The superior and inferior ganglia lie in the jugular foramen, the otic ganglion in the neck below the foramen ovale.

Clinical examination (see page 17)

Disorders of the glossopharyngeal nerve

Glossopharyngeal palsy from either medullary or nerve root lesions does not occur in isolation. When associated with X and XI cranial nerve lesions, this constitutes the *jugular foramen syndrome*. Lesions producing this syndrome are listed on page 177.

GLOSSOPHARYNGEAL NEURALGIA

Short, sharp, lancinating attacks of pain, identical to trigeminal neuralgia in nature but affecting the posterior part of the pharynx or tonsillar area. The pain often radiates towards the ear and is triggered by swallowing. Reflex bradycardia and syncope occur due to stimulation of vagal nuclei by discharges from glossopharyngeal. As with trigeminal neuralgia, carbamazepine often provides effective relief – if not microvascular decompression or section of the IX nerve roots or nerve give good results.

DISORDERS OF THE LOWER CRANIAL NERVES

TENTH (VAGUS) CRANIAL NERVE

This is a mixed nerve with motor, sensory and parasympathetic functions.

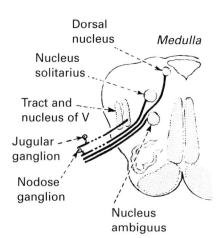

The central connections are complex though similar to those of the glossopharyngeal nerve.

1. Motor fibres supplying the pharynx, soft palate and larynx arise in the nucleus ambiguus.
2. Preganglionic parasympathetic fibres arise in the dorsal motor nucleus. Postganglionic fibres supply the thoracic and abdominal viscera.
3. Afferent fibres from the pharynx, larynx and external auditory meatus have cell bodies in the jugular ganglion and end in the nucleus and tract of the trigeminal nerve.
4. Afferent fibres from abdominal and thoracic viscera have cell bodies in the nodose ganglion and end in the nucleus solitarius. Taste perception in the pharynx ends similarly.

The nerve emerges from the brain stem as a series of converging rootlets. It exits from the cranial cavity by the jugular foramen where both ganglia lie.

Extracranial branches:

Motor and sensory supply to the pharynx

Superior laryngeal branch to the laryngeal muscles

Recurrent laryngeal branch

Supply to thoracic and abdominal viscera

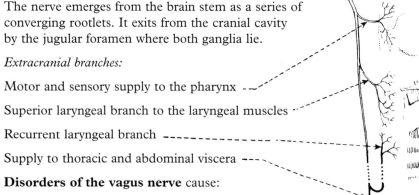

Disorders of the vagus nerve cause:

Palatal weakness
Unilateral – minimal symptoms.
Bilateral – nasal regurgitation of fluid, nasal quality of speech.
Pharyngeal weakness
Pharyngeal muscles are represented by the middle part of the nucleus ambiguus.
Unilateral – pharyngeal wall droops on the affected side.
Bilateral – marked dysphagia.
Laryngeal weakness
Motor fibres arise in the lowest part of the nucleus ambiguus.
Fibres to *tensors of the vocal cords* pass in *superior laryngeal nerves.*
Fibres to *adductors and abductors of the vocal cords* are supplied by the *recurrent laryngeal nerves.*

DISORDERS OF THE LOWER CRANIAL NERVES

Clinical examination (see page 17)

Direct examination of the vocal cords helps identification of the lesion site.

At rest

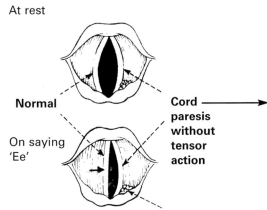

Normal

On saying 'Ee'

Cord paresis without tensor action ⟶ *Vagus nerve lesion above the origin of the superior and recurrent laryngeal nerves.*

Unilateral damage produces mild dysphagia, hoarseness and reduced vocal strength.

Bilateral damage at this level causes bilateral cord paresis. The cough is weak. Pharyngeal and palatal involvement cause marked dysphagia and nasal regurgitation. Breathlessness and stridor do not occur.

Mucus pools on affected side

At rest

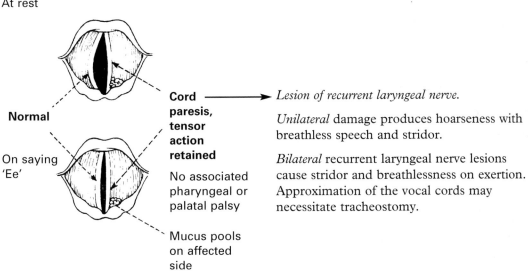

Normal

On saying 'Ee'

Cord paresis, tensor action retained ⟶ *Lesion of recurrent laryngeal nerve.*

Unilateral damage produces hoarseness with breathless speech and stridor.

No associated pharyngeal or palatal palsy

Bilateral recurrent laryngeal nerve lesions cause stridor and breathlessness on exertion. Approximation of the vocal cords may necessitate tracheostomy.

Mucus pools on affected side

Causes (see page 177)

175

DISORDERS OF THE LOWER CRANIAL NERVES

ELEVENTH (ACCESSORY) CRANIAL NERVE

This is a purely motor nerve supplying the sternomastoid and trapezius muscles.

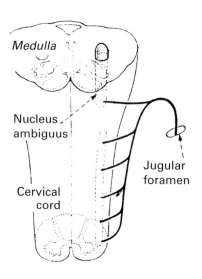

The cranial portion of the accessory nerve arises from the lowest part of the nucleus ambiguus in the medulla. The spinal part arises in the ventral grey matter of the upper five cervical segments, ascends alongside the spinal cord and passes through the foramen magnum. After joining with the cranial portion it exits as the accessory nerve through the jugular foramen.

The *supranuclear connections* act on the ipsilateral sternomastoid (turning the head to the contralateral side) and on the contralateral trapezius. This results in:
– head turning away from the relevant hemisphere during the seizure
– head turning towards the relevant hemisphere with cerebral infarction.

Unilateral lower motor neuron weakness produces a lower shoulder on the affected side (trapezius) and weakness in turning the head to the opposite side (sternomastoid).

Clinical examination (see page 17) *Causes* (see page 177)

TWELFTH (HYPOGLOSSAL) CRANIAL NERVE

This is a purely motor nerve which supplies the intrinsic muscles of the tongue.

The nucleus lies in the floor of the IV ventricle and fibres pass ventrally to leave the brain stem lateral to the pyramidal tract.

Since each nucleus is bilaterally innervated, a unilateral supranuclear lesion will not produce signs or symptoms. A bilateral supranuclear lesion results in a thin pointed (spastic) tongue which cannot be protruded.

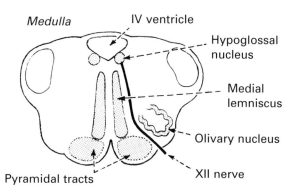

A lesion of the hypoglossal nerve results in atrophy and deviation of the tongue to the weak side

Clinical examination (see page 18) *Causes* (see page 177)

CAUSES OF LOWER CRANIAL NERVE PALSIES

Lower cranial nerve palsies seldom occur in isolation. Investigations include CT or MR imaging of the skull base. If negative, specific tests for systemic causes and EMG (for nerve and muscle disease) may be required.

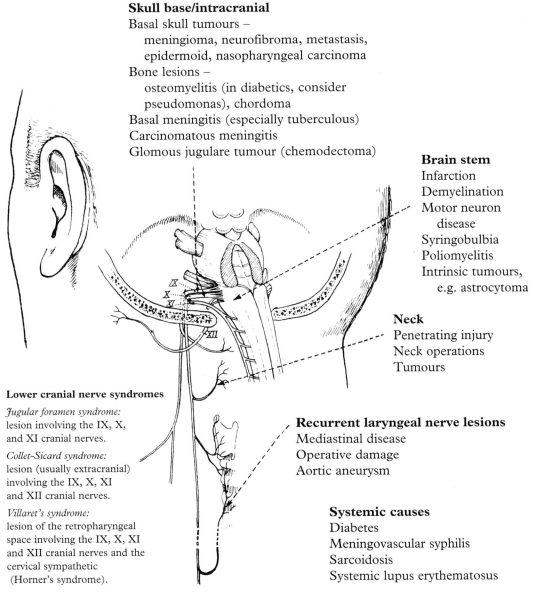

Skull base/intracranial

Basal skull tumours –
  meningioma, neurofibroma, metastasis,
  epidermoid, nasopharyngeal carcinoma
Bone lesions –
  osteomyelitis (in diabetics, consider
  pseudomonas), chordoma
Basal meningitis (especially tuberculous)
Carcinomatous meningitis
Glomous jugulare tumour (chemodectoma)

Brain stem

Infarction
Demyelination
Motor neuron
  disease
Syringobulbia
Poliomyelitis
Intrinsic tumours,
  e.g. astrocytoma

Neck

Penetrating injury
Neck operations
Tumours

Lower cranial nerve syndromes

Jugular foramen syndrome:
lesion involving the IX, X,
and XI cranial nerves.

Collet-Sicard syndrome:
lesion (usually extracranial)
involving the IX, X, XI
and XII cranial nerves.

Villaret's syndrome:
lesion of the retropharyngeal
space involving the IX, X, XI
and XII cranial nerves and the
cervical sympathetic
  (Horner's syndrome).

Recurrent laryngeal nerve lesions

Mediastinal disease
Operative damage
Aortic aneurysm

Systemic causes

Diabetes
Meningovascular syphilis
Sarcoidosis
Systemic lupus erythematosus

Polyneuritis cranialis

Multiple cranial nerve palsies of unknown aetiology which spontaneously remit. The diagnosis is dependent upon exclusion of other possible causes. Occasionally it occurs in association with or as a variant of postinfectious polyneuropathy.

Myasthenia gravis may present with a weakness of the bulbar musculature (see page 479).

CEREBELLAR DYSFUNCTION

Anatomy

The cerebellum lies in the posterior fossa, posterior to the brain stem, separated from the cerebrum above by the tentorium cerebelli.

The cerebellum consists of two laterally placed hemispheres and the midline structure – the vermis.

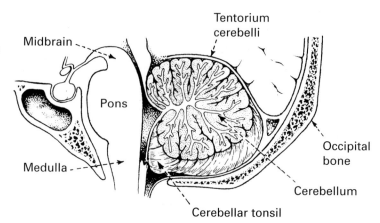

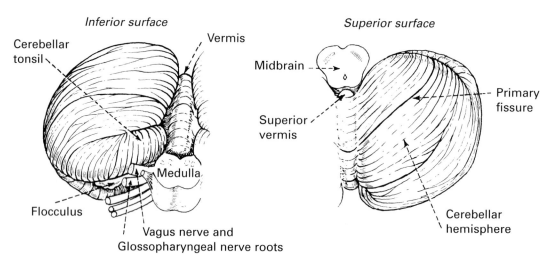

Three major phylogenetic subdivisions of the cerebellum are recognised.

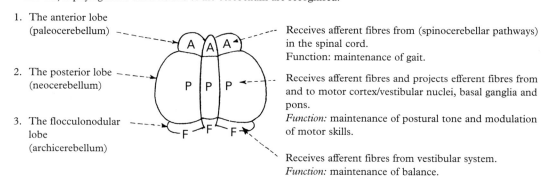

1. The anterior lobe (paleocerebellum)

Receives afferent fibres from (spinocerebellar pathways) in the spinal cord.
Function: maintenance of gait.

2. The posterior lobe (neocerebellum)

Receives afferent fibres and projects efferent fibres from and to motor cortex/vestibular nuclei, basal ganglia and pons.
Function: maintenance of postural tone and modulation of motor skills.

3. The flocculonodular lobe (archicerebellum)

Receives afferent fibres from vestibular system.
Function: maintenance of balance.

CEREBELLAR DYSFUNCTION

The cerebellar cortex is made up of three cell layers. The middle or Purkinje layer contains Purkinje cells. These are the only neurons capable of transmitting efferent impulses. Deep within the cerebellar hemispheres in the roof of the 4th ventricle, lie four paired nuclei separated by white matter from the cortex.

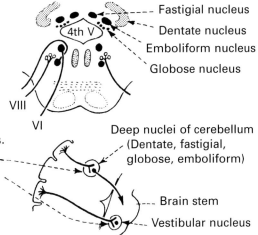

The efferent system

The Purkinje cells give rise to all efferent axons. These pass either to the deep nuclei of the cerebellum and thence to the brain stem, or to the vestibular nuclei of the brain stem. From there fibres relay back to the cerebral cortex and thalamus, or project into the spinal cord, influencing motor control.

The afferent system

Connections between the vestibular system and the cerebellum are described on page 171.

The spinocerebellar pathways form a major afferent input. These transmit 'subconscious' proprioception from muscles, joints and skin – especially of the lower limbs.

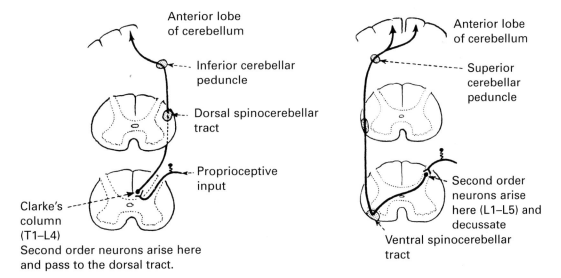

THE DORSAL SPINOCEREBELLAR TRACT

Anterior lobe of cerebellum

Inferior cerebellar peduncle

Dorsal spinocerebellar tract

Proprioceptive input

Clarke's column (T1–L4)
Second order neurons arise here and pass to the dorsal tract.

THE VENTRAL SPINOCEREBELLAR TRACT

Anterior lobe of cerebellum

Superior cerebellar peduncle

Second order neurons arise here (L1–L5) and decussate

Ventral spinocerebellar tract

The cerebellar peduncles: Three peduncles connect the cerebellum to the brain stem:
Superior peduncle – afferent and efferent fibres.
Middle peduncle – afferent fibres only.
Inferior peduncle – afferent and efferent fibres.

SYMPTOMS AND SIGNS OF CEREBELLAR DYSFUNCTION

The close relationship of structures within the posterior fossa makes the identification of exclusively cerebellar symptoms and signs difficult. Disease of the brain stem and its connections may produce identical results.

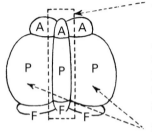

Damage to midline structures
– vermis (and flocculonodular lobe)

Results in: disturbance of equilibrium with unsteadiness on standing, walking and even sitting (truncal ataxia). The patient's gait is broad based and reeling. Eye closure does not affect balance (see Romberg's test). Tests of vestibular function, e.g. calorics, may be impaired.

Damage to hemisphere structures
– always produces signs *ipsilateral to the side of the lesion.*

Results in: a loss of the normal capacity to modulate fine voluntary movements. Errors or inaccuracies cannot be corrected. The patient complains of impaired limb co-ordination and certain signs are recognised:

Ataxia of extremities with unsteadiness of gait towards the side of the lesion.

Dysmetria: a breakdown of movement with the patient 'overshooting' the target when performing a specific motor task, e.g. finger-to-nose test.

Dysdiadochokinesia: a failure to perform a rapid alternating movement.

Intention tremor: a tremor which increases as the limb approaches its target.

Rebound phenomenon: the outstretched arm swings excessively when displaced.

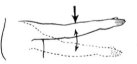

'Pendular' reflexes: the leg swings backwards and forwards when the knee jerk is elicited.

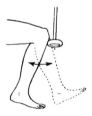

Eye movements
Nystagmus results from disease affecting cerebellar connections to the vestibular nuclei.

In unilateral disease, amplitude and rate increase when looking towards the diseased side.

Other ocular signs may occur, e.g. ocular dysmetria – an 'overshoot' when the eyes voluntarily fixate.

SYMPTOMS AND SIGNS OF CEREBELLAR DYSFUNCTION

Disturbance of speech
Scanning dysarthria may occur with speech occasionally delivered with sudden unexpected force – *explosive speech*. Whether dysarthria results from hemisphere or midline vermis disease remains debatable.
Dysarthria, like nystagmus, is an inconsistent finding in cerebellar disease.

Titubation
Titubation is a rhythmic 'nodding' tremor of the head from side to side or to and fro, usually associated with distal limb tremor. It appears to be of little localising value.

Head tilt
Abnormal head tilt suggests a lesion of the anterior vermis. Note that a IV (trochlear) cranial nerve palsy and tonsillar herniation also produce this abnormal posture.

Involuntary movements
Myoclonic jerks and choreiform involuntary movements occur with extensive cerebellar disease involving the deep nuclei.

ASSOCIATED NON-CEREBELLAR SIGNS AND SYMPTOMS: These arise from:

- obstructive hydrocephalus
- cranial nerve involvement
- brain stem involvement.

(Extensor spasms from brain stem damage may be wrongly described as 'cerebellar fits'.)

CLASSIFICATION OF CEREBELLAR DYSFUNCTION

The following disorders are dealt with in their specific sections.

Developmental
- agenesis
- Dandy-Walker malformation
- Arnold-Chiari malformations
- Von Hippel Lindau disease.

Demyelinative
- multiple sclerosis.
- acute disseminated encephalomyelitis (ADEM)

Degenerative/Hereditary
- cerebellar degeneration
- multi-system atrophy (MSA)
- spino-cerebellar ataxias (SCA)

Neoplastic
- astrocytoma, medulloblastoma, haemangioblastoma, metastasis

Paraneoplastic
- subacute cerebellar degeneration

Infectious
- abscess formation
- acute cerebellitis (viral)
- Creutzfeldt-Jacob disease

Metabolic
- myxoedema
- hypoxia, hypoglycaemia.
- alcohol (vitamin B_1 deficiency)
- inborn disorders of metabolism. (lipid or amino acid metabolism)

Vascular
- cerebellar haemorrhage
- cerebellar infarction.

Drugs/toxins
- alcohol
- phenytoin.

NYSTAGMUS

Nystagmus is defined as an involuntary 'to and fro' movement of the eyes in a horizontal, vertical, rotary or mixed direction. The presence and characteristics of such movements help localise to the site of neurological disease.

Nystagmus may be *pendular* – equal velocity and amplitude in all directions,
    or *jerk* – with a fast phase (specifying the direction) and a slow phase.

The normal maintenance of ocular posture and alignment of the eyes with the environment depends upon:

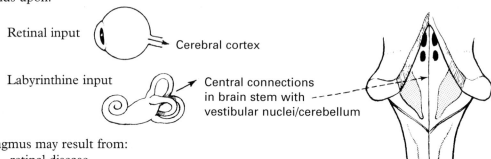

Retinal input → Cerebral cortex

Labyrinthine input → Central connections in brain stem with vestibular nuclei/cerebellum

Nystagmus may result from:
    – retinal disease
    – labyrinthine disease, or
    – disorders affecting the cerebellum or a substantial portion of the brain stem.

Examination for nystagmus
'Nystagmoid' movements of the eyes are present in many people at extremes of gaze. Nystagmus present with the eyes deviated less than 30° from the midline is abnormal.

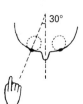

30°

When nystagmus is present only with the eyes deviated to one side
– *1st degree nystagmus.*
With eyes deviated to one side and in the midline position also
– *2nd degree nystagmus.*
When present in all directions of gaze – *3rd degree nystagmus.*
If nystagmus is detected, note the type (jerk or pendular), direction (of fast phase) and degree.
Nystagmus suppressed by visual fixation may appear in darkness, but this requires specialised techniques (electronystagmography – see page 63) to demonstrate.

RETINAL OR OCULAR nystagmus
Physiological: following moving objects beyond the limits of gaze – opticokinetic nystagmus.
Pathological: occurs when vision is defective. Fixation is impaired and the eyes vainly search.

Nystagmus is:

Rapid
Pendular (lacks slow and fast phase)
Increased when looking to sides
Persistent throughout lifetime

Occurs in *congenital cataract, congenital macula defect, albinism.*

NYSTAGMUS

VESTIBULAR nystagmus

Nystagmus arises from:

- natural stimulation of the vestibular apparatus – rotational or linear acceleration.
- artificially removing or increasing the stimulus from one labyrinth (e.g. caloric testing).
- damage to vestibular apparatus or the vestibular nerve.

Creates an imbalance between each side resulting in a slow drift of the eyes towards the damaged side (or side with the reduction in stimulus) followed by a fast compensatory movement to the opposite side.

Physiological

(i) Rotational acceleration produces nystagmus in the plane of rotation.

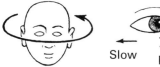 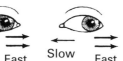

Slow Fast Slow Fast

> Slow phase in a direction tending to maintain the visual image.
> Fast phase in the opposite direction.

(ii) Caloric testing sets up convection currents in the lateral semicircular canal producing a horizontal nystagmus (see page 63).

Pathological

Damage to labyrinth or vestibular nerve.

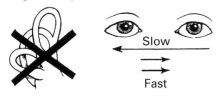

Slow

Fast

> Slow phase to side of lesion.
> Quick or fast phase to normal side.
> Rotatory component often present.
> Turning eyes away from the side of the lesion increases amplitude but does not change direction of nystagmus.
> In severe cases, the nystagmus is 3rd degree and gradually settles to 1st degree with recovery.
> Enhanced by loss of ocular fixation.
> Vertigo accompanies nystagmus.

Often associated with tinnitus and hearing loss. Vertigo and nystagmus settle simultaneously.

Occurs in acute labyrinthine disease – *Menière's disease, vestibular neuronitis, vascular disease.*

POSITIONAL nystagmus: this may occur in labyrinthine disease in association with vertigo when the patient assumes a certain posture.

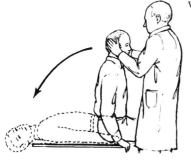

To elicit, suddenly reposition the patient:

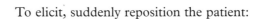

> After a delay of several seconds, nystagmus develops often with a rotatory component.
> With repeated testing, the nystagmus fatigues.

NYSTAGMUS

CENTRAL NERVOUS SYSTEM nystagmus

Central nystagmus arises from damage to the central vestibular connections in the vestibular nuclei and brain stem. The nystagmus may be horizontal, vertical, rotatory or dissociated (present in one eye only).

> The direction (fast phase) is determined by direction of gaze (multidirectional).
> Vertigo is seldom present.
> Signs of other nuclear or tract involvement in brain stem should be evident.

Central nystagmus occurs in *vascular disease, demyelination, neoplasms, nutritional disease (Wernicke's encephalopathy), alcohol intoxication and drug toxicity, e.g. phenytoin.*

Posterior fossa lesions may produce positional nystagmus. This may be distinguished from labyrinthine disease by:

> Absence of delay before onset, lack of fatiguing with repetitive testing, and a tendency to occur with any rather than one specific head movement.

Although nystagmus often occurs in cerebellar disease, the role of the cerebellum in its production remains unclear. *The fast phase tends to occur to the side of the cerebellar damage (i.e. the opposite of labyrinthine disease).*

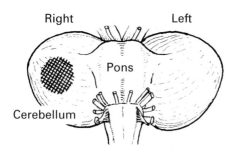

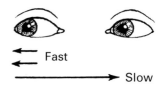

Rebound nystagmus occurs where the eyes 'overshoot' on return to the midline.

INTERNUCLEAR OPHTHALMOPLEGIA (Ataxic nystagmus)

The median longitudinal fasciculus links, among other structures, the innervation of the lateral rectus with the contralateral medial rectus muscle in order to coordinate horizontal gaze. A lesion of this fasciculus will cause *dissociate nystagmus.*

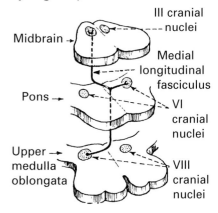

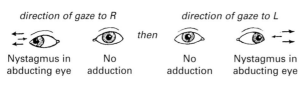

direction of gaze to R   *direction of gaze to L*

then

| Nystagmus in abducting eye | No adduction | No adduction | Nystagmus in abducting eye |

Eyes no longer move as one and nystagmus is present in one eye but not the other.

NYSTAGMUS

In unilateral medial longitudinal fasciculus lesions the eye fails to adduct on the affected side.

N.B. Internuclear ophthalmoplegia differs from a bilateral III nerve or nuclear lesion in that the pupil is not affected and when testing eye movements individually, some adduction occurs.

The disorder characteristically occurs in multiple sclerosis but also in brainstem infarction, haemorrhage, trauma, syringobulbia and drug toxicity (phenytoin).

OTHER VARIETIES OF CENTRAL NERVOUS SYSTEM NYSTAGMUS

1. **Downbeat nystagmus** 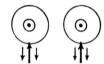 Occurs with lesions around the aqueduct of Sylvius or cervicomedullary junction. Fast phase is downwards (downbeating nystagmus).

2. **Convergence nystagmus** 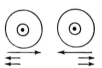 Occurs with lesions in upper midbrain region.

3. **See-saw nystagmus** 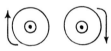 One eye intorts and moves up while the other extorts and moves down.
Occurs with sellar or parasellar mass lesion.

A group of confusing terms are used to describe abnormal, involuntary eye movements seen in cerebellar/brain stem disease:

Ocular bobbing – fast drift downwards, slow drift upwards; seen with large pontine lesions. (Horizontal eye movements are absent.)

Opsoclonus – rapid conjugate jerks of eyes; made worse by head movements. The eye movements are random.

Oscillopsia is a term used to describe the patient's awareness of jumping of the environment as a consequence of rapid jerking eye movements.

TREMOR

Tremor is a rhythmic involuntary movement normally affecting the limbs. Diagnosis depends on examination of the character of the tremor as well as the presence of other specific features.

Note the presence of tremor:

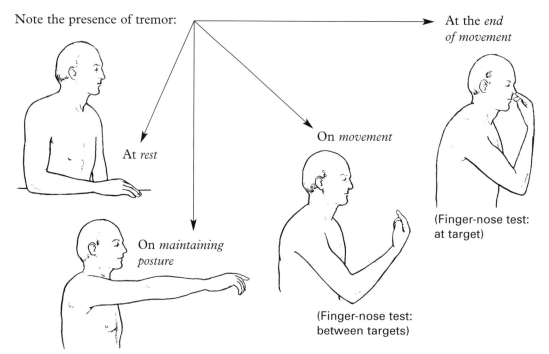

At the *end*
of movement

At *rest*

On *movement*

(Finger-nose test:
at target)

On *maintaining*
posture

(Finger-nose test:
between targets)

Observe:
  – the *rate* (slow, 4–6 Hz), (rapid, 6–12 Hz)
  – the *amplitude* (fine or coarse)
  – the *distribution:* head, trunk or limbs (distal or proximal)
  – *associated features* e.g. disorder of gait or balance
Most tremors disappear during sleep.

Physiological tremor is evident on maintaining a fixed posture, fast in rate (8–12 Hz), fine in character, distal in distribution and non-disabling. It is enhanced by fatigue, anxiety and drugs e.g. caffeine, steroids.

Pathological tremor occurs at rest or with movement, slow in rate, coarse in character, proximal or distal and often asymmetrical in distribution. This tremor is socially and physically disabling.

TREMOR

CHARACTERISTICS OF PATHOLOGICAL TREMOR

Tremor at rest

'Pill-rolling' tremor, decreasing
with movement.
Rate: 3–7 per second.
Amplitude: coarse.
Distribution: distal limbs.
Usually associated with bradykinesia
and rigidity.

PARKINSON'S DISEASE
OR DRUG INDUCED
PARKINSONISM

Tremor on maintaining posture and throughout range of movement

Tremor absent at rest, when the limb is relaxed,
but present on maintaining a fixed posture and
during movement.
Rate: 6–12 Hz
Amplitude: fine
Slow insidious onset
Distribution: Upper limbs involved,
        lower limbs rarely.
        Titubation (tremor of the head
        on the trunk) often present.

POSTURAL TREMOR

Specific types of postural tremor are recognised

FAMILIAL TREMOR   – often Mendelian dominant.
ESSENTIAL TREMOR – no family history
SENILE TREMOR   – develops in old age.

The tremor may progress until handwriting becomes impossible and feeding difficult.
Alcohol may temporarily abort the tremor; beta blockers may produce an improvement.

Tremor during and maximal at the end of movement

Tremor absent at rest; present during
movement and maximal on approaching
target, e.g. finger-nose test.
Rate: 4–6 per second.
Amplitude: coarse.
Distribution: Proximal and distal.
        Titubation may occur.
Usually associated with other cerebellar signs.

CEREBELLAR TREMOR
('intention tremor')

Extremely severe tremor – sufficient to interrupt ⟶ MIDBRAIN TREMOR due to disease
movement and throw patient off balance.   involving the cerebellar/red nucleus
                        connections, e.g. *multiple sclerosis*.

MYOCLONUS

Myoclonus is a shock-like contraction of muscles which occur irregularly and asymmetrically. Such jerks occur repetitively in the same muscle groups and range from a flicker in a single muscle to contraction in a group of muscles sufficient to displace the affected limb.

Pathophysiology

The precise nature of myoclonus remains unclear. Several forms exist, some clearly related to epilepsy; others may be associated with damage to inhibitory mechanisms in the brainstem reticular formation. Myoclonus may result from pathological changes affecting a variety of different sites including the motor cortex, cerebellum and spinal cord.

Clinical features

Myoclonic movements when repetitive vary in frequency between 5–60/minute. The muscles of the face, oral cavity and limbs are preferentially affected. The movements may be accentuated or precipitated by visual, auditory or tactile stimulation. Repetitive stimulation may result in a crescendo of myoclonus which resembles a seizure.

Physiological myoclonus occurs in sleep (hypnic jerks), with anxiety and in infants when feeding.

Causes

Myoclonus occurs in many rare conditions of the nervous system. Four groups of disorder are recognised:

Progressive myoclonus
Familial disorders:
- Lafora body disease
- Tay Sach's disease
- Gaucher's disease
- Ramsay Hunt syndrome
- Benign polymyoclonus

Degenerative disease:
- Subacute sclerosing panencephalitis
- Alzheimer's disease
- Pick's disease
- Diffuse Lewy body disease
- Huntington's disease
- Prion disease
- Creutzfeldt-Jacob disease

Metabolic disease associated with transient myoclonus
- Hyponatraemia
- Hypocalcaemia
- Renal, hypoxic, hepatic encephalopathy
- Non ketotic hyperglycaemia
- Hypoglycaemia

Epileptic disorders in which myoclonus occurs
Generalised seizures: – associated with petit mal
      – during prodrome of grand mal
      – photosensitive myoclonus
Juvenile myoclonic epilepsy
Lennox Gastaut syndrome (atypical petit mal, drop attacks and mental retardation)
West's syndrome

Miscellaneous disorders
- Cerebral anoxia
- Vasculitides
- Sarcoidosis
- Paraneoplastic disease
- Mitochondrial disease
- HIV encephalopathy
- Whipple's disease

Palatal myoclonus – an unusual myoclonic disorder with rapid regular movements of the soft palate and occasionally of the pharyngeal and facial musculature. Palatal movements occur at a rate of 120–140/minute. This disorder is associated with degenerative changes in the olivary and dentate nuclei.

Treatment
Benzodiazepine drugs such as clonazepam may suppress myoclonic movements. Piracetam (G.A.B.A. analogue) and levodopa or dopamine agonists are also used.

An exaggerated startle response can be confused with myoclonus. This is often physiological but can be disabling – hyperekplexia (Startle disease).

DISORDERS OF STANCE AND GAIT

The normal gait is characterised by an erect posture, moderately sized steps and the medial malleoli of the tibia 'tracing' a straight line.

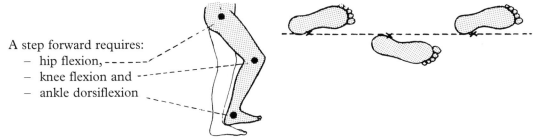

A step forward requires:
- hip flexion,
- knee flexion and
- ankle dorsiflexion

Co-ordination ensures fluidity of movement.
Antigravity reflexes maintain the erect posture. They depend upon spinal cord and brain stem connections to produce extension.

ASSESSMENT OF STANCE AND GAIT

In a patient complaining of disturbance of walking, careful assessment indicates the likely site of the causative lesion.

Watch the patient:
- walking
- performing *tandem gait* – heel to toe walking,
- standing with heels together with (a) eyes open, (b) eyes closed – this (Romberg's test) distinguishes cerebellar from sensory ataxia.

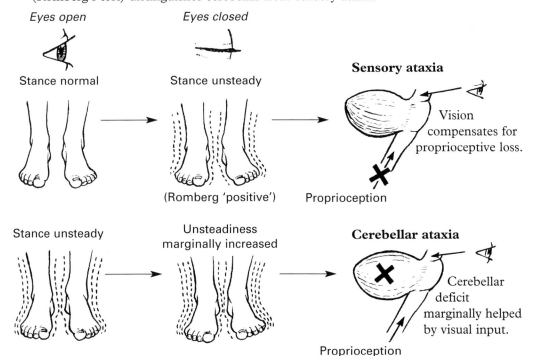

Eyes open   Eyes closed

Stance normal   Stance unsteady

Sensory ataxia

Vision compensates for proprioceptive loss.

(Romberg 'positive')   Proprioception

Stance unsteady   Unsteadiness marginally increased   **Cerebellar ataxia**

Cerebellar deficit marginally helped by visual input.

Proprioception

SPECIFIC DISORDERS OF STANCE AND GAIT

ATAXIC GAIT

1. Cerebellar The feet are separated widely when standing or walking.
Steps are jerky and unsure, varying in size.
The trunk sways forwards.
In mild cases: Tandem gait (heel-toe walking) is impaired; the patient falling to one or both sides.

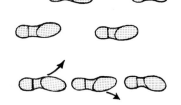

2. Sensory

Disturbed conscious or unconscious proprioception due to interruption of afferents in peripheral nerves or spinal cord (posterior columns, spinocerebellar tracts).
The gait appears normal when the eyes are open although the feet usually 'stamp' on the ground. Examination reveals a positive Romberg's test and impaired joint position sensation.

HEMIPLEGIC GAIT

The leg is extended and the toes forced downwards. When walking, abduction and circumduction at the hip prevent the toes from catching on the ground.
In paraplegia, strong adduction at the hips can produce a scissor-like posture of the lower limbs. In mild weakness, the gait may appear normal, but excessive wear occurs at the outer front aspect of the patient's shoe sole.

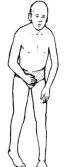

Hemiplegic gait

PARKINSONIAN (festinating) GAIT

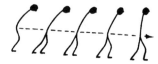

The patient adopts a flexed, stooping posture. To initiate walking, he leans forwards and then hurries (festinates) to 'catch up' on himself. The steps are short and shuffling.

STEPPAGE GAIT

Lower motor neuron weakness of pretibial and peroneal muscles produces this gait disorder. The patient lifts the affected leg high so that the toes clear the ground. When bilateral, it resembles a high-stepping horse.

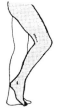

MYOPATHIC (waddling) GAIT

Characteristic of muscle disease. Trunk and pelvic muscle weakness result in a sway-back, pot-bellied appearance with difficulty in pelvic 'fixation' when walking.

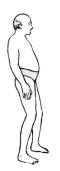

FRONTAL LOBE GAIT

Disturbance of connections between frontal cortex, basal ganglia and cerebellum produces this characteristic disturbance. The gait is wide based (feet wide apart). Initiation is difficult, the feet often seem 'stuck' to the floor. There is a tendency to fall backwards. Power and sensation are normal.

HYSTERICAL GAIT

Characterised by its bizarre nature.
Numerous variations are seen. The hallmark is inconsistency supported by the lack of neurological signs. Close observation is essential.

LIMB WEAKNESS

Limb weakness results from damage to the **motor system** at any level from the motor cortex to muscle.

UPPER MOTOR NEURON WEAKNESS

MUSCLE TONE
Hypertonicity develops after a period (a few days or weeks) of 'neural shock'. Passive movements produce a 'clasp knife' quality, i.e. sudden 'give' towards the end of movement. *Clonus* – present.

MUSCLE FASCICULATION
Absent.

MUSCLE WASTING
Absent – but, in the long term, disuse atrophy results.

REFLEXES
– **Tendon** – exaggerated.
– **Superficial** – depressed or absent (abdominal, cremasteric).
– **Plantar response** – extensor.

DISTRIBUTION
In general, whole limb or limbs are involved, e.g. monoplegia, hemiplegia, paraplegia.

Weakness shows a PREDILECTION for certain muscle group in a PYRAMIDAL DISTRIBUTION, i.e.

upper limbs   –   extensor   >   flexor
                  weakness   weakness

lower limbs   –   flexor   >   extensor
                  weakness   weakness

MOTOR CORTEX

Corticobulbar tract

MIDBRAIN

PONS
VII nerve

Somatotopic arrangement

MEDULLA
X, XI, XII
nerves

Decussation

SPINAL CORD

Lateral corticospinal tract

The anterior corticospinal tract carries only 20% of the descending fibres and decussates at segmental level.

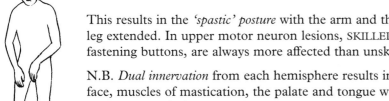

This results in the *'spastic' posture* with the arm and the wrist flexed and the leg extended. In upper motor neuron lesions, SKILLED movements, e.g. fastening buttons, are always more affected than unskilled movements.

N.B. *Dual innervation* from each hemisphere results in sparing of the upper face, muscles of mastication, the palate and tongue with a unilateral upper motor neuron lesion.

LIMB WEAKNESS

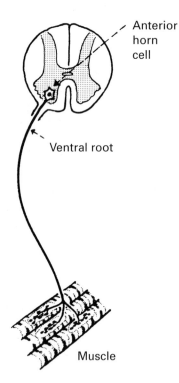

Anterior horn cell

Ventral root

Muscle

LOWER MOTOR NEURON WEAKNESS

MUSCLE TONE
Hypotonicity with diminished resistance to passive stretch.
Clonus – absent.

MUSCLE FASCICULATION
Present – irregular, non-rhythmical contractions of groups
of motor units. More prevalent in anterior horn cell disease
than in nerve root damage.

MUSCLE WASTING
Wasting becomes evident in the paretic muscle within 2–3
weeks of the onset.

REFLEXES

– **Tendon** – depressed or absent.
– **Superficial** – rarely affected
                (abdominal, cremasteric).
– **Plantar response** – flexor.

DISTRIBUTION

Either – muscle groups involved in distribution of a spinal
segment/root, plexus or peripheral nerve,

  or – generalised limb involvement affecting proximal or
distal muscles or following a specific distribution, e.g.
facioscapulohumeral dystrophy.

LIMB WEAKNESS

LESION LOCALISATION

The foregoing clinical features readily distinguish weakness of an upper motor neuron, lower motor neuron or mixed pattern. Combining these findings with other neurological signs enables localisation of the lesion site.

UPPER MOTOR NEURON LIMB WEAKNESS – UNILATERAL

Useful localising features (not always present)	Lesion site

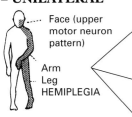

Face (upper motor neuron pattern)
Arm
Leg
HEMIPLEGIA

Impairment of conscious level.
Visual field deficit.
Dysphasia (if dominant hemisphere).

CONTRALATERAL HEMISPHERE LESION

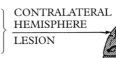

Alert.
No dysphasia (if dominant hemisphere).
Visual field deficit rare.

CONTRALATERAL INTERNAL CAPSULE LESION

Contralateral III nerve palsy.

CONTRALATERAL MIDBRAIN LESION

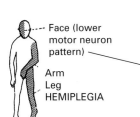

Face (lower motor neuron pattern)
Arm
Leg
HEMIPLEGIA

Conjugate gaze deviation towards the weak limbs (impaired movement towards the 'normal' limb).
Lower motor neuron facial weakness on side opposite the weak limbs.

CONTRALATERAL PONTINE LESION

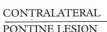

Arm

Visual field deficit.
Discriminatory sensory deficit.

CONTRA-LATERAL CORTEX LESION

Pain and temperature loss on the same side as the weakness and a Horner's syndrome and weak palate and tongue on the opposite side.

CONTRALATERAL MEDULLARY LESION

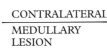

Leg
HEMIPLEGIA

Arm ± Face

Pain and temperature loss on the opposite side to the limb weakness and a Horner's syndrome and proprioception loss on the same side.

IPSILATERAL SPINAL LESION

C1
|
C4

Visual field deficit.
Dysphasia (if dominant hemisphere).
Discriminatory sensory deficit.

CONTRALATERAL CORTEX LESION

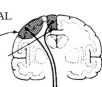

MONOPLEGIA

Leg

Discriminatory sensory deficit.

Pain and temperature loss in the opposite leg, proprioception loss on the same side.

IPSILATERAL SPINAL LESION

T1
|
L1

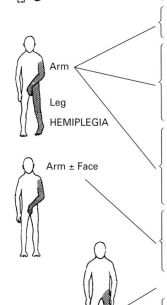

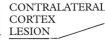
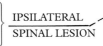

LIMB WEAKNESS

UPPER MOTOR NEURON LIMB WEAKNESS – LATERAL

Useful localising features (not always present)

Lesion site

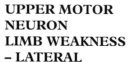

Face (lower motor neuron)

Arm — Arm

Leg — Leg

{ Facial movements lost but vertical eye movements retained – 'locked-in' syndrome. }

BILATERAL PONTINE LESION

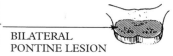

TETRAPLEGIA (syn. QUADRAPARESIS)

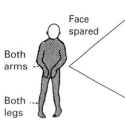

Face spared

Both arms

Both legs

{ Facial movements retained, but no tongue or palate movement or speech – a variant of the 'locked-in' syndrome. }

BILATERAL MEDULLARY LESION

C1
|
C3

{ Ventilatory support required (no cranial nerve lesion). }

BILATERAL CERVICAL SPINE LESION

Diaphragmatic respiration. ⟶

C4

PARAPLEGIA

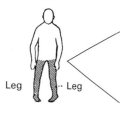

Leg — Leg

{ Discriminatory sensory loss. 'Frontal' incontinence. (Pain and temperature sensation intact.) }

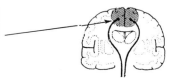

{ 'Sensory level' – impairment or loss of *all* sensory modalities. Hesitancy of micturition or acute urinary retention. }

BILATERAL THORACIC SPINE LESION

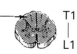

T1
|
L1

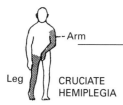

— Arm

Leg   CRUCIATE HEMIPLEGIA

{ Weakness of the palate and tongue on the side of the arm weakness. }

'leg' fibres   'arm' fibres

MEDULLARY LESION (below 'arm' fibre decussation above 'leg' fibre decussation)

LIMB WEAKNESS

MIXED UPPER AND LOWER MOTOR NEURON WEAKNESS – UNILATERAL OR BILATERAL

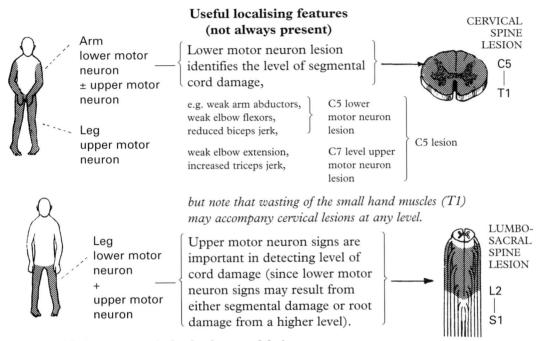

Useful localising features (not always present)

CERVICAL SPINE LESION

Arm lower motor neuron ± upper motor neuron

{ Lower motor neuron lesion identifies the level of segmental cord damage, }

C5
|
T1

e.g. weak arm abductors, weak elbow flexors, reduced biceps jerk,

} C5 lower motor neuron lesion

} C5 lesion

Leg upper motor neuron

weak elbow extension, increased triceps jerk,

C7 level upper motor neuron lesion

but note that wasting of the small hand muscles (T1) may accompany cervical lesions at any level.

Leg lower motor neuron + upper motor neuron

{ Upper motor neuron signs are important in detecting level of cord damage (since lower motor neuron signs may result from either segmental damage or root damage from a higher level). }

LUMBO-SACRAL SPINE LESION

L2
|
S1

N.B. Dual lesions, e.g. cervical + lumbar spondylosis may cause mixed (umn and lmn) signs in both arm and leg.

LOWER MOTOR NEURON LIMB WEAKNESS – UNILATERAL OR BILATERAL

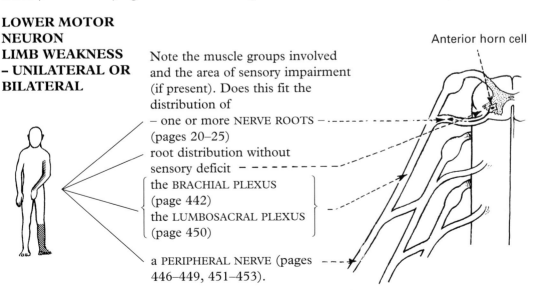

Note the muscle groups involved and the area of sensory impairment (if present). Does this fit the distribution of

– one or more NERVE ROOTS (pages 20–25)
root distribution without sensory deficit
the BRACHIAL PLEXUS (page 442)
the LUMBOSACRAL PLEXUS (page 450)

a PERIPHERAL NERVE (pages 446–449, 451–453).

Anterior horn cell

LIMB WEAKNESS

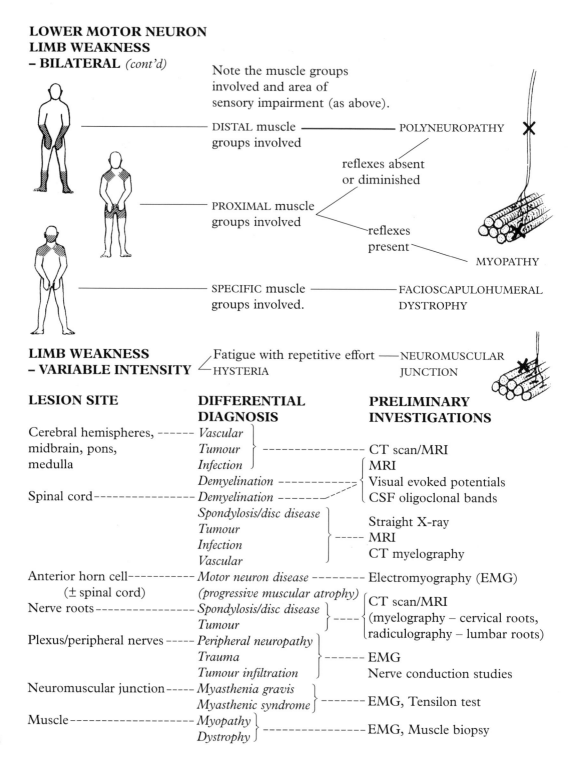

**LOWER MOTOR NEURON
LIMB WEAKNESS
– BILATERAL** *(cont'd)*

Note the muscle groups
involved and area of
sensory impairment (as above).

DISTAL muscle ——————— POLYNEUROPATHY
groups involved

reflexes absent
or diminished

PROXIMAL muscle
groups involved

reflexes
present

MYOPATHY

SPECIFIC muscle ——————— FACIOSCAPULOHUMERAL
groups involved. DYSTROPHY

**LIMB WEAKNESS
– VARIABLE INTENSITY** Fatigue with repetitive effort ——NEUROMUSCULAR
HYSTERIA JUNCTION

LESION SITE	**DIFFERENTIAL DIAGNOSIS**	**PRELIMINARY INVESTIGATIONS**
Cerebral hemispheres, midbrain, pons, medulla	*Vascular* *Tumour* *Infection*	CT scan/MRI
	Demyelination	MRI Visual evoked potentials CSF oligoclonal bands
Spinal cord	*Demyelination*	
	Spondylosis/disc disease *Tumour* *Infection* *Vascular*	Straight X-ray MRI CT myelography
Anterior horn cell (± spinal cord)	*Motor neuron disease* *(progressive muscular atrophy)*	Electromyography (EMG)
Nerve roots	*Spondylosis/disc disease* *Tumour*	CT scan/MRI (myelography – cervical roots, radiculography – lumbar roots)
Plexus/peripheral nerves	*Peripheral neuropathy* *Trauma* *Tumour infiltration*	EMG Nerve conduction studies
Neuromuscular junction	*Myasthenia gravis* *Myasthenic syndrome*	EMG, Tensilon test
Muscle	*Myopathy* *Dystrophy*	EMG, Muscle biopsy

SENSORY IMPAIRMENT

ANATOMY AND PHYSIOLOGY

The sensory system relays information from both the external and the internal environment.

Receptors
convert this information into
electrical action potentials.
- *Specialised* – smell, vision, hearing
- *Visceral* – viscera, smooth muscle
  (unconscious or autonomic) } considered separately
- *Somatic* – skin, striated muscle, joints

Cutaneous receptors are of several types and, while overlap does occur, each has some specific purpose.

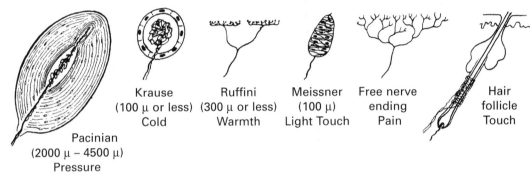

Pacinian
(2000 μ – 4500 μ)
Pressure

Krause
(100 μ or less)
Cold

Ruffini
(300 μ or less)
Warmth

Meissner
(100 μ)
Light Touch

Free nerve
ending
Pain

Hair
follicle
Touch

Muscle and tendon receptors
These receptors along with those of
pressure and touch provide information
on body and limb position –
proprioception.
Continual stimulation of most receptors
results in a reduction in the action
potential frequency – ADAPTATION

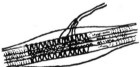

Muscle spindle

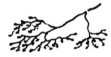

Golgi tendon
organ

CENTRAL CONNECTIONS

Sensory neurons (bipolar cells) relay information to
the spinal cord via the dorsal root to the dorsal root
entry zone. The anatomical and physical
characteristics of the neurons vary depending on the
information they carry, as do the central pathways:

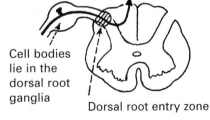

Cell bodies
lie in the
dorsal root
ganglia

Dorsal root entry zone

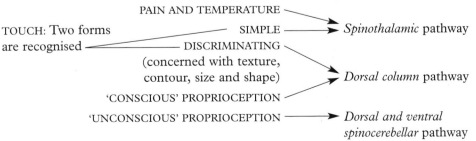

PAIN AND TEMPERATURE ⟶ *Spinothalamic* pathway

TOUCH: Two forms
are recognised — SIMPLE ⟶
DISCRIMINATING
(concerned with texture,
contour, size and shape)

'CONSCIOUS' PROPRIOCEPTION

Dorsal column pathway

'UNCONSCIOUS' PROPRIOCEPTION ⟶ *Dorsal and ventral
spinocerebellar* pathway

197

SENSORY IMPAIRMENT

SPINOTHALAMIC PATHWAY

1. Fibres enter the root entry zone and pass up or down for several segments in *Lissauer's* tract before terminating in the dorsal aspect of the dorsal horn.

2. *Second order neurons* synapse locally, cross the midline and run up the *spinothalamic* tract and *lateral lemniscus* to terminate in the posterolateral nucleus of the *thalamus*. Throughout its course, the fibres lie in a *somatotopic arrangement* with sacral fibres outermost. In the brain stem the lateral lemniscus gives off collateral branches to the *reticular formation*, which projects widely to the cerebral cortex and limbic system and is joined by fibres from the contralateral nucleus and tract of the trigeminal nerve.

3. From the thalamus, *third order neurons* project to the *parietal cortex*.

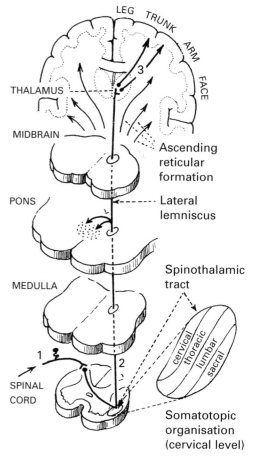

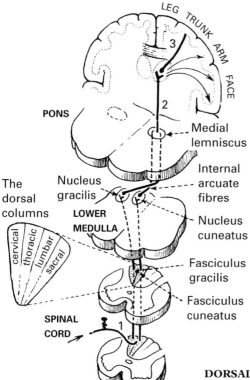

DORSAL COLUMN PATHWAY

1. Fibres enter in the root entry zone and run upwards in the *dorsal columns* to the *lower medulla* where they terminate in the *nucleus gracilis* and *nucleus cuneatus*.

2. *Second order neurons* decussate as the *internal arcuate fibres* and pass upwards in the *medial lemniscus*. Maintaining a *somatotopic arrangement*, they terminate in the ventral posterolateral thalamus.

3. *Third order neurons* arise in the thalamus and project to the *parietal cortex*.

DORSAL AND VENTRAL SPINOCEREBELLAR PATHWAYS: see Cerebellar dysfunction, page 178.

SENSORY IMPAIRMENT

EXAMINATION OF THE SENSORY SYSTEM: see page 21

CLINICAL FEATURES

Sensory disturbance may result in:

NEGATIVE symptoms: 'a loss of feeling'
'a deadness'.

POSITIVE symptoms: 'a pins and needles sensation'
'a burning feeling'.

Lesions of the PERIPHERAL NERVES or NERVE ROOTS may produce 'negative' or 'positive' symptoms.

SPINOTHALAMIC TRACT lesions –
seldom produce pain but usually a *lack of awareness of pain and temperature.*
This may result in:
– trophic changes: cold, blue extremities
hair loss
brittle nails
– painless burns
– joint deformation (Charcot's joints).

DORSAL COLUMN lesions –
produce a *discriminatory type of sensory loss.*
– impaired two point discrimination
– astereognosis (failure to discriminate objects held in the hand).
– sensory ataxia
(disturbed proprioception).

Lesions of the PARIETAL CORTEX also produce a *discriminatory type of sensory loss.* Minor lesions produce *sensory inattention* (perceptual rivalry) – with bilateral simultaneous limb stimulation, the stimulus is only perceived on the unaffected side.

LESION LOCALISATION

The pattern of the sensory deficit aids lesion localisation.

Sensory deficit	Useful localising features (if present)	Lesion site

HEMISENSORY LOSS

'Discriminatory' sensory deficit.
Sensory inattention
(perceptual rivalry)
Only minimal pain and
temperature loss

LESION OF CONTRALATERAL
PARIETAL
CORTEX

or selective deficit in face, arm,
trunk or leg.

SELECTIVE
CORTICAL
LESION

Loss of all sensory modalities
including pain and temperature
in the face, arm, trunk and leg.

CONTRALATERAL
THALAMIC LESION

SENSORY IMPAIRMENT

LESION LOCALISATION (*cont'd*)

Sensory deficit	Useful localising features (if present)	Lesion site

FACIAL SENSORY LOSS

HEMISENSORY LOSS

Loss of all modalities in the limbs (depending on the extent of the lesion)
Loss of pain and temperature on the opposite side of the face with or without 'muzzle' area sparing and a lateral gaze palsy towards that side.

CONTRALATERAL PONTINE LESION

(Ipsilateral to the facial sensory loss)

As above – but lateral gaze normal.
Weakness of palate and tongue on side opposite to the limb sensory deficit.

CONTRALATERAL MEDULLARY LESION

Loss of pain, temperature and light touch below a specific dermatome level (may spare sacral sensation).

CONTRALATERAL SPINOTHALAMIC TRACT LESION

(Partial spinothalamic tract lesion)

CERVICAL
THORACIC
LUMBAR
SACRAL

Loss of all modalities at one or several dermatome levels.

Loss of pain and temperature below a specific dermatome level.

BROWN-SEQUARD SYNDROME

Loss of proprioception and 'discriminatory' touch up to similar level and limb weakness.

(Partial cord lesion)

Bilateral loss of all modalities.
Bilateral leg weakness.

COMPLETE CORD LESION

Bilateral loss of pain and temperature.
Preservation of proprioception and 'discriminatory' sensation.

'SUSPENDED' SENSORY LOSS

CENTRAL CORD LESION

SENSORY IMPAIRMENT

LESION LOCALISATION (*cont'd*)

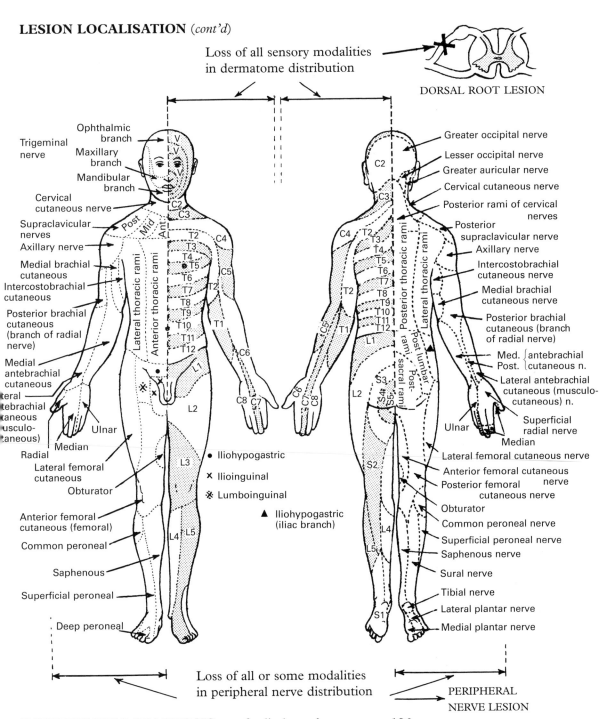

Loss of all sensory modalities in dermatome distribution

DORSAL ROOT LESION

Loss of all or some modalities in peripheral nerve distribution

PERIPHERAL NERVE LESION

DIFFERENTIAL DIAGNOSIS – as for limb weakness – page 196

PAIN

Peripheral receptors of pain – free nerve endings lying in skin or other organs – are the distal axons of sensory neurons. Such unmyelinated or only thinly myelinated axons are of small diameter. The termination and central connections of these axons are described on page 198.

The type of stimulus required to activate free endings varies, e.g. in muscle – ischaemia, in abdominal viscera – distension.

Certain substances – bradykinins, prostaglandins, histamine – may stimulate free nerve endings. These substances are released in damaged tissue.

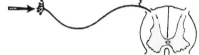

CONTROL OF SENSORY (PAIN) INPUT

The gate control theory

A relay system in the posterior horn of the spinal cord modifies pain input. This involves interneuronal connections within the substantia gelatinosa (a layer of the posterior horn which extends throughout the whole length of the spinal cord on each side).

An afferent impulse arriving at the posterior horn in *thick myelinated fibres* has an inhibitory effect in the region of the substantia gelatinosa.
An afferent impulse arriving in *thin myelinated or unmyelinated fibres* (i.e. transmitting pain) has an excitatory effect in the region of the substantia gelatinosa.
The overall interaction of these inhibitory or excitatory effects determines the activity of second order neurons of the spinothalamic pathway.
A reduction in activity of large sensory fibres 'opens' the gate.
Stimulation of large sensory fibres theoretically 'closes' the gate.
In addition to these segmental influences, higher centres also control the gate region and form part of a feed-back loop.

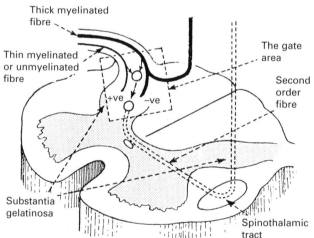

Cross section of the spinal cord: the gate area connections

Pain perception

The awareness of pain is brought about by projection from the thalamus to cerebral cortex. Personality, mood and neuroticism all influence the intensity of pain perception. Diffuse projections through Lissauer's tract and the reticular core of the spinal cord white matter to the reticular formation and limbic system probably contribute to the unpleasant, emotionally disturbing aspects of pain.

PAIN

NEUROTRANSMITTER SUBSTANCES

Evidence based on both human and animal studies has shown that an endogenous system, lying within the central nervous system can induce a degree of analgesia. Electrical stimulation of certain sites, such as the periaqueductal grey matter, can inhibit pain perception.

Receptor sites for endogenous opiates have been found in the posterior horns and thalamus as well as at several other sites. The endogenous substances which bind to these sites are called *encephalins* or *endorphins*.

Substance P, a polypeptide, found predominantly around free nerve ending receptors and in the spinal cord posterior horns, glutamate and calcitonin gene related peptide are the likely primary transmitters of pain.

DRUG TREATMENT

Sites of potential drug action:

Block transmission in nerves?

Block pain transmission centrally; opiates/narcotics

Block receptors at periphery, e.g. aspirin, non-steroidal anti-inflammatory drugs

Drug selection in pain treatment depends on the severity, cause and the expected duration of the pain, i.e. *acute* pain – less than 2 weeks duration, e.g. postoperative, post-traumatic, renal colic.

chronic pain – *benign* origin, e.g. postherpetic neuralgia phantom limb pain chronic back pain.

– *malignant* origin.

1. In acute pain, drug therapy ranges from *mild analgesics* – aspirin, paracetamol – to *narcotic agents* – morphine, heroin. *Tranquillisers* may also help.

2. In chronic pain of benign origin, narcotics and sedatives must be avoided. In these patients, depression usually plays a rôle and the clinician must not underestimate the value of *tricyclic antidepressants*.
Anticonvulsants – gabapentin and carbamazepine appear to benefit many patients, probably due to their membrane stabilizing effect.
Topical treatment – capsaicin blocks substance P and inhibits pain transmission in the skin. Used for postherpetic neuralgia.

3. In chronic pain from terminal malignancy, patients often require *strong narcotics* – morphine, heroin. Frequent administration of small doses provides the greatest effect.

PAIN – TREATMENT

PERIPHERAL TECHNIQUES

Generally used for more benign conditions and before resorting to central techniques.

NERVE BLOCKS: Injections of agents into peripheral nerves or roots abolishes pain in the appropriate dermatome; motor and sympathetic function are also lost. Local anaesthetics produce a temporary effect; neurolytic agents, e.g. phenol, alcohol, give permanent results.

– *Intraspinal* phenol or hypertonic saline for chronic pain usually used in patients with terminal malignancy.

– *Epidural* local anaesthetic produces temporary analgesia. Narcotic infusion appears useful for controlling postoperative pain and intractable pain in patients with terminal malignancy.

– *Sympathetic Ganglion or Trunk*
– anaesthetics or neurolytic agent often helps causalgic pain. (see page 206).

– *Paravertebral or Peripheral Nerve*
– local anaesthetics may benefit temporary pain states, e.g. fractured rib, but neurolytic agents often cause a painful neuritis.

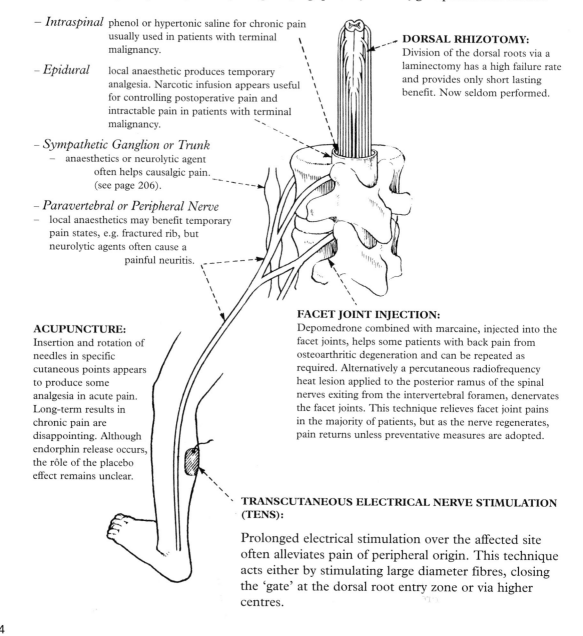

DORSAL RHIZOTOMY:
Division of the dorsal roots via a laminectomy has a high failure rate and provides only short lasting benefit. Now seldom performed.

ACUPUNCTURE:
Insertion and rotation of needles in specific cutaneous points appears to produce some analgesia in acute pain. Long-term results in chronic pain are disappointing. Although endorphin release occurs, the rôle of the placebo effect remains unclear.

FACET JOINT INJECTION:
Depomedrone combined with marcaine, injected into the facet joints, helps some patients with back pain from osteoarthritic degeneration and can be repeated as required. Alternatively a percutaneous radiofrequency heat lesion applied to the posterior ramus of the spinal nerves exiting from the intervertebral foramen, denervates the facet joints. This technique relieves facet joint pains in the majority of patients, but as the nerve regenerates, pain returns unless preventative measures are adopted.

TRANSCUTANEOUS ELECTRICAL NERVE STIMULATION (TENS):

Prolonged electrical stimulation over the affected site often alleviates pain of peripheral origin. This technique acts either by stimulating large diameter fibres, closing the 'gate' at the dorsal root entry zone or via higher centres.

PAIN – TREATMENT

CENTRAL TECHNIQUES

Used primarily in patients with intractable pain from malignancy

PRECENTRAL (MOTOR) CORTEX STIMULATION:
Promising technique in patients suffering hyperpathic pain after stroke or trigeminal territory neuropathic pain.

MESENCEPHALOTOMY:
A radiofrequency heat lesion in a stereotactically implanted electrode inserted into the midbrain reticular formation may help patients with head and neck malignancy.

DEEP BRAIN STIMULATION: Stimulation of implanted electrodes inserted in the periventricular grey matter or sensory relay nucleus of the thalamus may produce relief in patients with neuropathic pain. If successful, a radiocontrolled stimulator is implanted subcutaneously.

HYPOPHYSECTOMY:
By transphenoidal excision or with radioactive yttrium may help pain from metastatic deposits. The mechanism of relief remains uncertain; this is not merely due to tumour regression.

DORSAL ROOT ENTRY ZONE LESIONS
Following cord exposure, multiple radiofrequency heat lesions of the dorsal root entry zone are produced with a hand held electrode. This may help deafferentation pain, i.e. brachial plexus avulsion, but ipsilateral leg weakness is a potential complication.

PERCUTANEOUS ANTEROLATERAL CORDOTOMY: A percutaneous radiofrequency heat lesion of the spinothalamic tract now replaces open cordotomy. This produces pain relief in 90% of patients in the contralateral limbs. It is usually applicable in malignant states where simple methods of pain control have failed. Risks (ipsilateral limb weakness and respiratory difficulties) are small.

MYELOTOMY: Exposure of the cord and division of the decussating pain fibres produces pain relief on a temporary basis, restricting use to patients with terminal malignancy.

SPINAL CORD STIMULATION: Stimulation of electrodes inserted percutaneously or by open surgery into the epidural space may benefit patients with chronic pain, unresponsive to non-invasive techniques, provided the dorsal columns remain at least partially functional e.g. when lesions are distal to the dorsal root ganglion.

205

PAIN SYNDROMES

Pain is not primarily a pathological phenomenon, but serves a protective function. Conditions with loss of pain perception exemplify this, resulting in frequent injuries, burns and subsequent mutilations, e.g. syringomyelia, hereditary sensory neuropathy, congenital insensitivity to pain.

Pathological conditions do, however, cause pain – as a symptom of cancer, injury or other disease.

The following conditions produce characteristic pain syndrome.

CAUSALGIA

Causalgia is an intense, continuous, burning pain produced by an incomplete peripheral nerve injury. Touching the limb aggravates the pain, and the patient resents any interference or attempt at limb mobilisation. The skin becomes red, warm and swollen.

Theoretical mechanism

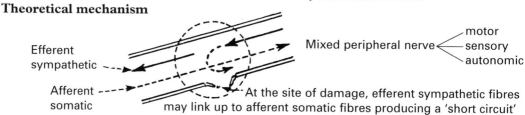

Efferent sympathetic

Afferent somatic

Mixed peripheral nerve — motor, sensory, autonomic

At the site of damage, efferent sympathetic fibres may link up to afferent somatic fibres producing a 'short circuit'

Causalgia only occurs with damage to peripheral nerves containing a large number of sympathetic fibres and responds in part to sympathetic blockade (pharmacological or surgical).

POSTHERPETIC NEURALGIA

Following activation of a latent infection with varicella zoster virus lying dormant in the dorsal root or gasserian ganglion, the patient develops a burning, constant pain with severe, sharp paroxysmal twinges over the area supplied by the affected sensory neurons. Touch exacerbates the pain. Thick myelinated fibres are preferentially damaged, possibly opening the 'gate'.

Treatment of postherpetic neuralgia is particularly difficult. Carbamazepine and/or antidepressants may help. Ethylchloride spray over the affected area provides temporary relief. Capsaicin, a topical NSAID can be an effective treatment.

THALAMIC PAIN

Thalamic stimulation may produce or abolish pain depending upon the electrode site. A vascular accident which involves the inhibitory portion of the thalamus may result in pain – the thalamic syndrome.

Clinical features: Hemianaesthesia at onset contralateral to the lesion precedes the development of pain. This is burning and diffuse, and exacerbated by the touch of clothing.

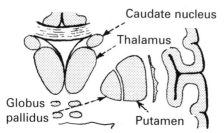

Caudate nucleus

Thalamus

Globus pallidus

Putamen

Treatment: Drug treatment gives poor results. A stereotactic procedure although increasing the sensory deficit may help.

Paradoxically the thalamic syndrome may occur following a thalamic stereotactic procedure for movement disorders.

PAIN SYNDROMES

PHANTOM LIMB PAIN

Following amputation of a limb, 10% of patients develop pain with a continuous persistent burning quality, caused by neuroma formation in the stump. The patient 'feels' the pain arising from some point on the missing limb (the pain input projects through pathways which retain the topographical image of the absent limb).

Treatment: Often responds to simple measures e.g. tricyclic antidepressants.

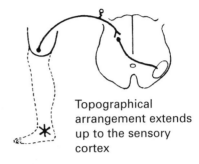

Topographical arrangement extends up to the sensory cortex

VISCERAL AND REFERRED PAIN

Deep visceral pain is dull and boring; it is the consequence of distension or traction on free nerve endings.
Referred pain of a dull quality relates to a specific area of the body surface – often hypersensitive to touch.

The basis of referred pain

The visceral afferents converge upon the same cells in the posterior horns as the somatic efferents. The patient 'projects' pain from the viscera to the area supplied by corresponding somatic afferent fibres.

A knowledge of the source of referred pain is important in diagnosis and treatment.

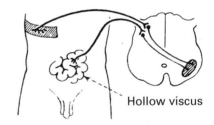

Hollow viscus

SITES OF REFERRED PAIN FROM SPECIFIC ORGANS

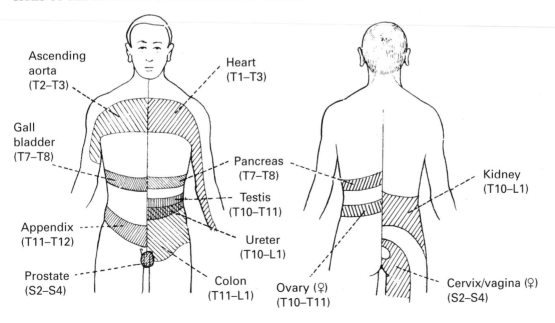

Ascending aorta (T2–T3)

Heart (T1–T3)

Gall bladder (T7–T8)

Pancreas (T7–T8)

Kidney (T10–L1)

Testis (T10–T11)

Appendix (T11–T12)

Ureter (T10–L1)

Prostate (S2–S4)

Colon (T11–L1)

Ovary (♀) (T10–T11)

Cervix/vagina (♀) (S2–S4)

LIMB PAIN

Pain may arise from any anatomical structure within the limb. Each produces characteristic features:

BONE – diffuse, aching pain
± palpable mass.

JOINTS – pain localised to affected joint.
– tenderness on palpation.
– movements restricted and painful.
– wasting of surrounding muscles may follow.

MUSCLES – pain localised to specific muscle
± wasting and weakness
± palpable mass.

TENDONS – pain localised to swollen, tender tendon sheath.

BLOOD VESSELS – pain brought on by exertion (claudication), relieved by rest.
– pain at rest in pale, pulseless limb (occlusion).
– pain associated with paraesthesia and digital pallor (Raynaud's).

NERVE ROOT – pain increased by coughing or by movement
± associated neurological deficit

PLEXUS OR PERIPHERAL NERVE – burning pain
± sweating, cyanosis and oedema of extremity,
± associated neurological deficit.

CAUSES OF UPPER LIMB PAIN

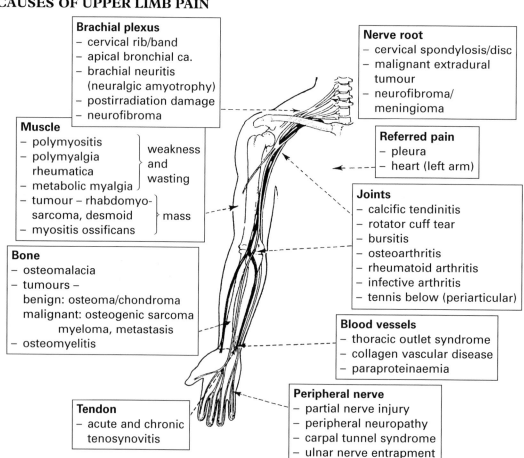

Brachial plexus
– cervical rib/band
– apical bronchial ca.
– brachial neuritis (neuralgic amyotrophy)
– postirradiation damage
– neurofibroma

Muscle
– polymyositis
– polymyalgia rheumatica
– metabolic myalgia
} weakness and wasting
– tumour – rhabdomyosarcoma, desmoid
– myositis ossificans
} mass

Bone
– osteomalacia
– tumours –
benign: osteoma/chondroma
malignant: osteogenic sarcoma myeloma, metastasis
– osteomyelitis

Tendon
– acute and chronic tenosynovitis

Nerve root
– cervical spondylosis/disc
– malignant extradural tumour
– neurofibroma/meningioma

Referred pain
– pleura
– heart (left arm)

Joints
– calcific tendinitis
– rotator cuff tear
– bursitis
– osteoarthritis
– rheumatoid arthritis
– infective arthritis
– tennis below (periarticular)

Blood vessels
– thoracic outlet syndrome
– collagen vascular disease
– paraproteinaemia

Peripheral nerve
– partial nerve injury
– peripheral neuropathy
– carpal tunnel syndrome
– ulnar nerve entrapment

LIMB PAIN

CAUSES OF LOWER LIMB PAIN

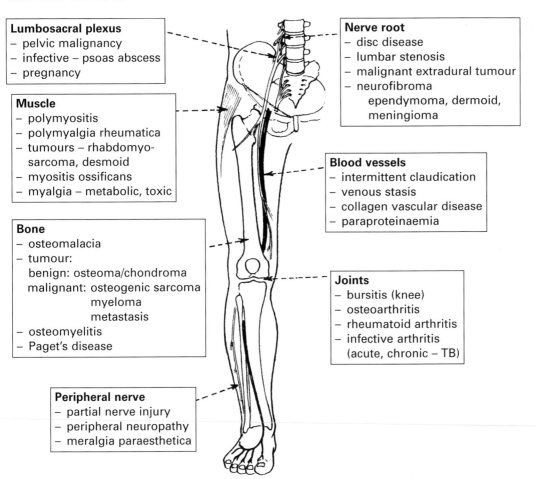

Lumbosacral plexus
– pelvic malignancy
– infective – psoas abscess
– pregnancy

Muscle
– polymyositis
– polymyalgia rheumatica
– tumours – rhabdomyo-
   sarcoma, desmoid
– myositis ossificans
– myalgia – metabolic, toxic

Bone
– osteomalacia
– tumour:
   benign: osteoma/chondroma
   malignant: osteogenic sarcoma
                myeloma
                metastasis
– osteomyelitis
– Paget's disease

Peripheral nerve
– partial nerve injury
– peripheral neuropathy
– meralgia paraesthetica

Nerve root
– disc disease
– lumbar stenosis
– malignant extradural tumour
– neurofibroma
   ependymoma, dermoid,
   meningioma

Blood vessels
– intermittent claudication
– venous stasis
– collagen vascular disease
– paraproteinaemia

Joints
– bursitis (knee)
– osteoarthritis
– rheumatoid arthritis
– infective arthritis
   (acute, chronic – TB)

Meralgia paraesthetica: burning, tingling pain over the outer aspect of the thigh, increased when standing or by walking, due to a localised neuritis of the lateral cutaneous nerve of the thigh. A patch of sensory impairment may be evident over the outer aspect of the thigh.

Ekbom's syndrome: (syn. restless legs syndrome): intolerable tingling, burning sensation or pain in both legs, occurring only when sitting or lying down and relieved by walking; no associated neurological abnormality.

Investigation of limb pain depends on the suspected cause and may include straight X-rays, CT scan, MRI, nerve conduction studies and EMG.

MUSCLE PAIN (MYALGIA)

Muscle pain is a common medical complaint. There are many causes and clinical evaluation and appropriate investigation is often difficult. The physiological mechanisms producing such a symptom are limited.

Mechanical pain results from excessive muscle tension or contraction and is 'cramp like'.

Inflammatory pain results from disruption of muscle fibres, inflammatory exudate and fibre swelling.

Ischaemic pain results from metabolic change, usually in response to exercise and is deep and aching.

Muscle pain may be physiological – as a consequence of extreme exercise or pathological – as a consequence of muscle, soft tissue or systemic illness.

DIAGNOSTIC APPROACH TO MUSCLE PAIN

History

Is muscle pain – present at rest?
– Polymyalgia rheumatica
– Fibromyalgia
– Parkinson's disease
– Collagen vascular disease

present with exercise?
– Physiological
– Metabolic myopathies
– Benign myalgic encephalomyelitis (ME)

localised?
– Muscle haematoma, abscess, tumour or fibromyalgia

generalised?
– Polymyalgia rheumatica
– Parkinson's disease
– Metabolic myopathies
– Inflammatory myopathies
– Benign myalgic encephalomyelitis (ME)

family history?
– Metabolic myopathies

exposure to toxins?
– Drug induced myopathies
– Alcoholic myopathy

Examination

Is there – wasting/weakness?
– Inflammatory myopathies
– Metabolic myopathies
– Drug induced myopathies
– Alcoholic myopathy

skin rash?
– Inflammatory myopathy (dermatomyositis)
– Collagen vascular disease

stiffness or spasms?
– Tetanus
– Tetany
– Spasticity
– Neuroleptic malignant syndrome
– Malignant hyperthermia

muscle swelling?
– Muscle abscess, tumour
– Metabolic myopathy

MUSCLE PAIN (MYALGIA)

DIAGNOSTIC APPROACH TO MUSCLE PAIN (*cont'd*)

Investigations

Serum creatine kinase (muscle enzyme)
  – elevated in muscle necrosis, high levels result in myoglobinuria

Imaging (occasionally used)
  Ultrasound, MR or CT in suspected
                    muscle haematoma,
                    abscess or tumour.
  Radionuclide (Gallium or in suspected muscle abscess, Technitium)

Electromyography (EMG)
  Will confirm presence of myopathy (rarely more specific)

Muscle biopsy (needle or open)
  Essential in diagnosis of
    – inflammatory myopathies
    – metabolic myopathies
  Helpful in collagen vascular disease

Ischaemic lactate test
  Measurement of post exercise changes in serum lactate
  Reduced response in – metabolic myopathies (disorders of glycolytic pathway)

Following extensive investigation, in a significant number of cases no cause of myalgia is found.

Most disorders are covered in relevant sections. Those that are not are briefly described.

Fibromyalgia
A common condition of uncertain pathology in which generalised muscle pain with localised tender areas occurs without objective clinical or laboratory abnormalities. Psychiatric symptoms commonly co-exist.

Malignant hyperpyrexia
Characterised by a sudden rise in body temperature whilst undergoing general anaesthesia, usually with halothane or succinylcholine. Certain hereditary myopathic disorders, e.g. myotonic dystrophy, central core disease – are unduly prone to this condition.

Muscle abscess
Commonly Staphylococcal due to local trauma or blood-borne in debilitated persons.

Polymyalgia rheumatica
Proximal muscle pain encountered in the elderly and often associated with giant cell arteritis. The ESR is elevated and the EMG is normal. Muscle biopsy shows type 2 fibre loss. Steroids are effective.

Muscle tumours
These are rare. Mixed pathological and of varying degrees of malignancy

Benign myalgic encephalomyelitis (ME)
Characterised by exercise induced muscle pain. A puzzling disorder often occurring after viral illness, associated with fatigue, without clear diagnostic criteria and merging with depressive symptoms.

OUTCOME AFTER BRAIN DAMAGE

Outcome after brain damage has major social and financial implications for both patients and their families. In a welfare state, society may carry most, if not all of the financial burden, particularly with more severe disability. The greater the disability, the greater the support required. Conditions causing brain damage do not respect age; survivors may need long-term care.

A variety of methods have been devised to categorise outcome. Such classifications provide end-points for audit and research, and a means of assessing therapeutic intervention. They permit prediction based on clinical and investigative findings early in the course of the disease. Most outcome scales have been developed with a particular disease in mind (e.g. Bartel/Rankin – stroke, Karnofsky – tumour). In 1975 Jennett and Bond developed the Glasgow Outcome Scale (GOS) for the assessment of head injured patients, and this is now widely applied in the assessment of patients with other causes of brain damage.

The Glasgow Outcome Scale   Five categories exist –
1. Death
2. Persistent Vegetative State   – see below.
3. Severe Disability   – *dependent* for some support in every 24 hour period.
4. Moderate Disability   – *independent* but disabled. May or may not be capable
  of return to work.
5. Good recovery   – *good*, but not necessarily complete recovery. e.g. cranial nerve deficit.
  Could (although may not) return to work.

The Vegetative State
Severe bilateral hemisphere damage may result in a state in which the patient has no awareness of themselves or of their environment. Although periods of eye opening and closure may occur suggesting sleep/wake cycles, along with spontaneous movements of the face, trunk and limbs, the patient does not communicate or interact with others in any way.

The vegetative state becomes 'permanent' when irreversibility can be established with a high degree of certainty, i.e. > 6 months after non-traumatic coma and > 12 months after traumatic coma. At one month after *trauma*, about 1/3 of patients in the vegetative state will show some improvement over the subsequent year. After *non-traumatic coma*, outcome is much worse; only about 7% show some improvement and have severe disability.

Outcome Prediction
Outcome from **non-traumatic** coma depends on a variety of factors including the patient's *age*, the *duration* and *depth* of the coma, and the *cause* of the damage provided this is not drug induced.

		Poor outcome (GOS 1–3)	Favourable outcome (GOS 4–5)
	Infective metabolic	65%	35%
	Hypoxic – ischaemic	90%	10%
Duration	> 6 hours	85%	15%
Depth	Absent pupillary response at 24 hours	100%	0%
	Speaking, eye movements and reactive pupils at 2 hours	0%	100%

Outcome from **traumatic coma** see page 235.

BRAIN DEATH

The advent of improved intensive care facilities and more aggressive resuscitation techniques has led to an increase in numbers of patients with irreversible brain damage in which tissue oxygenation is maintained by a persistent heart beat and artificial ventilation.

A government working party has published guidelines for the diagnosis of brain death which, when fulfilled, indicate that recovery is impossible. In these patients, organs may be removed for transplantation before discontinuing ventilation.

The tests are designed to detect failure of *brain stem* function, but certain *preconditions* must first be met.

Preconditions

Depressant drugs must not contribute towards the patient's clinical state – if in doubt allow an adequate time interval to elapse to eliminate any possible persistent effect.

Hypothermia must not be a primary cause – ensure that temperature is not less than 35°C.

Severe *metabolic* or *endocrine* disturbance must be excluded as a possible cause of the patient's condition.

The patient must be on a ventilator as a result of inadequate spontaneous respiration or respiratory arrest – if a neuromuscular blocking drug has been used, exclude a prolonged effect by observing a muscle twitch on nerve stimulation, e.g. electrical stimulation of the median nerve should cause a thumb twitch.

The cause of the patient's condition must be established and this must be compatible with irreversible brain damage, e.g. severe head injury, spontaneous intracerebral haematoma. *If in doubt, delay brain death testing.*

BRAIN DEATH TESTS

PUPIL
RESPONSE

No pupil reaction to light

N.B. Ensure light intensity is adequate.

CORNEAL REFLEX

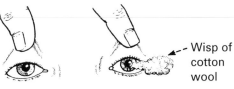

←– Wisp of cotton wool

No orbicularis oculi contraction in response to corneal stimulation.

VESTIBULO-OCULAR REFLEX

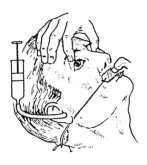

No eye movements occur when 50 ml of iced water are slowly injected into the external meatus. (Ensure that the external meatus is not occluded with wax or blood.) In coma with preserved brain stem function, the eyes tonically deviate towards the tested ear after a delay of 20 seconds. Maximal response is obtained with the head raised 30° from the horizontal.

GAG REFLEX

Suction tube

Bronchial stimulation (with a suction tube) fails to produce a 'cough' response.

213

BRAIN DEATH

MOTOR RESPONSE
No motor response in the face or in the muscle supplied by cranial nerves in response to a painful stimulus, e.g. supraorbital pain.

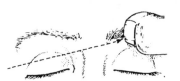

N.B. Limb responses are of no value in testing brain stem integrity. Movements can occur in response to limb or trunk stimulation (especially in the legs), and tendon reflexes may persist in a patient with brain stem death but intact cord function. Conversely, limb movements and reflexes may be absent in a patient with an intact brain stem and spinal cord damage.

RESPIRATORY MOVEMENTS
No respiratory movements are observed when the patient is disconnected from the ventilator. During this test, anoxia is prevented by passing 6 litres O_2 per minute down the endotracheal tube. This should maintain adequate PO_2 levels for up to 10 minutes. N.B. Ensure that apnoea is not a result of a low PCO_2. This should be greater than 6.65 kPa (50 mmHg).

Clinician's status
The British recommendations state that these tests should be carried out by two doctors, both with expertise in the field; one of consultant status, the other of consultant or senior trainee status. The doctors may carry out the tests individually or together.

Test repetition and timing
The test should be repeated but the interval should be left to the discretion of the clinician. The initial test may be performed within a few hours of the causal event, but in most instances is delayed for 12–24 hours, or longer if there is any doubt about the preconditions.

Timing of death
Certification of death occurs when brain death is established, i.e. at the time of the second test. Old concepts of death occurring at the time the heart ceases to beat are no longer applicable.

Supplementary investigations
Electroencephalography (EEG) is of no value in diagnosing brain death. Some patients with the potential to recover show a 'flat' trace; in others with irreversible brain stem damage, electrical activity can occasionally be recorded from the scalp electrodes.

Similarly, angiography or cerebral blood flow measurement are of no additional value to the clinical tests described above, provided the preconditions are fulfilled.

LOCALISED NEUROLOGICAL DISEASE AND ITS MANAGEMENT

A. INTRACRANIAL

HEAD INJURY

INTRODUCTION

Many patients attend accident and emergency departments with head injury. Approximately 300 per 100 000 of the population per year require hospital admission; of these 9 per 100 000 die, i.e. 5000 patients per year in Britain. Some of these deaths are inevitable, some are potentially preventable.

The principal causes of head injury include road traffic accidents, falls, assaults and injuries occurring at work, in the home and during sports. The relative frequency of each cause varies between different age groups and from place to place throughout the country.

Head injuries from road traffic accidents are most common in young males; alcohol is frequently involved. Road traffic accidents, although only constituting about 25% of all patients with head injury, are the cause of more serious injuries. This cause contributes to 60% of the deaths from head injury; of these, half die before reaching hospital.

In many countries preventative and punitive measures controlling alcohol levels and the use of seat belts, air bags and crash helmets have reduced the incidence. Once a head injury has occurred, nothing can alter the impact damage. The aim of head injury management is to minimise damage arising from secondary complications.

PATHOLOGY

Imaging permits the categorisation of brain damage into *focal* and *diffuse*, although often both types co-exist. Alternatively brain damage can be classified as *primary* occurring at impact, or *secondary* from ongoing neuronal damage, haematoma, brain swelling, ischaemia or infection.

FOCAL DAMAGE

Cortical contusions and lacerations

These may occur under or opposite (contre-coup) the site of impact, but most commonly involve the frontal and temporal lobes. Contusions are usually multiple and may occur bilaterally. Multiple contusions do not in themselves contribute to depression of conscious level, but this may arise when bleeding into the contusions produces a space-occupying haematoma.

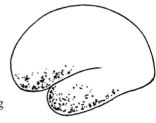

Intracranial haematoma

Intracranial bleeding may occur either outside (extradural) or within the dura (intradural).

Intradural lesions usually consist of a mixture of both subdural and intracerebral haematomas although pure subdurals occur in a proportion. Brain damage is caused directly or indirectly as a result of tentorial or tonsillar herniation.

Incidence of haematoma:
Extradural – 27%
Intradural:
Pure subdural – 26%
Intracerebral.
± subdural – 38%
Extra- + Intradural – 8%

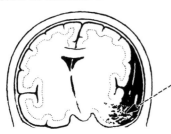

Intracerebral ± subdural (burst lobe)

Contusions in the frontal and temporal lobes often lead to bleeding into the brain substance, usually associated with an overlying subdural haematoma.

'Burst lobe' is a term sometimes used to describe the appearance of intracerebral haematoma mixed with necrotic brain tissue, rupturing out into the subdural space.

HEAD INJURY

FOCAL DAMAGE (*cont'd*)

Subdural

In some patients impact may rupture bridging veins from the cortical surface to the venous sinuses producing a pure subdural haematoma with no evidence of underlying cortical contusion or laceration.

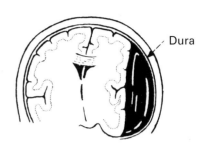

Dura

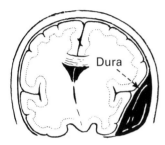

Dura

Extradural

A skull fracture tearing the middle meningeal vessels bleeds into the extradural space. This usually occurs in the temporal or temporoparietal region. Occasionally extradural haematomas result from damage to the sagittal or transverse sinus.

Tentorial/tonsillar herniation (syn. 'cone')

It is unlikely that high intracranial pressure alone directly damages neuronal tissue, but brain damage occurs as a result of tonsillar or tentorial herniation (see page 79). A progressive increase in intracranial pressure due to a supratentorial haematoma initially produces midline shift. Herniation of the medial temporal lobe through the tentorial hiatus follows (*lateral tentorial herniation*), causing midbrain compression and damage. Uncontrolled lateral tentorial herniation or diffuse bilateral hemispheric swelling will result in *central tentorial herniation*. Herniation of the cerebellar tonsils through the foramen magnum (*tonsillar herniation*) and consequent lower brainstem compression may follow central tentorial herniation or may result from the infrequently occurring traumatic posterior fossa haematoma.

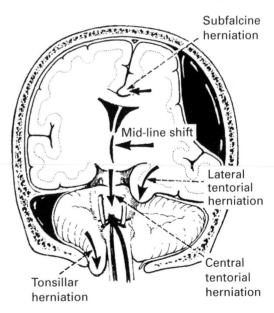

Subfalcine herniation

Mid-line shift

Lateral tentorial herniation

Central tentorial herniation

Tonsillar herniation

Infection

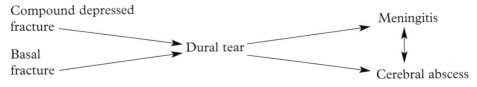

Compound depressed fracture

Basal fracture

Dural tear

Meningitis

Cerebral abscess

The presence of a dural tear provides a potential route for infection. This seldom occurs within 48 hours of injury. Meningitis may develop after several months or years.

HEAD INJURY

DIFFUSE DAMAGE

Diffuse axonal injury

Shearing forces cause immediate mechanical damage to axons. Over the subsequent 48 hours, further damage results from release of excitotoxic neurotransmitters which cause Ca^{2+} influx into cells and triggers the phospholipid cascade (page 243). Genetic susceptibility conferred by the presence of the APOE ε4 gene may also play a part. Depending on the severity of the injury, effects may range from mild coma to death.

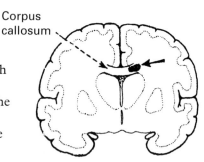

Corpus callosum

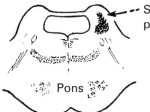

Superior cerebellar peduncle

Pons

The *macrosopic* appearance may appear entirely normal but in some patients pathological sections reveal small haemorrhagic tears, particularly in the corpus callosum or in the superior cerebellar peduncle.

Microscopic evidence of neuronal damage depends on the duration of survival and on the severity of the injury. After a few days, retraction balls and microglial clusters are seen in the white matter.

Retraction balls reflect axonal damage. Note only axons in one plane are involved, indicating the direction of the 'shear'

Microglial clusters (hypertrophied microglia) are found diffusely throughout the white matter

If the patient survives 5 weeks or more after injury then appropriate staining demonstrates Wallerian degeneration of the long tracts and white matter of the cerebral hemispheres. Even a minor injury causing a transient loss of consciousness produces some neuronal damage. Since neuronal regeneration is limited, the effects of repeated minor injury are cumulative.

Cerebral swelling

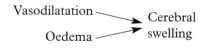

Vasodilatation
Oedema
→ Cerebral swelling

This may occur with or without focal damage. It results from either vascular engorgement or an increase in extra- or intracellular fluid. The exact causative mechanism remains unknown

Cerebral ischaemia

Cerebral ischaemia commonly occurs after severe head injury and is caused by either hypoxia or impaired cerebral perfusion. In the normal subject, a fall in blood pressure does not produce a drop in cerebral perfusion since 'autoregulation' results in cerebral vasodilatation. After head injury, however, autoregulation is often defective and hypotension may have more drastic effects. Glutamate excess and free radical accumulation may also contribute to neuronal damage (see page 243).

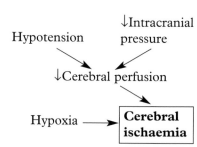

Hypotension ↓Intracranial pressure
↓Cerebral perfusion
Hypoxia → **Cerebral ischaemia**

HEAD INJURY – CLINICAL ASSESSMENT

MULTIPLE INJURY – PRIORITIES OF ASSESSMENT

Patients admitted in coma with multiple injuries require urgent care and the clinician must be aware of the priorities of assessment and management.

Airway
Check for obstruction and use oropharyngeal airway or endotracheal tube. ⟶

Breathing
Administer oxygen and check respiratory movements are adequate; if not, ventilate.

↓

Chest/abdominal injury
Examine chest for possible flail segment ⟵ or haemo/pneumothorax. Examine abdomen for possible bleeding; if in doubt, use peritoneal lavage. (X-ray chest and abdomen.)

Circulation
Check pulse and blood pressure. If patient is hypotensive, replace blood loss with IV fluids followed by whole blood if Hb <10 g/l.

↓

Head/spinal injury
Assess conscious level and focal signs. ⟶ Consider possibility of spinal injury. (X-ray skull and spine, CT scan.)

Limb injury
Examine limbs for lacerations and fractures. (X-ray.)

When intracranial haematoma is suscepted, a CT scan is essential, especially before clinical signs are masked by a general anaesthetic required for the management of limb or abdominal injuries. However, if difficulty occurs in maintaining blood pressure, then urgent laparotomy or thoracotomy would take precedence over further investigation of a possible intracranial haematoma.

HEAD INJURY – ASSESSMENT

Some patients may describe the events leading to and following head injury, but often the doctor depends on descriptions from witnesses.

Points to determine:

Period of loss of consciousness: Relates to severity of diffuse brain damage and may range from a few seconds to several weeks.

Period of post-traumatic amnesia: This is the period of permanent amnesia occurring after head injury. It also reflects the severity of damage and in severe injuries may last several weeks. (Period of retrograde amnesia, i.e. amnesia for events before the injury is of less value since it bears no relation to the severity of injury and may improve with time.)

Cause and circumstances of the injury: The patient may collapse, or crash his vehicle as a result of some preceding intracranial event, e.g. subarachnoid haemorrhage or epileptic seizure. The more 'violent' the injury, the greater the risk of associated extracranial injuries.

Presence of headache and vomiting: These are common symptoms after head injury. If they persist, the possibility of intracranial haematoma must be considered.

HEAD INJURY – CLINICAL ASSESSMENT

EXAMINATION

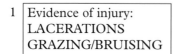

1 | Evidence of injury:
LACERATIONS
GRAZING/BRUISING

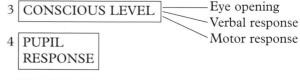

3 | CONSCIOUS LEVEL — Eye opening / Verbal response / Motor response

4 | PUPIL RESPONSE

2 | BASAL FRACTURE SIGNS   5 | LIMB WEAKNESS   6 | EYE MOVEMENTS

1. Lacerations and bruising

The presence of these features confirms the occurrence of a head injury, but traumatic intracranial haematoma can occur in patients with no external evidence of injury.

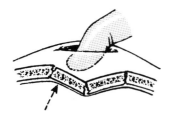

Always explore deep lacerations with a gloved finger for evidence of a *depressed fracture*.

Beware of falling into the trap of diagnosing a depressed fracture when only scalp haematoma is present.

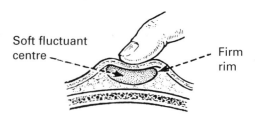

Soft fluctuant centre ---   Firm rim

Consider the possibility of a hyperextension injury to the cervical spine if frontal laceration or bruising is present.

2. Basal skull fracture

Clinical features indicate the presence of a basal skull fracture which may not be evident on routine skull X-ray or even on specific views of the skull base. If present, a potential route of infection exists with the concomitant risk of meningitis.

ANTERIOR FOSSA FRACTURE

CSF rhinorrhoea

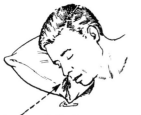

If the nasal discharge contains glucose, then the fluid is CSF rather than mucin.

Bilateral periorbital haematoma

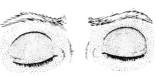

Bruising limited to the orbital margins indicates blood tracking from behind.

Subconjunctival haemorrhage

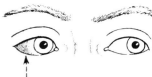

Bruising under conjunctiva extending to posterior limits of the sclera indicates blood tracking from orbital cavity.

HEAD INJURY – CLINICAL ASSESSMENT

Basal skull fracture (*cont'd*)

PETROUS FRACTURE

Bleeding from the external auditory meatus or CSF otorrhoea:

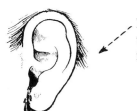

Blood or *CSF* leaking through a torn tympanic membrane must be differentiated from a laceration of the external meatus.

Battle's sign:
Bruising over the mastoid
may take 24–48 hours to develop.

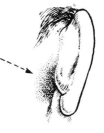

3. Conscious level

Assess patient's conscious level in terms of *eye opening*, *verbal* and *motor response* on admission (see page 5) and record at regular intervals thereafter. An observation chart incorporating these features is essential and clearly shows the trend in the patient's condition. Deterioration in conscious level indicates the need for immediate investigation and action where appropriate.

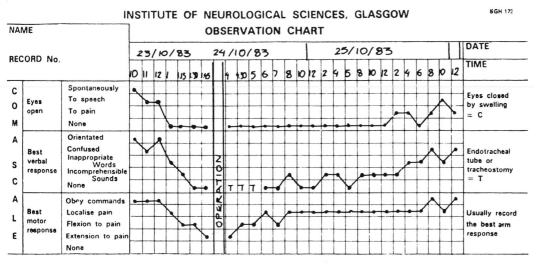

Reproduced by permission of the Nursing Times

HEAD INJURY – CLINICAL ASSESSMENT

4. Pupil response
The light reflex (page 140) tests optic (II) and oculomotor (III) nerve function. Although II nerve dysfunction after head injury is important to record and may result in permanent visual impairment, it is the III nerve function which is the most useful indicator of an expanding intracranial lesion. Herniation of the medial temporal lobe through the tentorial hiatus directly damages the III nerve resulting in pupil dilatation with impaired or absent reaction to light. The *pupil dilates on the side of the expanding lesion* and is an important localising sign. With a further increase in intracranial pressure, bilateral III nerve palsies may occur.

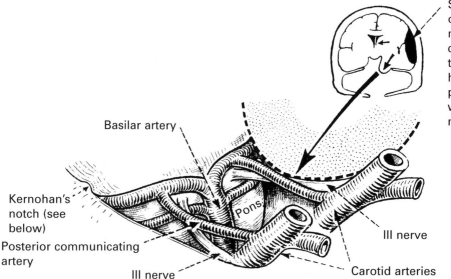

Space-occupying mass causing tentorial herniation presents with a III nerve palsy

Basilar artery

Kernohan's notch (see below)

Posterior communicating artery

III nerve

Pons

III nerve

Carotid arteries

5. Limb weakness
Determine limb weakness by comparing the response in each limb to painful stimuli (page 30). Hemiparesis or hemiplegia usually occurs in the limbs contralateral to the side of the lesion but may also occur in the ipsilateral limbs. This is due to indentation of the contralateral cerebral peduncle by the edge of the tentorium cerebelli (Kernohan's notch). Limb deficits are therefore of limited value in localising the site of the lesion.

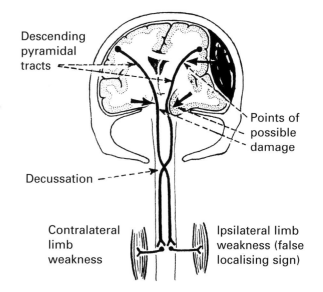

Descending pyramidal tracts

Points of possible damage

Decussation

Contralateral limb weakness

Ipsilateral limb weakness (false localising sign)

HEAD INJURY – CLINICAL ASSESSMENT

6. Eye movements

Evaluation of eye movements does not help in immediate management, but provides a useful prognostic guide.

Eye movements may occur spontaneously, or can be elicited reflexly (page 30) by head rotation (oculocephalic reflex) or by caloric stimulation (oculovestibular reflex).

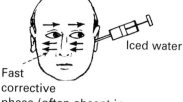

SPONTANEOUS   OCULOCEPHALIC (Doll's eye) REFLEX   OCULOVESTIBULAR REFLEX

Iced water

Fast corrective phase (often absent in the comatose patient)

Abnormal eye movements may result from: brainstem dysfunction, damage to the nerves supplying the extraocular muscles or damage to the vestibular apparatus. Absent eye movements relate to low levels of responsiveness and indicate a gloomy prognosis.

Vital signs

At the beginning of the century, the eminent neurosurgeon Harvey Cushing noted that a rise in intracranial pressure led to a rise in blood pressure and a fall in pulse rate and produced abnormal respiratory patterns. In the past, much emphasis has been placed on close observation of these vital signs in patients with head injury. These changes, however, may not occur and when present are usually preceded by deterioration in conscious level. This last observation is therefore more relevant.

Cranial nerve lesions

Basal skull fracture or extracranial injury can result in damage to the cranial nerves. Evidence of this damage must be recorded but, with the exception of a III nerve lesion, does not usually help immediate management. Full cranial nerve examination is difficult in the comatose patient and this can await patient co-operation.

Clinical assessment cannot reliably distinguish the type or even the site of intracranial haematoma, but is invaluable in indicating the need for further investigation and in providing a baseline against which any change can be compared.

HEAD INJURY – INVESTIGATION AND ADMISSION CRITERIA

IN THE ACCIDENT AND EMERGENCY DEPARTMENT

If an emergency CT scan is *not* planned –

X-ray the skull if:
(plus cervical spine, chest, abdomen, pelvis and limbs if required)

– conscious level is impaired at the time of examination or if the patient has lost consciousness at any time since the injury
– neurological symptoms or signs are present
– CSF leak from the nose (rhinorrhoea) or ear (otorrhoea)
– penetrating injury is suspect
– significant scalp bruising or swelling
– patient assessment is difficult (e.g. alcohol intoxication).

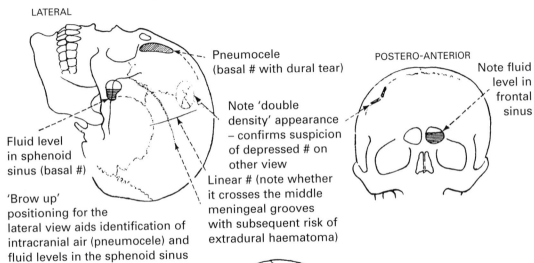

LATERAL

Pneumocele (basal # with dural tear)

Note 'double density' appearance – confirms suspicion of depressed # on other view

Linear # (note whether it crosses the middle meningeal grooves with subsequent risk of extradural haematoma)

Fluid level in sphenoid sinus (basal #)

'Brow up' positioning for the lateral view aids identification of intracranial air (pneumocele) and fluid levels in the sphenoid sinus

POSTERO-ANTERIOR

Note fluid level in frontal sinus

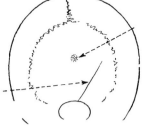

TOWNE'S
Pineal shift is occasionally observed, indicating the presence of a mass (but beware, a rotated film is misleading)

A Towne's view is essential, otherwise occipital # will be missed

Some units recommend CT scanning for all patients with head injury. Such resources are not always available. For patients in whom a CT scan is not immediately planned, a skull fracture identifies those at high risk of intracranial haematoma. In those patients, CT scan is essential (see page 225).

Risk of intracranial haematoma (requiring removal) in adults attending A & E departments after head injury.		
No skull #	– orientated	1 in 6000
No skull #	– not orientated	1 in 120
Skull #	– orientated	1 in 32
Skull #	– not orientated	1 in 4

Adapted with permission Mendelow et al 1983
ii: 1173–1176 British Medical Journal

HEAD INJURY – INVESTIGATION AND ADMISSION CRITERIA

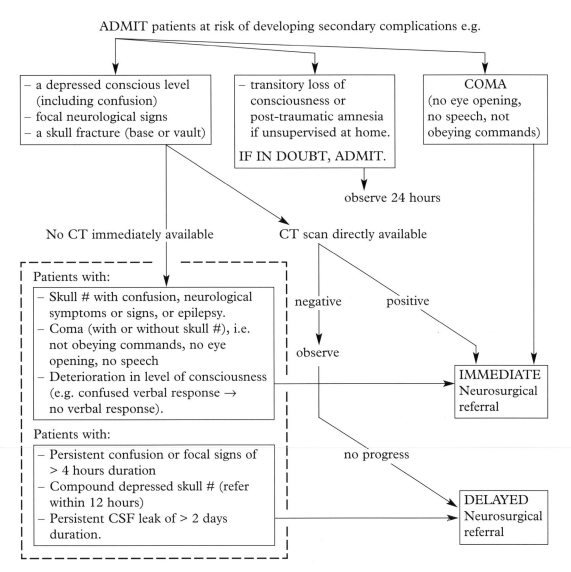

ADMIT patients at risk of developing secondary complications e.g.

- a depressed conscious level (including confusion)
- focal neurological signs
- a skull fracture (base or vault)

– transitory loss of consciousness or post-traumatic amnesia if unsupervised at home.

IF IN DOUBT, ADMIT.

COMA (no eye opening, no speech, not obeying commands)

observe 24 hours

No CT immediately available

CT scan directly available

Patients with:
- Skull # with confusion, neurological symptoms or signs, or epilepsy.
- Coma (with or without skull #), i.e. not obeying commands, no eye opening, no speech
- Deterioration in level of consciousness (e.g. confused verbal response → no verbal response).

Patients with:
- Persistent confusion or focal signs of > 4 hours duration
- Compound depressed skull # (refer within 12 hours)
- Persistent CSF leak of > 2 days duration.

negative   positive

observe

no progress

IMMEDIATE Neurosurgical referral

DELAYED Neurosurgical referral

Transfer to the neurosurgical unit

Prior to the transfer, ensure that resuscitation is complete, and that more immediate problems have been dealt with (see page 219). Insert an oropharyngeal airway. Intubate and ventilate if the patient is in coma or if the blood gases are inadequate ($PO_2 < 8\,kPa$ on air, $13\,kPa$ on O_2 or $CO_2 > 6\,kPa$). If the patient's conscious level is deteriorating, an intravenous bolus infusion of 100 ml of 20% mannitol should 'buy time' by temporarily reducing the intracranial pressure.

NOTE: for comatose patients with an unstable systemic state from multiple injuries, a negative CT scan in the local hospital may avoid a dangerous transfer to the neurosurgical unit.

HEAD INJURY – INVESTIGATION

CT scan in head injury

Scans must extend from the posterior fossa to the vertex, otherwise haematomas in these sites will be missed.

EXTRADURAL haematoma –
area of increased density,
convex inwards.
Spread limited by dural
adhesion to skull

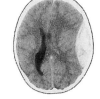

Midline shift with compression
of ipsilateral ventricle

SUBDURAL haematoma – area of increased
density spreading around surface of cerebral
hemisphere. Subdural haematomas become
isodense with brain 10–20 days following
injury and hypodense thereafter.

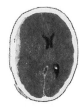

The contralateral
ventricle often dilates
due to obstruction at
the foramen of Munro

INTRACEREBRAL haematoma – 'BURST
LOBE' (± subdural haematoma) – appears
as an irregular area of increased density
(blood clot) surrounded by area of low
density (oedematous brain).

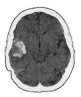

overlying
subdural
haematoma

'Burst'
temporal
lobe

Whether a haematoma is present or not, look at the *basal cisterns*.

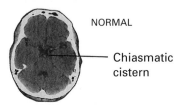

NORMAL

Chiasmatic
cistern

Obliteration of one
or both cisterns
indicates raised
intracranial pressure
with brain shift from
an expanding mass
or hemispheric
swelling

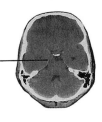

With *diffuse shearing injuries*, small haematomas may be seen on CT scan scattered throughout the white matter, particularly in the corpus callosum, the subcortical white matter and in the brainstem adjacent to the cerebellar peduncles.

If *hydrocephalus* is present on the upper scan cuts, look carefully for a haematoma (extradural, subdural or intracerebral) in the posterior fossa, compressing and obstructing the 4th ventricle.

Further investigation may be required to exclude other coincidental or contributory causes of the head injury, e.g. drugs, alcohol, postictal state, encephalitis (Cause of coma, see page 84).

HEAD INJURY – MANAGEMENT

Management aims at preventing the development of secondary brain damage from intracranial haematoma, ischaemia, raised intracranial pressure with tentorial or tonsillar herniation and infection.

– Ensure the *airway is patent* and that *blood oxygenation is adequate. Intubation* is advisable in patients 'flexing to pain' or worse. *Ventilation* may be required if respiratory movements are depressed or lung function is impaired, e.g. 'flail' segment, aspiration pneumonia, pulmonary contusion or fat emboli. Hypoxia can cause direct cerebral damage, but in addition causes vasodilatation resulting in an increase in cerebral blood volume with subsequent rise in ICP.

– A *space-occupying haematoma requires urgent evacuation* (see over). If the patient's conscious level is deteriorating, give an initial or repeat i.v. bolus of mannitol (100 ml of 20%). Coagulation should be checked and any deficits corrected.

– Scalp *lacerations* require cleaning, inspection to exclude an underlying depressed fracture and suturing.

– *Correct hypovolaemia* following blood loss – but avoid fluid overload as this may aggravate cerebral oedema. In adults, 2 litres/day of fluid is sufficient. Commence nasogastric fluids or oral fluids when feasible.

– *Anticonvulsants* (e.g. fosphenytoin) must be given intravenously if seizures occur; further seizures and in particular status epilepticus significantly increase the risk of cerebral anoxia.

– *Monitor intracranial pressure (ICP), blood pressure and cerebral perfusion pressure (CPP)* in selected patients with diffuse swelling or after evacuation of an intracranial haematoma. Maintain CPP either by raising blood pressure or by treating raised intracranial pressure (see below).

– *Brain protective agents* include corticosteroids, free radical scavengers, calcium channel blockers, and glutamate antagonists. The evolution of axonal damage after a diffuse shearing injury may provide a window of opportunity for treatment and experimental animal studies have revealed encouraging results. Trials of these agents in head-injured patients however, have failed to show efficacy, perhaps due to insufficient patient numbers or a failure to target treatment at appropriate patients. An ongoing study of corticosteroids hopes to recruit 20 000 patients.

– *Operative repair of a dural defect* is required if the CSF leak persists for more than 7 days. (Many still use *prophylactic antibiotics* in patients with a CSF leak, but there is no conclusive evidence of their efficacy and they may do more harm than good by encouraging the growth of resistant organisms.) The development of meningitis requires prompt treatment with an empirical antibiotic.

HEAD INJURY – MANAGEMENT

INTRACRANIAL HAEMATOMA
Most intracranial haematomas require urgent evacuation – evident from the patient's clinical state combined with the CT scan appearance of a space-occupying mass.

Extradural haematoma
Using the CT scan the position of the extradural haematoma is accurately delineated and a 'horse shoe' craniotomy flap is turned over this area, allowing complete evacuation of the haematoma. For low temporal extradural haematomas, a 'question mark' flap may be more suitable. If patient deterioration is rapid, a burr hole and craniectomy positioned centrally over the haematoma may provide temporary relief, but this seldom provides adequate decompression.

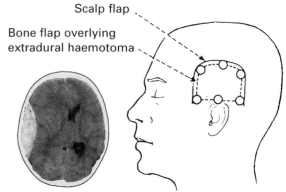

Scalp flap

Bone flap overlying extradural haemotoma

Subdural/intracerebral haematoma ('burst lobe')
Subdural and intracerebral haematomas usually arise from lacerations on the under-surface of the frontal and/or temporal lobes. Again the CT scan is useful in demonstrating the exact site. A 'question mark' flap permits good access to both frontal and temporal 'burst' lobes. The subdural collection is evacuated and any underlying intracerebral haematoma is removed along with necrotic brain.

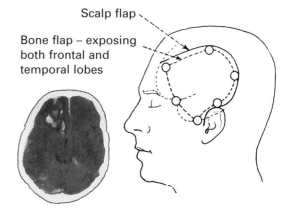

Scalp flap

Bone flap – exposing both frontal and temporal lobes

N.B. Burr holes are insufficient to evacuate an acute subdural haematoma or to deal with any underlying cortical damage.

Conservative management of traumatic intracranial haematomas
Not all patients with traumatic intracranial haematomas deteriorate. In some, the haematomas are small and clearly do not require evacuation. In others, however, the decision to operate or not proves difficult, e.g. the CT scan may reveal a moderate-sized haematoma with minimal or no mass effect in a conscious but confused patient.

If conservative management is adopted, careful observation in a neurosurgical unit is essential. Any deterioration indicates the need for immediate operation. In this group of patients, intracranial pressure monitoring may serve as a useful guide. An intracranial pressure of 30 mmHg or more suggests that haematoma evacuation is required as the likelihood of subsequent deterioration with continued conservative management would be high.

HEAD INJURY – MANAGEMENT

TREATMENT OF RAISED INTRACRANIAL PRESSURE (ICP)

Raised ICP in the absence of any easily treatable condition (e.g. intracranial haematoma or raised pCO_2) requires careful management. The various techniques used to lower ICP have already been described (page 81–82) but these must not be applied indiscriminately.

Studies have failed to confirm that active treatment of raised ICP following head injury improves outcome. Failure to show benefit from ICP treatment in the past may have resulted from a 'blind' use of hyperventilation. The vasoconstriction produced by lowering the pCO_2 reduces ICP by reducing intracranial blood volume. But vasoconstriction may reduce cerebral blood flow to ischaemic levels. Previous advice on the use of a jugular bulb O_2 saturation monitor to measure the amount of O_2 taken up by the brain (arteriovenous oxygen difference ($AVDO_2$)) and guide the safety of hyperventilation, no longer applies, since it is now established that hyperventilation of head injured patients does more harm (from cerebral ischaemia) than good.

Recent studies show that head injured patients nursed in a modern ITU are still at risk of sustaining potentially harmful 'insults' to the brain in the first few days after head injury including high ICP, low BP, low cerebral perfusion pressure (CPP), hypoxaemia or raised temperature. The maintenance of cerebral perfusion pressure is probably as important as treating raised ICP and this should be maintained at more than 70mmHg.

Patient selection for ICP monitoring: Monitoring ICP and CPP is most relevant in patients with a flexion response or worse to painful stimuli (a response of 'localising to pain' signifies a milder degree of injury and spontaneous recovery is likely). Such patients may have already undergone removal of an intracranial haematoma or may have had no mass lesion on CT scan (i.e. diffuse injury or contusional damage). Each neurosurgical unit is likely to have its own policy for ICP monitoring but the following outline may serve as a guide.

If **ICP high** (e.g. > 25 mmHg)
    & BP low (e.g. mean < 100 mmHg) → measure central venous pressure (CVP) or insert Swan Ganz catheter.

      – if CVP low → give plasma volume expanders e.g. haemacel (do not use mannitol)

      – if CVP normal → give inotropic agents (e.g. dobutamine)

      Aim for CPP > 65–70 mmHg

If **ICP high,**
    & BP normal → give hypnotics e.g. Propofol, Etomidate. (see page 82)

      Aim for CPP > 65–70 mmHg

      Do *not* hyperventilate

HEAD INJURY – MANAGEMENT

DIFFUSE BRAIN DAMAGE/NEGATIVE CT SCAN

A proportion of patients have no intracranial haematoma on CT scan or have only a small haematoma or contusion without mass effect.

In these patients, coma or impairment of conscious level may be due to:

– *diffuse axonal injury* – suspect if conscious level impaired from impact.

– *cerebral ischaemic damage*
– *cerebral swelling*   suspect if deterioration is delayed – a patient who talks
– *fat emboli*   after impact does not have a significant shearing injury.
– *meningitis*

Several of these factors may coexist and contribute to brain damage in patients with intracranial haematoma.

The management principles outlined above apply; in particular it is essential to ensure that respiratory function is adequate and that cerebral perfusion pressure is maintained.

Fat emboli usually occur a few days after injury and may be related to fracture manipulation; deterioration of respiratory function usually accompanies cerebral damage and most patients require ventilation.

Meningitis may occur several days after injury in the presence of basal fractures.

Cerebral swelling may occur at any time after injury and cause a rise in intracranial pressure.

REPEAT CT SCANNING

Indications:

Delayed deterioration in clinical state
Maintained rise in ICP   in patients with diffuse injury or following
            or   evacuation of an intracranial haematoma
Failure to improve after 48 hours

Occasionally, small areas of 'insignificant' contusion on an initial CT scan may develop into a space-occupying haematoma requiring evacuation. Following haematoma evacuation, recollection may occur in 5–10% of cases.

DEPRESSED SKULL FRACTURE

This injury is caused by a blow from a sharp object. Since diffuse 'deceleration' damage is minimal, patients seldom lose consciousness.

SIMPLE DEPRESSED FRACTURE (closed injury)
There is no overlying laceration and no risk of infection. Operation is not required except for cosmetic reasons. Removal of any bone spicules imbedded in brain tissue does not reverse neuronal damage.

COMPOUND DEPRESSED FRACTURE (open injury)
A scalp laceration is related to (but does not necessarily overlie) the depressed bone segments. A compound depressed fracture with an associated dural tear may result in meningitis or cerebral abscess.

Investigation
Double density appearance on *skull X-ray* suggests depression but tangential views may be required to establish the diagnosis. Impairment of conscious level or the presence of focal signs indicate the need for a *CT scan* to exclude underlying extradural haematoma or severe cortical contusion. Selecting bone window levels on CT scan will clearly demonstrate any depressed fragments.

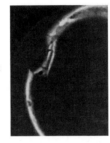

'Bony' window levels on CT scan clearly demonstrate the depressed fragments

Management

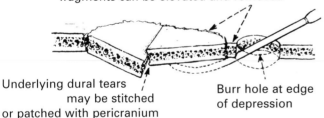

Bone edges nibbled away until fragments can be elevated and removed

Underlying dural tears may be stitched or patched with pericranium

Burr hole at edge of depression

Treatment aims to minimise the risk of infection. The wound is debrided and the fragments elevated within 24 hours from injury. Bone fragments are either removed or replaced after washing with antiseptic. Antibiotics are not essential unless the wound is excessively dirty.

If the venous sinuses are involved in the depressed fracture, then operative risks from excessive bleeding may outweigh the risk of infection and antibiotic treatment alone is given.

Complications
Most patients make a rapid and full recovery, but a few develop complications:

Infection: May lead to meningitis or abscess formation. Some believe that operation does not reduce the infection risk and advocate a conservative approach unless contamination is severe.

Epilepsy: Early epilepsy (in the first week) occurs in 10% of patients with depressed fracture. Late epilepsy develops in 15% overall, but is especially common when the dura is torn, when focal signs are present, when post-traumatic amnesia exceeds 24 hours or when early epilepsy has occurred (the risk ranges from 3 to 60%, depending on the number of the above factors involved). Elevation of the bone fragments does not alter the incidence of epilepsy.

231

DELAYED EFFECTS OF HEAD INJURY

POST-TRAUMATIC EPILEPSY

Early epilepsy (occurring within the first week from injury)

Early epilepsy occurs in 5% of patients admitted to hospital with non-missile (i.e. deceleration) injuries. It is particularly frequent in the first 24 hours after injury. Focal seizures are as common as generalised seizures. Status epilepticus occurs in 10%.

The risk of early epilepsy is high in

– children under 5 years.
– patients with prolonged post-traumatic amnesia
– patients with an intracranial haematoma
– patients with a compound depressed fracture.

Late epilepsy (occurring after the first week from injury)

Late epilepsy also occurs in about 5% of all patients admitted to hospital after head injury. It usually presents in the first year, but in some the first attack occurs as long as 10 years from the injury. Usually seizures are generalised, but temporal lobe epilepsy (complex partial seizures) occurs in 20%. Late epilepsy is prevalent in patients with

– early epilepsy (25%)
– intracranial haematoma (35%)
– compound depressed fracture (17%).

Prophylactic anticonvulsants appear to be of little benefit in preventing the development of an epileptogenic focus. Management is discussed on page 100.

CEREBROSPINAL FLUID (CSF) LEAK

After head injury a basal fracture may cause a fistulous communication between the CSF space and the paranasal sinuses or the middle ear. Profuse CSF leaks (rhinorrhoea or otorrhoea) are readily detectable, but brain may partially plug the defect and the leak may be minimal or absent. Patients risk developing meningitis particularly in the first week, but in some this occurs after several years. When this is associated with anterior fossa fractures, it is usually pneumococcal; when associated with fractures through the petrous bone, a variety of organisms may be involved.

Clinical signs of a basal fracture have previously been described (page 220). The patient may comment on a 'salty taste' in the mouth. Anosmia suggests avulsion of the olfactory bulb from the cribriform plate.

Management

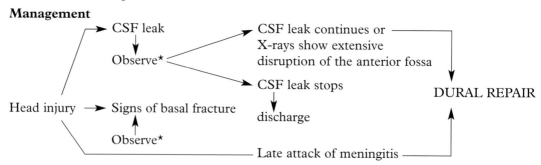

*A recent Working Party concluded that evidence does not support the use of prophylactic antibiotics (Lancet (1994) 344:1547–1551). Prophylactic antibiotics only encourage resistance and late attacks of meningitis may still occur despite their use.

DELAYED EFFECTS OF HEAD INJURY

CSF LEAK (*cont'd*)

Preoperative investigations

Coronal high definition CT scanning should identify the fracture site.

CT cisternography – CT scanning after running contrast injected into the lumbar theca, up to the basal cisterns may identify the exact site of the leak.

CSF isotope infusion studies combined with pledget insertion into the nasal recesses may also be of value, but results can be misleading.

Operation

As fractures of the anterior fossa often extend across the midline, a bifrontal exploration is required. The dural tear is repaired with fascia lata, pericranium or synthetic dural substitute. A CSF leak through the middle ear requires a subtemporal approach.

Failure to repair a CSF fistula may result from impaired CSF absorption with an intermittent or persistent elevation of ICP. In these patients a CSF shunt may be required.

POSTCONCUSSIONAL SYMPTOMS

Even after relatively minor head injury, patients may have persistent symptoms of:
- headache, dizziness and increased irritability
- difficulty in concentration and in coping with work
- fatigue and depression.

This condition was once thought to have a purely psychological basis, but it is now recognised that in an injury of sufficient severity to cause loss of consciousness, or a period of post-traumatic amnesia, some neuronal damage occurs; studies show a distinct delay in information processing in these patients, requiring several weeks to resolve. Vestibular 'concussion' (end-organ damage) may contribute to the symptomatology ('dizziness' and vertigo).

CUMULATIVE BRAIN DAMAGE

The effects of repeated neuronal damage are cumulative; when this exceeds the capacity for compensation, permanent evidence of brain damage ensues. The 'punch-drunk' state is well recognised in boxers; dementia may also occur from repeated head injury in jockeys.

DELAYED EFFECTS OF HEAD INJURY

CRANIAL NERVE DAMAGE

Cranial nerve damage occurs in about one-third of patients with severe head injury, but treatment is seldom of benefit. These lesions may contribute towards the patient's residual disability.

Nerve	Cause of damage	Clinical problem	Management	Prognosis
I	Usually associated with anterior fossa fracture and CSF rhinorrhoea	Anosmia	Nil	Recovery often occurs in a few months
II	Optic nerve usually damaged in the optic foramen Chiasmal damage occasionally occurs. [N.B. Visual loss may also occur from damage to the globe, occipital cortex or optic radiations]	Visual loss or field defect in one eye Bitemporal hemianopia.	Nil Local eye/orbital damage may need treatment	Recovery seldom occurs
III IV VI	III nerve damage usually results from tentorial herniation but can also occur in fractures involving the superior orbital fissure or cavernous sinus IV nerve damage is uncommon VI nerve damage is usually associated with fractures of the petrous or sphenoid bones	Pupil inequality, ptosis and disturbance of ocular movements	Nil [other than removing cause of tentorial herniation]	Recovery usually occurs
V	Occasionally follows petrous or sphenoid fractures	Facial numbness	Nil	Usually permanent
VII	Associated with petrous fracture	Immediate or delayed facial palsy	Otologists occasionally recommend decompression. Early steroid therapy may benefit	Immediate lesions have a poor prognosis; delayed lesions usually recover
VIII	Petrous fracture may damage: – nerve – cochlea – ossicles Haemotympanum may result	Vertigo, 'dizziness', hearing loss, tinnitus	Ossicular damage may benefit from operation	Vestibular symptoms usually improve after several weeks. Nerve deafness is usually permanent. Conductive deafness from haemotympanum should gradually improve
IX, X XI, XII	Associated with very severe basal fractures or extracranial injury	Patient seldom survives primary damage		

DELAYED EFFECTS OF HEAD INJURY

OUTCOME AFTER SEVERE HEAD INJURY

Head injury remains a major cause of disability and death, especially in the young. Of those patients who survive the initial impact and remain in coma for at least 6 hours, approximately 40% die within 6 months. The extent of recovery in the remainder depends on the severity of the injury. Residual disabilities include both mental (impaired intellect, memory and behavioural problems) and physical defects (hemiparesis and dysphasia). Most recovery occurs within the first 6 months after injury, but improvement may continue for years. *Physiotherapy* and *occupational therapy* play an important role not only in minimising contractures and improving limb power and function but also in stimulating patient motivation.

Outcome is best categorised with the *Glasgow Outcome Scale* (GOS – see page 212) which uses *dependence* to differentiate between intermediate grades. After severe injury, about 40% regain an independent existence and may return to premorbid social and occupational activities. Inevitably some remain severely disabled requiring long term care, but few (<2%) are left in a vegetative state with no awareness or ability to communicate with their environment (see page 212). Prognosis in this group is marginally better than for non-traumatic coma – with about one-third of those vegetative at *one month* regaining consciousness within one year; of those who regain consciousness, over two-thirds either subsequently die or remain severely disabled. Of those vegetative at *3 months* after the injury, none regain an independent existence.

Prognostic features following traumatic coma

The duration of coma relates closely to the severity of injury and to the final outcome, but in the early stages after injury the clinician must rely on other features – age, eye opening, verbal and motor responses, pupil response and eye movements.

	Poor outcome (GOS 1–3)	Favourable outcome (GOS 4–5)
Patients in coma for > 6 hours	61%	39%
Best *Glasgow Coma Score* > 11	18%	82%
Best *Glasgow Coma Score* 8–10	32%	68%
Best *Glasgow Coma Score* < 8	73%	27%
Pupillary response – reacting	50%	50%
Pupillary response – non-reacting	96%	4%
Age < 20 years	41%	59%
Age > 60 years	94%	6%

(from Jennett, B, Teasdale, G, Braakman, R. et al. (1979) Neurosurgery 4:283–289)

CHRONIC SUBDURAL HAEMATOMA

Subdivision of subdural haematomas into acute and subacute forms serves no practical purpose. Chronic subdural haematoma however is best considered as a separate entity, differing both in presentation and management.

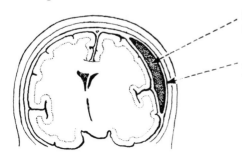

Chronic subdural haematoma – fluid may range from a faint yellow to a dark brown colour

A membrane grows out from the dura to envelop the haematoma

Chronic subdural haematomas occur predominantly in *infancy* and in the *elderly*. Trauma is the likely cause, although a history of this is not always obtained.

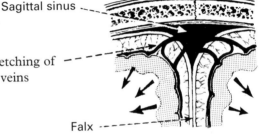

Sagittal sinus

Falx

Predisposing factors

- Cerebral atrophy
- Low CSF pressure (after a shunt or fistula)

} cause stretching of bridging veins

- Alcoholism
- Coagulation disorder

Breakdown of protein within the haematoma and a subsequent rise in osmotic pressure was originally believed to account for the gradual enlargement of the untreated subdural haematoma. Studies showing equality of osmotic pressures in blood and haematoma fluid cast doubt on this theory and recurrent bleeding into the cavity is now known to play an important role.

Clinical features tend to be non-specific.

- Dementia.
- Deterioration in conscious level, occasionally with fluctuating course.
- Symptoms and signs of raised ICP.
- Focal signs occasionally occur, especially limb weakness. This may be ipsilateral to the side of the lesion, i.e. a false localising sign (see page 222).

CHRONIC SUBDURAL HAEMATOMA

Diagnosis

CT Scan appearances depend on the time between the injury and the scan.

With injuries 1–3 weeks old, the subdural haematoma may be isodense with brain tissue. In this instance, i.v contrast enhancement may delineate the cortical margin.

Beyond 3 weeks subdural haematomas appear as a low density lesion.

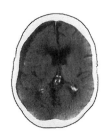

Injury > 3 weeks old: low density lesion seen over hemisphere convexity.

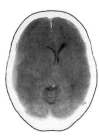

Isodense lesion causing midline shift. Note the shape of the ventricles

If CT scan shows midline shift without any obvious extra- or intracerebral lesion, look at the shape of the ventricles.

Separation of the frontal and occipital horns suggests an intrinsic lesion, e.g. encephalitis rather than a surface collection

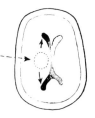
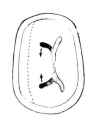

Extracerebral collection, i.e. chronic subdural haematoma, causes approximation of frontal and occipital horns

Management

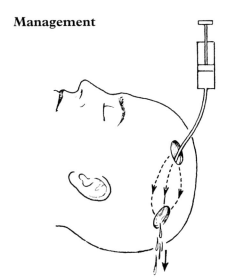

Adult

The haematoma is evacuated through two or three burr holes and the cavity is irrigated with saline. Drains may be left in the subdural space and nursing in the head-down position may help prevent recollection.

Craniotomy with excision of the membrane is seldom required.

In patients who have no depressed conscious level, conservative treatment with steroids over several weeks may result in resolution.

Infants

The haematoma is evacuated by repeated needle aspiration through the anterior fontanelle. Persistent subdural collections require a subdural peritoneal shunt. As in adults, craniotomy is seldom necessary.

CEREBROVASCULAR DISEASES

Vascular diseases of the nervous system are amongst the most frequent causes of admission to hospital. The annual incidence in the UK varies regionally between 150–200/100 000, with a prevalence of 600/100 000 of which one-third are severely disabled.

Better control of hypertension, reduced incidence of heart disease and a greater awareness of all risk factors have combined to reduce mortality from stroke. Despite this, stroke still ranks third behind heart disease and cancer as a cause of death in affluent societies.

RISK FACTORS

Prevention of cerebrovascular disease is more likely to reduce death and disability than any medical or surgical advance in management. Prevention depends upon the identification of risk factors and their correction.

Hypertension

Hypertension is a major factor in the development of thrombotic cerebral infarction and intracranial haemorrhage.

There is no critical blood pressure level; the risk is related to the height of blood pressure and increases throughout the whole range from normal to hypertensive. A 6 mmHg fall in diastolic blood pressure is associated in relative terms with a 40% fall in the fatal and non-fatal stroke rate.

Systolic hypertension (frequent in the elderly) is also a significant factor and not as harmless as previously thought.

Cardiac disease

Cardiac enlargement, failure and arrhythmias, as well as rheumatic heart disease, patent foramen ovale and, rarely, cardiac myxoma are all associated with an increased risk of stroke.

Diabetes

The risk of cerebral infarction is increased twofold in diabetes. More effective treatment of diabetes has not reduced the frequency of atherosclerotic sequelae.

Heredity

Close relatives are at only slightly greater risk than non-genetically related family members of a stroke patient. Diabetes and hypertension show familial propensity thus clouding the significance of pure hereditary factors.

Blood lipids, cholesterol, smoking, diet/obesity, soft water

These factors are much less significant than in the genesis of coronary artery disease.

Race

Alterations in life style, diet and environment probably explain the geographical variations more than racial tendencies.

Haematocrit

A high blood haemoglobin concentration (or haematocrit level) is associated with an increased incidence of cerebral infarction. Other haematological factors, such as decreased fibrinolysis, are important also.

Oral contraceptives

The evidence of pill-related stroke is inconclusive. A recent prospective study has suggested an increased risk of subarachnoid haemorrhage rather than thromboembolic stroke.

CEREBROVASCULAR DISEASE – MECHANISMS

'Stroke' is a generic term, lacking pathological meaning. Cerebrovascular diseases can be defined as those in which brain disease occurs secondary to a pathological disorder of blood vessels (usually arteries) or blood supply.

1. Occlusion by thrombus or embolus

Whatever the mechanism, the resultant effect on the brain is either:
   ischaemia/infarction, or
   haemorrhagic disruption.

2. Rupture of vessel wall

3. Disease of vessel wall

4. Disturbance of normal properties of blood

Of all strokes: – 85% are due to INFARCTION
                  – 15% are due to HAEMORRHAGE

CEREBROVASCULAR DISEASE – NATURAL HISTORY

Approximately one-third of all 'strokes' are fatal. The age of the patient, the anatomical size of the lesion, the degree of deficit and the underlying cause all influence the outcome.

Immediate outcome
In cerebral haemorrhage, mortality approaches 50%.

Cerebral infarction fares better, with an immediate mortality of less than 20%, fatal lesions being large with associated oedema and brain shift.

Embolic infarction carries a better outcome than thrombotic infarction.

Fatal cases of infarction die either at onset or else, more commonly, after the first week from cardiovascular or respiratory complications.

The level of consciousness on admission to hospital gives a good indication to immediate outcome. The deeper the conscious level the graver the prognosis.

Long-term outcome
The prognosis following infarction due to thrombosis or embolisation from diseased neck vessels or heart is dependent on the progression of the underlying atherosclerotic disease. Recurrent cerebral infarction rates vary between 5%–15% per year. Symptoms of coronary artery disease and/or peripheral vascular disease may also ensue. Five year mortality is 44% for males and 36% for females.

The long-term prognosis following survival from haemorrhage depends upon the cause and the treatment.

CEREBROVASCULAR DISEASE – CAUSES

OCCLUSION (50%)

Atheromatous/thrombotic

1. Large vessel occlusion or stenosis (e.g. carotid artery)

2. Branch vessel occlusion or stenosis (e.g. middle cerebral artery)

3. Perforating vessel occlusion (lacunar infarction)

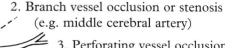

Non-atheromatous diseases of the vessel wall

1. Collagen disease e.g.   rheumatoid arthritis
   systemic lupus erythematosis (SLE)
2. Vasculitis e.g. polyarteritis nodosa
   temporal arteritis
3. Granulomatous vasculitis e.g. Wegener's granulomatosis
4. Miscellaneous e.g. syphilitic vasculitis
   fibromuscular dysplasia
   sarcoidosis
   trauma

EMBOLISATION (25%) from:

1. Atheromatous plaque in the intracranial or extracranial arteries or from the aortic arch.

2. The heart:
   – valvular heart disease
   – arrhythmias
   – ischaemic heart disease
   – bacterial and non-bacterial endocarditis
   – atrial myxoma
   – prosthetic valves
   – patent foramen ovale
   – cardiomyopathy

3. Miscellaneous:
   – fat emboli
   – air emboli
   – tumour emboli.

DISEASES OF BLOOD

e.g. Coagulopathies
Haemoglobinopathies

VENOUS THROMBOSIS

Venous thrombosis may occur with infection and dehydration or in association with arterial occlusion when related to oestrogen excess.

DECREASED CEREBRAL PERFUSION

Infarction between arterial territories may result from impaired perfusion from e.g. cardiac dysrhythmia
GI blood loss

HAEMORRHAGE (20%)

Into the brain substance – parenchymal (15%) and/or subarachnoid space (5%)
Hypertension
Amyloid vasculopathy
Aneurysm
Arteriovenous malformation

Neoplasm
Coagulation disorder e.g. haemophilia
Anticoagulant therapy
Vasculitis
Drug abuse e.g. cocaine
Trauma

OCCLUSIVE AND STENOTIC CEREBROVASCULAR DISEASE

PATHOLOGY
The normal vessel wall comprises:

Intima: a single endothelial cell lining.

Media: fibroblasts and smooth muscle with collagen support and elastic tissue.

Adventitia: mainly composed of thick collagen fibres.

Within brain and spinal cord tissue the adventitia is usually very thin and the elastic lamina between media and adventitia less apparent.

The intima is an important barrier to leakage of blood and constituents into the vessel wall. In the development of the atherosclerotic plaque, damage to the endothelium of the intima is the primary event.

The atherosclerotic plaque
Following intimal damage:

Intimal cells
Smooth muscle cells laden with cholesterol, lipids, phospholipids } build up subintimally.
Collagen and elastic fibres

Haemorrhage may occur within the plaque or the plaque may ulcerate into the lumen of the vessel forming an intraluminal mural thrombus. Either way, the lumen of the involved vessel is narrowed (stenosed) or blocked (occluded).

The plaque itself may give rise to emboli. Cholesterol is present partly in crystal form and fragments following plaque rupture may be sufficiently large to occlude the lumen of distal vessels. The cholesterol esters, lipids and phospholipids each play a role in the aggregation of such emboli.

The carotid bifurcation in the neck is a frequent site at which the antheromatous plaque causes stenosis or occlusion.

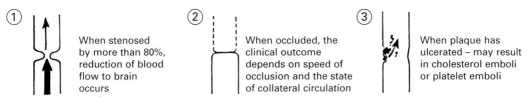

① When stenosed by more than 80%, reduction of blood flow to brain occurs

② When occluded, the clinical outcome depends on speed of occlusion and the state of collateral circulation

③ When plaque has ulcerated – may result in cholesterol emboli or platelet emboli

Platelet emboli arise from thrombus developed over the damaged endothelium. This thrombus is produced partly by platelets coming into contact with exposed collagen fibres. Endothelial cells synthesise PROSTACYCLIN which is a potent vasodilator and inhibitor of platelet aggregation. THROMBOXANE A2, synthesised by platelets, has opposite effects. In thrombus formation these two PROSTAGLANDINS actively compete with each other.

CEREBROVASCULAR DISEASE – PATHOPHYSIOLOGY

Standard techniques of cerebral blood flow (CBF) measurement provide information on both global and regional flow in patients with cerebral ischaemia or infarction. Recent availability of positron emission tomography (PET), recording oxygen and glucose metabolism, as well as blood flow and blood volume, gives a more detailed and accurate understanding of pathophysiological changes after stroke.

Changes in cerebral infarction

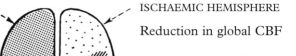

NON-ISCHAEMIC HEMISPHERE

ISCHAEMIC HEMISPHERE

Mild reduction in global CBF – perhaps due to transneuronal depression of metabolism in the unaffected hemisphere – diaschisis.

Reduction in global CBF

In the infarcted area and its surroundings, more subtle changes of regional cerebral blood flow (rCBF) are detected.

In the normal brain, cerebral blood flow to a particular part varies depending on the metabolic requirements, i.e. the supply of O_2 and glucose is 'coupled' to the tissue needs. After infarction, between areas of reduced flow and areas of luxury perfusion, lie areas of *relative luxury perfusion* where reduced flow exceeds the tissue requirements, i.e. 'uncoupling' of flow and metabolism has occurred. Studies with SPECT imaging suggest that 40% of infarcts are reperfused with blood within 48 hrs.

Areas of *reduced flow* are bordered by areas of increased flow – *luxury perfusion* – due to vasodilatation of arteriolar bed in response to lactic acidosis.

These changes in rCBF are transient and revert to normal within days of the onset. The degree of disturbance of rCBF correlates with outcome. Flow of < 28 ml/min/100 g results in the development of the morphological changes of infarction.

Pathophysiology of ischaemia

Progression from reversible ischaemia to infarction depends upon the degree and duration of the reduced blood flow.

THRESHOLDS OF CEREBRAL ISCHAEMIA

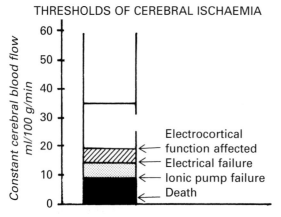

Constant cerebral blood flow ml/100 g/min

← Electrocortical function affected
← Electrical failure
← Ionic pump failure
← Death

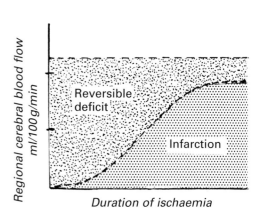

Regional cerebral blood flow ml/100g/min

Reversible deficit

Infarction

Duration of ischaemia

CEREBROVASCULAR DISEASE – PATHOPHYSIOLOGY

Ischaemic cascade

A significant fall in cerebral blood flow produces a cascade of events which, if unchecked, lead to the production and accumulation of toxic compounds and apoptosis (programmed cell death).

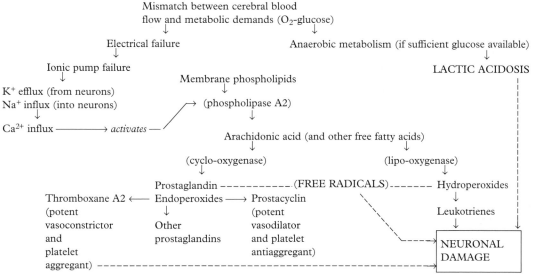

Role of neurotransmitters

Recent research has shown that one of the amino acid excitatory neurotransmitters, Glutamate, in *excess* is a powerful neurotoxin, playing an important role in ischaemic brain damage.

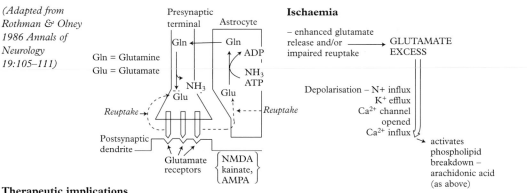

Therapeutic implications

Identification of harmful neurotransmitters and of the pathways involved in the ischaemic cascade has led to a surge of interest in *brain protective agents* –

Ca^{2+} antagonists: studies of Nimodipine in patients with SAH have shown a significant reduction in ischaemic complications. This drug acts by opening up the collateral circulation and by blocking Ca^{2+} influx, however there is no evidence of efficacy in acute infarction.

Glutamate antagonists (e.g. NMDA antagonist – 'MK801', CGS 1975S): significantly reduces ischaemia in animal studies. Toxicity has prevented clinical trials.

Barbiturates: these reduce cerebral metabolism, thereby reducing neuronal requirements. They also block free radical production. The dosage required to lower metabolism produces significant hypotension and benefits remain unproven.

Free radical scavengers: Early studies suggest that these agents may produce some benefit in reducing ischaemia.

TRANSIENT ISCHAEMIC ATTACKS (TIAs)

Transient ischaemic attacks are episodes of focal neurological symptoms due to inadequate blood supply to the brain. Attacks are sudden in onset, resolve within 24 hours or less and leave no residual deficit. These attacks are important as warning episodes or precursors of cerebral infarction.

Before diagnosing TIAs, consider other causes of transient neurological dysfunction – migraine, partial seizures, hypoglycaemia, syncope and hyperventilation.

The pathogenesis of transient ischaemic attacks

A reduction of cerebral blood flow below 20–30 ml/100 g/min produces neurological symptoms. The development of infarction is a consequence of the *degree* of reduced flow and the *duration* of such a reduction. If flow is restored to an area of brain within the critical period, ischaemic symptoms will reverse themselves. TIAs may be due to:

1. Reduced flow through a vessel:

a fall in perfusion pressure, e.g. cardiac dysrhythmia associated with localised stenotic cerebrovascular disease

– the *haemodynamic* explanation.

2. Blockage of the passage of flow by embolism:

arising from plaques in aortic arch/extracranial vessels or from the heart

– the *embolic* explanation.

Both mechanisms occur. Emboli are accepted as the cause of the majority of TIAs.

The symptomatology of TIAs

Anterior (90%)
  Carotid territory
  hemiparesis,
  hemisensory disturbance,
  dysphasia,
  monocular blindness
  (amaurosis fugax)

Posterior (7%)
  Vertebrobasilar territory
  loss of consciousness
  bilateral limb motor/sensory dysfunction
  binocular blindness
  vertigo, tinnitus,   ⎫ not singly, but in
  diplopia, dysarthria ⎭ combination
                         with each other

A small number of transient ischaemic attacks are difficult to fit convincingly into either anterior or posterior circulation, e.g. dysarthria with hemiparesis.

The natural history of TIAs

Following a TIA, between 5–10% of patients will develop infarction in each year of follow-up, irrespective of the territory involved. The risk of infarction is probably at its greatest in the first 3–6 months after the initial TIA. Not all patients who develop cerebral infarction have had a warning TIA.

CLINICAL SYNDROMES – LARGE VESSEL OCCLUSION

OCCLUSION OF THE INTERNAL CAROTID ARTERY – may present in a 'stuttering' manner due to progressive narrowing of the lumen or recurrent emboli.

The degree of deficit varies – occlusion may be asymptomatic and identified only at autopsy, or a catastrophic infarction may result.

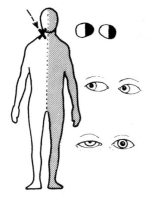

In the most extreme cases there may be:
> Deterioration of conscious level
> Homonymous hemianopia of the contralateral side
> Contralateral hemiplegia
> Contralateral hemisensory disturbance
> Gaze palsy to the opposite side – eyes deviated to the side of the lesion

A partial Horner's syndrome may develop on the side of the occlusion (involvement of sympathetic fibres on the internal carotid wall).

Occlusion of the dominant hemisphere side will result in a global aphasia.

Examination of the neck will reveal:

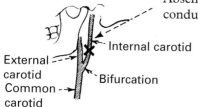

Absent carotid pulsation at the angle of the jaw with poorly conducted heart sounds along the internal carotid artery.

Prodromal symptoms prior to occlusion may take the form of monocular blindness – AMAUROSIS FUGAX and transient hemisensory or hemimotor disturbance (see page 255).

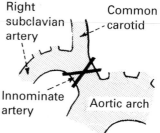

The origins of the vessels from the aortic arch are such that an *innominate artery occlusion* will result not only in the clinical picture of carotid occlusion but will produce diminished blood flow and hence blood pressure in the right arm.

The outcome of carotid occlusion depends on the collateral blood supply primarily from the circle of Willis, but, in addition, the external carotid may provide flow to the *anterior and middle cerebral arteries* through meningeal branches and retrogradely through the ophthalmic artery to the *internal carotid artery*.

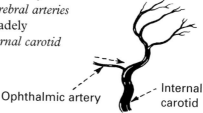

CLINICAL SYNDROMES – LARGE VESSEL OCCLUSION

ANTERIOR CEREBRAL ARTERY

Anatomy

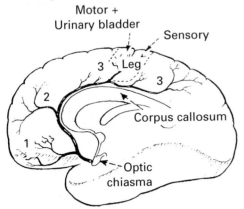

Medial surface of right cerebral hemisphere

The anterior cerebral artery is a branch of the internal carotid and runs above the optic nerve to follow the curve of the corpus callosum. Soon after its origin the vessel is joined by the anterior communicating artery. Deep branches pass to the anterior part of the internal capsule and basal nuclei.

Cortical branches supply the medial surface of the hemisphere:
1. Orbital
2. Frontal
3. Parietal

Clinical features

The anterior cerebral artery may be occluded by embolus or thrombus. The clinical picture depends on the site of occlusion (especially in relation to the anterior communicating artery) and anatomical variation, e.g. both anterior cerebral arteries may arise from one side by enlargement of the anterior communicating artery.

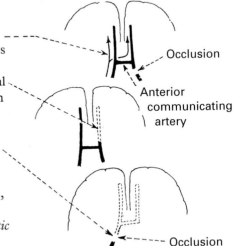

Occlusion proximal to the anterior communicating artery is normally well tolerated because of the cross flow.

    Distal occlusion results in weakness and cortical sensory loss in the contralateral lower limb with associated incontinence. Occasionally a contralateral grasp reflex is present.

    Proximal occlusion when both anterior cerebral vessels arise from the same side results in 'cerebral' paraplegia with lower limb weakness, sensory loss, incontinence and presence of grasp, snout and palmomental reflexes.

Bilateral frontal lobe infarction may result in *akinetic mutism* (page 109) or deterioration in conscious level.

CLINICAL SYNDROMES – LARGE VESSEL OCCLUSION

MIDDLE CEREBRAL ARTERY

Anatomy

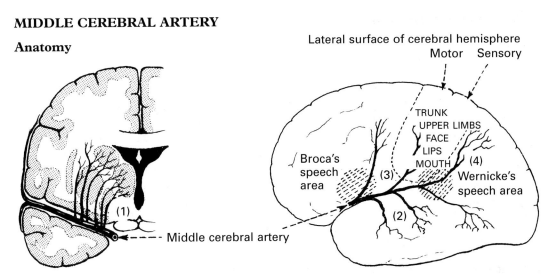

The middle cerebral artery is the largest branch of the internal carotid artery. It gives off (1) deep branches (perforating vessels – lenticulostriate) which supply the anterior limb of the internal capsule and part of the basal nuclei. It then passes out to the lateral surface of the cerebral hemisphere at the insula of the lateral sulcus. Here it gives off cortical branches (2) temporal, (3) frontal, (4) parietal.

Clinical features

The middle cerebral artery may be occluded by embolus or thrombus. The clinical picture depends upon the site of occlusion and whether dominant or non-dominant hemisphere is affected.

Occlusion at the insula

All cortical branches are involved –
- Contralateral hemiplegia (leg relatively spared)
- Contralateral hernianaesthesia and hemianopia
- Aphasia (dominant)
- Neglect of contralateral limbs ⎫
- Dressing difficulty ⎬ (non-dominant)

When cortical branches are affected individually, the clinical picture is less severe, e.g. involvement of parietal branches alone may produce Wernicke's dysphasia with no limb weakness or sensory loss.

The deep branches (perforating vessels) of the middle cerebral artery may be a source of haemorrhage or small infarcts (lacunes – see later).

CLINICAL SYNDROMES – LARGE VESSEL OCCLUSION

VERTEBRAL ARTERY OCCLUSION

Anatomy

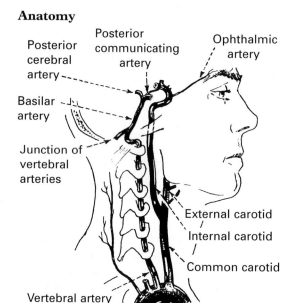

The vertebral artery arises from the subclavian artery on each side. Underdevelopment of one vessel occurs in 10%.

The vertebral artery runs from its origin through the foramen of the transverse processes of the mid-cervical vertebrae. It then passes laterally through the transverse process of the axis, then upwards to the atlas accompanied by a venous plexus and across the suboccipital triangle to the vertebral canal. After piercing the dura and arachnoid matter, it enters the cranial cavity through the foramen magnum. At the lower border of the pons, it unites with its fellow to form the basilar artery.

The vertebral artery and its branches supply the medulla and the inferior surface of the cerebellum before forming the basilar artery.

Clinical features

Occlusion of the vertebral artery, when low in the neck, is compensated by anastomotic channels.

When one vertebral artery is hypoplastic, occlusion of the other is equivalent to basilar artery occlusion.

Only the posterior inferior cerebellar artery (PICA) depends solely on flow through the vertebral artery. Vertebral artery occlusion may therefore present as a PICA syndrome (page 252).

The close relationship of the vertebral artery to the cervical spine is important. Rarely, damage at intervertebral foramina or the atlanto-axial joints following subluxation may result in intimal damage, thrombus formation and embolisation.

Vertebral artery compression during neck extension may cause symptoms of intermittent vertebrobasilar insufficiency.

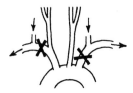

X Stenosis of the proximal left or right subclavian artery may result in retrograde flow down the vertebral artery on exercising the arm. This is commonly asymptomatic and demonstrated incidentally by Doppler techniques or angiography. Occasionally symptoms of vertebrobasilar insufficiency arise – *subclavian 'steal' syndrome*. Surgical reconstruction or bypass of the subclavian artery may be indicated.

CLINICAL SYNDROMES – LARGE VESSEL OCCLUSION

BASILAR ARTERY OCCLUSION

Anatomy

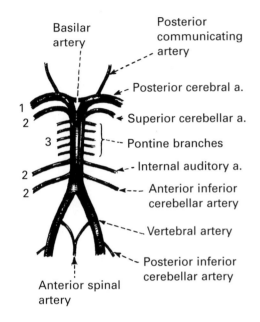

Basilar artery

Posterior communicating artery

- Posterior cerebral a.

- Superior cerebellar a.

- Pontine branches

- Internal auditory a.

- Anterior inferior cerebellar artery

- Vertebral artery

- Posterior inferior cerebellar artery

Anterior spinal artery

The basilar artery supplies the brain stem from medulla upwards and divides eventually into posterior cerebral arteries as well as posterior communicating arteries which run forward to join the anterior circulation (circle of Willis).

Branches can be classified into:
1. Posterior cerebral arteries
2. Long circumflex branches
3. Paramedian branches.

Clinical features

Prodromal symptoms are common and may take the form of diplopia, visual field loss, intermittent memory disturbance and a whole constellation of other brain stem symptoms:
– vertigo
– ataxia
– paresis
– paraesthesia

The *complete basilar syndrome* following occlusion consists of:
– impairment of consciousness → coma
– bilateral motor and sensory dysfunction
– cerebellar signs
– cranial nerve signs indicative of the level of occlusion.
The clinical picture is variable. Occasionally basilar thrombosis is an incidental finding at autopsy.

'Top of basilar' occlusion: This results in lateral midbrain, thalamic, occipital and medial temporal lobe infarction. Abnormal movements (hemiballismus) are associated with visual loss, pupillary abnormalities, gaze palsies, impaired conscious level and disturbances of behaviour.

Paramedian perforating vessel occlusion gives rise to the 'LOCKED-IN' SYNDROME (page 253) and LACUNAR infarction (page 254).

CLINICAL SYNDROMES – LARGE VESSEL OCCLUSION

POSTERIOR CEREBRAL ARTERY

Anatomy

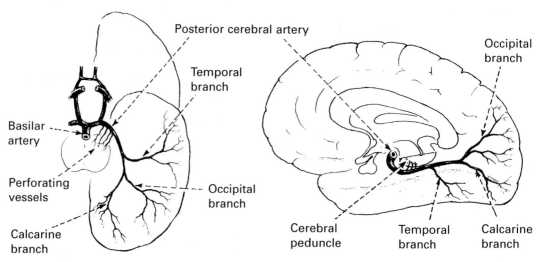

Undersurface of left cerebral hemisphere   Medial surface of right hemisphere

The posterior cerebral arteries are the terminal branches of the basilar artery. Small perforating branches supply midbrain structures, choroid plexus and posterior thalamus. Cortical branches supply the undersurface of the temporal lobe – temporal branch; and occipital and visual cortex – occipital and calcarine branches.

Clinical features

Proximal occlusion by thrombus or embolism will involve perforating branches and structures supplied:

> *Midbrain syndrome* – III nerve palsy with contralateral hemiplegia
> > – WEBER'S SYNDROME

> *Thalamic syndromes* – chorea or hemiballismus with hemisensory disturbance.

Occlusion of cortical vessels will produce a different picture with visual field loss (homonymous hemianopia) and sparing of macular vision (the posterior tip of the occipital lobe, i.e. the macular area, is also supplied by the middle cerebral artery).

Posterior cortical infarction in the dominant hemisphere may produce problems in naming colours and objects.

CLINICAL SYNDROMES – BRANCH OCCLUSION

BASILAR ARTERY – LONG CIRCUMFLEX BRANCH OCCLUSION

Anatomy

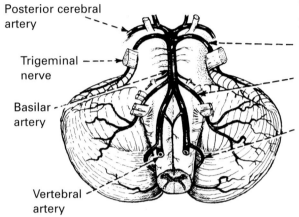

Posterior cerebral artery

Trigeminal nerve

Basilar artery

Vertebral artery

The cerebellum is supplied by three paired blood vessels:

1. Superior cerebellar artery ⎫
2. Anterior inferior cerebellar artery ⎬ arise from basilar artery

3. Posterior inferior cerebellar artery (PICA) which arises from the vertebral artery.

It can be seen that a vascular lesion in the territory of these vessels will produce, not only cerebellar, but also brain stem symptoms and signs localising to:

      (a) superior pontine,
      (b) inferior pontine and
      (c) medullary levels.

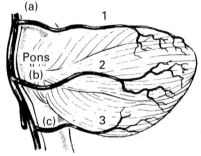

(a)

Pons

(b)

(c)

1

2

3

Clinical features

Superior cerebellar artery syndrome results in:

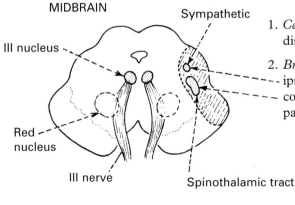

MIDBRAIN

III nucleus

Red nucleus

III nerve

Sympathetic

Spinothalamic tract

1. *Cerebellum* –
   disturbed gait, limb ataxia.

2. *Brain stem* –
   ipsilateral Horner's syndrome,
   contralateral sensory loss –
   pain/temperature (including face).

251

CLINICAL SYNDROMES – BRANCH OCCLUSION

Clinical features *(cont'd)*

Anterior inferior cerebellar artery syndrome results in:

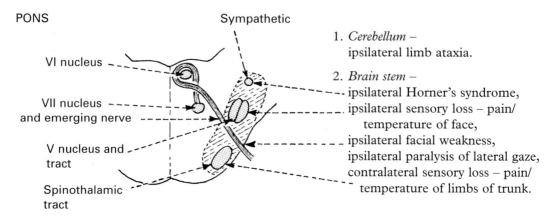

PONS

VI nucleus

VII nucleus and emerging nerve

V nucleus and tract

Spinothalamic tract

Sympathetic

1. *Cerebellum –*
   ipsilateral limb ataxia.

2. *Brain stem –*
   ipsilateral Horner's syndrome,
   ipsilateral sensory loss – pain/
   temperature of face,
   ipsilateral facial weakness,
   ipsilateral paralysis of lateral gaze,
   contralateral sensory loss – pain/
   temperature of limbs of trunk.

Posterior inferior cerebellar artery syndrome (lateral medullary syndrome) results in:

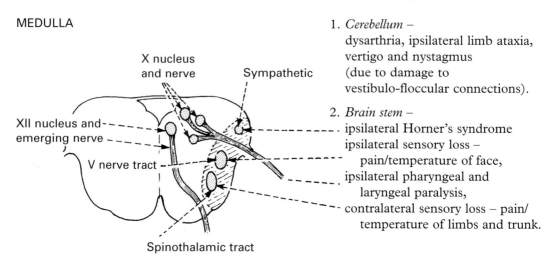

MEDULLA

X nucleus and nerve

Sympathetic

XII nucleus and emerging nerve

V nerve tract

Spinothalamic tract

1. *Cerebellum –*
   dysarthria, ipsilateral limb ataxia,
   vertigo and nystagmus
   (due to damage to
   vestibulo-floccular connections).

2. *Brain stem –*
   ipsilateral Horner's syndrome
   ipsilateral sensory loss –
   pain/temperature of face,
   ipsilateral pharyngeal and
   laryngeal paralysis,
   contralateral sensory loss – pain/
   temperature of limbs and trunk.

CLINICAL SYNDROMES – BRANCH OCCLUSION

BASILAR ARTERY – PARAMEDIAN BRANCH OCCLUSION

MIDBRAIN

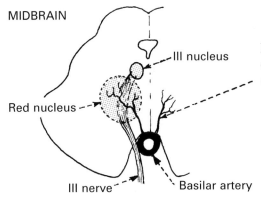

Paramedian branch occlusion is produced by occlusion of the penetrating midline branches of the basilar artery.

At the midbrain level damage to the nucleus or the fasciculus of the oculomotor nerve (III) will result in a complete or partial III nerve palsy; damage to the red nucleus (outflow from opposite cerebellar hemisphere) will also produce contralateral tremor – referred to as BENEDIKT'S SYNDROME.

PONS

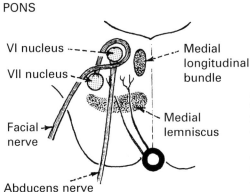

At the pontine level an abducens nerve (VI) palsy will occur with ipsilateral facial (VII) weakness and contralateral sensory loss – light touch, proprioception (medial lemniscus damage) when the lesion is more basal.

Abducens and facial palsy may be accompanied by contralateral hemiplegia – MILLARD-GUBLER SYNDROME.

MEDULLA

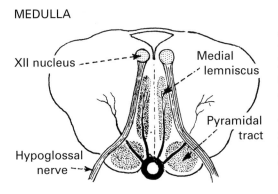

At the medullary level, bilateral damage usually occurs and results in the 'LOCKED-IN' SYNDROME. The patient is paralysed and unable to talk, although some facial and eye movements are preserved.

Spinothalamic sensation is retained, but involvement of the medial lemniscus produces loss of 'discriminatory' sensation in the limbs. The syndrome usually follows basilar artery occlusion and carries a grave prognosis.

CLINICAL SYNDROMES – LACUNAR STROKE (LACI)

Occlusion of deep penetrating arteries produces subcortical infarction characterised by *preservation* of cortical function – language, other cognitive and visual functions.

Clinical syndromes are distinctive and normally result from long-standing hypertension. In 80%, infarcts occur in periventricular white matter and basal ganglia, the rest in cerebellum and brain stem. Areas of infarction are 0.5–1.5 cm in diameter and occluded vessels demonstrate lipohyalinosis, microaneurysm and microatheromatous changes. Lacunar or subcortical infarction accounts for 17% of all thromboembolic strokes and knowledge of commoner syndromes is essential.

1. Pure motor hemiplegia

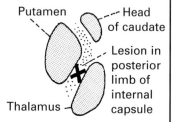

Putamen — Head of caudate

Lesion in posterior limb of internal capsule

Thalamus

Clinical: Equal weakness of contralateral face, arm and leg with dysarthria
Vessel(s): Lenticulostriate A.

2. Pure sensory stroke

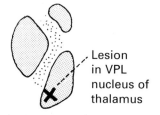

Lesion in VPL nucleus of thalamus

Clinical: Numbness and tingling of contralateral face and limbs. Sensory examination may be normal
Vessel(s): Thalamogeniculate A.

3. Dysarthria/clumsy hand

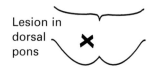

Lesion in dorsal pons

Clinical: Dysarthria due to weakness of ipsilateral face and tongue associated with clumsy but strong contralateral arm.
Vessel(s): Perforating branch of Basilar A.

4. Ataxic hemiparesis

Lesion in ventral pons (interruption of pontocerebellar fibres)

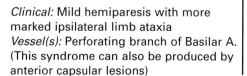

Clinical: Mild hemiparesis with more marked ipsilateral limb ataxia
Vessel(s): Perforating branch of Basilar A. (This syndrome can also be produced by anterior capsular lesions)

5. Severe dysarthria with facial weakness

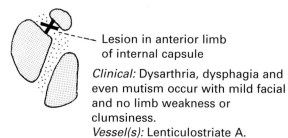

Lesion in anterior limb of internal capsule

Clinical: Dysarthria, dysphagia and even mutism occur with mild facial and no limb weakness or clumsiness.
Vessel(s): Lenticulostriate A.

Sensorimotor syndromes are common although anatomical basis is obscure. A recent Stroke Data Bank survey showed the commonest presentations to be:

Pure motor hemiplegia 57%
Sensorimotor 20%
Ataxic hemiparesis 10%
Pure sensory 7%
Dysarthria/Clumsy hand 6%

Investigations MRI is superior to CT demonstrating lacunae, although either may occasionally misdiagnose a small resolving haematoma. Confirmation of lacunar stroke may save patients from unnecessary investigations for carotid and cardiac embolic source.

Prognosis For all syndromes this is encouraging. Careful control of blood pressure and the use of aspirin usually prevents recurrence. Multiple lacunar infarctions – 'état lacunaire' – results in shuffling gait, pseudobulbar palsy and subcortical dementia.

CLASSIFICATION OF SUBTYPES OF CEREBRAL INFARCTION

A recently devised classification of infarction has proved simple and of practical value in establishing *diagnosis* and in *predicting outcome* –

	Clinical features	**Outcome**
Total Anterior Circulation Syndrome (TACS)	motor and sensory deficit, hemianopia and disturbance of higher cerebral function	Poor
Partial Anterior Circulation Syndrome (PACS)	any two of above or isolated disturbance of cerebral function	Variable
Posterior Circulation Syndrome (POCS)	signs of brainstem dysfunction or isolated hemianopia	Variable
Lacunar Anterior Circulation Syndrome (LACS)	pure motor stroke or pure sensory stroke or pure sensorimotor stroke or ataxic hemiparesis	Good

EMBOLISATION

Emboli consist of friable atheromatous material, platelet-fibrin clumps or well formed thrombus.

The **diagnosis** of embolic infarction depends on:
- The identification of an embolic *source*, e.g. cardiac disease.
- The clinical picture of *sudden onset.*
- Infarction in the territory of a major vessel or large branch.

Clinical picture – depends on the vessel involved. Emboli commonly produce *transient ischaemic attacks (TIA)* as well as *infarction.*

Symptoms are referable to the eye (retinal artery) and to the anterior and middle cerebral arteries, and take the form of:

Visual loss – transient, i.e. *amaurosis fugax* or permanent.
Hemisensory and hemimotor disturbance.
Disturbance of higher function, e.g. dysphasia.
Focal or generalised seizures – may persist for some time after the ischaemic episode.
Depression of conscious level if major vessel occlusion occurs.

Emboli less frequently affect the posterior circulation.

EMBOLI FROM THE INTERNAL CAROTID ARTERY AND AORTA

Emboli from these sources are commonest outwith the heart. The majority of all cerebral emboli arise from ulcerative plaques in the carotid arteries (see page 241).

Emboli arising from the aorta (atheromatous plaque or aortic aneurysm) often involve both hemispheres and systemic embolisation (e.g. affecting limbs) may coexist.

EMBOLISATION

EMBOLI OF CARDIAC ORIGIN

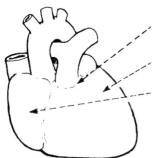

The heart represents a major source of cerebral emboli.
Valvular heart disease: rheumatic heart disease e.g. mitral stenosis with atrial fibrillation or mitral value prolapse.
Ischaemic heart disease: myocardial infarction with mural thrombus formation.
Arrhythmias: Non-rheumatic (non-valvular) atrial fibrillation is the most common cause of cardioembolic stroke
Bacterial endocarditis may give rise to septic cerebral embolisation with ischaemia → infection → abscess formation.
Neurological signs will occur in 30% of all cases of bacterial endocarditis, *S. aureus* and *streptococci* being the offending organisms in the majority.

Non-bacterial endocarditis (marantic endocarditis): associated with malignant disease due to fibrin and platelet deposition on heart valves.

Atrial myxoma is a rare cause of recurrent cerebral embolisation. Bihemisphere episodes with a persistently elevated ESR should arouse suspicion which may be confirmed by cardiac ultrasound.

Patent foramen ovale may result in paradoxical embolisation; suspect in patient with deep venous thrombosis who develops cerebral infarction. Emboli can also arise from intracardiac thrombus.

New cardiac imaging techniques especially Transoesophageal Echocardiography (TOE) allow a more accurate detection of potential embolic source. Transcranial Doppler (TCD) may characterise emboli by analysing their signals and help quantify risk of recurrence.

EMBOLI FROM OTHER SOURCES

Fat emboli: following fracture, especially of long bones and pelvis, fat appears in the bloodstream and may pass into the cerebral circulation, usually 3–6 days after trauma. Emboli are usually multiple and signs are diffuse.

Air emboli follow injury to neck/chest, or follow surgery. Rarely, air emboli complicate therapeutic abortion. Again the picture is diffuse neurologically. Onset is acute; if the patient survives the first 30 minutes, prognosis is excellent.

Nitrogen embolisation or decompression sickness (the 'bends') produces a similar picture, but if the patient survives, neurological disability may be profound.

Tumour emboli result in metastatic lesions; the onset is usually slow and progressive. Acute stroke-like presentation may occur, followed weeks or months later by the mass effects.

Lung
Melanoma
Testicular tumours
Lymphoblastic leukaemia } commonly metastasise to brain.
Prostate
Breast
Renal

STENOTIC/OCCLUSIVE DISEASE – INVESTIGATIONS

1. CONFIRM THE DIAGNOSIS

Computerised tomography (CT scan)

All patients should have a CT scan, urgently if
– conscious level depressed
– diagnosis uncertain
– on anticoagulants
– before commencing/resuming antithrombotics
– if thrombolysis is considered.

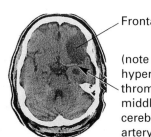

Frontal infarct

(note hyperdense thrombosed middle cerebral artery)

Infarction is evident as a low-density lesion which conforms to a vascular territory, i.e. usually wedge shaped. Subtle changes occur within 3 hours in some patients; most scans become abnormal within 48 hours.

CT scan also identifies:
– the site and size of the infarct, providing a prognostic guide
– the presence of haemorrhagic infarction where bleeding occurs into the infarcted area
– intracerebral haemorrhage or tumour.

Magnetic resonance imaging (MRI)

T2 prolongation (hyperintensity in relation to white and grey matter) occurs within hours of onset of ischaemic symptoms. Advanced techniques, diffusion weighted imaging (DWI) and perfusion imaging (PWI) show respectively early infarction (cytotoxic oedema) and ischaemic tissue at risk (the ischaemic penumbra). These advanced techniques are valuable predictors of outcome and guide treatments directed as 'ischaemic salvage' e.g. thrombolysis.

2. DEMONSTRATE THE SITE OF PRIMARY LESION

(a) Non-invasive investigation

Ultrasound – Doppler/Duplex scanning: assesses extra- and intracranial vessels (page 43). A normal study precludes the need for angiography.

Cardiac ultrasound (transthoracic or transoesophageal): this often reveals a cardiac embolic source in young people with stroke, e.g. prolapsed mitral valve, patent foramen ovale.

Magnetic resonance angiography (MRA)

'Time of flight' or contrast enhanced techniques are used. Whilst of value in patients with heavily calcified carotid plaques, resistant to Doppler, it tends to overestimate the severity of stenosis. When assessing the carotid arteries it is best used in combination with Doppler. Its non-invasive nature makes it helpful in investigating the intracranial circulation.

Computed tomographic angiography (CTA)

Dynamic helical CT, following bolus injection of non-ionic contrast, can be used to investigate both intracranial and extracranial vasculature. CTA compared with DSA correctly classifies the degree of carotid stenosis in 96% of cases but is insensitive to ulcerative plaque. Again it is best used in conjunction with Doppler.

(b) Digital intravenous subtraction angiography (DSA)

The combination of the above techniques has decreased the need for invasive investigation but often *cerebral angiography* is still required to make a definitive diagnosis. The role and safety of angiography *immediately* following infarction is uncertain. In the elderly or poor-risk patient, investigations to demonstrate the site of the primary lesion may be inappropriate.

STENOTIC/OCCLUSIVE DISEASE – INVESTIGATIONS

Indication for angiography

1. With suspected *extracranial* vascular disease
   - a recovered stroke patient ⎱ if ultrasound
     at further risk ⎰ positive.
   - following TIAs

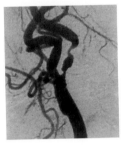

Carotid
stenosis
and
ulceration

2. With suspected *intracranial* vascular disease.
Angiography identifies the site and nature of the
disease in intra- and extracranial vessels, and
indicates the degree of collateral circulation.

Suspected carotid disease: demonstrate both carotids, intracranial vessels, the aortic arch and
origins of the vertebrals. Approximately two-thirds of patients with carotid territory attacks
will have angiographic abnormality.

Suspected vertebrobasilar disease: note the intracranial vessels and the course of the vertebral
artery through the cervical foramina where osteophytic encroachment may occur. Note that
proximal subclavian occlusion may result in retrograde flow down the vertebral arteries into
the subclavian arteries, and cause TIAs aggravated by arm exercise – *subclavian steal* (page 248).

3. IDENTIFY FACTORS WHICH MAY INFLUENCE TREATMENT AND OUTCOME

General investigations identify conditions which may predispose towards premature
cerebrovascular disease. These are essential in all patients.

Chest x-ray – cardiac enlargement – hypertension/valvular heart disease

ECG – ventricular enlargement and/or arrhythmias – hypertension/embolic disease
recent myocardial infarct – embolic disease
sinoatrial conduction defect – embolic disease/output failure

Blood glucose – diabetes mellitus

Serum lipids and cholesterol – hyperlipidaemia

ESR – ⎱
Auto-antibodies – ⎰ vasculitis/collagen vascular disease ⎱
Urine analysis – polyarteritis, thrombocytopenia ⎬ See inflammatory vasculitis
Full blood count – polycythaemia, thrombocytopenia ⎰ and blood diseases (pages 262–265)

VDRL-TPHA – neurosyphilis

Prothrombin time – circulating auto-anticoagulants

Partial thromboplastin time (PTT) – prolonged by lupus anticoagulant

Note drug history – oral contraceptives, amphetamines, opiates

Cervical spine X-ray – atlanto-axial subluxation

Following the interpretation of these preliminary investigations, more detailed studies may
be required, e.g.

- cardiac ultrasound — cardiac embolic source
- blood cultures ——— subacute bacterial endocarditis
- HIV screen ——— AIDS
- sickle cell screen ⎱
- plasma electrophoresis ⎬ haematological disorder
- viscosity studies ⎰
- anticardiolipin antibodies – antiphospholipid syndrome – muscle biopsy – mitochondrial
disease

CEREBRAL INFARCTION – MANAGEMENT

THE ACUTE STROKE
Clinical history, examination and investigation will separate infarction and haemorrhage.
Once the nature of the 'stroke' has been confidently defined, treatment should be instigated.

Treatment aims
- Prevent progression of present event
- Prevent immediate complication
- Prevent the development of subsequent events
- To rehabilitate the patient.

General measures

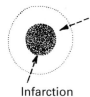

Infarction

Around the edge of an infarct, ischaemic tissue is at risk, but is potentially recoverable. This compromised but viable tissue must be protected by ensuring an adequate supply of glucose and oxygen. Factors which might affect this must be maintained – hydration, oxygenation, blood pressure. To this end, treat chest infections and cardiac failure/dysrhythmias. Paradoxically, hyperglycaemia adversely affects outcome.

Specific measures
The following are generally ineffective, or are as yet inadequately evaluated.

Anticoagulant therapy
In patients with a known cardiac source of emboli, the risk of recurrent embolic infarction is high and anticoagulant therapy should be commenced once CT scan has ruled out haemorrhagic infarction. In chronic valvular disease, treatment is long term; following myocardial infarction (with mural thrombus) – 6 months. With mitral valve prolapse, antiplatelet drugs will suffice. In atrial fibrillation the overall annual risk of stroke is 5%. Several recent trials show highly significant benefit from long term oral anticoagulation with warfarin.

Trials have shown no net benefit of heparin treatment in patients with acute infarction. Despite this, heparin is often used in the management of 'stroke in evolution'. The neurological deficit fluctuates but gradually worsens over some hours. The gradual progression is considered due to increasing thrombus formation with progressive 'silting' of collateral vessels. Studies of anticoagulant therapy produce conflicting results probably because of other potential mechanisms, e.g. collateral perfusion failure.

Thrombolytic agents
Recent experience with thrombolytic agents, especially recombinant tissue plasminogen activator (IVrTPA) suggests a sustained, significant neurological improvement when initiated within a few hours of infarction. Such agents are associated with rapid recanalisation of occluded vessels. Randomised clinical trials of rTPA and other thrombolytics are currently underway. Experience with streptokinase shows unacceptable risk of intracranial haemorrhage and studies have been suspended.

CEREBRAL INFARCTION – MANAGEMENT

Specific measures (*cont'd*)

Decreasing blood viscosity

Improving hydration and venesection lower the haematocrit and reduce blood viscosity, thereby increasing cerebral blood flow (to a greater extent than the oxygen carrying capacity is reduced). Studies of venesection alone have produced disappointing results. Plasma expanders, low molecular weight dextran and drugs that effect red blood cell deformity (pentoxifylline) lower blood viscosity but similarly appear to be of little value.

Neuronal rescue

Experimental work indicates a pathological role for intracellular calcium influx in neuronal injury. Excitatory amino acids – glutamate and glycine – promote calcium influx by acting on receptor-mediated membrane channels (*N*-methyl-D-aspartate-NMDA channels.) The NMDA channel has at least 6 sites which may be pharmacologically blocked. Agents such as MK801, Mg^{2+}, CGS-19755 and d-Methorphan have been evaluated in animal models. To date none have been effective in human clinical trials although Mg^{2+} is still under evaluation. Voltage dependent calcium channel antagonists (Nimodipine, Diltiazem, Nifedipine and Verapamil) have been assessed, with, to date, disappointing results, in large multicentre studies of acute infarction.

Treatment of oedema

The degree of concomitant oedema relates to the magnitude of infarction. Oedema develops early and may cause ventricular displacement and transtentorial herniation with secondary brain stem damage. Controversy exists as to whether oedema is vasogenic or cytotoxic (as associated with metabolic encephalopathies), or a mixture of the two. Its effective treatment should lower morbidity and mortality but steroids and hyperosmolar agents (e.g. mannitol) have been used with little effect on outcome. The poor response probably reflects the 'mixed' nature of the oedema.

Prevention of further stroke

The recognition of risk factors and their correction to minimise the risk of further events forms a necessary and important step in long-term treatment.

- Control hypertension
- Emphasise the need to stop cigarette smoking
- Correct lipid abnormality
- Give platelet antiaggregation drugs (aspirin or in selected cases Dipyridamole or Clopidogrel) to reduce the rate of reinfarction
- Remove or treat embolic source (long term anticoagulation in atrial fibrillation)
- Treat inflammatory or vascular inflammatory diseases
- Stop thrombogenic drugs, e.g. oral contraceptives.

TIAs AND MINOR INFARCTION – MANAGEMENT

The aim of treatment is to prevent subsequent cerebral infarction:
Establish diagnosis and exclude other pathologies causing transient neurological
symptoms, e.g. migraine.
Establish which vessel is involved —————— carotid territory
                                                vertebrobasilar artery.

Correct predisposing condition.
Examine patient for evidence of extracranial vascular disease:
Palpate carotids, upper limb pulses. Auscultate the neck for bruits.
Check blood pressure in both arms. Examine heart.

Medical treatment

General   Reduce risk factors as described (page 238).

Antiplatelet agents: several studies indicate that aspirin is a useful prophylactic in
patients with TIAs. The UK TIA aspirin trial compared placebo with aspirin
1200 mg and aspirin 300 mg per day. Results showed no difference between
the high and low dose, but both treatment groups showed an 18% reduction in
end points (vascular and non-vascular events and mortality). Examination of
individual end points – disabling stroke and vascular deaths, showed no

Specific   significant benefit. Despite the possibility that aspirin might predispose to
haemorrhagic stroke, the authors recommend that a patient requiring
prophylaxis for cerebrovascular or cardiovascular disease should receive aspirin
(300 mg per day), provided no contraindications exist (e.g. peptic ulcer).
Clopidogrel, a new platelet antiaggregant has been compared with aspirin and
appears slightly more effective, especially in women whose TIAs persist on
aspirin.

Anticoagulation
In the absence of atrial fibrillation, there is no evidence that anticoagulated
TIA patients do more favourably than control groups.

Surgical treatment

Carotid endarterectomy was introduced in 1954. Recent trials – European Carotid Surgery
Trial (ECST) and North American Symptomatic Carotid Endarterectomy Trial (NASCET)
have defined its role in treatment. High grade (> 70%) stenosis should be operated on by an
experienced surgeon. Mild stenosis (< 30%) should be treated with antiplatelet drugs. The
place of surgery in moderate stenosis (30%–70%) remains unclear. The role of angioplasty
with or without 'stenting' is currently being assessed. Trials show surgery for asymptomatic
carotid disease produces negligible benefit. Most surgery is confined to the carotid territory,
though osteophytic vertebral artery compression, subclavian steal syndrome and vertebral
artery origin stenosis are all amenable to surgery.

Superficial temporal to middle cerebral artery anastomosis (anterior circulation)
Extracranial-intracranial (EC-IC) bypass aims at enhancing the collateral circulation in patients with carotid or
middle cerebral artery occlusion to lessen the likelihood of further ipsilateral infarction. A randomised multicentre
international study, however, demonstrated that 'bypass was not superior to conservative treatment'. Despite many
criticisms of the trial, this procedure has generally been abandoned. With the development of noninvasive
techniques for assessing the intracranial collateral circulation, it is still possible that, with improved patient selection,
this operation could gain favour in the future.

HYPERTENSION AND CEREBROVASCULAR DISEASE

Next to age, the most important factor predisposing to cerebral infarction or haemorrhage is hypertension. The risk is equal in males and females and is proportional to the height of blood pressure (diastolic and systolic).

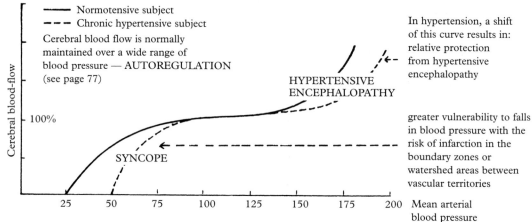

The pathological effects of sustained hypertension are:
– Charcot Bouchard microaneurysms → INTRACEREBRAL HAEMORRHAGE (from perforating vessels)
– Accelerated atheroma and thrombus formation → INFARCTION (large vessels)
– Hyalinosis and fibrin deposition → INFARCTION (lacunes – small vessels)

HYPERTENSIVE ENCEPHALOPATHY

An acute, usually transient, cerebral syndrome precipitated by sudden severe hypertension. The excessive blood pressure may be due to *malignant hypertension* from any cause, or uncontrolled hypertension in *glomerulonephritis*, *pregnancy* (eclampsia) or *phaeochromocytoma*.

The mechanism is complex: Cerebral resistance vessels

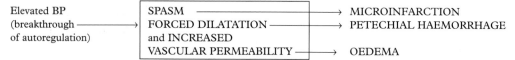

Clinical features: Headache and confusion precede convulsions and coma. Papilloedema with haemorrhages and exudates are invariably found. Proteinuria and signs of renal and cardiac failure are common.
Diagnosis: CT scanning shows a widespread white matter low attenuation and excludes other pathology. MRI confirms increased brain water content and SPECT shows hyperperfusion adjacent to these changes.
Treatment: a precipitous fall in blood pressure can result in retinal damage and watershed infarction. Gradually reduce blood pressure with i.v. nitroprusside or hydralazine. Reserve peritoneal dialysis for resistant cases.
N.B. *With treatment full recovery is usual. Without treatment death occurs.*

BINSWANGER'S ENCEPHALOPATHY (Subcortical arteriosclerotic encephalopathy – SAE)

A *rare* disorder in which progressive dementia and pseudobulbar palsy are associated with diffuse hemisphere demyelination. The CT scan shows areas of periventricular low attenuation, often also involving the external capsule. The pathological changes were previously attributed to chronic diffuse oedema, but the recent finding of a high plasma viscosity in these patients suggests that this, in conjunction with hypertensive small vessel disease, could produce chronic ischaemic change in central white matter.

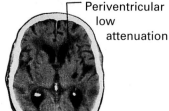

Subclinical forms of this disease may exist as this CT scan appearance is occasionally found in asymptomatic patients.

MRI appears more sensitive in establishing radiological diagnosis.

DISEASES OF THE VESSEL WALL

VASCULITIS AND COLLAGEN VASCULAR DISEASES

These disorders have systemic as well as neurological features. Occasionally only the nervous system is diseased.

Collagen vascular diseases:
– Systemic lupus erythematosus
– Rheumatoid arthritis
– Other connective tissue disorders.

Vasculitis
– Vasculitis associated with connective tissue disease.
– Micropolyangiitis (previously called polyarteritis nodosa).
– Allergic angiitis (hypersensitivity vasculitis).
– Takayasu's arteritis.
– Isolated angiitis of the central nervous system (IAC).
– Giant cell arteritis/Temporal arteritis
– Churg-Strauss angiitis.

All the above conditions can result in infarction or haemorrhage.

Granulomatous vasculitis e.g. Wegener's granulomotosis.

Mechanism
An immune basis for these disorders is likely.

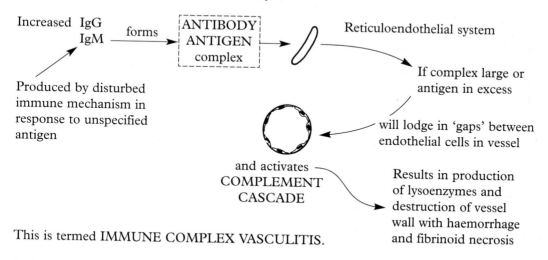

Increased IgG IgM — forms → ANTIBODY ANTIGEN complex → Reticuloendothelial system

Produced by disturbed immune mechanism in response to unspecified antigen

If complex large or antigen in excess

will lodge in 'gaps' between endothelial cells in vessel

and activates COMPLEMENT CASCADE

Results in production of lysoenzymes and destruction of vessel wall with haemorrhage and fibrinoid necrosis

This is termed IMMUNE COMPLEX VASCULITIS.

Indirect immunofluorescent microscopy on biopsy material will demonstrate the presence of immune complexes.

In giant cell arteritis and granulomatous vasculitis, cellular immune mechanisms are probably to blame and vessels are directly attacked. A reaction of antigen with sensitised lymphocytes results in lymphokine release – attracted mononuclear cells release lysosomal enzymes with resultant granuloma formation.

263

DISEASES OF THE VESSEL WALL

VASCULITIS AND COLLAGEN VASCULAR DISEASES (*cont'd*)

In all vasculitides affecting predominantly large and medium size vessels, angiography is important in establishing diagnosis. On MRI the presence of bilateral cortical and subcortical infarction is suggestive.

SYSTEMIC LUPUS ERYTHEMATOSUS: in 75% of patients nervous system involvement occurs and may predate systemic manifestation.

– Psychiatric change
– Dementia
– Seizures
– HEMIPLEGIA
– Cranial or peripheral
  nerve involvement
– SPINAL stroke
– Involuntary movements.

Investigations

Blood

Elevated ESR and C-reactive protein
Circulating antibodies to nucleoproteins e.g. anti-DNA(ANA)
Elevated immunoglobulins
Depressed serum complement levels
Prolonged prothrombin time and antiphospholipid antibodies (60%)

Other

EEG – diffuse disturbance
CT/MRI – multiple small intraparenchymal haemorrhages or infarcts
CSF – protein elevated (Ig), mononuclear cells
Angiography – vessels have beaded appearance

Pathology

The predominant CNS finding is microvascular injury with hyalinisation, perivascular lymphocytosis, endothelial proliferation and thrombosis. Active vasculitis is rare. Cardiogenic embolism and coagulopathy (antiphospholipid antibodies) are alternative mechanisms of stroke.

Treatment

Corticosteroids in moderate dosage. In patients with severe or fulminant disease, immunosuppressants and plasma exchange may help.

POLYARTERITIS NODOSA

Neurological involvement is common (80%): Small and medium size arteries are affected.

– HEMIPLEGIA – microinfarction
– INTRACRANIAL HAEMORRHAGE – aneurysm formation
– SPINAL INFARCTION or HAEMORRHAGE
– Peripheral nerve involvement (mononeuritis multiplex)

–'Cogan's' syndrome $\left\{\begin{array}{l}\text{Interstitial keratitis}\\\text{deafness}\\\text{vertigo}\end{array}\right\}$ $\begin{array}{l}\text{progressing to}\\\rightarrow \text{seizures/stroke/coma}\end{array}$

Hypertension and renal involvement are common.

Investigations

Blood

Elevated ESR and C-reactive protein
Anaemia
Leukocytosis
Eosinophilia
Antinuclear cytoplasmic antibodies (ANCA)
Circulating immune complexes
IgM rheumatoid factor

Other

Biopsy – renal or peripheral nerve
– necrotic vessel
– lumen diminished
– leucocytes and eosinophils in necrotic media and adventitia

CT/MRI as in systemic lupus erythematosus
Angiography. Multiple irregularities and micro-aneurysm formation. These changes can be visible on MRA

Treatment

Steroids and immunosuppressant therapy have dramatically improved outcome (60% 5-year survival). Plasmapheresis is successful in acute cases.

DISEASES OF THE VESSEL WALL

VASCULITIS AND COLLAGEN VASCULAR DISEASES (*cont'd*)

ALLERGIC ANGIITIS (Hypersensitivity vasculitis)

Intercurrent illnesses (infection or neoplasia) trigger immune complex deposition and basement membranes of capillaries and venules. Systemic symptoms – rash, fever and arthralgia are associated with multiorgan involvement. Neurological features – neuropathy, stroke-like syndromes – occur in 30% of patients. Investigations suggest systemic upset – elevated ESR, anaemia, leukopaenia. Skin biopsy confirms peri-venular inflammation. Treatment of underlying infection and steroids produce rapid improvement.

TAKAYASU'S (PULSELESS) DISEASE

A giant cell arteritis involving the aorta and its major branches. Predominantly affects Asian females in third or fourth decades.

Symptoms:
- Non-specific – fever, arthralgias and myalgia
- Vascular – myocardial ischaemia, peripheral vascular disease
- Neurological vascular TIAs (including subclavian steal), strokes and dementia.

Diagnosis:
Steroids are useful initially. The role of surgical reconstruction of occluded vessels is uncertain

ISOLATED ANGIITIS OF CENTRAL NERVOUS SYSTEM

Systemic symptoms and laboratory evidence of generalised vasculitis are absent.
Presentation with headaches/seizures/encephalopathy and stroke

Diagnosis:
Condition should be borne in mind in atypical stroke
- CSF shows lymphocytes
- MRI, multiple ischaemic changes
- Angiography, beading (multiple narrow segments) on intracranial arteries
- Meningeal biopsy.

Treatment:
Prognosis often dismal.
Steroids and cyclophosphamide may produce remission.

GIANT CELL ARTERITIS (see page 71)

CHURG STRAUSS ANGIITIS

A distinctive syndrome of eosinophilia, pulmonary infiltrates, neuropathy and encephalopathy or stroke. Related to polyarteritis nodosa, steroid responsive. Other immunosuppressants e.g. cyclophosphamide in resistant cases.

GRANULOMATOUS VASCULITIS/WEGENER'S GRANULOMATOSIS

A rare disorder, most frequent in males aged 20–50 years.

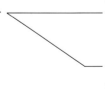

Upper or lower respiratory tract granuloma is associated with glomerulonephritis
Small arteries and capillaries are affected

Neurological involvement
- direct granulomatous invasion of skull base (cranial nerve palsies, visual failure from chiasmal compression)
- Stroke-like symptoms from vasculitis.

Diagnosis:
- Elevated ESR and C-reactive protein (CRP)
- Elevated immunoglobulins
- Impaired renal function
- Radiological findings: Chest and sinuses: granuloma mass
  MRI (cranium): granuloma mass or vasculitis.

Treatment:
- Immunosuppression: steroids and cyclophosphamide
- Surgical decompression of granulomas occasionally required.

DISEASES OF THE BLOOD

Disorders of the blood may manifest themselves as 'stroke-like' syndromes. Examination of the peripheral blood film is an important investigation in cerebrovascular disease. Where indicated, more extensive haematological investigation is necessary.

DISSEMINATED INTRAVASCULAR COAGULATION (DIC)
A consequence of:

Sepsis
Pregnancy   results in   Acute intravascular   leading to   A bleeding tendency with
Malignancy   ⟶   coagulation   ⟶   haemorrhage into skin and
Immune reactions   Consuming platelets   organs including the
                                        and clotting factor   NERVOUS SYSTEM.

Neurological involvement – a diffuse fluctuating encephalopathy, subarachnoid or subdural haemorrhage.

Diagnosis confirmed by – low platelet count – prolonged prothrombin time, elevated fibrin degradation products and reduced fibrinogen levels.

Treatment
Heparin. Fresh frozen plasma/vitamin K. Treatment of underlying cause.

HAEMOGLOBINOPATHIES
These are genetically determined disorders in which abnormal haemoglobin is present in red blood cells.

Sickle cell disease
This disorder is common in Negro populations and also occurs sporadically throughout the Mediterranean and Middle East region.
The patient is of small stature, usually with chronic leg ulcers, cardiomegaly and hepatosplenomegaly. When arterial oxygen saturation is reduced, 'sickling' will occur, manifested clinically by abdominal pain/bone pain.

Neurological involvement – hemiparesis, optic atrophy, subarachnoid haemorrhage.

Diagnosis is confirmed in vitro by the 'sickling' of cells when O_2 tension is reduced and by haemoglobin electrophoresis.

Treatment
Analgesics for pain
O_2 therapy, or hyperbaric O_2
exchange transfusion should
be carried out for those with
a severe or progressive deficit.

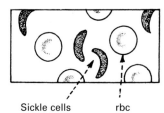

Sickle cells   rbc

ANTIPHOSPHOLIPID ANTIBODIES
These IgG or IgM antibodies prolong APTT and appear to be associated with thrombotic stroke. There remains uncertainty as to whether they are caused by or represent a transient non-specific 'acute phase' reaction to illness. Such antibodies can be found in patients with systemic lupus erythematosus.

ANTITHROMBIN III, PROTEIN C and PROTEIN S DEFICIENCY
Deficiency of any of these circulating antithrombotic fibrinolytic agents can result in deep venous thrombosis, pulmonary embolism or cerebral venous sinus thrombosis.

DISEASES OF THE BLOOD

POLYCYTHAEMIA

Both polycythaemia rubra vera (primary) and secondary polycythaemia may result in *neurological* involvement –
increased viscosity results in reduced cerebral blood flow and an increased tendency towards thrombosis.

Headaches, visual blurring and vertigo are common neurological symptoms.

Transient ischaemic attacks and thrombotic cerebral infarction occur.

Diagnosis

Hb and PCV are elevated.

Primary polycythaemia is confirmed by increased red cell count, white blood count and platelets.

Secondary polycythaemia – respiratory, renal or congenital heart disease are causal.

Treatment

Venesection with replacement of volume with low molecular weight dextran.

Antimitotic drugs may also be used when polycythaemia is due to myeloproliferative disease.

HYPERGAMMAGLOBULINAEMIA

An increase in serum gamma globulin may arise as a primary event or secondary to leukaemia, myeloma, amyloid.

Neurological involvement develops in 20% of cases – due to increased viscosity.

Clinical features are similar to those of polycythaemia – peripheral nervous system involvement may also occur.

Diagnosis is confirmed by protein electrophoresis.

Treatment – underlying cause – plasmapheresis.

THROMBOTIC THROMBOCYTOPENIC PURPURA (syn: Moschkowitz's syndrome)

This is a fibrinoid degeneration of the subintimal structures of small blood vessels. Lesions occur in all organs
including the brain.

Clinical features – fever with purpura and multiorgan involvement and neurological features of diffuse
encephalopathy or massive intracranial haemorrhage.

Haemolytic anaemia, haematuria and thrombocytopenia are the main laboratory features.

Treatment

Heparin, steroids and platelet inhibitors may be of value.

THROMBOCYTOPENIA

Whether idiopathic, drug-induced or due to myeloproliferative disorders, this condition may be associated with
intracranial haemorrhage.

THROMBOCYTOSIS

This is an elevation in platelet count above 600 000 per mm^3. It may be part of a myeloproliferative disorder, or
'reactive' to chronic infection. Patients present with recurrent thrombotic episodes.

Treatment

Aspirin in mild cases; plasmapheresis and antimitotic drugs if more severe.

HYPERFIBRINOGENAEMIA

Serum fibrinogen is occasionally elevated in people with cerebrovascular disease. This enhances coagulation and
raises blood viscosity. Infection, pregnancy, malignancy and smoking all raise fibrinogen and may explain in part the
increased risk of cerebral infarction. Arvin (Malayan viper venom) acutely lowers serum levels.

CEREBROVASCULAR DISEASE – VENOUS THROMBOSIS

The venous sinuses are important in CSF absorption, with arachnoid villi invaginating the sagittal sinus in particular. Thrombotic occlusion of the venous system occurs with
— head trauma
— infection
— dehydration
— pregnancy, puerperium and pill
— coagulation disorders
— malignant meningitis
— miscellaneous disorders
    e.g. sarcoid, Behçets

Improved imaging (MRI) has resulted in increased recognition. Venous infarction accounts for 1% of all 'strokes'.

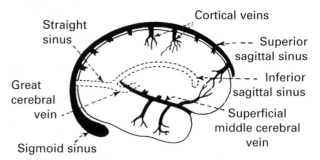

The cerebral venous system

Superior sagittal and lateral sinus thrombosis (85% of cases)
Impaired CSF drainage results in headache, papilloedema and impaired consciousness. Venous infarction produces seizures and focal deficits (e.g. hemiplegia).

Diagnosis is suggested by venous (nonarterial territory) infarction and 'empty delta' sign (following contrast the wall of the sinus enhances but not the central thrombus on CT) and confirmed by occlusion of filling deficit on MR angiography/ venography. Outcome is variable; benign intracranial hypertension may develop (p. 374). A thorough search for causation – coagulation screen, drug history and underlying systemic illness – essential.

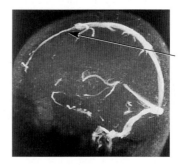

MR angiogram showing virtual occlusion of the superior sagittal sinus

Treatment:
The role of heparin remains uncertain and is currently being evaluated.

Deep cerebral venous thrombosis (10% of cases)
This produces venous infarction of the basal ganglion and other subcortical structures. Presentation with similar features; diagnosis can only be established by imaging (CT/MRI and MRV). The role of heparin is again uncertain.

Cavernous sinus thrombosis (5% of cases)

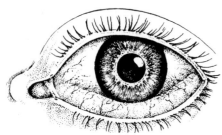

Commonly results from infection spreading from the jaw through draining veins or paranasal sinuses. Painful ophthalmoplegia, proptosis and chemosis with oedema of periorbital structures are associated with facial numbness and fever. The disorder may be bilateral. Base diagnosis on clinical suspicion supported by venography. Treatment with antibiotics and if indicated, sinus drainage.

CEREBROVASCULAR DISEASE – UNUSUAL FORMS

ABNORMALITIES OF EXTRACRANIAL VESSELS

FIBROMUSCULAR DYSPLASIA

This disease involves intracranial as well as extracranial vessels which appear like a 'string of beads'. The patient presents with infarction as a result of thrombotic occlusion or from an associated saccular aneurysm, of which there is an increased risk. Transluminal angioplasty can be used to dilate a stenotic segment.

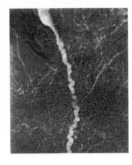

Dilated and narrowed segments of vessel. Produced by fibrosis of the lamina media.

SPONTANEOUS ARTERIAL DISSECTION

Extracranial and intracranial dissections are an underdiagnosed cause of stroke in young persons. Spontaneous dissections occur in Marfan's syndrome, fibromuscular dysplasia, migraine and hypertension. Pathological examination often reveals cystic degeneration or necrosis of the media.

TRAUMA TO CAROTID AND VERTEBRAL VESSELS

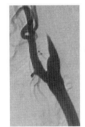

Internal carotid artery dissection

A direct blow to the neck, a sustained tight grip around the neck or a hyperextension injury may produce an intimal tear of the extracranial vessels. This may lead to dissection and occlusion.

The vertebral arteries are particularly susceptible to trauma in view of their close relationship to the cervical spine at intervertebral foramina, the atlanto-axial joint and the occipito-atlantal joint. Carotid dissection may present with a painful isolated Horner's syndrome or lower cranial nerve palsies.

Angiography will confirm, and exploration and/or anticoagulant therapy may halt thrombus formation.

CERVICAL RIB

Pressure from a cervical rib can result in aneurysmal formation in the subclavian artery with endothelial damage, thrombus formation and embolisation down the arm or retrograde thrombus spread and embolisation to the vertebral and common carotid arteries.

INFLAMMATION VESSEL OCCLUSION

Infection in structures close to the carotid artery can result in inflammatory change in the vessel wall and secondary thrombosis. In children, infection in the retropharyngeal fossa (tonsillar infection) may cause cerebral infarction. Meningitis (especially pneumococcal) may result in secondary arteritis and occlusion of intracerebral vessels as they cross the subarachnoid space.

MOYAMOYA DISEASE

Bilateral occlusion of the carotid artery at the siphon is followed by the development of a fine network of collateral arteries and arterioles at the base of the brain. This may be a congenital or acquired disorder associated with previous meningitis, oral contraception or granulomatous disease (e.g. sarcoidosis). Children present with alternating hemiplegia, adults with subarachnoid haemorrhage. There is no specific treatment though some use surgical revascularisation procedures.

HOMOCYSTINURIA

A recessively inherited disorder. Accumulation of homocystine in blood damages endothelium and induces premature occlusive arterial disease. The significance of the heterozygote state is uncertain.

MELAS

See Mitochondrial disorders (page 478).

CEREBROVASCULAR DISEASE – INTRACEREBRAL HAEMORRHAGE

By definition, 'intracerebral haemorrhage' occurs within the brain substance, but rupture through to the cortical surface may produce associated 'subarachnoid' bleeding. When the haemorrhage occurs deep in the hemisphere, rupture into the ventricular system is common.

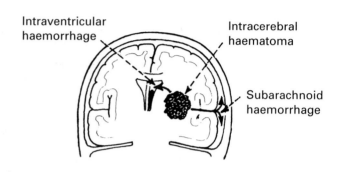

CAUSES

Hypertension ⎫	Anticoagulants
Cerebral amyloid angiopathy ⎬ 80%	Vasculitis
Aneurysm	Drug abuse e.g. cocaine
Arteriovenous malformation	Trauma
Neoplasm	Haemorrhagic infarction
Coagulation disorders e.g. haemophilia	Idiopathic

In autopsy series, hypertension accounts for 40–50% of patients dying from non-traumatic haematomas. In hypertensive patients, degenerative changes weaken the walls of small intraparenchymal perforating vessels. Rupture usually occurs near a vessel bifurcation. The 'microaneurysms' originally described by Charcot and Bouchard are more likely to be small subadventitial haemorrhages or extravascular clots. In normotensive patients without any evident underlying pathology the cause remains unknown, but cryptic arteriovenous malformations are suspect especially in younger patients (i.e. less than 40 years) and when the haematoma is 'lobar' (i.e. frontal, temporal, parieto-occipital). In these patients, the haematoma may temporarily or permanently obliterate the lesion. Reinvestigation following haematoma resolution occasionally reveals previously undetected malformations. In the normotensive elderly patient, subcortical haematomas are commonly associated with amyloid vasculopathy, a degenerative disorder affecting the walls of arteries.

PATHOLOGICAL EFFECTS

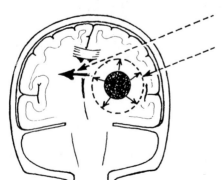

Space-occupying effect – brain shift.

The haematoma may continue to expand beyond the first few hours due to continued bleeding.

Within 48 hours the blood and plasma act on surrounding brain causing disruption of the blood–brain barrier, vasogenic and cytotoxic oedema, neuronal damage and necrosis.

Haematoma resolution occurs in 4–8 weeks, leaving a cystic cavity.

INTRACEREBRAL HAEMORRHAGE

SITES

In *hypertensive* patients, up to 70% occur in the basal ganglia/thalamic region.

In *normotensive* patients:

Frontal — 15%
Basal ganglia/thalamus —— 37%
Parieto-occipital — 15%
Temporal —— 21%
Cerebellar — 8%
Pontine —— 4%

CLINICAL EFFECTS

SUPRATENTORIAL HAEMATOMA

Mass effect: Sudden onset of headache followed by either a rapid loss of consciousness or a gradual deterioration in conscious level over 24–48 hours.

Focal signs: Hemiparesis, hemisensory loss and homonymous hemianopia are common. The patient may be aware of limb weakness developing prior to losing consciousness. A III nerve palsy indicates transtentorial herniation.

CEREBELLAR HAEMATOMA
– Sudden onset of headache with subsequent effects developing either acutely or subacutely –
Cerebellar and brainstem symptoms and signs, e.g. severe ataxia, dysarthria, nystagmus, vertigo and vomiting
CSF obstruction → hydrocephalus with symptoms and signs of ↑ICP.

PONTINE HAEMATOMA
– Sudden loss of consciousness
Quadraplegia
Respiratory irregularities → slowed respiration
Pinpoint pupils, pyrexia
Skewed/dysconjugate eye movements
Death often follows.

INVESTIGATIONS

A CT scan determines the exact site and size of the haematoma and excludes other pathologies.

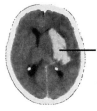
Intracerebral haematoma (basal ganglia)

High density area without contrast enhancement

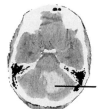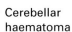
Look for hydrocephalus on higher cuts

Cerebellar haematoma

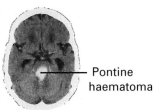
Pontine haematoma

Angiography/CT angiography

– Performed immediately if clinical state requires urgent operation, to identify a secondary cause i.e. arteriovenous malformation, aneurysm or vasculitis.
– Otherwise delayed until condition improves and the haematoma resolves, unless age and medical condition preclude further management.

In patients with negative angiography, a late MRI may demonstrate a CAVERNOUS ANGIOMA (see page 296).

INTRACEREBRAL HAEMORRHAGE

MANAGEMENT

Supratentorial haematoma
In 1961 a controlled study of conservative versus operative evacuation of intracerebral haematomas (through a craniotomy flap) showed no difference in outcome (McKissock et al) and as a result many surgeons adopted a conservative approach.

More recent studies suggest that in selected patients, operative decompression is worthwhile. In general, haematoma evacuation is indicated in patients who deteriorate gradually from the 'mass' effect, especially when the lesion lies superficially; operation will not benefit moribund patients, i.e. patients extending to painful stimuli with no pupil reaction.

PROGNOSIS

Poor prognostic features
– Large, deep lesions (basal ganglia/thalamic)
– Intraventricular blood
– Depth of conscious level (flexion or extension to painful stimuli).

Good prognostic factors
– small superficial lesions (i.e. frontal, temporal or parieto-occipital)
– conscious patients or patients localising to painful stimuli.

The overall mortality ranges from 25–60% (90% if the patient is in coma) and is improved by an integrated 'Stroke Unit'

Cerebellar haematoma:
Small haematomas causing minimal effects may be managed conservatively. Otherwise, urgent evacuation through a suboccipital craniectomy is required. Relief of brain stem compression may be life saving and operative morbidity is low.

The overall mortality is approximately 30%.

Pontine haemorrhage
The mortality from pontine haemorrhage is high. A conservative approach is usually adopted although some advocate operative exploration.

INTRAVENTRICULAR HAEMORRHAGE
Haemorrhage into the ventricles causes a sudden loss of consciousness. With a large bleed, death may follow from the pressure transmission from within the ventricular system. Blood in the ventricles does not in itself cause damage and, following clot resolution, complete recovery may occur.

No treatment is required; attempts at flushing out the ventricles usually fail. If the blood 'cast' causes obstructive hydrocephalus, then ventricular drainage (although hampered by the presence of blood) is indicated. Infusion of thrombolytic agents awaits evaluation.

SUBARACHNOID HAEMORRHAGE (SAH)

Intracranial vessels lie in the *subarachnoid* space and give off small perforating branches to the brain tissue. Bleeding from these vessels or from an associated aneurysm occurs primarily into this space. Some intracranial aneurysms are embedded within the brain tissue and their rupture causes intracerebral bleeding with or without subarachnoid haemorrhage.

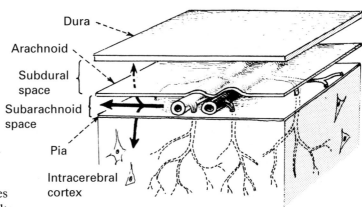

Occasionally the arachnoid layer gives way and a subdural haematoma results.

INCIDENCE
Subarachnoid haemorrhage occurs in approximately 10–15 per 100 000 per year.

CAUSE
Cerebral aneurysms are the most frequent cause of subarachnoid haemorrhage, with arteriovenous malformations accounting for 6%.

In some patients detailed investigation fails to reveal a source of the haemorrhage. Hypertension may account for some. Cryptic arteriovenous malformations or small thrombosed aneurysms may contribute to the remainder.

CAUSES OF SAH	
	Approx. Incidence
Aneurysm	70–75%
A-V malformations	5%
Bleeding diathesis Anticoagulants Tumours Vasculitis	< 5%
Undefined	15%

SYMPTOMS AND SIGNS
The severity of the symptoms is related to the severity of the bleed.

Usually the *headache* is severe and the onset instantaneous (often described as a 'blow to the head'). A transient or prolonged *loss of consciousness* or *epileptic seizure* may immediately follow. Nausea and *vomiting* commonly occur. Symptoms continue for many days.

Occasionally, the headache is mild (although still instantaneous) and may represent a 'warning leak' of blood before a major bleed.

Signs of meningism develop after 3–12 hours

Neck stiffness is present in most patients on passive neck flexion.

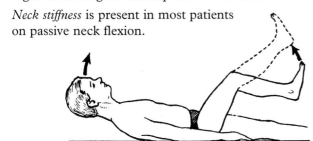

Kernig's sign: stretching nerve roots by extending the knee causes pain.

SUBARACHNOID HAEMORRHAGE (SAH)

SYMPTOMS AND SIGNS (*cont'd*)

Coma or depression of conscious level may result from the direct effect of the subarachnoid haemorrhage or from the mass effect of an associated intracerebral haematoma.

Focal damage from a haematoma will produce *focal signs*, e.g. limb weakness, dysphasia. The presence of a III nerve palsy indicates either transtentorial herniation or direct nerve damage from a posterior communicating artery aneurysm (or rarely from a basilar artery aneurysm).

Epilepsy frequently occurs and may mask other features.

Fundus examination may reveal *papilloedema* or a *subhyaloid or vitreous haemorrhage* caused by the sudden rise in intracranial pressure.

A *'reactive hypertension'* commonly develops, i.e. a rise in BP in patients with no evidence of pre-existing hypertension, and takes several days to return to normal levels.

Pyrexia is also a common finding; if severe and fluctuating, it may reflect ischaemic hypothalamic damage.

INVESTIGATIVE APPROACH

Lumbar puncture establishes the diagnosis of subarachnoid haemorrhage, but in patients with a mass lesion, lumbar puncture could precipitate transtentorial herniation.

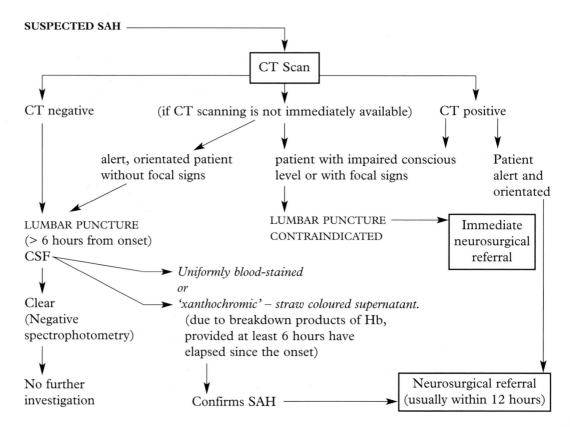

SUBARACHNOID HAEMORRHAGE

INVESTIGATIVE APPROACH (*cont'd*)

Age limit for neurosurgical referral: Although mortality and morbidity increase with age, with the option of endovascular aneurysm treatment, age limitations no longer apply provided the patient's clinical state is satisfactory.

CT scan

Confirms the diagnosis of SAH in 95% (if within 48 hours of the bleed).

Blood may be *widely distributed*
– throughout the
   basal cisterns,
   Sylvian and
   interhemispheric ————
   fissures

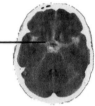

– over the
   cortical sulci ————

– within the
   ventricular
   system ————

or *more localised* aiding identification of the site of the ruptured aneurysm

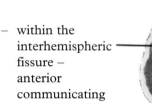

e.g. – within ————
   a Sylvian fissure –
   middle cerebral
   aneurysm

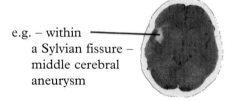

– within the
   interhemispheric ————
   fissure –
   anterior
   communicating
   aneurysm

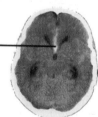

CT also identifies other associated lesions
– hydrocephalus
– intracerebral haematoma
– tumour
– arteriovenous malformation

Blood restricted to the interpeduncular region and not extending ———— into the lateral Sylvian or interhemispheric fissures (i.e. a *'perimesencephalic' pattern*) is usually associated with a negative angiogram, but angiography is still required to exclude a basilar aneurysm.

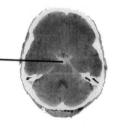

MRI scan

Not routinely used, but in patients with multiple aneurysms, MRI performed several days after the bleed may provide greater sensitivity than CT in detecting small areas of subarachnoid clot and help determine the particular lesion responsible.

N.B. Spinal arteriovenous malformations can also cause SAH – if the patient's pain begins in the back before spreading to the head, or if any features of cord compression exist, then MRI of the cervical or thoracic spine should be the preliminary investigation (see page 419).

SUBARACHNOID HAEMORRHAGE

CT/MR angiography

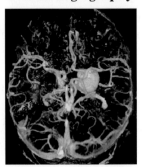

These non invasive techniques, particularly when combined with 3-D or 4-D imaging (colour as the 4th dimension), will detect up to 95% of intracranial aneurysms, but those < 3 mm in diameter may be missed. Both MRA and in particular CTA can provide more information than conventional angiography about the aneurysm shape and size of the neck.

Demonstration of an aneurysm which matches the distribution of blood on standard CT, permits planning of treatment on the assumption that this is the source of the haemorrhage.

CT angiogram showing carotid aneurysm

Digital angiography

Four-vessel angiography is usually performed in all patients to ensure detection of all aneurysms, even those under 3 mm in size. In patients where initial treatment was based on CTA or MRA, or for those in poor clinical condition, the clinician may delay this investigation until a later date.

Antero-posterior, lateral and oblique views are required for each vessel.

Look for *aneurysms* at vessel bifurcations around the circle of Willis, on the middle cerebral and pericallosal vessels, and on the vertebral artery at the posterior inferior cerebellar artery origin.
(Mycotic aneurysms lie more peripherally.)

Carotid angiogram – lateral view

Look for *arteriovenous malformations* – an abnormal leash of blood vessels demonstrated in the arterial phase. N.B. Small AVMs are difficult to detect and only early filling of a vein may draw attention to their presence.

Note '*spasm*' of an arterial segment, usually near a ruptured aneurysm, although it may be distant or diffuse.

Beware mistaking a vessel loop seen end-on for an aneurysm – an aneurysm will be evident on more than one view, e.g. lateral and oblique.

Negative angiography

Angiography fails to reveal a source of the subarachnoid haemorrhage in approximately 20% of patients. In the presence of arterial spasm, reduction in flow may prevent the demonstration of an aneurysm and repeat angiography may be required at a later date.

Prognosis: In patients with a 'perimesencephalic' pattern of haemorrhage on CT scan and with negative angiography, the outlook is excellent; those patients with an 'aneurysmal' pattern with blood lying in the interhemispheric or Sylvian fissure still run a risk of rebleeding.

CEREBRAL ANEURYSMS

INCIDENCE

At autopsy intracranial aneurysms are found in approximately 2% of the population.

Aneurysm rupture occurs in 6–12 per 100 000 per year

Female:male = 3.2; but this ratio varies with age: < 40 years, male > females
> 40 years, females > males

Risk factors: atherosclerotic diseases (2.3x), family history (4x),
polycystic kidney disease (4.4x).

Inheritance: investigations reveal aneurysms in 10% of relatives with two or more affected 1st degree family members. The genetic basis remains unknown. Procollagen III deficiency may play a role in some patients.

MORPHOLOGY

Intracranial aneurysms are usually *saccular,* occurring
at vessel bifurcations.
Size varies from a few millimetres to several centimetres.
Those over 2.5 cm are termed 'giant' aneurysms.

Fusiform dilatation and ectasia of the carotid and the basilar artery may follow atherosclerotic damage. These aneurysms seldom rupture.
Mycotic aneurysms, secondary to vessel wall infection, arise from haematogenous spread, e.g. subacute bacterial endocarditis.

Aneurysm rupture: usually occurs at the fundus of the aneurysm and the risk appears to be related to size. Smoking, hypertension and alcohol excess also play a part. In some patients, rupture occurs during exertion, straining or coitus, but in most there is no associated relationship.

Sites of saccular aneurysm

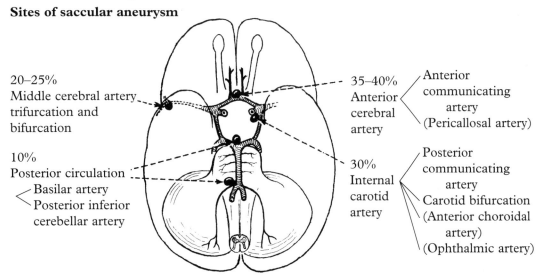

20–25%
Middle cerebral artery
trifurcation and
bifurcation

10%
Posterior circulation
Basilar artery
Posterior inferior
cerebellar artery

35–40%
Anterior
cerebral
artery

Anterior
communicating
artery
(Pericallosal artery)

30%
Internal
carotid
artery

Posterior
communicating
artery
Carotid bifurcation
(Anterior choroidal
artery)
(Ophthalmic artery)

Multiple aneurysms: in approximately 30% of patients with aneurysmal SAH, more than one aneurysm is demonstrated on angiography.

CEREBRAL ANEURYSMS

PATHOGENESIS

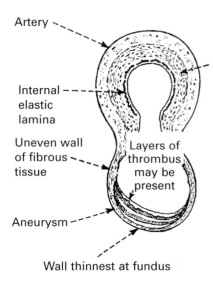

Artery

Internal elastic lamina

Uneven wall of fibrous tissue

Layers of thrombus may be present

Aneurysm

Wall thinnest at fundus

The exact cause of aneurysm formation may be multifactorial.

Aneurysms were once thought to be 'congenital' due to the finding of *developmental defects in the tunica media*. These defects occur at the apex of vessel bifurcation as do aneurysms, but they are also found in many extracranial vessels as well as intracranial vessels; saccular aneurysms in contrast are seldom found outwith the skull. Tunica media defects are often evident in children, yet aneurysms are rare in this age group. It now appears that *defects of the internal elastic lamina* are more important in aneurysm formation and these are probably related to arteriosclerotic damage.

Aneurysms often form at sites of *haemodynamic stress* where for example, a congenitally hypoplastic vessel leads to excessive flow in an adjacent artery. It is not known whether they form rapidly over the space of a few minutes, or more slowly over days, weeks, or months.

Hypertension may play a role; more than half the patients with ruptured aneurysm have pre-existing evidence of raised blood pressure. (Aneurysm formation is common in patients with hypertension from coarctation of the aorta.)

CLINICAL PRESENTATION

Of those patients with intracranial aneurysms presenting acutely, most have had a subarachnoid haemorrhage. A few present with symptoms or signs due to compression of adjacent structures. Others present with an aneurysm found incidentally.

1. Rupture

The features of SAH have already been described in detail (page 273); they include sudden onset of headache, vomiting, neck stiffness, loss of consciousness, focal signs and epilepsy.

Since the severity of the haemorrhage relates to the patient's clinical state and this in turn relates to outcome, much emphasis has been placed on categorising patients into 5 level grading systems, e.g. Hunt and Hess, Nishioka. A scale incorporating the Glasgow Coma scale (page 29) has been adopted by the World Federation of Neurosurgical Societies:

WFNs Grade	Glasgow Coma Score	Motor deficit
I	15	absent
II	14–13	absent
III	14–13	present
IV	12–7	present or absent
V	6–3	present or absent

Glasgow Coma Score
eye opening 1–4   e.g. no eye opening (1)
verbal response 1–5   no verbal response (1)
motor response 1–6   spastic flexion to pain (3)
3–15   = 5

This grading scale correlates well with final outcome and provides a prognostic index for the clinician. In addition, it enables matching of patient groups before comparing the effects of different management techniques.

CEREBRAL ANEURYSMS

CLINICAL PRESENTATION *(cont'd)*

2. Compression from aneurysm sac

A large *internal carotid artery aneurysm (or anterior communicating artery aneurysm)* may compress –

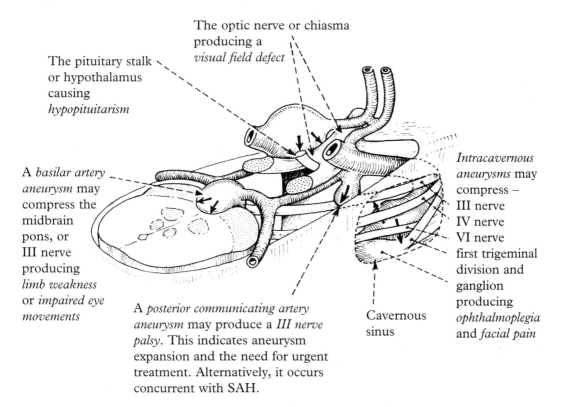

The pituitary stalk or hypothalamus causing *hypopituitarism*

The optic nerve or chiasma producing a *visual field defect*

Intracavernous aneurysms may compress – III nerve IV nerve VI nerve first trigeminal division and ganglion producing *ophthalmoplegia* and *facial pain*

A *basilar artery aneurysm* may compress the midbrain pons, or III nerve producing *limb weakness* or *impaired eye movements*

A *posterior communicating artery aneurysm* may produce a *III nerve palsy*. This indicates aneurysm expansion and the need for urgent treatment. Alternatively, it occurs concurrent with SAH.

Cavernous sinus

3. Incidental finding

The improved availability of sensitive high quality, non-invasive MR or CT imaging techniques has greatly increased the number of patients in whom an intracranial aneurysm is detected incidentally, during investigation for other disease.

CEREBRAL ANEURYSMS

NATURAL HISTORY OF RUPTURED ANEURYSM

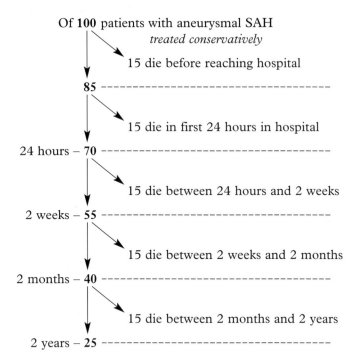

Of **100** patients with aneurysmal SAH
treated conservatively

15 die before reaching hospital

85 -

15 die in first 24 hours in hospital

24 hours – **70** -

15 die between 24 hours and 2 weeks

2 weeks – **55** -

15 die between 2 weeks and 2 months

2 months – **40** -

15 die between 2 months and 2 years

2 years – **25** -

SAH from ruptured aneurysm carries a high initial mortality risk which gradually declines with time. Of those who survive the initial bleed, rebleeding and cerebral infarction (see below) are the major causes of death.

These figures are based on studies of conservative treatment carried out in the 1960s, at a time when the risks of operation were greater and benefits uncertain.

COMPLICATIONS OF ANEURYSMAL SAH

INTRACRANIAL
- Rebleeding
- Cerebral ischaemia/infarction
- Hydrocephalus
- 'Expanding' haematoma
- Epilepsy.

EXTRACRANIAL
- Myocardial infarction
- Cardiac arrhythmias
- Pulmonary oedema
- Gastric haemorrhage (stress ulcer).

CEREBRAL ANEURYSMS – COMPLICATIONS

REBLEEDING

Rebleeding is a major problem following aneurysmal SAH. In the first 28 days (in *untreated* patients), approximately 30% of patients would rebleed; of these 70% die. In the following few months the risk gradually falls off but it never drops below 3.5% per year.

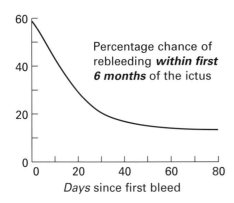

Percentage chance of rebleeding **within first 6 months** of the ictus

Days since first bleed

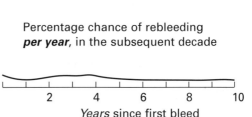

Percentage chance of rebleeding **per year**, in the subsequent decade

Years since first bleed

Adapted from Winn, Richardson, Jane 1977
Annals of Neurology

If, for example, a patient survives the first 30 days after a bleed, there is still a 20% chance of a rebleed occurring in the next 5 months. Even if patients survive the 'high risk' period in the first 6 months, there is still a considerable chance of rebleeding and death in the subsequent years.

The clinical picture of rebleeding is that of SAH, but usually the effects are more severe than the initial bleed. Most patients lose consciousness; the risk of death from a rebleed is more than twice that from the initial bleed.

Investigation

All patients deteriorating suddenly require a CT scan. This helps in establishing the diagnosis of rebleeding and excludes a remediable cause of the deterioration, e.g. acute hydrocephalus.

281

CEREBRAL ANEURYSMS – COMPLICATIONS

CEREBRAL ISCHAEMIA/INFARCTION

Following subarachnoid haemorrhage, patients are at risk of developing cerebral ischaemia or infarction and this is an important contributory factor to mortality and morbidity. Cerebral ischaemia/infarction may occur as an immediate and direct result of the haemorrhage, but more often develops 4–12 days after the onset, either before or after operation – hence the term 'delayed cerebral ischaemia'. Approximately 25% of patients develop clinical evidence of delayed ischaemia/infarction; of these 25% die as a result. About 10% of the survivors remain permanently disabled.

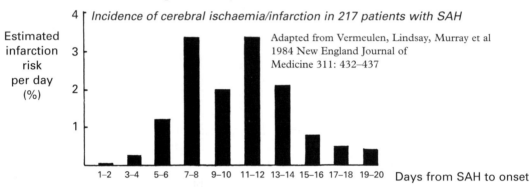

Incidence of cerebral ischaemia/infarction in 217 patients with SAH

Estimated infarction risk per day (%)

Adapted from Vermeulen, Lindsay, Murray et al 1984 New England Journal of Medicine 311: 432–437

Days from SAH to onset

Aetiology of cerebral ischaemia/infarction

Several factors probably contribute to the development of cerebral ischaemia or infarction: '*Vasospasm*': arterial narrowing on angiography occurs in up to 60% of patients after SAH and is either focal or diffuse. The development of 'vasospasm' shows a similar pattern of delay to that of cerebral ischaemia.

The angiogram appearance was initially thought to result from arterial constriction; this may be so, but the pathogenesis of 'vasospasm' now seems more complex. Many vasoconstrictive substances either released from the vessel wall or from the blood clot appear in the CSF after SAH, e.g. serotonin, prostaglandin, oxyhaemoglobin, but numerous studies with vasoconstrictor antagonists have failed to reverse the angiographic narrowing or to reduce the incidence of ischaemia. This failure may be a result of the *arteriopathic changes* which have been observed in the vessel wall. Only calcium antagonists appear to have a beneficial effect (see page 243).

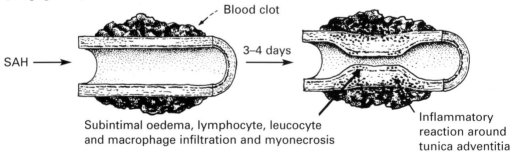

Blood clot

SAH →

3–4 days

Subintimal oedema, lymphocyte, leucocyte and macrophage infiltration and myonecrosis

Inflammatory reaction around tunica adventitia

The greater the amount of blood in the basal cisterns (as shown on CT scan), the higher the incidence of arterial narrowing and associated ischaemic deficits.

CEREBRAL ANEURYSMS – COMPLICATIONS

Hypovolaemia
Hyponatraemia develops after SAH in many patients due to excessive renal secretion of sodium rather than a dilutional effect from inappropriate antidiuretic hormone secretion. Fluid loss and a fall in plasma volume follow.

These patients are particularly at risk of developing cerebral ischaemic deficits, probably as a result of increased blood viscosity.

Reduced cerebral perfusion pressure
Following SAH, intracranial haematoma or hydrocephalus may cause a rise in intracranial pressure (ICP). Since cerebral perfusion pressure = mean BP – ICP, a subsequent reduction in cerebral perfusion may occur.

Clinical effects of cerebral ischaemia/infarction
This may affect one particular arterial territory producing characteristic signs:

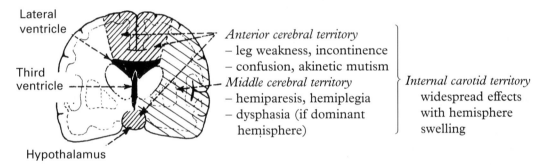

Commonly the ischaemia occurs in multiple areas, often in both hemispheres. This correlates with the pattern of arterial 'spasm'.

Transcranial Doppler: a significant increase in flow velocity within an intracranial vessel may indicate developing 'vasospasm', even before clinical problems develop, and allow the early introduction of prophylactic measures (see page 288).

HYDROCEPHALUS
Following SAH, cerebrospinal fluid drainage may be impaired by:
– blood clot within the basal cisterns ⎱ 'communicating' hydrocephalus (see page 370)
– obstruction of the arachnoid villi ⎰
– blood clot within the ventricular system – 'obstructive' hydrocephalus.

Acute hydrocephalus occurs in about 20% of patients, usually in the first few days after the ictus; occasionally this is a late complication. In only one-third are symptoms of headache, impaired conscious level, dementia, incontinence, or gait ataxia severe enough to warrant treatment.

In a further 10% of patients, hydrocephalus develops late – months or even years after the haemorrhage.

CEREBRAL ANEURYSMS – COMPLICATIONS

'EXPANDING' INTRACEREBRAL HAEMATOMA

Brain swelling around an intracerebral haematoma may aggravate the mass effect of the haematoma; this may cause a progressive deterioration in conscious level or progression of focal signs.

EPILEPSY

Epilepsy may occur at any stage after SAH, especially if a haematoma has caused cortical damage.

Seizures may be generalised or partial (focal).

EXTRACRANIAL COMPLICATIONS

Myocardial infarction/cardiac arrhythmias: electrocardiographic and pathological changes in the myocardium are occasionally evident after SAH, and ventricular fibrillation has been recorded. These problems are likely to occur secondarily to catecholamine release following ischaemic damage to the hypothalamus.

Pulmonary oedema: this occasionally occurs after SAH, probably as a result of massive sympathetic discharge; note the 'pink, frothy' sputum and typical auscultatory and chest X-ray findings.

Gastric haemorrhage: bleeding from gastric erosions occasionally occurs after SAH but rarely threatens life.

CEREBRAL ANEURYSMS – MANAGEMENT FOLLOWING SAH

Headache requires *analgesia* – codeine or dihydrocodeine. Stronger analgesics may depress conscious level and mask neurological deterioration. Management is otherwise aimed at preventing complications –

PREVENTION OF REBLEEDING

Bed rest: Usually enforced after SAH, although there is no evidence that this reduces the rebleed risk. Allowing the patients to use the toilet may induce less 'stress' than using a bedpan.

Antifibrinolytic agents: tranexamic acid, epsilon aminocaproic acid.

These agents prevent rebleeding by delaying clot dissolution around the aneurysm fundus. Past studies have shown that this beneficial effect has been offset by an increased incidence of cerebral ischaemia. A recent study has suggested that a very short course (12–24 hours) of tranexamic acid, given *immediately* after diagnosis, reduces rebleeding within this high-risk period without increasing cerebral ischaemia. When combined with prompt aneurysm repair, tranexamic acid may still have potential therapeutic benefit.

Fibrinolytic mechanism

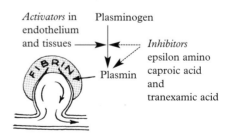

CEREBRAL ANEURYSMS – MANAGEMENT FOLLOWING SAH

OPERATIVE TECHNIQUES

Direct clipping of the aneurysm neck: Through a craniotomy and using the operating microscope, the surgeon dissects out the aneurysm and applies a clip across the neck without compromising the proximal or distal vessels. Clipping prevents rebleeding; clip slippage rarely occurs. If any part of the neck lies outwith the clip, this may occasionally lead to recurrent growth.

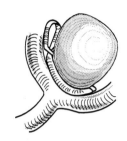

Wrapping: If the width of the aneurysm neck or its involvement with adjacent vessels prevents clipping, then muslin gauze may be wrapped around the fundus. This provides some protection, but rebleeding may still occur.

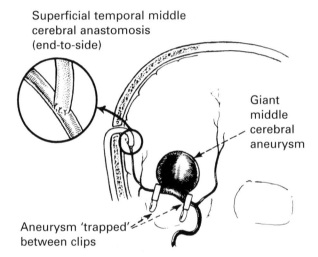

Superficial temporal middle cerebral anastomosis (end-to-side)

Giant middle cerebral aneurysm

Aneurysm 'trapped' between clips

Trapping: Used for giant aneurysms (>25 mm diameter) where other methods have failed due to the width of the aneurysm neck. Should be combined with cerebral revascularisation to minimize the risk of ischaemia. Techniques include either superficial temporal–middle cerebral artery anastomosis or insertion of a saphenous vein or radial artery bypass graft from the carotid to the middle cerebral artery.

Proximal occlusion – common carotid ligation: Reserved for aneurysms arising directly from the carotid artery where other techniques have failed or were not attempted e.g. an intracavernous or 'giant' ophthalmic artery aneurysm. Most patients tolerate common carotid occlusion; collateral circulation through the Circle of Willis and reverse flow in the external carotid artery usually provide sufficient hemispheric flow to prevent ischaemic complications.

Temporary occlusion under local anaesthesia can help predict patients who fail to tolerate this, but despite these methods, late ischaemic deficits occasionally occur.

Carotid occlusion provides protection from rebleeding in the 'high risk' period. *Beyond the first 6 months, the risk reverts to that of an untreated aneurysm i.e. 3.5% per year.* As other techniques have improved, proximal occlusion has become less popular.

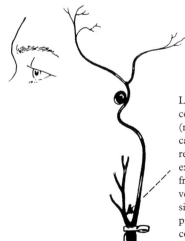

Ligation of the common carotid artery (rather than the internal carotid artery) permits retrograde flow in the external carotid artery from anastomosis with vessels on the opposite side and may help prevent ischaemic complications.

CEREBRAL ANEURYSMS – MANAGEMENT FOLLOWING SAH

ENDOVASCULAR TECHNIQUES

Coil embolisation: this endovascular technique where multiple helical platinum coils are packed into the aneurysm fundus, has been developed and refined over the last decade. A tracker catheter is inserted via a femoral puncture and guided up through the arterial system into the aneurysm sac.

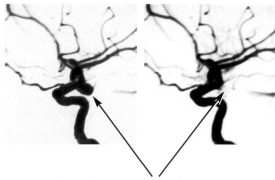

The coil attached to the end of a delivery wire is then guided into the fundus and after accurate placement, the passage of an electric current causes electrochemical release. On average, 4–5 coils are required to pack each aneurysm.

Posterior communicating aneurysm before and after coil embolisation

The radiologist aims to completely obliterate the fundus, but this is not always feasible and to avoid occluding the adjacent vessel, a portion of the neck may remain. In either case, a small risk of rebleeding persists, even when completely obliterated. Thrombotic complications may also occur during the procedure.

Balloon remodelling: the wider the aneurysm neck, the greater the risk that coils will project into and occlude the vessel lumen. A balloon is attached to a second catheter and periodically inflated across the aneurysm neck during coil insertion to preserve the vessel lumen.

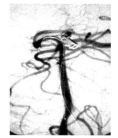 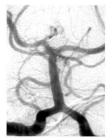

Basilar bifurcation aneurysm with wide neck – before coiling (note vasospasm)   during coil embolisation with inflatable balloon in situ   and after coiling

Balloon occlusion: intra-arterial inflation of a detachable balloon can serve as an alternative method of proximally occluding a carotid or a vertebral artery (see page 285). Temporary occlusion can provide intra-operative protection or when carried out under local anaesthetic can test a patient's tolerance before making occlusion permanent.

Stents: although routinely used for extracranial vessels, stents have only recently been developed for intracranial use. These may help maintain flow across the neck of giant aneurysms and allow the fundus to be packed off with coils, or filled with onyx.

Onyx: a liquid polymer which solidifies on contact with blood, used on a trial basis to inject into the fundus of giant aneurysms.

CEREBRAL ANEURYSMS – MANAGEMENT FOLLOWING SAH

SELECTION OF TREATMENT

Direct surgical clipping has been the standard method of aneurysm treatment for many years with trapping/proximal ligation reserved for those patients where direct repair fails. Since coil embolisation was introduced over the last 10 years and despite the lack of evidence of benefit, radiological referral for this treatment has increased, particularly for patients with posterior circulation aneurysms. It would appear that this technique could be used for at least 80% of aneurysms.

Preliminary results of a large multicentre randomized trial of clipping vs. endovascular treatment (the International Subarachnoid Aneurysm Trial – ISAT) demonstrated a 23% reduction in the proportion of patients with a poor outcome (dependent or dead) at one year in those patients undergoing coil embolisation, despite more rebleeds occurring in this group. The trial was almost exclusively restricted to anterior circulation aneurysms. We await longer-term follow up, but until then a crucial question remains – does coil embolisation prevent late rebleeding? Even without this information, release of this data in the UK resulted in an increase from 35% to 55% of patients receiving endovascular treatment.

Aneurysm treatment now requires a team approach, with the interventional radiologists playing a role in management decisions. Some patients e.g. those with basilar bifurcation aneurysms, difficult anterior circulation aneurysms, the elderly or those in poor clinical condition are more likely to require coil embolisation, whereas others, such as those with large middle cerebral aneurysms are more likely to require direct operative treatment. Unfortunately aneurysms that are difficult to treat with one technique are often difficult to treat with both methods.

TIMING OF TREATMENT

Pioneers of *aneurysm surgery* found that operation within a day or two of the haemorrhage carried an unacceptable risk. Operative mortality rates fell dramatically when operation was delayed for several weeks, but the longer the delay, the greater the possibility of death from rebleeding. The clinical condition or 'grade' of the patient also played a major part, the worse the grade the worse the outcome.

In recent years, with improved operative and anaesthetic techniques, 'early' operation within a few days of the haemorrhage has become feasible. Most surgeons now advocate operation within 2–3 days if possible, at least for those in grade I or II, if not for all patients. The additional risks appear small and are outweighed by the benefit of preventing rebleeding. Once the aneurysm is clipped, aggressive methods of treating ischaemia with induced hypertension can be applied.

It is not yet known whether the timing of *coil embolisation* is relevant, but since this technique avoids potentially harmful effects of brain retraction and vessel dissection, early treatment may not only be feasible, but may improve endovascular access if carried out before the onset of vasospasm. If coil embolisation were planned, it would seem appropriate to perform this whenever manpower and facilities permitted.

CEREBRAL ANEURYSMS – MANAGEMENT FOLLOWING SAH

PREVENTION OF CEREBRAL ISCHAEMIA/INFARCTION

Despite considerable clinical and experimental research, cerebral ischaemia is still a major cause of morbidity and mortality after subarachnoid haemorrhage. In recent years some advances have proved beneficial.

Calcium antagonists: several large studies have confirmed that Nimodipine (and Nicardipine) reduce the incidence of cerebral infarction by about one third and improve outcome. Whether these act by improving collateral circulation, by reducing the harmful effect of calcium flooding into brain cells or by reducing cerebral 'vasospasm' remains uncertain.

Avoidance of antihypertensive therapy: after SAH, autoregulation (page 77) is often impaired; a drop in BP causes a reduction in cerebral blood flow with a subsequent risk of cerebral ischaemia. Patients on long-term antihypertensive treatment can continue with this therapy, but 'reactive' hypertension should not be treated.

High fluid intake (haemodilution): maintenance of a high fluid input (3 litres per day) may help prevent a fall in plasma volume from sodium and fluid loss. If hyponatraemia develops do *not* restrict fluids (this significantly increases the risk of cerebral infarction). If sodium levels fall below 130 mmol/1, give hypertonic saline or fludrocortisone.

Plasma volume expansion (hypervolaemia): expanding the plasma volume with colloid, e.g. plasma proteins, dextran 70, Haemacel, increases blood pressure and improves cerebral blood flow. This should be given either prophylactically in high risk patients (heavy cisternal blood load on CT scan or with high Doppler velocities) or at the first clinical sign of ischaemia. If clinical evidence of ischaemia develops despite this treatment, then combine with:

Hypertensive therapy: treatment with inotropic agents, e.g. dobutamine, increases cardiac output and blood pressure. Since cerebral autoregulation commonly fails after subarachnoid haemorrhage, increasing blood pressure increases cerebral blood flow. Up to 70% of ischaemic neurological deficits developing after aneurysm operations can be reversed by inducing hypertension; often a critical level of blood pressure is evident.

Early recognition and treatment of a developing neurological deficit may prevent progression from ischaemia to infarction. Delayed treatment may merely aggravate vasogenic oedema in an ischaemic area. This technique of induced hypertension is now widely applied, with good results, but requires careful, intensive monitoring. In view of the risk of precipitating aneurysm rupture, it is reserved until after aneurysm repair.

CEREBRAL ANEURYSMS – MANAGEMENT FOLLOWING SAH

PREVENTION OF CEREBRAL ISCHAEMIA/INFARCTION (*cont'd*)

Transluminal angioplasty/papaverine infusion: this involves balloon dilatation of the vasospastic segment of the vessel. It is usually combined with an intra-arterial infusion of the antispasmodic agent papaverine. Although no controlled studies exist, many small studies report a beneficial effect on cerebral blood flow and on clinical state. Timing is difficult. If used too early, the patient may be unnecessarily exposed to an invasive procedure; if too late, the ischaemia may be irreversible. Consider angiography and angioplasty if other measures (haemodilution/hypervolaemia/hypertension) have failed to reverse a significant clinical deterioration within a few hours.

Brain protective agents: to date, studies of neuroprotective drugs (antioxidants and anti-inflammatory agents) other than calcium antagonists, have failed to demonstrate a beneficial effect after subarachnoid haemorrhage.

HYDROCEPHALUS

Hydrocephalus causing acute deterioration in conscious level requires urgent CSF drainage with a ventricular catheter (in 'communicating' hydrocephalus lumbar puncture may provide temporary benefit).

Gradual deterioration or failure to improve in the presence of enlarged ventricles indicates the need for permanent CSF drainage with either a ventriculoperitoneal or lumboperitoneal shunt.

EXPANDING INTRACEREBRAL HAEMATOMA

Intracerebral haematomas from ruptured aneurysms do not require specific treatment unless the 'mass' effect causes a deterioration of conscious level. This necessitates urgent CT or digital angiography followed by evacuation of the haematoma with or without simultaneous clipping of the aneurysm; under these circumstances, operative mortality is high.

OUTCOME AFTER SUBARACHNOID HAEMORRHAGE

Of patients surviving the initial bleed and admitted within 3 days to the neurosurgical unit, approximately 10% die within the following 30 days. Over half make a good recovery and regain former employment, although in a proportion, minor personality change and intellectual deficit persist.

Factors providing a prognostic guide are: age, quantity of subarachnoid blood on CT scan, loss of consciousness at the ictus, clinical condition on admission and the presence of pre-existing hypertension or arterial disease.

Operative mortality ranges from 5–26% depending on the patient's clinical condition and the timing of operation.

Management mortality takes into account all patients, including those not undergoing operation due to premature death or poor clinical condition. These figures are of more value when comparing results of different management regimes. Management mortality from coil treatment is only available for selected patient groups e.g. Grades I/II = 8%.

Operative mortality at 6 months
Nos. undergoing operation – 439

Grade (Hunt & Hess)	Mortality (%)	Good recovery/ Moderate disability (%)
I/II	5	88
III	14	64
IV/V	26	33

Management mortality at 6 months
Nos. admitted – 471

Grade (Hunt & Hess)	Mortality (%)	Good recovery/ Moderate disability (%)
I/II	6	86
III	17	62
IV/V	37	28

Adapted from Cesarini, Hardemark and Persson
1999 Journal of Neurosurgery 90:664–672

Comparing different operative or management policies: Comparison of different treatments for ruptured aneurysms is difficult, unless conducted under the confines of a randomised controlled trial. 'Operative mortality' provides limited information unless patient groups are carefully matched for age, clinical condition and timing of operation. 'Management mortality' (e.g. outcome of all admitted patients up to 3 months from the ictus) is of more practical value, but even then, admission policies require careful scrutiny.

CEREBRAL ANEURYSMS – UNRUPTURED

UNRUPTURED ANEURYSMS

Identification of unruptured aneurysms may result from –

- Investigation of unrelated neurological symptoms with CT, MRI or angiography
- Investigation of symptoms arising as a result of aneurysmal compression of adjacent structures
- Investigation of patients with a family history of aneurysmal SAH (see page 292)
- Investigation of SAH when multiple aneurysms exist (about 25% of patients)

Management: depends on the above circumstances and on balancing the risk of rupture (and death) in future years against the risk of aneurysm repair; the decision is often difficult. The recently reported International Study of Unruptured Intracranial Aneurysms (ISUIA), by far the largest study of its kind, examined both the *natural history* and the *results of treatment* of unruptured aneurysms. The data suggested that the risk of rupture related to the size, site and the occurrence of a SAH from a previously treated source. For small aneurysms < 7 mm in diameter and no previous SAH, the annual risk of rupture was 0.1% (far lower than the 1–2% suggested from previous smaller studies). Only aneurysms > 10 mm in diameter and those in certain sites (basilar bifurcation) had an annual risk of rupture from 1–3.5%. The study also reported a combined operative mortality and morbidity of 10–15%, a figure higher than surgeons had previously liked to admit. The operative risk increased with age, aneurysm size and a site on the posterior circulation. All these factors must also be taken into account when determining appropriate management.

Aneurysms found coincidentally with a ruptured aneurysm appear to be at higher risk than other incidental aneurysms and the surgeon may clip both the ruptured and unruptured aneurysms if accessible through the same craniotomy flap.

When aneurysms present with compressive symptoms such as a III nerve palsy, it is assumed that recent expansion has occurred and that rupture could be imminent. Such patients normally receive urgent treatment.

CEREBRAL ANEURYSMS – SCREENING

SCREENING FOR INTRACRANIAL ANEURYSMS

When two or more members of a family have a history of cerebral aneurysms or SAH, then other members of that family (over the age of 25 years) have an increased risk of harbouring an intracranial aneurysm (about 8% or 4x greater than the rest of the population). A similar increased risk occurs for patients with a genetic predisposition, e.g. polycystic kidney disease, Type IV Ehlers-Danlos. Before undergoing screening to detect whether such an aneurysm exists, several important facts should be considered –

– We do not know how rapidly aneurysms form. They may develop over a few hours, days or weeks. A negative screening investigation will fail to provide the reassurance that a subarachnoid haemorrhage from a ruptured aneurysm will never occur.

– The ISUIA study described above, suggests that for small aneurysms, the rupture risk is extremely low. Even if a small aneurysm is found, treatment risks may preclude any action.

– Aneurysm repair, either by direct operation or by coil embolisation, carries a risk of death or disability, which depends on the patient's age and the size and site of the aneurysm.

– The presence of an aneurysm may carry implications for life insurance, mortgage applications and even for future pregnancies (since the risk of aneurysm rupture is increased during pregnancy).

If after consultation and consideration of these issues the patient wishes to proceed with screening, then CT angiography would be the most appropriate technique, accepting that this may fail to detect aneurysms 3 mm or less in diameter. For those who decide not to undergo screening, other measures may minimise the risk of aneurysm formation in the future – avoid smoking and treat elevated blood pressure and cholesterol.

ARTERIOVENOUS MALFORMATIONS

Arteriovenous malformations (AVMs) are developmental anomalies of the intracranial vasculature; they are not neoplastic despite their tendency to expand with time and the descriptive term 'angioma' occasionally applied.

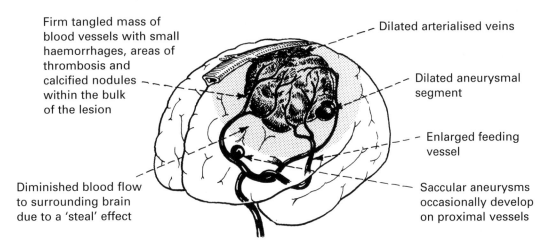

Firm tangled mass of blood vessels with small haemorrhages, areas of thrombosis and calcified nodules within the bulk of the lesion

Diminished blood flow to surrounding brain due to a 'steal' effect

Dilated arterialised veins

Dilated aneurysmal segment

Enlarged feeding vessel

Saccular aneurysms occasionally develop on proximal vessels

Dilated arteries feed directly into a tangled mass of blood vessels of varying calibre; they bypass the capillary network and shunt oxygenated blood directly into the venous system. As a result of raised intraluminal pressure, veins may adopt an 'aneurysmal' appearance. Arteriovenous malformations may occur at any site but are commonest in the middle cerebral artery territory.

Vascular malformations vary in size and different forms exist:

Capillary telangiectasis: an area of dilated capillaries, like a small petechial patch on the brain surface – especially in the pons. These lesions are often only revealed at autopsy.

Cavernous malformation/angioma: plum coloured sponge-like mass composed of a collection of blood filled spaces, but without enlargement of feeding or draining vessels.

CLINICAL PRESENTATION

Haemorrhage

About 40–60% of patients with an AVM present with haemorrhage – often with an intracerebral or intraventricular component. In comparison with saccular aneurysms, AVMs tend to bleed in younger patients, i.e. 20–40 years, and are less likely to have a fatal outcome. Vasospasm and delayed ischaemic complications rarely develop. Small AVMs, those with high intranidal pressure and those draining exclusively to deep veins have an increased risk of haemorrhage.

Annual risk of haemorrhage: patients with no history of haemorrhage have an annual risk of bleeding of 2–4%. For those presenting with haemorrhage, the risk of rebleeding may be higher, particularly in the first year. One study reported an annual risk of 17%.

Mortality from haemorrhage: in contrast to the high mortality following aneurysm rupture, haemorrhage from an AVM carries the relatively low mortality rate of approximately 10–15%.

293

ARTERIOVENOUS MALFORMATIONS

CLINICAL PRESENTATION (*cont'd*)

Epilepsy

Generalised or partial seizures commonly occur in patients with arteriovenous malformation, especially if the lesion involves the cortical surface. Of patients presenting with haemorrhage, 30% have a history of epilepsy.

Neurological deficit

Large AVMs, especially those involving the basal ganglia, may present with a slowly progressive dementia, hemiparesis or visual field defect, probably as a result of a 'steal' effect. The infrequent brain stem AVM may also produce a motor or sensory deficit, with or without cranial nerve involvement.

Headache

Attacks of well localised headache – unilateral and throbbing – occur in a proportion of patients subsequently shown to have a large AVM.

Cranial bruit

Auscultation, especially over the eyeball, occasionally reveals a bruit.

INVESTIGATIONS

CT scan

Most AVMs are evident on CT scan unless masked by the presence of an intracranial haematoma. A double dose of intravenous contrast may aid visualisation, especially with small 'cryptic' lesions.

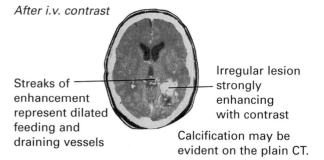

After i.v. contrast

Streaks of enhancement represent dilated feeding and draining vessels

Irregular lesion strongly enhancing with contrast

Calcification may be evident on the plain CT.

MRI

Conventional MRI will clearly demonstrate the AVM as a region of flow voids, with associated signal change within or around the lesion from areas of old haemorrhage or gliosis.

The MRI provides exact anatomical detail and helps surgical planning. Functional MRI (page 42) aids identification of any adjacent eloquent areas.

MRI is the investigation of choice in identifying a *cavernous malformation*, often missed on CT scanning and rarely seen on angiography. Most lesions show marked signal change around this lesion due to a rim of haemosiderin deposition.

T2 weighted MRI showing relationship of AVM (flow voids) to surrounding structures

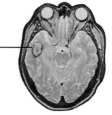

Cavernous malformation

ARTERIOVENOUS MALFORMATIONS

INVESTIGATIONS *(cont'd)*

Angiography

Four-vessel angiography confirms the presence of an AVM and delineates the feeding and draining vessels. Occasionally small AVMs are difficult to detect and only *early venous filling* may draw attention to their presence.

N.B. In the presence of a haematoma, angiography should be delayed until the haematoma resolves, otherwise local pressure may mask demonstration of an AVM. If the angiogram is subsequently negative, then MRI is required to exclude the presence of a cavernous malformation.

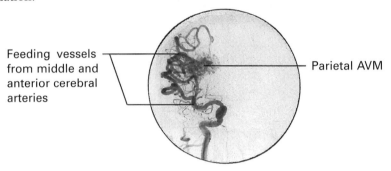

Feeding vessels from middle and anterior cerebral arteries

Parietal AVM

MANAGEMENT

Various methods of treating arteriovenous malformations are available. All risk further damage and a team comprised of the neurosurgeon and neuroradiologist should decide on the optimal method or combination of methods for each patient. The urgency of the patient's clinical condition and the risks of treatment must be weighed against the risk of a conservative approach.

Indications for intervention

– 'Expanding' haematoma associated with AVM
– Progressive neurological deficit
– Risk of haemorrhage especially
    – young patients with many years at risk
    – AVMs < 3 cm

Consider operative risk
low in – AVMs in 'non eloquent' sites
    – AVMs < 3 cm diameter
    – with superficial venous drainage
high in – AVMs > 3 cm diameter
    – AVMs in 'eloquent' sites
    – with drainage to deep veins

ARTERIOVENOUS MALFORMATIONS

Methods of treatment

Operation: *Excision* – complete excision of the AVM (confirmed by per- or postoperative angiography) is the most effective method of treatment particularly for small AVMs in non-eloquent areas. Image guidance (page 382) may aid localisation. Larger lesions (> 6 cm) have a greater risk of postoperative hyperperfusion syndrome and brain swelling and carry a 40% risk of permanent neurological deficit.

Stereotactic radiosurgery: Focused beams from multiple cobalt sources or from a linear accelerator (25 Gy) obliterates about 75% of AVMs < 3 cm in diameter, but this may take *up to 3 years during which time the risk of haemorrhage persists.* Smaller lesions < 1 cm can receive a higher dose (50 Gy) and in those, the cure rate is 90%. For lesions greater than 3 cm, the lower dose required to minimise the damaging effect of local tissue destruction, makes obliteration unlikely. Pre-treatment with embolisation helps only if this produces a segmental reduction in size. Suboptimal embolisation may merely hinder radiosurgical treatment. Despite the delay in action, radiosurgery may prove ideal for small deeply seated lesions.

Embolisation: Skilled catheterisation permits selective embolisation of feeding vessels with isobutyl-cyanoacrylate, although this technique is not without risk. Embolisation may cure up to 10% of AVMs when small and supplied by a single feeding vessel, but usually filling persists from collateral supply. When used preoperatively, it may significantly aid operative removal.

CAVERNOUS MALFORMATIONS (syn. cavernous angioma)

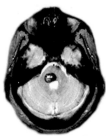

T2 weighted MRI showing dark haemosiderin ring around brainstem cavernous malformation

With the appearance of improved imaging, in particular MRI, cavernous malformations are now identified as a source of intracranial haemorrhage in some patients with an otherwise normal CT scan and angiogram. They occur in 0.5% of the population, are occasionally multiple and in a few patients, have a familial basis. A cavernous malformation may present with epilepsy, haemorrhage or with focal neurological signs. Once diagnosed, the annual risk of haemorrhage is about 1% per year, but this varies depending on whether the lesion lies deeply (i.e. brainstem or basal ganglia) or superficially. With deep lesions in critical sites, a small bleed causes damage more readily. For deep lesions the risk of a bleed sufficiently severe to cause neurological signs is about 5%, whereas for a superficial lesion, this is almost zero. Unfortunately the high risk, deep lesions are more hazardous to surgically remove, although this may be the appropriate management in selected patients.

ARTERIOVENOUS MALFORMATIONS

ANEURYSM OF THE VEIN OF GALEN

This is a type of arteriovenous malformation in which arteries feed directly into the great vein of Galen causing massive aneurysmal dilatation. Patients present either in the neonatal period with severe high output cardiac failure due to the associated arteriovenous shunt, in infancy with cranial enlargement due to an obstructive hydrocephalus, or in childhood with subarachnoid haemorrhage. A cranial bruit is always evident. Cardiac failure usually develops in the neonatal period and is usually fatal. In the other groups the treatment of choice is now endovascular obliteration of the feeding vessels combined with ventricular drainage if required. As a result, the high mortality and morbidity experienced with direct operative repair has considerably reduced.

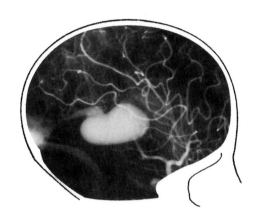

STURGE-WEBER SYNDROME

Angiomatosis affecting the facial skin, eyes and leptomeninges produces the characteristic features of the Sturge-Weber syndrome – a capillary naevus over the forehead and eye, epilepsy and intracranial calcification. (See page 559.)

DURAL ARTERIOVENOUS FISTULA

In contrast to AVMs these fistulous communications are usually acquired rather than developmental in origin. Arterial blood drains directly into either a venous sinus, cortical veins or a combination of both (see carotid-cavernous fistula page 298). The aetiology remains unknown, but sinus thrombosis or trauma may play a part. In a benign form, no reversal of flow occurs and no treatment is required. When retrograde venous flow occurs, venous hypertension results and haemorrhage may follow. For this type, treatment requires ligation and division of the draining vein, often combined with endovascular occlusion.

ARTERIOVENOUS MALFORMATIONS

CAROTID–CAVERNOUS FISTULA

A fistulous communication between the internal carotid artery and the cavernous sinus may follow skull base trauma either immediately or after a delay of several days or weeks. Less often carotid-cavernous fistulae occur spontaneously, perhaps from rupture of a small intracavernous meningeal artery or a saccular carotid aneurysm.

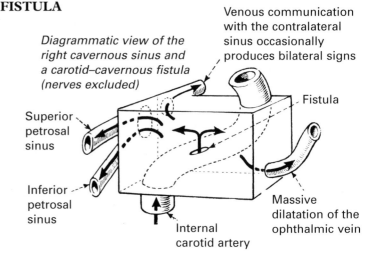

Diagrammatic view of the right cavernous sinus and a carotid–cavernous fistula (nerves excluded)

Venous communication with the contralateral sinus occasionally produces bilateral signs

Fistula

Superior petrosal sinus

Inferior petrosal sinus

Internal carotid artery

Massive dilatation of the ophthalmic vein

Clinical features

Symptoms develop *suddenly* (cf. cavernous sinus thrombosis) – the patient becomes aware of pulsating tinnitus as a 'noise' inside the head. Pain may follow. Examination reveals characteristic signs:

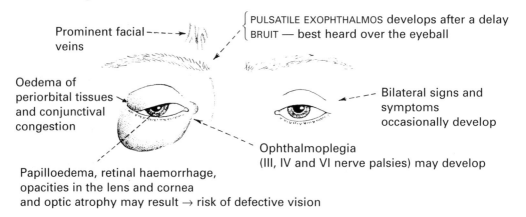

Prominent facial veins

PULSATILE EXOPHTHALMOS develops after a delay
BRUIT — best heard over the eyeball

Oedema of periorbital tissues and conjunctival congestion

Bilateral signs and symptoms occasionally develop

Ophthalmoplegia (III, IV and VI nerve palsies) may develop

Papilloedema, retinal haemorrhage, opacities in the lens and cornea and optic atrophy may result → risk of defective vision

Methods of fistula repair

Spontaneous closure occurs in up to 60%. Provided symptoms do not progress, for the first few months, treatment should be conservative.

Embolisation: with *detachable balloon* catheterization, either through the transvenous or intra-arterial route, is usually the first line of treatment.

Other methods include – *Embolisation with muscle emboli or plastic beads* introduced into the internal carotid artery.

– *Trapping:* ligation of the supraclinoid carotid and ophthalmic arteries intracranially, followed by ligation of the internal carotid artery in the neck.

– Direct operative repair: repair of the fistula within the cavernous sinus with the aid of cardiopulmonary bypass.

INTRACRANIAL TUMOURS

INCIDENCE
Primary brain tumours occur in approximately 6 persons per 100 000 per year. Fewer patients with metastatic tumours reach a neurosurgical centre, although the actual incidence must equal, if not exceed that of primary tumours. About 1 in 12 primary brain tumours occur in children under 15 years.

SITE
In adults, the commonest tumours are gliomas, metastases and meningiomas; most lie in the supratentorial compartment.

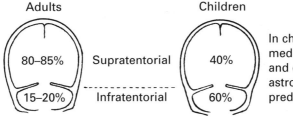

Adults   80–85% Supratentorial   15–20% Infratentorial

Children   40%   60%

In children, medulloblastomas and cerebellar astrocytomas predominate.

PATHOLOGY
Intracranial tumours are often described as 'benign' or 'malignant', but these terms cannot be directly compared with their extracranial counterparts:

A *benign* intracranial tumour may have devastating effects if allowed to expand within the rigid confines of the skull cavity. A benign astrocytoma may infiltrate widely throughout brain tissue preventing complete removal, or may occupy a functionally critical site preventing even partial removal.

A *malignant* intracranial tumour implies rapid growth, poor differentiation, increased cellularity, mitosis, necrosis and vascular proliferation, but metastases to extracranial sites rarely occur.

Pathological classification
In 2000, the World Health Organisation drew up an internationally agreed classification of intracranial tumours based on the tissue of origin. This system avoids the term 'glioma' – previously encompassing astrocytoma, oligodendroglioma, ependymoma and glioblastoma multiforme. The cell origin of the highly malignant glioblastoma is now recognizable as astrocytic rather than embryonal as previously classified.

INTRACRANIAL TUMOURS – PATHOLOGICAL CLASSIFICATION

NEUROEPITHELIAL

Astrocytes → **Astrocytoma:** The most common primary brain tumour. Histological features permit separation into four grades depending on the degree of malignancy. Grading only reflects the features of the biopsy specimen and not necessarily those of the whole tumour. The most malignant type – glioblastoma (grade IV) – occurs most frequently and widely infiltrates surrounding tissue.

Other types range from the less common low-grade astrocytomas including the pilocytic type (grade I) and diffuse types (fibrillary, protoplasmic and gemistocytic) (grade II) to the anaplastic astrocytomas (grade III).

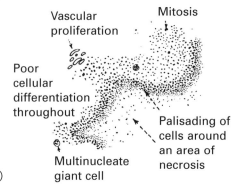

Composite diagram showing the characteristic features of a glioblastoma.

Vascular proliferation

Mitosis

Poor cellular differentiation throughout

Palisading of cells around an area of necrosis

Multinucleate giant cell

Oligodendrocytes → **Oligodendroglioma:** Usually a slowly growing, sharply defined tumour (grade II). Variants include an anaplastic form (grade III) and a 'mixed' oligoastrocytoma (grade II).

Ependymal cells and choroid plexus → **Ependymoma:** Occurs anywhere throughout the ventricular system or spinal canal, but is particularly common in the 4th ventricle and cauda equina. It infiltrates surrounding tissue and may spread throughout the CSF pathways. Variants include an anaplastic type and a subependymoma arising from subependymal astrocytes.

→ **Choroid plexus papilloma:** Rare tumours and an uncommon cause of hydrocephalus due to excessive CSF production. They are usually benign but occasionally occur in a malignant form.

Neurons → **Ganglioglioma/gangliocytoma/neurocytoma:** Rare tumours containing ganglion cells and abnormal neurons occurring in varying degrees of malignancy. This classification includes the very low grade dysembryoplastic neuroepithelial tumour (DENT).

Pineal cells → **Pineocytoma/pineoblastoma:** Extremely rare tumours. The latter are less well differentiated and show more malignant features.

Poorly differentiated and embryonal cells → **Glioblastoma:** A highly malignant astrocytic tumour (see above).

→ **Medulloblastoma:** A malignant tumour of childhood arising from the cerebellar vermis. Small closely packed cells are often arranged in rosettes surrounding abortive axons. May seed through the CSF pathways.

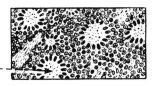

INTRACRANIAL TUMOURS – PATHOLOGICAL CLASSIFICATION

MENINGES → **Meningioma:** Arises from the arachnoid granulations, usually closely related to the venous sinuses but also found over the hemispheric convexity.

The tumours compress rather than invade adjacent brain. They also occur in the skull base, spinal canal and orbit. Most are benign (despite their tendency to invade adjacent bone) but some undergo sarcomatous change.

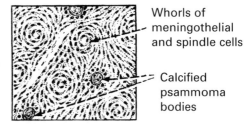

Whorls of meningothelial and spindle cells

Calcified psammoma bodies

Histological types – meningothelial, transitional, fibroblastic and angioblastic.

The haemangio-pericytoma is poorly differentiated, aggressive in nature and of uncertain histogenesis.

→ **Meningeal sarcoma** and primary **Meningeal melanoma:** Exceedingly rare tumours.

NERVE SHEATH CELLS → **Schwannoma** (Syn. neurilemmoma/neurinoma): a non-invasive, slowly growing tumour of the Schwann cells, surrounding the vestibular part of the VIII cranial nerve roots or the peripheral nerves.

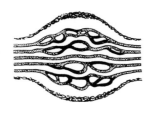

Different histological types exist:

Antoni type A
Antoni type B $\Big\}$ see page 329

→ **Neurofibroma:** tumour of Schwann cells, fibroblasts and perineural-like cells producing a fusiform expansion through which nerve fibres run. It involves the spinal nerve roots or peripheral nerves but rarely affects cranial nerves and has a greater tendency to undergo malignant change than schwannoma. This tumour is the type associated with Von Recklinghausen's disease, although schwannomas and mixed tumours also occur (see page 557).

N.B. Many tumours have mixed characteristics in varying proportions.

BLOOD VESSELS **Haemangioblastoma:**

Occurs within the cerebellar parenchyma or spinal cord. In 1926, Lindau described a syndrome relating cerebellar and/or spinal haemangioblastomas with similar tumours in the retina and cystic lesions in the pancreas and kidney (Von Hippel-Lindau disease).

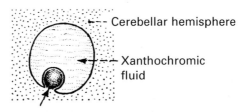

Cerebellar hemisphere

Xanthochromic fluid

Reddish-brown tumour nodule lying in the wall of the cyst. Histology shows a mass of blood vessels separated by clear, foamy vacuolated (stromal) cells

301

INTRACRANIAL TUMOURS – PATHOLOGICAL CLASSIFICATION

GERM CELLS

→ **Germinoma:** Primitive spheroidal cell tumour comparable to seminoma of the testis.

→ **Teratoma:** A tumour containing a mixture of well differentiated tissues – dermis, muscle, bone.

} uncommon tumours of the *pineal region* (not arising from pineal cells)

TUMOURS OF THE SELLAR REGION

→ **Craniopharyngioma:** Arises from cell rests of buccal epithelium and lies in close relation to the pituitary stalk. Usually a nodular tumour with cystic areas containing greenish fluid and cholesteatomatous material.

→ **Pituitary adenoma:** Benign tumour, usually secreting excessive quantities of prolactin, growth hormone, adrenocorticotrophic hormone, thyrotropin or gonadotropin.

CYSTS AND TUMOUR LIKE CONDITIONS

→ **Epidermoid/dermoid cysts:** Rare cystic tumours arising from cell rests predetermined to form epidermis or dermis.

→ **Colloid cyst:** A cystic tumour arising from an embryological remnant in the anterior roof of the 3rd ventricle.

LOCAL EXTENSION FROM ADJACENT TUMOURS

→ **Chordoma:** Rare tumour arising from cell rests of the notochord. May occur anywhere from the sphenoid to the coccyx – but commonest in the basi-occipital and the sacrococcygeal region, invading and destroying bone at these sites.

→ **Glomus jugulare tumour** (syn. chemodectoma): Vascular tumour arising from 'glomus jugulare' tissue lying either in the bulb of the internal jugular vein or in the mucosa of the middle ear. The tumour invades the petrous bone and may extend into the posterior fossa or neck.

→ Other local tumours include **chondroma, chondrosarcoma** and **cylindroma**.

Primary central nervous system lymphoma (PCNSL): Forms around periventricular parenchymal blood vessels. May be solitary or multifocal. It generally occurs in immuno-compromised patients, e.g. AIDS. Metastatic spread from systemic lymphoma (e.g. non-Hodgkin's lymphoma) is less common, involves the meninges and is rarely intraparenchymal.

Metastatic tumours: May arise from any primary site but most commonly spread from the bronchus or breast. Nervous system metastases occur in 25% of patients with disseminated cancer.

Tumour markers

Immunohistochemical techniques permit identification of antigens specific for certain cell or tissue characteristics and aid the histological diagnosis of tumours.

e.g. *Glial fibrillary acidic protein (GFAP)* – for astrocytic tumours
Cytokeratin – for metastatic carcinoma
Synaptophysin – for neuronal tumours
HMB 45 – for malignant melanoma

Some markers also indicate the degree of proliferation in various tumours (e.g. *Ki-67*). The identification of growth factors (e.g. *Epidermal growth factor (EGRF)*) may help distinguish between a primary glioblastoma (arising de novo) from a secondary glioblastoma (dedifferentiating from a previous lower grade tumour). Molecular techniques are increasingly used to identify *loss of heterozygosity* e.g. 1p,19q in oligodendroglioma.

INTRACRANIAL TUMOURS – CLASSIFICATION ACCORDING TO SITE

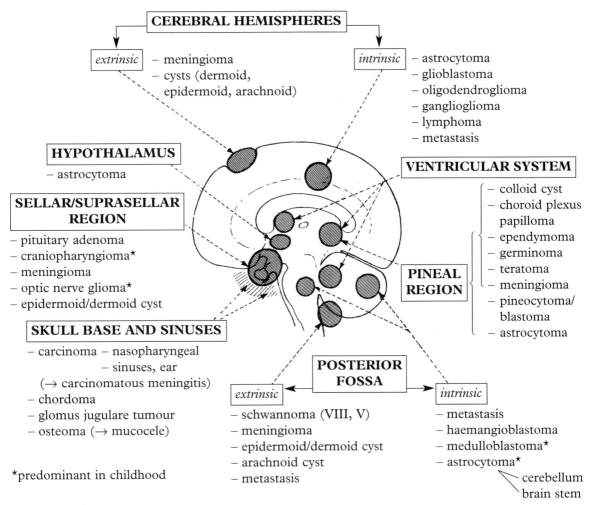

CEREBRAL HEMISPHERES

extrinsic
– meningioma
– cysts (dermoid,
   epidermoid, arachnoid)

intrinsic
– astrocytoma
– glioblastoma
– oligodendroglioma
– ganglioglioma
– lymphoma
– metastasis

HYPOTHALAMUS
– astrocytoma

SELLAR/SUPRASELLAR REGION
– pituitary adenoma
– craniopharyngioma★
– meningioma
– optic nerve glioma★
– epidermoid/dermoid cyst

VENTRICULAR SYSTEM
– colloid cyst
– choroid plexus
   papilloma
– ependymoma
– germinoma
– teratoma
– meningioma
– pineocytoma/
   blastoma
– astrocytoma

PINEAL REGION

SKULL BASE AND SINUSES
– carcinoma – nasopharyngeal
              – sinuses, ear
   (→ carcinomatous meningitis)
– chordoma
– glomus jugulare tumour
– osteoma (→ mucocele)

POSTERIOR FOSSA

extrinsic
– schwannoma (VIII, V)
– meningioma
– epidermoid/dermoid cyst
– arachnoid cyst
– metastasis

intrinsic
– metastasis
– haemangioblastoma
– medulloblastoma★
– astrocytoma★

⟍ cerebellum
   brain stem

★predominant in childhood

AETIOLOGY

Genetic factors: Over recent years, the role of genetic factors in tumour development has gained increasing prominence. Transformation of normal cells to malignant growth probably results from a variety of different processes –

(a) Normal cell growth and
    differentiation controlled by – *proto-oncogenes*
                                        ↓
                               expression altered
                                        ↓
                                   oncogenes
                                        ↓
                        alters encoded proteins transforming
                               cell into malignant state

303

INTRACRANIAL TUMOURS – AETIOLOGY/INCIDENCE

AETIOLOGY (*cont'd*)

(b) Inactivation of expression of *tumour suppressor genes* (e.g. loss of the p53 gene in many patients with low grade astrocytoma).

(c) Over expression of genes controlling growth factor (e.g. amplification of EGFR in primary glioblastoma).

Clearly defined inherited factors play a minor role. Only 5% of patients have a family history of brain tumour and with the exception of **tuberous sclerosis** (related to the formation of subependymal astrocytomas) and **neurofibromatosis** (linked to an increased incidence of optic nerve glioma and meningioma) do not fall into an obvious autosomal recessive or dominant pattern. Others include von Hippel-Lindau disease, Cowden's disease and Li-Fraumeni syndrome.

Cranial irradiation: long term follow-up of patients undergoing whole head irradiation for treatment of tinea capitis and childhood leukemia shows an increased incidence of both benign and malignant tumours – astrocytoma, meningioma.

Immunosuppression: increased incidence of lymphoma.

INCIDENCE

The table below details the incidence of intracranial tumours examined by the Neuropathology Department, Institute of Neurological Sciences, Glasgow (population 2.7 million) over a 5 year period.

SUPRATENTORIAL	Adults		Children (< 15 years)	
Anaplastic astrocytoma (including glioblastoma)	347	(40%)	5	(7%)
Meningioma	134	(15%)	–	
Metastasis	105	(12%)	–	
Astrocytoma	73	(8%)	5	(7%)
Pituitary adenoma	31	(4%)	–	
Craniopharyngioma	13	(1%)	9	(13%)
Oligodendroglioma	9	(1%)	1	(1%)
Colloid cyst	4	(<1%)	–	
Lymphoma	2	(<1%)	–	
Others	11	(1%)	6	(9%)
INFRATENTORIAL				
Schwannoma	50	(6%)	–	
Metastasis	39	(4%)	–	
Haemangioblastoma	17	(2%)	–	
Astrocytoma	12	(1%)	19	(27%)
Meningioma	12	(1%)	–	
Medulloblastoma	6	(<1%)	17	(24%)
Dermoid/epidermoid	3	(<1%)	1	(1%)
Ependymoma			4	(6%)
Others	8	(1%)	3	(4%)
	Total 876		70	

– As a result of AIDS and immuno-suppression, the incidence of primary cerebral lymphoma has significantly increased.

(Adapted from Adams, Graham and Doyle, 1981 Brain Biopsy)

INTRACRANIAL TUMOURS – CLINICAL FEATURES

Symptoms tend to develop insidiously, gradually progressing over a few weeks or years, depending on the degree of malignancy (cf. acute onset of a cerebrovascular accident followed by a gradual improvement if the patient survives). Occasionally tumours present acutely due to haemorrhage or the development of hydrocephalus.

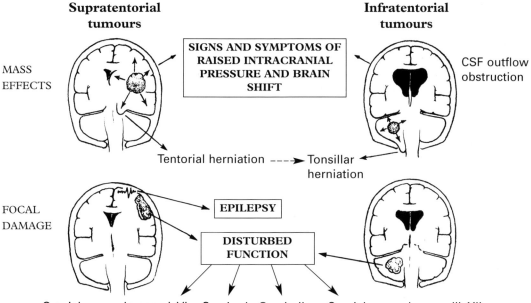

CLINICAL EFFECTS

RAISED INTRACRANIAL PRESSURE – headache, papilloedema $\rbrace$ (see pages
BRAIN SHIFT – vomiting, deterioration of conscious level, pupillary dilatation $\rbrace$ 79–81)

EPILEPSY (see page 90)

– generalised
– partial
  (simple or
  complex)
– partial
  progressing
  to generalised

(occur in 30% of patients with brain tumours)

Partial motor seizures arise in the motor cortex
– tonic or clonic movements in the contralateral face or limbs.

Partial seizures help localise the tumour site.

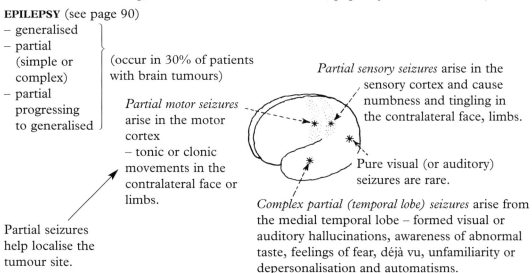

Partial sensory seizures arise in the sensory cortex and cause numbness and tingling in the contralateral face, limbs.

Pure visual (or auditory) seizures are rare.

Complex partial (temporal lobe) seizures arise from the medial temporal lobe – formed visual or auditory hallucinations, awareness of abnormal taste, feelings of fear, déjà vu, unfamiliarity or depersonalisation and automatisms.

305

INTRACRANIAL TUMOURS – CLINICAL FEATURES

DISTURBED FUNCTION

Supratentorial – see higher cortical dysfunction, pages 107–115

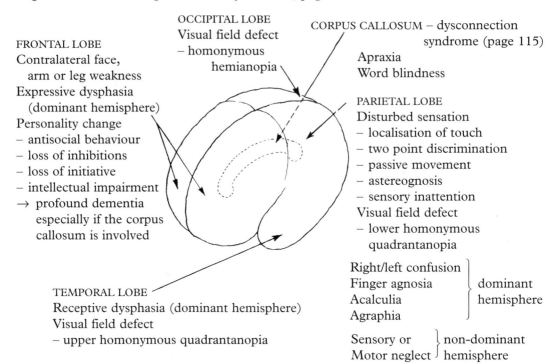

OCCIPITAL LOBE
Visual field defect
– homonymous
    hemianopia

CORPUS CALLOSUM – dysconnection
                syndrome (page 115)
Apraxia
Word blindness

FRONTAL LOBE
Contralateral face,
    arm or leg weakness
Expressive dysphasia
    (dominant hemisphere)
Personality change
– antisocial behaviour
– loss of inhibitions
– loss of initiative
– intellectual impairment
→ profound dementia
    especially if the corpus
    callosum is involved

PARIETAL LOBE
Disturbed sensation
– localisation of touch
– two point discrimination
– passive movement
– astereognosis
– sensory inattention
Visual field defect
– lower homonymous
    quadrantanopia

Right/left confusion
Finger agnosia   } dominant
Acalculia   } hemisphere
Agraphia

TEMPORAL LOBE
Receptive dysphasia (dominant hemisphere)
Visual field defect
– upper homonymous quadrantanopia

Sensory or   } non-dominant
Motor neglect   } hemisphere
(e.g. dressing
apraxia)

HYPOTHALAMUS/PITUITARY
Endocrine dysfunction.

Supratentorial tumours may directly
damage the I and II cranial nerves.
Cavernous sinus compression or invasion
may involve the III–VI cranial nerves.

Infratentorial

MIDBRAIN/BRAIN STEM
Cranial nerve lesions III–XII
Long tract signs
    – motor and sensory
Deterioration of conscious level
Tremor (red nucleus)
Impaired eye movements
Pupillary abnormalities
Vomiting, hiccough (medulla)

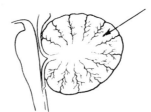

CEREBELLUM – see cerebellar
    dysfunction, pages 178–181
Ataxic gait
Intention tremor
Dysmetria
Dysarthria
Nystagmus

N.B. Intrinsic brain stem tumours in contrast to
    extrinsic tumours are more likely to produce
    long tract (motor and sensory) signs early in
    the course of the disease.

INTRACRANIAL TUMOURS – INVESTIGATION

Chest X-ray } The high incidence of metastatic tumour makes these tests mandatory in
ESR, CRP } patients with suspected intracranial tumour.

Skull X-ray (if performed) Note:

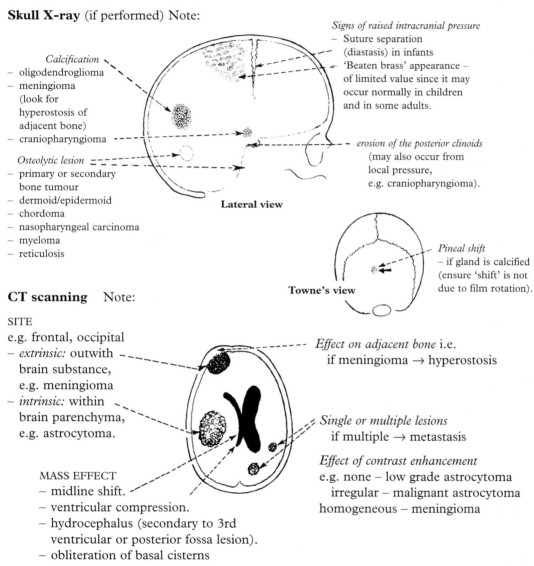

Signs of raised intracranial pressure
– Suture separation
   (diastasis) in infants
– 'Beaten brass' appearance –
   of limited value since it may
   occur normally in children
   and in some adults.

Calcification
– oligodendroglioma
– meningioma
   (look for
   hyperostosis of
   adjacent bone)
– craniopharyngioma

Osteolytic lesion
– primary or secondary
   bone tumour
– dermoid/epidermoid
– chordoma
– nasopharyngeal carcinoma
– myeloma
– reticulosis

erosion of the posterior clinoids
   (may also occur from
   local pressure,
   e.g. craniopharyngioma).

Lateral view

Pineal shift
   – if gland is calcified
   (ensure 'shift' is not
   due to film rotation).

Towne's view

CT scanning Note:

SITE
e.g. frontal, occipital
– *extrinsic:* outwith
   brain substance,
   e.g. meningioma
– *intrinsic:* within
   brain parenchyma,
   e.g. astrocytoma.

Effect on adjacent bone i.e.
   if meningioma → hyperostosis

Single or multiple lesions
   if multiple → metastasis

Effect of contrast enhancement
e.g. none – low grade astrocytoma
   irregular – malignant astrocytoma
homogeneous – meningioma

MASS EFFECT
– midline shift.
– ventricular compression.
– hydrocephalus (secondary to 3rd
   ventricular or posterior fossa lesion).
– obliteration of basal cisterns

HIGH DEFINITION SCANS (1 mm slice width) – useful in the detection of pituitary, orbital
and posterior fossa tumours.

CORONAL AND SAGITTAL
RECONSTRUCTION
DIRECT CORONAL SCANNING
} – useful in demonstrating the vertical extent of a tumour
   and its relationship with other structures, especially
   when intraventricular or arising from the pituitary
   fossa or skull base.

307

INTRACRANIAL TUMOURS – INVESTIGATION

MRI Note: SITE, MASS EFFECT and LESION MULTIPLICITY as for CT scanning.

Of particular value in demonstrating tumours around the skull base, cranio-cervical junction and the brainstem.

Flow voids show the relationship of adjacent blood vessels to the tumour.

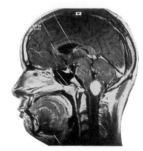

Coronal and sagittal scanning provide additional information, showing the exact anatomical relationship of the tumour to the sulci and gyri, the ventricles, the falx and the tentorium cerebelli.

T1 weighted MRI with gadolinium showing a haemangioblastoma involving the medulla.

Paramagnetic enhancement: intravenous gadolinium increases sensitivity of detection and clarifies the site of origin, i.e. intrinsic or extrinsic, and may delineate the border between tumour and surrounding oedema.

Single or multiple lesions: MRI appears more sensitive than CT scanning in identifying small tumours and improves the detection of multiple lesions, e.g. metastasis.

Angiography/CTA/MRA: although angiography may reveal a tumour 'blush' or vessel displacement, it is only occasionally required to supplement other investigations. In some patients, it provides useful preoperative information, e.g. identifies feeding vessels to a vascular tumour or tumour involvement and constriction of major vessels.

CSF examination: lumbar puncture is contraindicated if the clinician suspects intracranial tumour. If CSF is obtained by another source, e.g. ventricular drainage or during shunt insertion, then cytological examination may reveal tumour cells.

Tumour markers: although useful as an aid to histological diagnosis (see page 302), attempts to find a substance in blood or CSF which reflects growth of a specific tumour have been limited – only the link between elevated alpha fetoprotein and human chorionic gonadotrophins with yolk sac tumours and choriocarcinoma of the third ventricle helps diagnosis.

DIFFERENTIAL DIAGNOSIS OF INTRACRANIAL MASS LESIONS (other than tumour)

Vascular – haematoma
– giant aneurysm
– arteriovenous malformation
– infarct with oedema
– venous thrombosis.

Trauma – haematoma
– contusion.

Infection – abscess
– tuberculoma
– sarcoidosis
– encephalitis.

Cysts – arachnoid
– parasitic (hydatid).

INTRACRANIAL TUMOURS – MANAGEMENT

STEROID THERAPY

Steroids dramatically reduce oedema surrounding intracranial tumours, but do not affect tumour growth.

A loading dose of 12 mg i.v. dexamethasone followed by 4 mg q.i.d. orally or by injection often reverses progressive clinical deterioration within a few hours. After several days treatment, gradual dose reduction minimises the risk of unwanted side effects.

Sellar/parasellar tumours occasionally present with steroid insufficiency. In these patients, steroid cover is an essential prerequisite of any anaesthetic or operative procedure.

OPERATIVE MANAGEMENT

Most patients with intracranial tumours require one or more of the following approaches:

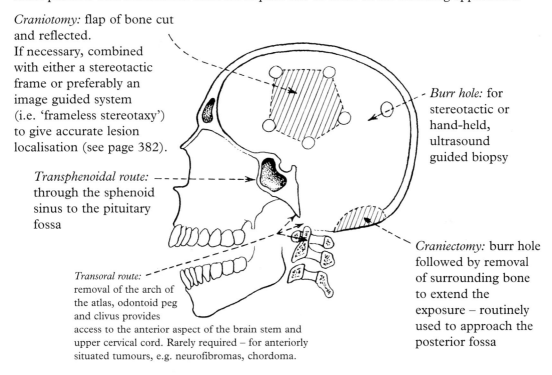

Craniotomy: flap of bone cut and reflected.
If necessary, combined with either a stereotactic frame or preferably an image guided system (i.e. 'frameless stereotaxy') to give accurate lesion localisation (see page 382).

Transphenoidal route: through the sphenoid sinus to the pituitary fossa

Transoral route: removal of the arch of the atlas, odontoid peg and clivus provides access to the anterior aspect of the brain stem and upper cervical cord. Rarely required – for anteriorly situated tumours, e.g. neurofibromas, chordoma.

Burr hole: for stereotactic or hand-held, ultrasound guided biopsy

Craniectomy: burr hole followed by removal of surrounding bone to extend the exposure – routinely used to approach the posterior fossa

The subsequent procedure – *biopsy, partial tumour removal/internal decompression or complete removal* – depends on the nature of the tumour and its site. The infiltrative nature of primary malignant tumours prevents complete removal and often operation is restricted to biopsy or tumour decompression. Prospects of complete removal improve with benign tumours such as meningioma or craniopharyngioma; if any tumour tissue is overlooked, or if fragments remain attached to deep structures, then recurrence will result.

INTRACRANIAL TUMOURS – MANAGEMENT

RADIOTHERAPY
Treatment of intracranial tumours with radiotherapy utilises one of the following:
- *megavoltage* X-rays
- electron beam from a *linear accelerator* (which can also produce megavoltage X-rays)
- *accelerated particles from a cyclotron*, e.g. nuclei of helium, protons (awaits full evaluation)
- γ rays from *cobalt*[60].

In contrast to older methods, these modern techniques produce greater tissue penetration and avoid radiation damage to the skin surface. The effect of radiotherapy depends on the total dose – usually up to 60 Gy, and the treatment duration. This must be balanced against the risk to normal structures. Treatment aims to provide the highest possible dose to a specified region whilst minimising irradiation to adjacent normal brain. Various methods have been developed to achieve this –

- *Conformal therapy* where standard radiotherapy is administered, but the beams are shaped by the use of variable collimators or blocks which conform with the shape of the tumour, thereby eliminating normal brain.
- *Stereotactic radiosurgery (SRS)* where multiple converging beams from a linear accelerator or from multiple cobalt[60] sources are focused on a selected target in a *single* treatment. *Stereotactic radiotherapy (SRT)* uses the same localisation method but with fractionated treatment as used in conventional radiotherapy (see page 381).
- *Interstitial techniques* where the tumour is treated from within (brachytherapy) by the implantation of multiple radioactive seeds, e.g. iodine[125].
- *Beam intensity modulated radiotherapy (IMRT)* uses non-uniform beams of varying intensity (in contrast to the conventional uniform dose intensity) to complex tumour volumes. This helps protect surrounding structures, yet allows a higher dose.
- *Proton therapy* is available in only a few centres. It allows the delivery of high doses of radiation to very localised regions adjacent to vital structures such as the skull base.

Radiotherapy is of particular value in the management of malignant tumours – malignant astrocytoma, metastasis, medulloblastoma and germinoma, but also plays an important part in the management of some benign tumours – pituitary adenoma, craniopharyngioma. With some tumours that seed throughout the CSF pathways, e.g. medulloblastoma, *whole neural axis irradiation* minimises the risk of a distant recurrence.

Complications of radiotherapy: following treatment, deterioration in a patient's condition may occur for a variety of reasons:

- Increased oedema – during treatment – reversible.
- Demyelination – after weeks, months – usually reversible.
- *Radionecrosis* – in usually 1–2 years (range 6 months–10 years) – irreversible.
- Cognitive impairment – whole brain irradiation causes dementia, ataxia and incontinence in over 10% at one year. Radiotherapy should be avoided in children under 3 years of age.
- Radiation induced tumours e.g. meningioma, may result many years after the treatment.

Oedema, demyelination and radionecrosis may involve the spinal cord after irradiation of spinal tumours.

INTRACRANIAL TUMOURS – MANAGEMENT

CHEMOTHERAPY

Chemotherapeutic agents have been used for many years in the management of malignant brain tumours, but their benefits remain limited. Drugs most commonly used include nitroso-ureas (e.g. BCNU, CCNU, methyl-CCNU), procarbazine, vincristine and methotrexate.

Studies with *Temozolomide,* an oral alkylating agent that penetrates the blood–brain barrier, have produced encouraging results when used in patients with recurrent anaplastic astrocytomas and glioblastoma. One promising aspect of this drug is its apparent low toxicity. Trials examining its use as an adjuvant chemotherapeutic agent in various tumours are underway. In *anaplastic astrocytomas* and *glioblastomas* the role of chemotherapy as a primary treatment is questionable. Meta-analysis has shown a small but significant increase in survival, but chemotherapy is usually reserved for tumour recurrence after resection and radiotherapy. Carmustine impregnated wafers may also be considered both as a primary treatment or for tumour recurrence (see below).

Recent studies have shown that patients with *anaplastic oligodendrogliomas,* particularly those with allelic loss of 1p and 19q (almost 50%), respond well to procarbazine, lomustine and vincristine chemotherapy and in future this treatment may take precedence over radio-therapy. Other tumours where chemotherapy plays an important role include *medullo-blastomas, primary CNS lymphomas* and *germ cell tumours.*

Chemotherapy has no role in low grade astrocytomas, but some recommend using chemotherapy rather than radiotherapy for *low grade oligodendrogliomas.*

Problems of drug administration

Toxicity: The ideal cytotoxic drug selectively kills tumour cells; but tumour cell response relates directly to the dose. High drug dosage frequently causes bone marrow suppression which may limit cytotoxic activity before an adequate therapeutic dose is reached.

Drug access: 'Toxic' doses are usually required before sufficient amounts penetrate the blood–brain barrier and gain access to the tumour cells.

Intrinsic resistance: Some tumour cells appear to have an inbuilt resistance to certain drugs. The vast array of available cytotoxic drugs and the infinite permutations of combined therapy creates difficulties in drug selection.

IMPROVING ACCESS: Modifying the blood–brain barrier with mannitol or preliminary binding with liposomes may improve the passage of cytotoxic drugs to tumour tissue. Similarly direct intra-carotid injection may improve access over conventional routes. One study has reported a 2–3 month increase in survival in patients undergoing intraoperative placement of 'slow release' carmustine polymers in high grade gliomas.

GENE THERAPY

Gene therapy is the manipulation of the genetic material of tumour cells for therapeutic benefit. Various vectors (usually viral) are used to introduce genes
- to either replace a missing gene (e.g. a tumour suppressor gene),
- to counteract a harmful overactive gene (e.g. Epidermal Growth Factor Receptor (EGFR) gene),
- to stimulate apoptosis, to block angiogenesis and invasion or more commonly,
- to kill the cell directly (Herpes Simplex virus) or indirectly via a pro-drug (e.g. Herpes Simplex Thymidine kinase/Ganciclovir.

All treatments remain experimental. Although results of some preliminary trials have been disappointing, gene therapy generates considerable research interest and future potential.

TUMOURS OF THE CEREBRAL HEMISPHERES – INTRINSIC

Intrinsic tumours arise within the brain substance.

ASTROCYTOMA (and glioblastoma multiforme)
Astrocytomas may occur in any age group, but are commonest between 40 and 60 years.

Male:female = 2:1

Primary sites: Found in equal incidence throughout the frontal, temporal, parietal and thalamic regions, but less often in the occipital lobe. Microscopic classification defines 4 grades (Kernohan I–IV), but this is of limited accuracy. A more practical description for the clinician divides tumours into either 'malignant' or 'low grade'.

Anaplastic astrocytoma/glioblastoma multiforme

Anaplastic astrocytomas (grade III) and glioblastoma multiforme (grade IV) constitute about 40% of all primary intracranial tumours. Glioblastoma occurs 4x more commonly than anaplastic astrocytoma. Peak age incidence is 53 years and 40 years respectively. These tumours widely infiltrate adjacent brain; growth is rapid. At autopsy, microscopic examination often reveals direct spread to multiple distant sites.

Genetic analysis differentiates 'primary' glioblastoma arising de novo (e.g. amplification of EGFR gene, loss of p16, mutation of PTEN and loss of heterozygosity of 10q), from a 'secondary' glioblastoma where dedifferentiation has occurred from a lower grade tumour (loss of p53).

MALIGNANT ASTROCYTOMA

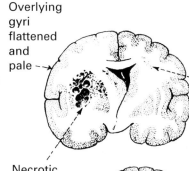

Overlying gyri flattened and pale ~

At autopsy 75% show microscopic spread to the contralateral hemisphere. Some patients may present with a bilateral corpus callosal tumour or 'butterfly' astrocytoma

Necrotic areas may coalesce and form cystic cavities

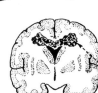

'Low grade' astrocytoma

Grade I/II astrocytomas make up 14% of all primary intracranial tumours. The more frequent grade II tumours occur on average around 35 years. They are diffuse and slowly growing, and composed of well differentiated astrocytic cells subdivided into fibrillary, protoplasmic and gemistocytic types. Up to 90% show loss of the p53 gene. Although benign, these tumours widely infiltrate surrounding brain and lack of definitive edge or capsule.

The pilocytic (grade I) astrocytoma occurs in children and young adults in the hypothalamic region, the optic nerve in association with NF1 (page 557) and in the cerebellum and brainstem (pages 327, 328). They grow very slowly, can often stabilise and even regress. Even partial resection can result in a cure.

FIBRILLARY ASTROCYTOMA

Firm, rubbery texture with or without cystic regions

Infiltrates surrounding brain with minimal mass effect and neuronal damage

TUMOURS OF THE CEREBRAL HEMISPHERES – INTRINSIC

ASTROCYTOMA (cont'd)

CLINICAL FEATURES

Astrocytomas may present with:

– epilepsy – more common with low grade tumours
– signs and symptoms of focal brain damage – dysphasia, hemiparesis, personality change
– signs and symptoms of raised intracranial pressure – headache, vomiting, depression of conscious level.

Symptoms usually develop gradually, progressing over several weeks, months or years, the rate depending on the degree of malignancy. Sudden deterioration suggests haemorrhage into a necrotic area. In a patient with long standing epilepsy, the rapid development of further symptoms may result from malignant change within a previously 'low grade' lesion.

INVESTIGATIONS

CT scan: appearances vary considerably; in general, malignant and low grade lesions show different characteristics:

Anaplastic astrocytoma/glioblastoma

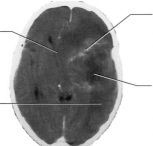

Note site and associated mass effect
– ventricular compression
– midline shift

Areas of mixed density, *irregularly enhance with contrast.* No clear plane exists between tumour and brain

Surrounding low density indicates either oedema or infiltrative tumour

Central, low density regions represent necrotic areas or cystic cavities; neither enhances with contrast

Low grade astrocytoma

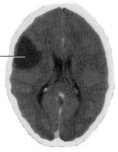

A low density region, *usually unenhancing with contrast* suggests a low grade infiltrative lesion; detection is often difficult in early stages.
Calcification occasionally occurs.

MRI: with and without gadolinium identifies the tumour location, size and degree of surrounding oedema more clearly. MRI is a more sensitive investigation for detecting low grade astrocytomas.

The *MR spectroscopy* profile (page 42) may suggest a pathological diagnosis.

MRI with gadolinium enhancement showing a glioblastoma invading the corpus callosum

313

TUMOURS OF THE CEREBRAL HEMISPHERES – INTRINSIC

ASTROCYTOMA (*cont'd*)

MANAGEMENT

The management of glial tumours varies depending on a number of factors –
- the lesion site
- the degree of malignancy
- the presence or absence of a raised ICP
- the degree of disability and the effect of steroid therapy
- the suspected nature of the tumour on imaging
- the patient's age
- the patient's wishes

TREATMENT OPTIONS

Steroid therapy: For patients presenting with symptoms of raised intracranial pressure and/or focal neurological signs, a loading dose of dexamethasone 12 mg i.v. followed by 4 mg q.i.d., by injection or orally, reduces surrounding oedema and leads to rapid improvement. Steroid treatment is an essential prerequisite to operation. Its introduction has significantly reduced the perioperative mortality. After several days, a gradual reduction in dosage avoids side effects.

Biopsy: Imaging is insufficient to conclusively establish the diagnosis. If not proceeding to an open operation, failure to confirm the nature of the lesion risks omitting treatment in benign conditions such as abscess, tuberculoma or sarcoidosis. Identification of tumour type and grade gives a prognostic guide and aids further management.

METHODS:

Framed or frameless stereotactic methods (see page 380) – permit accurate placement of a fine cannula at a predetermined site selected on CT scan or MRI. Stereotactic guidance is essential for small and/or deep inaccessible lesions (e.g. hypothalamus) and enables biopsy of specific regions in larger tumours e.g. enhancing areas on the MRI or CT scan. Prior selection of the needle path avoids vessels and important structures, thus minimising the risks. Since the degree of malignancy varies from region to region within a single lesion, several samples are taken from different sites to increase accuracy. If findings vary, then the region of greatest malignancy dictates the tumour grade. These techniques are now frequently used, even for more accessible lesions, due to the low mortality and morbidity. Provided patients receive preoperative steroid cover the risks are small, but occasionally biopsy produces or increases a focal deficit or causes a fatal haemorrhage.

Ultrasound guided – a brain cannula inserted into the abnormal region permits aspiration of a small quantity of tissue for immediate (smear and frozen section) and later (paraffin section) examination.

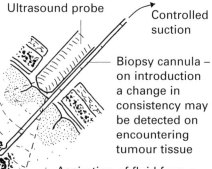

Ultrasound probe

Controlled suction

Biopsy cannula – on introduction a change in consistency may be detected on encountering tumour tissue

Aspiration of fluid from a cystic cavity may provide a temporary decompression.

TUMOURS OF THE CEREBRAL HEMISPHERES – INTRINSIC

ASTROCYTOMA

TREATMENT OPTIONS (*cont'd*)

Tumour resection: perhaps combined with ultrasound or with *framed* or *frameless stereotaxy* to aid tumour localisation.

Through a craniotomy, the surgeon performs an 'open' biopsy under direct vision, or resects as much tumour tissue as is safely feasible without damaging eloquent regions. The difficulty lies in the absence of a plane of cleavage between tumour tissue and brain. Stereotactic methods can identify the boundaries seen on CT scan or MRI but this is limited by the resolution of the imaging. Large resections are most safely performed in the frontal, occipital or non-dominant temporal lobes. Most believe that the greater the reduction of the tumour mass, the greater the effect of adjuvant therapy. Ideally the extent of the resection can be monitored with real-time MRI (i.e. MR scanning within the operating theatre), but this is still only available in a few centres.

Radiotherapy: Most effective in rapidly growing tumours – grade III and IV. Radiotherapy extends survival, but does not cure. Studies show a dose–effect relationship – the greater the dose to the tumour area, the longer the survival. Usually up to 60 Gy is delivered in fractionated doses (see page 310). Methods of 'conformal' therapy and 'interstitial radiotherapy' (see page 310) aim to achieve this. The use of radiosurgery for grade III/IV tumours awaits the results of randomised trials.

Chemotherapy: Various chemotherapeutic agents (usually nitrosoureas and more recently temozolomide) have been used in the management of anaplastic astrocytoma and glioblastoma. A proportion of tumours undoubtedly respond and survival times are increased by approximately 2 months, but side effects may reduce the quality of life. Treatment is usually reserved for recurrent tumours. Alternatives include inserting carmustine impregnated wafers in the tumour bed which improves survival by 2–3 months.

TUMOURS OF THE CEREBRAL HEMISPHERES – INTRINSIC

Treatment selection and prognosis

Since treatment cannot cure, the clinician must consider quality of survival as well as the duration.

Malignant astrocytoma/glioblastoma multiforme: Despite modern techniques, these tumours still carry a grave prognosis, irrespective of the selected treatment.

Median survival (months)	
Burr hole biopsy	3–4
Tumour resection	6
Burr hole biopsy + radiotherapy	6–8
Tumour resection + radiotherapy	9–10

Extensive tumour resection extends average survival by 2 months; at 1 year, the percentage of patients surviving varies little, irrespective of whether burr hole biopsy or tumour resection is performed. Complete removal is impossible; even the formidable 'hemispherectomy' fails due to interhemispheric spread. Radiotherapy appears to have the greatest effect, extending the mean survival period by 3–4 months.

Management policies vary widely, but in general, *tumour resection with radiotherapy* is considered in:

– younger patients
– patients with 'accessible' lesions
– patients with symptoms of raised ICP from the mass effect
– patients without severe disability

Tumour recurrence in these patients may warrant *chemotherapy* or even reoperation with or without interstitial radiotherapy.

A *diagnostic biopsy* may be appropriate in the elderly, and in patients with marked disability (e.g. severe dysphasia) unlikely to improve after resection.

Low grade astrocytoma: A poorly defined region of low density on CT scan without contrast enhancement suggests a low grade tumour (grade I or II) with a better prognosis. In such patients who often present with epilepsy without other symptoms, there is no evidence that active intervention with operation and/or radiotherapy changes outcome. In this instance, both clinician and patient may prefer to follow a conservative approach. If subsequent CT or MR scanning shows definitive tumour progression (expansion or contrast enhancement, or if clinical symptoms supervene, then surgical treatment and radiotherapy can follow as appropriate.

About 50–60% of patients with grade II astrocytomas survive 5 years; about 40% survive 10 years. Of those patients with pilocytic (grade I) astrocytomas, 80% survive 20 years.

TUMOURS OF THE CEREBRAL HEMISPHERES – INTRINSIC

OLIGODENDROGLIOMA

Oligodendrogliomas are far less common than astrocytomas. They occur in a slightly younger age group – 30–50 years, and usually involve the frontal lobes. Occasionally involvement of the ventricular wall results in CSF seeding. Calcification occurs in 40%.

Oligodendroglioma

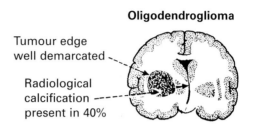

Tumour edge well demarcated

Radiological calcification present in 40%

Some tumours involve the ventricular wall – CSF seeding may occur

In contrast to astrocytomas, the tumour margin often appears well defined. Both low grade and anaplastic forms exist. Genetic analysis of anaplastic oligodendrogliomas has revealed that almost 50% have 1p and 19q allelic losses (i.e. loss of heterozygosity) and this group responded well to chemotherapy.

Management and prognosis: the approach is similar to astrocytomas with most delaying treatment of low grade tumours until symptoms appear. Patients can expect to survive for 12–16 years. For patients with anaplastic oligodendrogliomas, resection followed by chemotherapy is combined with either immediate or delayed radiotherapy. Ideally treatment should depend on the patient's genetic profile. The 50% patients with loss of 1p and 19q alleles respond well to chemotherapy and survive over 10 years. The 27% with a genetic profile similar to primary glioblastoma (page 312) seldom respond to chemotherapy and survive on average about 16 months.

Mixed oligoastrocytoma: those with a mixed form of astrocytoma/oligodendroglioma have a prognosis lying between that for each type.

HYPOTHALAMIC ASTROCYTOMA

Hypothalamic tumours usually occur in children; they are usually astrocytomas of the pilocytic (juvenile) type. The clinical effect of hypothalamic damage takes different forms. Initially the child *fails to thrive* and becomes *emaciated*. Signs of *panhypopituitarism* may develop. Eventually an anabolic phase results in *obesity* accompanied by *diabetes insipidus* and *delayed puberty*. Disturbance of affect and of sleep–wake rhythms may occur.

Upward tumour extension may obstruct the foramen of Munro and cause hydrocephalus.

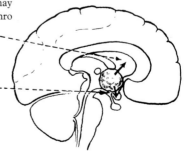

Involvement of the tuberal region may result in the rare presentation of *precocious puberty* with secondary sexual characteristics developing in children perhaps only a few years old. Downward extension invades the optic chiasma and impairs vision.
Management: The site of the lesion prevents operative removal; a stereotactic biopsy may aid tumour identification. If hydrocephalus is present, a bilateral ventriculoperitoneal shunt relieves pressure symptoms. Radiotherapy is of doubtful value.

317

TUMOURS OF THE CEREBRAL HEMISPHERES – INTRINSIC

METASTATIC TUMOURS

Common primary sites

Any malignant tumour may metastasise to the brain. Malignant melanomas show the highest frequency (66% of patients); this contrasts with tumours of the cervix and uterus where < 3% develop intracranial metastasis. The most commonly encountered metastatic intracranial tumours arise from the bronchus and the breast; of patients with carcinomas at these sites, 25% develop intracranial metastasis.
In over 50% of patients, metastases are multiple.

– bronchus
– breast
– kidney
– thyroid
– stomach
– prostate
– testis
– melanoma

Spread is usually haematogenous to the grey/white matter junction. Occasionally a metastasis to the skull vault may result in a nodule or plaque forming over the dural surface from direct spread.

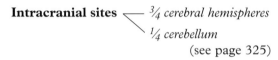

Intracranial sites — ¾ *cerebral hemispheres*
¼ *cerebellum*
(see page 325)

Involvement of the ventricular wall or encroachment into the basal cisterns may result in tumour cells seeding through the CSF pathways – malignant meningitis.

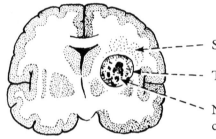

------ Surrounding oedema is often marked.

----- Tumour margin – well defined.

----- Necrotic areas may break down to form cystic cavities containing a pus-like fluid.

Clinical features

Patients with supratentorial metastatic tumours may present with epilepsy, or with signs and symptoms occurring from focal damage or raised intracranial pressure. Cerebellar metastases are discussed on page 325. Malignant meningitis causes single or multiple cranial nerve palsies and may obstruct CSF drainage (see page 513).

TUMOURS OF THE CEREBRAL HEMISPHERES – INTRINSIC

METASTATIC TUMOURS (*cont'd*)

Investigations

A **CT scan** shows single or multiple well demarcated lesions of variable size. Often an extensive low density area, representing oedema, surrounds the lesion.

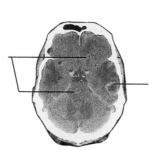

Metastatic lesions usually enhance with contrast. A ring-like appearance may resemble an abscess – but the wall is irregular and thickened.

MRI scanning, with and without paramagnetic enhancement, is even more sensitive than CT in detecting small metastatic lesions.

The search for a primary lesion if not already established must include a thorough clinical examination and a chest X-ray. Other investigations including barium studies, intravenous pyelogram (IVP), abdominal CT scans, ultrasound and sputum and urine cytology have questionable value, unless clinically indicated.

Management and prognosis:

Corticosteriods (dexamethasone) have a dramatic, rapid effect, producing clinical improvement in most patients.

– *Solitary lesions:* If the tumour lies in an accessible site, complete excision followed by radiotherapy provides good results – survival usually depends on the extent of extracranial disease and its ability to respond to treatment rather than on intracranial recurrences. Stereotactic radiosurgery provides a valuable alternative, particularly for lesions less than 3 cm in diameter and for deep-seated lesions. In patients with no other evidence of systemic cancer, the median survival period approaches 2 years. In patients with other evidence of systemic disease, results are less good with a median survival of 8 months.

– *Multiple lesions:* Operative removal is seldom practical. Provided no doubt exists about the diagnosis (abscesses or tuberculomata may resemble metastasis) radiosurgery may be administered to two or even three lesions. For other patients whole brain irradiation may be considered.

TUMOURS OF THE CEREBRAL HEMISPHERES – INTRINSIC

PRIMARY CNS LYMPHOMA (PCNSL) (syn. HIGH GRADE NON HODGKIN'S B-CELL LYMPHOMA) Single or multiple lymphomas usually lie deep within the basal ganglia or in the periventricular region. Some are discrete lesions, others extensively invade surrounding brain. Histology shows sleeves of primitive reticulum cells extending outwards from the blood vessels. The incidence is significantly increased in AIDS and in immunocompromised patients.

CSF examination is important; 30% of patients with PCNSL show positive cytology. A positive Epstein-Barr test within tumour cells in CSF is diagnostic of AIDS lymphoma.

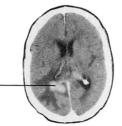

Multiplicity also suggests lymphoma.

CT scan: shows an enhancing homogeneous hyperdense region, often in a periventricular location

Same patient after 7 days steroid treatment

Management: In AIDS patients, CT and MRI finding of PCNSL appear similar to toxoplasmosis; antiprotozoal therapy should be tried first. Failure to respond indicates the need for *biopsy*. *Steroids* can cause dramatic shrinkage, and the CT scan should be repeated if any delay occurs prior to biopsy. *Radiotherapy* also has dramatic effects, but with this treatment alone, the median survival period is only 10–12 months. Recent studies show that methotrexate based *chemotherapy* (in patients with a normal immune system) can increase median survival to up to 44 months. Some now advocate delaying radiotherapy treatment until a recurrence occurs. AIDS patients, who receive radiotherapy, have a median survival of about 4 months, but chemotherapy can improve this in selected patients.

GANGLIOGLIOMA
This a rare tumour occurring in the younger age group (< 30 years), composed of abnormal neuronal growth mixed with a glial component. The proportion of each component varies from patient to patient. Growth is slow and malignant change uncommon; when this occurs it probably develops in the glial component.
Management follows that of low grade astrocytomas.

NEUROBLASTOMA
Rarely occurs intracranially in children < 10 years. Highly cellular, malignant lesion composed of small round cells, some showing neuronal differentiation.

TUMOURS OF THE CEREBRAL HEMISPHERES – EXTRINSIC

Extrinsic tumours arise outwith the brain substance.

MENINGIOMA

Meningiomas constitute about one-fifth of all primary intracranial tumours. They are slow growing and arise from the arachnoid granulations. These lie in greatest concentration around the venous sinuses, but they also occur in relation to surface tributary veins. Meningiomas may therefore develop at any meningeal site. Occasionally they are multiple.

Meningiomas present primarily in the 40–60 age group and have a slight female preponderance. They are principally benign tumours, although 1–2% show malignant change.

Pathology

Various histological types are described – syncytial, transitional, fibroblastic and angioblastic; different types may coexist within the same tumour. These distinctions serve little clinical value, although it is important to identify the anaplastic (malignant) form, as this indicates the likelihood of rapid growth and a high rate of recurrence following removal.

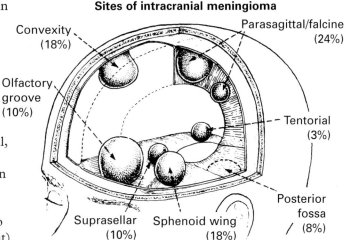

Sites of intracranial meningioma

Convexity (18%)

Parasagittal/falcine (24%)

Olfactory groove (10%)

Tentorial (3%)

Suprasellar (10%)

Sphenoid wing (18%)

Posterior fossa (8%)

The remainder arise from the middle fossa, orbital roof and lateral ventricle

Macroscopic appearance
The dural origin usually incorporates the main arterial supply.
The tumour surface, although often lobulated, is well demarcated from the surrounding brain and attached only by small bridging vessels. Marked *oedema* often develops in the surrounding brain.

A reactive *hyperostosis* develops in adjacent bone, forming a swelling on the inner table. Hyperostosis affecting the outer table may produce a palpable lump. Tumour tissue may infiltrate adjacent bone.

Parasagittal tumours may invade and obstruct the sagittal sinus.

Tumour texture and vascularity varies considerably from patient to patient – some are firm and fibrous, others soft. *Calcified deposits* (psammoma bodies) are often found.

En-plaque meningioma: In some patients, rather than developing a spherical form, the meningioma spreads 'en-plaque' over the dural surface. This type often arises from the outer aspect of the sphenoid wing.

TUMOURS OF THE CEREBRAL HEMISPHERES – EXTRINSIC

MENINGIOMA Clinical features:

Approximately a quarter of patients with meningioma present with epilepsy – often with a focal component. In the remainder, the onset is insidious with pressure effects (headache, vomiting, papilloedema) often developing before focal neurological signs become evident.

Notable characteristic features occur, dependent on the tumour site – PARASAGITTAL/ PARAFALCINE tumours lying near the vertex affect the 'foot' and 'leg' area of the motor or sensory strip. *Partial seizures* or a *'pyramidal' weakness* may develop in the leg (i.e. primarily affecting foot dorsiflexion, then knee and hip flexion). Extension of the lesion through the falx can produce *bilateral leg weakness*. Posteriorly situated parasagittal tumours may present with a *homonymous hemianopia*. Tumours arising anteriorly may grow to extensive proportions before causing focal signs; eventually minor *impairment of memory, intellect* and *personality* may progress to a *profound dementia*.

INNER SPHENOIDAL WING tumours may compress the optic nerve and produce *visual impairment*. Examination may reveal a central *scotoma* or other *field defect* with *optic atrophy*.

N.B. The FOSTER KENNEDY syndrome denotes a tumour causing optic atrophy in one fundus from direct pressure and papilloedema in the other due to increased intracranial pressure.

Involvement of the cavernous sinus or the superior orbital fissure may produce *ptosis* and *impaired eye movements* (III, IV and VI nerve palsies) or *facial pain and anaesthesia* (V_1 nerve damage) – see diagram on page 151. *Proptosis* occasionally results from venous obstruction from tumour extension into the orbit.

OLFACTORY GROOVE tumours destroy the olfactory bulb or tract causing unilateral followed by bilateral *anosmia*. Often unilateral loss passes unnoticed by the patient; with tumour expansion, dementia may gradually ensue.

SUPRASELLAR tumours – see page 344.

Investigations:

SKULL X-RAY – note:
Associated signs of long-standing increased ICP, i.e. posterior clinoid erosion.

Bony hyperostosis – radiating spicules occasionally seen ('sunray' effect).

15% show calcification.

Dilated middle meningeal groove.

CT SCAN

Before i.v. contrast

Meningioma – well circumscibed lesions of a density usually greater than, or equal to brain with a surrounding area of low attenuation (oedema). Calcification may be evident.

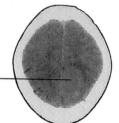

After i.v. contrast

A dense, usually homogeneous enhancement occurs after contrast injection.
N.B. Unenhanced CT is more sensitive than unenhanced MRI in detecting meningiomas.

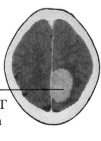

TUMOURS OF THE CEREBRAL HEMISPHERES – EXTRINSIC

MENINGIOMA Investigations (*cont'd*)

MRI: On T1 weighted images most meningiomas are isointense with brain, but after gadolinium injection, they diffusely and strikingly enhance. T2 weighted images give useful preoperative information by identifying major vessels and showing their relationship with the tumour.

ANGIOGRAPHY: Characteristically shows a highly vascular lesion with a typical tumour 'blush', but with the availability of CT angiography, its main value is in selective catheterisation and embolisation of external carotid feeding vessels to reduce tumour vascularity and diminish operative risks from excessive haemorrhage.

3-D CT ANGIOGRAPHY: can show the relationship of surrounding blood vessels to the tumour.

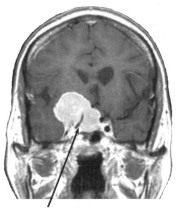

Coronal MRI with gadolinium enhancement showing meningioma invading cavernous sinus and sella turcica and encasing the carotid artery

Management

Management aims at complete removal of both the tumour and its origin without damaging adjacent brain; but this depends on the tumour site and its nature. Even with 'convexity' tumours, where complete excision of the dural origin is possible, overlooking a small fragment of tumour may result in recurrence. This is more likely with malignant meningiomas where the plane of cleavage is often obscured.

Parasagittal meningioma

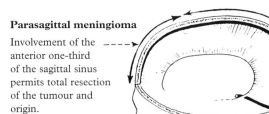

Involvement of the anterior one-third of the sagittal sinus permits total resection of the tumour and origin.

Resection of the posterior two-thirds of the sagittal sinus carries an unacceptably high risk of bilateral venous infarction; in this region every effort is made to spare (or repair) the sinus and its draining veins.

Tumours arising from the skull base seldom permit excision of the origin. Occasionally the patient's age or the tumour site prevents operation or allows only a limited removal; in these patients, a conservative approach may be more appropriate, only intervening if tumour progression causes disabling symptoms. Alternatively stereotactic radiosurgery could be considered particularly for tumours < 3 cm. Standard radiotherapy is unlikely to help unless histology reveals evidence of malignant change.

Operative results: with modern techniques, operative mortality has fallen to less than 3%, but this varies depending on the size and position of the tumour.

Although *in vitro* studies have demonstrated numerous hormonal receptors (e.g. progesterone and oestrogen) in meningioma tissue, clinical studies of hormonal therapy have failed to show any benefit.

Tumour recurrence: depends predominantly on the completeness of removal and on the duration of follow-up. With 'total' resection, about 20% recur after 10 years. With sub-total resection over 50% require a further operation within 10 years.

TUMOURS OF THE CEREBRAL HEMISPHERES – EXTRINSIC

HAEMANGIOPERICYTOMA

A tumour arising from the meninges, but of uncertain cell of origin. It presents with similar clinical features and CT/MRI appearance to meningiomas, but is fifty times less common. Angiography may show a more prominent vascular supply. Calcification does not occur. Haemangiopericytomas tend to invade adjacent bone and to recur even after apparent complete surgical removal. Post-operative radiotherapy should delay recurrence.

ARACHNOID CYSTS

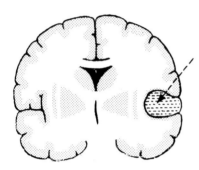

These cystic collections of CSF-like fluid of developmental origin occur in about 0.3% of the population and are usually asymptomatic. About ¾ lie above the tentorium; of these ⅔ occur in the Sylvian fissure, then often associated with temporal lobe hypoplasia.

Arachnoid cysts may gradually increase in size, either due to CSF being driven in through a valve-like opening or by active secretion of fluid from the cyst wall. Occasionally patients present with mass effects, or in children with asymmetric cranial enlargement, macrocephaly and/or psychomotor retardation. More often they are discovered incidentally on CT or MRI.

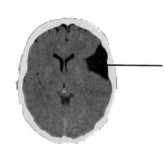

CT scan: shows a low density (CSF density) well demarcated lesion, occasionally producing expansion of the overlying bone.

Treatment: usually *cystoperitoneal shunting* or *marsupialisation* (via a craniotomy) is reserved for those patients presenting with mass effect, but some believe that prophylactic treatment in young children aids normal brain development.

EPIDERMOID/DERMOID CYSTS

These cysts, more commonly found in the posterior fossa (page 333), occasionally develop in the Sylvian or interhemispheric fissure. They are either of congenital or acquired origin due to implantation and sequestration of ectoderm. They may present with epilepsy, features of raised intracranial pressure or with focal neurological signs. Rupture into the subarachnoid space causes a chemical meningitis.

On CT scan, the extreme low attenuation of the cyst contents is characteristic. Symptoms may necessitate operative evacuation of the cyst contents. Complete removal of the cyst wall is difficult and reaccumulation may occur.

Lipomas

Rarely occur intracranially. They are usually found incidentally on imaging or at autopsy and are often associated with other developmental anomalies such as agenesis of the corpus callosum. They are located in midline structures e.g. corpus callosum, dorsal midbrain and cerebellar vermis. They require no treatment.

TUMOURS OF THE POSTERIOR FOSSA – INTRINSIC

CEREBELLAR METASTASIS

In adults, metastasis is the commonest tumour of the cerebellar hemisphere. Primary tumour sites match those of supratentorial lesions (page 318).

Clinical features: may present acutely or progress over several months.

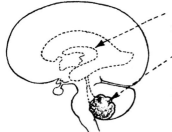

CSF obstruction *hydrocephalus* – signs and symptoms of raised intracranial pressure.
Cerebellar signs – ataxia, nystagmus, dysarthria, inco-ordination.

Extension into the cerebellopontine angle may damage cranial nerves V–XII – especially if a *malignant plaque* develops.

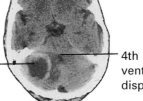

4th ventricle displaced

Investigations

CT scan shows a well-defined solid or cystic lesion lying within the cerebellar hemisphere and enhancing irregularly with contrast.

Obstructive hydrocephalus is often evident on higher scan cuts. As with cerebral metastases MRI is more sensitive in detecting small lesions.

Management

Operative removal of a single metastasis through a suboccipital craniectomy is worthwhile, provided the patient has a reasonable prognosis from the primary tumour. Risks are small – extensive cerebellar hemisphere resection (on one side) seldom produces any significant permanent deficit. A course of *radiotherapy* can follow operation if resection is incomplete. Radiosurgery provides a possible alternative to surgical resection. Persistence of obstructive hydrocephalus requires a ventriculoperitoneal shunt.

HAEMANGIOBLASTOMA

This benign tumour of vascular origin occurs primarily in the middle-aged; it is slightly more prevalent in males and is the commonest primary cerebellar tumour of adults. In some patients, haemangioblastomas occur at other sites, e.g. the spinal cord and retina and may be associated with other pathologies e.g. polycythaemia and cysts in the pancreas and kidneys – *Von Hippel-Lindau disease* (page 559).

The tumour is usually highly vascular. In 70% there is an associated cyst, the lining of which does not contain tumour.

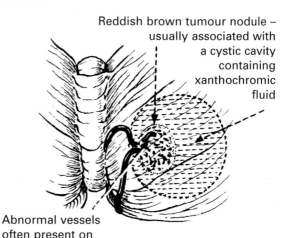

Reddish brown tumour nodule – usually associated with a cystic cavity containing xanthochromic fluid

Abnormal vessels often present on cerebellar surface

325

TUMOURS OF THE POSTERIOR FOSSA – INTRINSIC

HAEMANGIOBLASTOMA (*cont'd*)

Clinical features

Cerebellar signs and symptoms or the effects of CSF obstruction usually develop insidiously. Occasionally subarachnoid haemorrhage occurs. In female patients, symptoms often appear during pregnancy. Polycythaemia due to increased erythropoietin production is common.

Investigations

CT scan shows a well defined low density cystic region in the cerebellum with a strongly enhancing nodule in the wall. Occasionally, multiple lesions are evident.

MRI also shows intense enhancement of the solid component with tortuous flow voids reflecting the high vascularity.

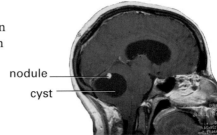

nodule

cyst

Management

In some patients *operative removal* of the tumour nodule is straightforward, but recurrences (or further tumours at other sites, e.g. spine) develop in 20%. Patients with highly vascular solid tumours can present a formidable surgical challenge, particularly if they involve the medulla. Pre-operative embolisation may significantly reduce the surgical risks.

MEDULLOBLASTOMA

Medulloblastomas are primitive neuroectodermal tumours (PNETs), which occur predominantly in childhood, with a peak age incidence of about 5 years. They arise in the cerebellar vermis and usually extend into the 4th ventricle. They are highly malignant. In 30%, spread occurs throughout the CSF, often seeding to the lateral ventricles or the spinal theca. The origin is uncertain but appears to arise from primitive embryonic cells.

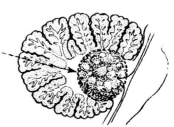

Clinical features

Destruction of the cerebellar vermis causes truncal and gait ataxia often developing over a few weeks.

Alternatively, the patient presents with signs and symptoms of raised intracranial pressure due to blockage of CSF drainage. In the very young, failure to recognise these features has resulted in permanent visual loss from severe papilloedema.

Investigations

CT scan shows an isodense midline lesion in the cerebellar vermis, compressing and displacing the 4th ventricle and enhancing strongly with contrast.

MRI may provide more anatomical detail and more readily detects supratentorial CSF seedlings.

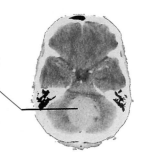

Higher cuts show dilated ventricles, sometimes containing CSF tumour seedlings.

TUMOURS OF THE POSTERIOR FOSSA – INTRINSIC

MEDULLOBLASTOMA (*cont'd*)

Management
Staging is essential because of the high incidence of leptomeningeal spread and bone marrow involvement. Assess this with spinal MRI with gadolinium, CSF analysis and bone marrow examination. CSF obstruction may require urgent relief, preferably by endoscopic 3rd ventriculostomy.

Operation: The aim is to remove as much tumour as possible (particularly if staging has excluded disseminated disease), without damaging crucial structures in the floor of the 4th ventricle.

Radiotherapy: the most effective post-operative treatment. Whole neural axis irradiation (unacceptable in children < 3 years), attempts to cover any CSF seeding.

Chemotherapy: routinely used, but the extent to which chemotherapy alters the quality or duration of survival is less certain.

Prognosis
Five-year survival ranges from 50–85% depending on the extent of tumour removal, dissemination and age (< 3 years poor risk).

CEREBELLAR ASTROCYTOMA
In contrast to astrocytomas of the cerebral hemispheres, cerebellar astrocytomas are usually low grade tumours of the fibrillary or pilocytic types. They are particularly common in children and carry an excellent prognosis. Occasionally a more diffuse or anaplastic type occurs with a less favourable outcome. They usually lie in the cerebellar hemisphere or vermis but occasionally extend through a peduncle into the brain stem. Many have cystic components.

Clinical features
Cerebellar signs and symptoms tend to develop gradually over many months; if CSF obstruction occurs, the patient may present acutely with headache, papilloedema and deteriorating conscious level.

Investigations
CT scan – density changes and the degree of contrast enhancement are variable.

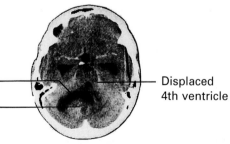

Often a low density cystic area abuts or encircles the tumour mass

Displaced 4th ventricle

MRI – may provide more anatomical definition.

Management
Ideally, complete *operative removal* is attempted provided the brain stem is not involved. With pilocytic tumours, 80% survive 20 years. Even after partial removal 'cures' have been reported. Persistent hydrocephalus may require 3rd ventriculostomy or a ventriculoperitoneal shunt.

TUMOURS OF THE POSTERIOR FOSSA – INTRINSIC

BRAIN STEM ASTROCYTOMA

Rarely, astrocytomas arise within the brain stem. Most are of the fibrillary or pilocytic types and diffusely expand the pontine region although they can be malignant. They develop mainly in children or young adults.

Clinical features

Cranial nerve palsies and long tract signs gradually develop as the tumour progresses. Eventually conscious level is impaired. More malignant gliomas are associated with a rapidly progressing course, often with signs of raised intracranial pressure.

Investigations

CT scan may show low density within the brainstem, with absence of surrounding cisterns and posterior displacement of the 4th ventricle.

MRI scanning is superior to CT scanning in the detection and evaluation of brain stem astrocytoma.

Management

Operative exploration is rarely indicated. Radiotherapy is often administered, usually after a stereotactic biopsy, with occasional palliation of symptoms and uncertain effect on survival. Chemotherapy is of no value.

Prognosis

At best, the 5-year survival following radiotherapy is 35%, although some patients may survive for up to 20 years with minimum disability.

TUMOURS OF THE POSTERIOR FOSSA – EXTRINSIC

ACOUSTIC SCHWANNOMA

Nerve sheath tumours are the commonest infratentorial tumours, constituting 6% of all primary intracranial tumours and 80% of cerebellopontine angle lesions. They usually present in middle age (40–50 years) and occur more frequently in women. Bilateral schwannomas occur in 5% of patients and are characteristic of type 2 neurofibromatosis (NF 2) (page 557).

They are benign, slowly growing tumours which arise primarily from the *vestibular* portion of the VIII cranial nerve and lie in the cerebellopontine angle – a wedge shaped area bounded by the petrous bone, the pons and the cerebellum. Rarely these tumours arise from the V cranial nerve.

Schwannomas expand at an average rate of 2 mm/year, but up to 40% show no growth on serial investigation.

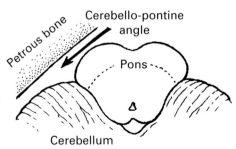

TUMOURS OF THE POSTERIOR FOSSA – EXTRINSIC

ACOUSTIC SCHWANNOMA (*cont'd*)

Pathology: The other type of nerve sheath tumour – neurofibroma (page 301) – does not occur intracranially.

Different histological types exist, often within the same tumour:

Antoni type A – shoals and whorls of tightly packed cells in groups or palisades

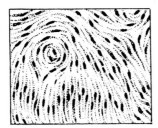

Antoni type B – a meshwork of interlinked loosely packed stellate cells.

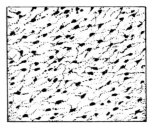

Clinical features

Patients with acoustic tumours often complain of *occipital pain* on the side of the tumour. In addition:

VIII nerve damage causes a *gradually progressive sensorineural deafness* noted over many months or years. *Vertigo* is rarely troublesome since slow tumour growth readily permits compensation. Similarly *tinnitus* is usually minimal.

V nerve damage can occur with tumours > 2 cm and causes *facial pain, numbness* and *paraesthesia*. *Depression of the corneal reflex* is an important early sign.

Compression of the aqueduct and the 4th ventricle may result in hydrocephalus with *symptoms and signs of raised intracranial pressure.*

N.B. Left cerebellar hemisphere removed to expose the divided cerebellar peduncles.

Facial weakness is surprisingly *uncommon* despite marked VII nerve compression.

IX, X and XI nerve damage seldom occurs but occasionally large tumours cause *swallowing difficulty, voice change* and *palatal weakness.*

Cerebellar and pontine damage – large tumours (> 4 cm) may compress the cerebellum causing *ataxia, ipsilateral inco-ordination* and *nystagmus*. Pontine damage may produce a *contralateral hemiparesis.*

329

TUMOURS OF THE POSTERIOR FOSSA – EXTRINSIC

ACOUSTIC SCHWANNOMA (*cont'd*)

Investigations

Neuro-otological test (see pages 61–63) } help differentiate deafness due to:
– audiometry — conductive deficit
– speech audiometry — cochlear deficit
– stapedial reflex decay — sensorineural — retrocochlear deficit
(e.g. acoustic tumour)

– *brainstem auditory evoked potential (BAEP)* – perhaps the most sensitive of these tests shows a delay of the wave V latency on the affected side.

CT scan

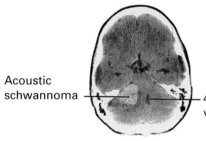

Acoustic schwannoma — — 4th ventricle

I.V. contrast is essential, since acoustic tumours are often isodense. After contrast the tumour, lying adjacent to the IAM enhances strongly. Low density cystic areas are occasionally seen. Patients with 4th ventricle compression may show associated dilatation of the 3rd and lateral ventricles.

CT scanning also demonstrates the size of the mastoid air cells – useful information for operation.

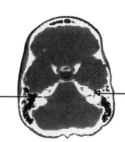

Bone window levels usually show dilation of the internal auditory meatus. — Normal internal auditory meatus

MRI

The investigation of choice, particularly for small intracanalicular tumours. On a T1 weighted image, the lesion enhances strongly after i.v. gadolinium.

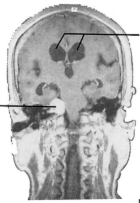

Coronal section showing an acoustic schwannoma indenting the pons and extending into the internal auditory meatus. — dilated ventricles

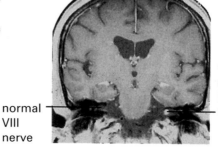

normal VIII nerve — Coronal section showing small intracanalicular tumour

TUMOURS OF THE POSTERIOR FOSSA – EXTRINSIC

ACOUSTIC SCHWANNOMA Management

Treatment aims at – tumour removal with minimal risk,
  – preservation of facial nerve function,
  – retention of useful hearing unless this is already lost.

Some patients presenting with small tumours may prefer to adopt a *conservative approach*, only intervening if serial MR imaging shows significant growth.

Technique

Middle fossa approach: temporal lobe retraction exposes acoustic tumour and facial nerve from above. The tentorium cerebelli and the superior petrosal sinus are divided if necessary.

TRANSLABYRINTHINE APPROACH: approaching the tumour through the mastoid air cells and the labyrinth, permits early identification of the facial nerve; tumour decompression and removal follows.

SUBOCCIPITAL APPROACH: the cerebellopontine angle is approached from below by removing occipital bone and retracting the cerebellum.

Tumour debulking aids dissection of the tumour capsule from the surrounding structures, including the facial nerve. Drilling away the posterior wall of the internal meatus exposes the tumour and facial nerve lying within the canal.

Some surgeons prefer a joint translabyrinthine/suboccipital approach.

All methods have their advocates. Limited visualisation of the brain stem structures through a translabyrinthine approach makes this inappropriate for large tumours. Inevitably this approach damages hearing. With very small tumours, careful removal via the suboccipital route may preserve the cochlear nerve as well as facial nerve function. Peroperative monitoring is essential to aid preservation of the facial nerve. Auditory evoked potential monitoring may help hearing preservation in appropriate patients. All tumour tissue must be removed; incomplete removal results in late recurrence.

Results

Outcome relates to tumour size. With a tumour diameter of 5 mm or less, some hearing can be preserved in > 50% and facial nerve function in > 95%. With tumours of 2–3 cm, all lose hearing and 25–50% lose facial nerve function, and this may take many months to recover. Incomplete eye closure may require *tarsorrhaphy* to prevent corneal ulceration. When facial nerve palsy persists, *hypoglossal-facial anastomosis* may improve the cosmetic result. Swallowing difficulty from lower cranial nerve damage seldom persists.

Mortality ranges from 1–3% and usually results from damage to important vascular structures (e.g. anterior inferior cerebellar artery), haemorrhage, aspiration pneumonia or pulmonary embolus.

Stereotactic radiosurgery: this single dose technique (see page 310), initially reserved for elderly patients, is now used more widely for schwannomas < 3 cm in size. Centres report 'control' of tumour growth in up to 90%, with preservation of hearing in about 50% and facial nerve function in 90%, but eradication is exceptional. No long term follow-up results are yet available.

TUMOURS OF THE POSTERIOR FOSSA – EXTRINSIC

TRIGEMINAL SCHWANNOMA

Rarely schwannomas arise from the trigeminal ganglion or nerve root. These lie in the middle fossa or extend into the cerebellopontine angle, compress surrounding structures – cavernous sinus, midbrain and the pons – and erode the apex of the petrous bone.

Clinical features are usually long-standing – facial pain, paraesthesia and numbness. Compression of posterior fossa structures results in nystagmus, ataxia and hemiparesis.

CT scan or MRI with contrast demonstrates an enhancing lesion eroding the petrous apex and extending into the middle and/or posterior fossa.

Management: Operative removal, even if subtotal, should provide long-lasting benefit. The tumour is approached either from above via a subtemporal route across the middle fossa floor, from below via a suboccipital craniectomy, or via a combination of these approaches.

MENINGIOMA

Approximately 8% of all intracranial meningiomas arise in the posterior fossa.

Clinical features

These depend on the exact tumour site. Those arising over the *cerebellar convexity* may not present until the mass obstructs CSF drainage. Meningiomas arising in the *cerebellopontine angle* may involve any cranial nerve from V to XII. A *clivus* meningioma may cause bilateral VI nerve palsies before pontine pressure causes long tract signs.

Tumours growing at the *foramen magnum*, compressing the cervico-medullary junction, produce characteristic effects – pyramidal weakness initially affecting the ipsilateral arm, followed by the ipsilateral leg, spreading to the contralateral limbs with further tumour growth.

Investigations

CT scan with intravenous contrast will identify the tumour site, but *MRI* with gadolinium enhancement shows more anatomical detail.

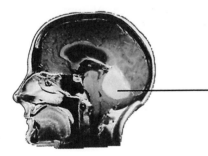

TI weighted *MRI* with gadolinium showing a large tumour arising from the tentorium and straight sinus, compressing the cerebellar vermis and the 4th ventricle.

Management

As with supratentorial meningiomas, treatment aims at complete tumour removal. In the posterior fossa, cranial nerve involvement makes this difficult and exacting; excision of the tumour origin is seldom possible. For some, stereotactic radiosurgery is an alternative method of controlling tumour growth.

TUMOURS OF THE POSTERIOR FOSSA – EXTRINSIC

EPIDERMOID/DERMOID CYSTS

These rare cysts of embryological origin develop from cells predestined to become either epidermis or dermis. They most commonly arise in the cerebellopontine angle but may also occur around the suprasellar cisterns, in the lateral ventricles and in the Sylvian fissures, often extending deeply into brain tissue.

Pathology: Depends on cell of origin:

Epidermoid (epidermis) – a thin transparent cyst wall often adheres firmly to surrounding tissues; the contents – keratinised debris and cholesterol crystals – produce a 'pearly' white appearance.

Dermoid (dermis) – as above, but thicker walled and, in addition, containing hair follicles and glandular tissue. Midline dermoid cysts lying in the posterior fossa often connect to the skin surface through a bony defect. This presents a potential route for infection.

Clinical features
When lying in the cerebellopontine angle, epidermoid/dermoid cysts often cause *trigeminal neuralgia* (see page 161). Neurological findings may range from a depressed corneal reflex to multiple cranial nerve palsies. Rupture and release of cholesterol into the subarachnoid space produces a severe and occasionally fatal *chemical meningitis*. The presence of a *suboccipital dimple* combined with an attack of *infective meningitis* should raise the possibility of a posterior fossa dermoid cyst with a cutaneous fistula.

Investigations
CT scan shows a characteristic low density (often 'fat' density) lesion, unchanged after contrast enhancement or showing only slight peripheral enhancement. Calcification may be evident.

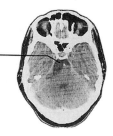

T2 weighted *MRI* appears more sensitive than CT in detecting an abnormality, but the hyperintense signal does not differentiate an arachnoid cyst from an epidermoid.

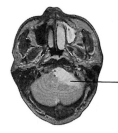

T2 weighted MRI showing lower cranial nerves traversing the lesion.

Treatment
Adherence of the cyst wall to important structures often prevents complete removal, but evacuation of the contents provides symptomatic relief. Aseptic meningitis in the postoperative period requires prompt treatment with steroids. Even when removal is incomplete, recollection of the keratinised debris is uncommon and may take many years.

SELLAR/SUPRASELLAR TUMOURS – PITUITARY ADENOMA

Tumours of the pituitary gland constitute about 5–10% of intracranial tumours. They arise from the anterior portion of the gland and are usually benign.

'CLASSIC' classification
Previously based on the light microscopic appearance of the tumour cell type.

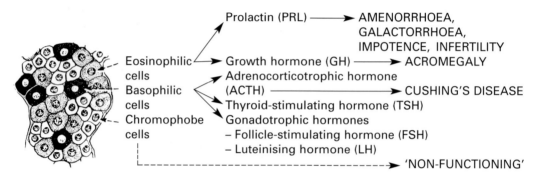

PRL text:
- Prolactin (PRL) ⟶ AMENORRHOEA, GALACTORRHOEA, IMPOTENCE, INFERTILITY
- Eosinophilic cells
- Growth hormone (GH) ⟶ ACROMEGALY
- Basophilic cells
- Adrenocorticotrophic hormone (ACTH) ⟶ CUSHING'S DISEASE
- Thyroid-stimulating hormone (TSH)
- Chromophobe cells
- Gonadotrophic hormones
  – Follicle-stimulating hormone (FSH)
  – Luteinising hormone (LH)
- ⟶ 'NON-FUNCTIONING'

PRESENT classification

Immunohistochemical techniques permit a classification based on the hormone type secreted, but this does not necessarily reflect the active form of the hormone. About half of the 'non-functioning' chromophobe adenomas are shown to secrete prolactin.

	Incidence
– GH secreting tumour	20–25%
– Prolactinoma	25–50%
– ACTH secreting tumour	5–10%
– TSH secreting tumour	} rare
– FSH/LH secreting tumour	
– Inactive	25–40%

CLINICAL PRESENTATION

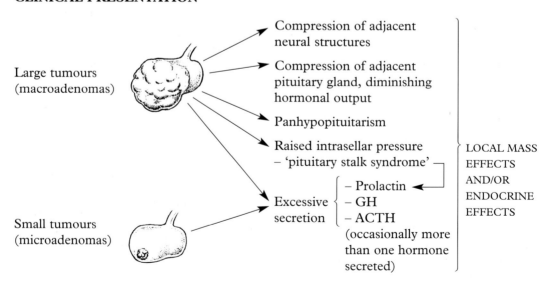

Large tumours (macroadenomas)

Small tumours (microadenomas)

- Compression of adjacent neural structures
- Compression of adjacent pituitary gland, diminishing hormonal output
- Panhypopituitarism
- Raised intrasellar pressure – 'pituitary stalk syndrome'
- Excessive secretion
  – Prolactin
  – GH
  – ACTH
  (occasionally more than one hormone secreted)

LOCAL MASS EFFECTS AND/OR ENDOCRINE EFFECTS

SELLAR/SUPRASELLAR TUMOURS – PITUITARY ADENOMA

LOCAL MASS EFFECT

Headache
Occurs in most patients with enlargement of the pituitary fossa. It is not specific in site or nature.

Visual field defects
Pressure on the inferior aspect of the optic chiasma usually causes *superior temporal quadrantanopia* initially, with progression to bitemporal hemianopia, but any pattern can occur.

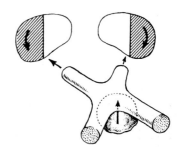

Cavernous sinus compression

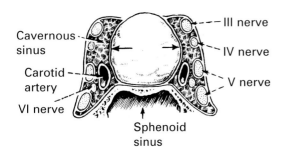

Cavernous sinus
Carotid artery
VI nerve
Sphenoid sinus
III nerve
IV nerve
V nerve

In some pituitary tumours, lateral expansion may compress nerves lying within the walls of the cavernous sinus. The III nerve is especially vulnerable.

Rarely vertical expansion obstructs the foramen of Munro causing hydrocephalus and/or hypothalamic compression (page 342).

ENDOCRINE EFFECT

1. HYPERSECRETION
The clinical syndrome produced is dependent on the hormone secreted.

Growth hormone (GH)
Stimulates growth and plays a part in control of protein, fat and carbohydrate metabolism. Excess GH in the adult causes ACROMEGALY.

In childhood, prior to fusion of bone epiphyses, GH excess causes GIGANTISM.

GH levels are usually increased to > 10 mU/l. Increased serum levels of insulin growth factor-1 enhances the effect of growth hormone on target organs.

Hyperglycaemia normally suppresses GH secretion. GH samples are taken in conjunction with blood glucose during a glucose tolerance test. The lack of GH suppression after glucose administration confirms the presence of a tumour.

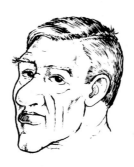

Enlargement of soft tissues, cartilage and bones in face, hands and feet

Coarse skin

Sweating
Hypertension
Diabetes in 10%
Increased risk of bowel cancer

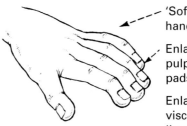

'Soft, doughy' hands

Enlarged finger pulps and heel pads.

Enlarged viscera – heart, liver, thyroid.

SELLAR/SUPRASELLAR TUMOURS – PITUITARY ADENOMA

HYPERSECRETION (*cont'd*)

Prolactin

This hormone helps promote lactation. Prolactinoma is the commonest type of pituitary tumour. Immunoassay techniques aid early detection. Female:male ratio – 4:1

This tumour may present with
- INFERTILITY
- AMENORRHOEA
- GALACTORRHOEA

In males, the tumour may present with IMPOTENCE or remain undetected until local pressure effects occur.

In most centres, a serum prolactin of 500 mU/l is considered abnormal, but before assuming the presence of a prolactin secreting tumour, other causes must be excluded.

Causes of hyperprolactinaemia

- Stress
- Pregnancy
- Drugs (phenothiazines, oestrogens)
- Hypothyroidism
- Renal disease
- Pituitary adenoma
- Hypothalamic lesion (e.g. sarcoid, craniopharyngioma) or the pituitary stalk syndrome
- Seizures

Prolactin differs from other anterior pituitary hormones in that it is under tonic *inhibitory* control from the hypothalamus. Hypothalamic lesions or raised intrasellar pressure, compromising hypothalamic–pituitary perfusion (i.e. the *'pituitary stalk syndrome'*) produce a rise in serum prolactin, but levels seldom exceed 2000 mU/l. Prolactin levels above 4000 mU/l invariably indicate prolactinoma.

SELLAR/SUPRASELLAR TUMOURS – PITUITARY ADENOMA

Adrenocorticotrophic hormone (ACTH)

ACTH stimulates secretion of cortisol and androgens. Hypersecretion from a pituitary adenoma or hyperplasia causes CUSHING'S DISEASE (bilateral adrenal hyperplasia) which presents with the characteristic features of CUSHING'S SYNDROME.

This syndrome may also be caused by excessive oral corticosteroids, but also by an adrenal tumour or by ectopic secretion of ACTH from a bronchial carcinoma.

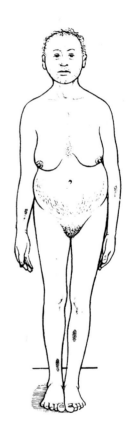

Features of Cushing's syndrome
- Moon face
- Acne
- Hirsutism and baldness
- Buffalo-type obesity
- Purple striae over flanks and abdomen
- Bruising
- Muscle weakness and wasting
- Osteoporosis
- Hypertension
- Increased susceptibility to infection
- Diabetes mellitus

A loss of normal diurnal variation of plasma free cortisol and an increase in 24 hour urinary free cortisol indicates excess secretion. The diagnosis of a pituitary cause is suggested by finding normal or moderately raised ACTH levels which suppress with high doses of dexamethasone.

Ectopic ACTH production does not suppress with dexamethasone and with adrenal tumours, ACTH levels are virtually undetectable.

Other tests include
- the effect of corticotrophin releasing factory
  ($\uparrow$ACTH and cortisol if pituitary origin)
- petrosal versus peripheral venous sampling
  to identity the source of the ACTH.

Bilateral adrenalectomy for Cushing's syndrome is sometimes followed by the development of *Nelson's syndrome* – high ACTH levels, pituitary enlargement and marked skin pigmentation.

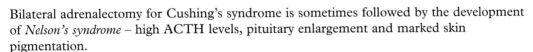

TSH – stimulates thyroid hormone secretion
FSH – controls growth of ovarian follicles/spermatogenesis
LH – induces ovulation/testosterone secretion

⎤ Hypersecreting
⎬ tumours
⎦ very rare.

337

SELLAR/SUPRASELLAR TUMOURS – PITUITARY ADENOMA

2. HYPOSECRETION

Many pituitary tumours are diagnosed before panhypopituitarism develops, but large tumours may cause gradual impairment of pituitary hormone secretion. Growth hormone and the gonadotrophins are first affected, followed by TSH and ACTH. Panhypopituitarism only occurs when more than 80% of the anterior pituitary is destroyed.

Impaired secretion	Adults	Children
GH –	'Adult GH deficiency syndrome' – weight gain, loss of libido, fatigue	Pituitary dwarfism – (diminished somatic
Gonadotrophins – ACTH –	Amenorrhoea, sterility, loss of libido Glucocorticoid and androgen deficiency, muscle weakness and fatigue	growth, retarded sexual development, hypoglycaemic
TSH –	Secondary hypothyroidism – sensitivity to cold, dry skin, physical and mental sluggishness, coarseness of hair	episodes, normal intelligence)
Prolactin* –	Failure of lactation	

* Prolactin secretion is most resistant to pituitary damage. Deficiency is seldom evident, usually only presenting after postpartum haemorrhage (Sheehan's syndrome) as a failure of lactation associated with the other features of panhypopituitarism.

Pituitary hormone assay cannot distinguish low 'normal' levels from impaired secretion, *but low levels of pituitary hormone in the presence of low target gland hormones* confirm hyposecretion, e.g. low TSH levels despite a low serum thyroxine. Basal levels guide replacement therapy.

The lack of response to tests designed to increase specific pituitary hormones provides additional confirmation of hypofunction:

1. GH } ACTH } – *Insulin tolerance test:* Hypoglycaemia acting via the hypothalamic pituitary axis should elevate GH and ACTH levels, the latter causing a significant rise in plasma cortisol.
2. Gonadotrophin – *Gonadotrophin releasing hormone (GnRH) injection* should produce a rapid rise in LH and a slower rise in FSH.
3. TSH } Prolactin } – *Thyrotrophin releasing hormone (TRH) injection* should increase plasma levels of both TSH and prolactin.

The above tests can be carried out simultaneously as the *Combined pituitary stimulation test.* Insulin, GnRH and TRH are injected intravenously and all anterior pituitary hormones measured from repeated blood samples taken over a 2-hour period. Glucose levels are also checked to ensure adequacy of the hypoglycaemia.

PITUITARY APOPLEXY
This is an uncommon complication of pituitary tumours due to the occurrence of infarction followed by haemorrhage into the tumour. Severe headache of sudden onset simulating subarachnoid haemorrhage, rapidly progressive visual failure and extraocular nerve palsies accompany acute pituitary insufficiency. Death may follow unless urgent steroid treatment is instituted.

SELLAR/SUPRASELLAR TUMOURS – PITUITARY ADENOMA

NEURORADIOLOGICAL INVESTIGATION

LARGE TUMOURS

Skull X-ray
Large tumours cause
expansion or 'ballooning'
of the pituitary fossa
and
may erode the floor

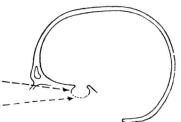

CT scan with contrast enhancement demonstrates tumours filling the pituitary fossa and expanding into the suprasellar compartment, but **MRI** gives more anatomical detail, clearly delineating any suprasellar extension and the effect on adjacent structures.

Sagittal T1
weighted MRI
with gadolinium
showing a large
pituitary tumour
of mixed intensity
with suprasellar
extension.

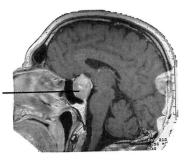

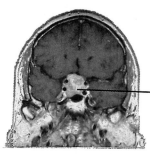

Coronal view
of same
patient
showing
relationships
of the tumour
to the carotid
arteries and
the cavernous
sinus.

MICROADENOMAS

Coronal **CT Scanning** with contrast may demonstrate a low density region within the gland tissue (or may show deviation of the pituitary stalk from the midline). Tumours > 5 mm diameter produce these characteristic appearances. Tumours under this size are difficult to detect.

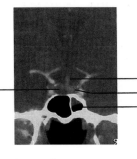

Pituitary stalk
(undeviated)
Normal gland
Sphenoid sinus

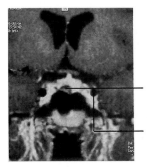

MRI is marginally better than CT scanning in the detection of microadenomas but both have false positives and false negatives.

Microadenoma

Carotid artery within
cavernous sinus

CT angiography or MR angiography may be required before transphenoidal operation to exclude the presence of an incidental medially projecting aneurysm.

SELLAR/SUPRASELLAR TUMOURS – PITUITARY ADENOMA

MANAGEMENT

A variety of different forms of treatment are available:

Drug therapy

Dopamine agonists lower abnormal circulating hormone concentrations, especially prolactin. In most patients with a prolactinoma, the prolactin levels fall and the tumour shrinks. These patients require long-term therapy as the source of the hyperprolactinaemia persists. Cessation of treatment can result in rapid tumour re-expansion. Agents used include bromocriptine and cabergoline, a long acting preparation.

Somatostatin analogues: e.g. octreotide, inhibit growth hormone production and cause some tumour shrinkage in a proportion of patients. It is no longer used as long-term therapy unless a specific contraindication to surgery exists.

Operative approach

From BELOW:

1. *Trans-sphenoidal*

Through an incision in the upper gum the nasal mucosa is stripped from the septum and the pituitary fossa approached through the sphenoid sinus. The microscope aids vision and either traditional intraoperative fluoroscopy or *'frameless'* *stereotaxy* (page 382) is used for guidance. In recent years, an alternative trans-sphenoidal technique has been developed using an *endoscopic approach*. This technique can also be combined with frameless three-dimensional image localization.

Through this route the pituitary gland can be directly visualised and explored for microadenomas. Even large tumours with suprasellar extensions may be removed from below, avoiding the need for craniotomy.

From ABOVE

2. *Transfrontal*

Through a craniotomy flap the frontal lobe is retracted to provide direct access to the pituitary tumour. This approach is usually reserved for tumours with large frontal or lateral extensions.

N.B. Patients may require steroid cover before any anaesthetic or operative procedure.

Radiotherapy

Pituitary adenomas are radiosensitive and external irradiation is commonly employed. Occasionally, radioactive seeds of yttrium or gold are implanted into the pituitary fossa, either via a trans-sphenoidal approach or stereotactically through a frontal burr hole.

Several months elapse before hormone levels begin to fall. Pituitary function gradually declines over a 5–10 year period after treatment and most patients eventually require replacement hormone therapy to prevent symptoms of hypopituitarism developing.

SELLAR/SUPRASELLAR TUMOURS – PITUITARY ADENOMA

MANAGEMENT (cont'd)

Treatment selection
Treatment choice depends on:
- presenting problems and patient's requirements,
  e.g. restoring fertility, halting visual deterioration.
- patient's age.
- preference and experience of the treatment centre.

Microadenomas

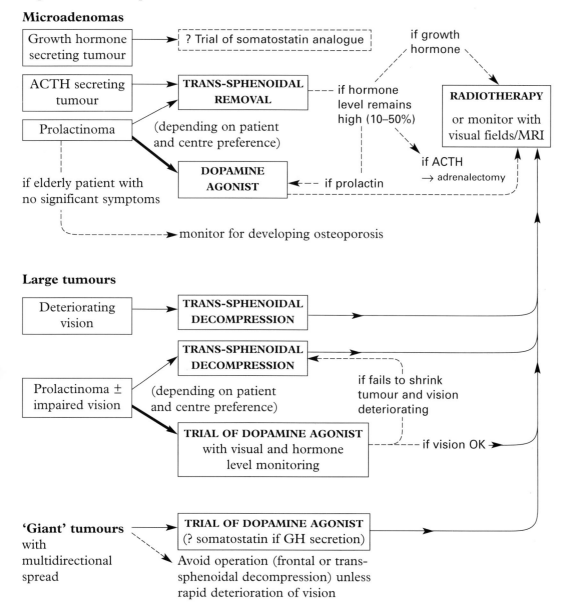

Large tumours

SELLAR/SUPRASELLAR TUMOURS

CRANIOPHARYNGIOMA

These cystic tumours constitute about 3% of all primary intracranial tumours. They present predominantly in children and in young adults but symptoms may develop at any age. Although benign, their proximity to crucial structures poses complex problems of management. About 40% of craniopharyngiomas have solid components of squamous epithelium with calcified debris and one or more cystic regions containing greenish cholesteatomatous fluid. In 20% the tumour is solid throughout. Although the tumour capsule appears well defined, histological examination reveals finger-like projections extending into adjacent tissue with marked surrounding gliosis.

Sites: Growth usually begins near the pituitary stalk, but may extend in many directions.

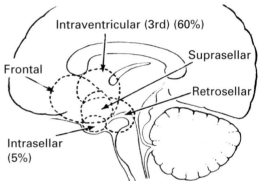

Clinical features: depend on the exact site and size of the tumour. Growth is slow and most signs and symptoms develop insidiously.

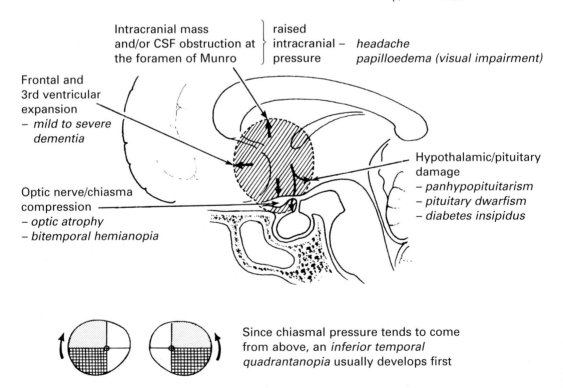

Intracranial mass and/or CSF obstruction at the foramen of Munro } raised intracranial pressure — *headache* *papilloedema (visual impairment)*

Frontal and 3rd ventricular expansion
– *mild to severe dementia*

Optic nerve/chiasma compression
– *optic atrophy*
– *bitemporal hemianopia*

Hypothalamic/pituitary damage
– *panhypopituitarism*
– *pituitary dwarfism*
– *diabetes insipidus*

Since chiasmal pressure tends to come from above, an *inferior temporal quadrantanopia* usually develops first

SELLAR/SUPRASELLAR TUMOURS

CRANIOPHARYNGIOMA *(cont'd)*

Investigations

Skull X-ray: shows calcification above or within the pituitary fossa in most children and in 25% of adults.

CT scan: shows a lesion of mixed density containing solid and cystic components — lying in the suprasellar region.

In children, CT scan invariably shows some calcification —

The cyst capsule often enhances with contrast.

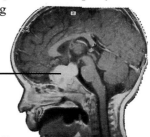

Coronal or sagittal *MRI* helps by demonstrating the exact relation- ships of the tumour — to the 3rd ventricle

MRI: provides greater anatomical detail

Pituitary function studies (page 338): often demonstrate the need for hormone replacement.

Management

Several options exist; the more aggressive the treatment, the higher the risks, but the lower the recurrence rate.

All patients require steroid cover before any anaesthetic or operative procedure.

Operative removal usually involves a subfrontal or subtemporal craniotomy, perhaps combined with a transcallosal approach (i.e. splitting the anterior corpus callosum from above and approaching the tumour through the 3rd ventricle). The trans-sphenoidal route may permit removal of purely intrasellar tumours.

Methods

1. *Total tumour excision (+ radiotherapy if recurrence develops)*
2. *Subtotal tumour excision + radiotherapy*
3. *Cyst drainage +* ——— *radiotherapy*
   (with an indwelling   *or*
   catheter and reservoir)   *implantation of yttrium-90 or chemotherapeutic agent (bleomycin)*

Attempted total excision carries a risk of life-threatening hypothalamic damage, but if successful avoids the immediate need and associated risks of radiotherapy to a developing brain. Operative mortality lies between 0–10% and depends on the tumour site and the extent of the attempted removal. Some report a recurrence rate of up to 30% within 10 years of an apparent 'total' removal. This presumably results from residual tumour extensions lying beyond the capsule.

Within subtotal removal the recurrence rate approaches 90%, but with radiotherapy this falls to 30–50% after 5 years.

The decision to aim for total or subtotal removal requires careful judgement.

Preoperative investigations help but the final decision often awaits direct exploration.

SELLAR/SUPRASELLAR TUMOURS

OPTIC NERVE (GLIOMA) ASTROCYTOMA

This rare tumour usually presents in children under 10 years. Up to one-third are associated with neurofibromatosis (NFI) where the tumour may be bilateral. Tumour growth expands the nerve in a fusiform manner. Some extend anteriorly into the orbit, others posteriorly to involve the optic chiasma. All are of the pilocytic type and growth is slow.

Optic nerve tumour may 'dumbell' though the optic foramen.

Clinical features

Visual field scotomas gradually progress to *complete visual loss.*

Orbital extension causes *proptosis.*

In some patients posterior expansion beyond the chiasma causes *hypothalamic damage (precocious puberty and other endocrine disturbance)* and/or hydrocephalus.

X-rays of the orbital foremen show dilatation and *CT scans* demonstrate an enhancing mixed attenuation mass within the orbit or lying in the suprasellar region. *MRI* is more sensitive for chiasmatic extensions.

Management		Prognosis
Unilateral within orbit	– Complete excision with orbital enucleation if necessary	– Long-term survival expected.
Lesion involving the optic chiasma	– Conservative approach (the value of radiotherapy is not known and may risk vasculitis and intellectual deterioration).	– Patients may retain vision for many years; survival is often long-term. Those with hypothalamic damage have a poor prognosis.

SUPRASELLAR MENINGIOMA

Meningiomas arising from the tuberculum sellae often present early as a result of chiasmal compression causing visual field defects – usually a *bitemporal hemianopia.*

Straight X-rays may show *hyperostosis* of the tuberculum sellae or planum sphenoidale.

CT scan shows a rounded, often partly calcified suprasellar mass homogeneously enhancing with contrast. *MRI* provides improved anatomical detail.

Unfortunately the visual defect often persists after operation, but attempted removal is essential to prevent further progression.

T1 weighted MRI with gadolinium

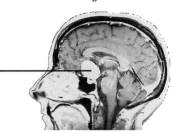

MENINGIOMA OF THE OPTIC NERVE SHEATH

Rarely, meningiomas arise from the optic nerve sheath, usually extending in dumbbell fashion through the optic foramen. Some penetrate the orbital dura and invade the orbital contents. Total excision is impossible without sacrificing the adjacent optic nerve.

SUPRASELLAR EPIDERMOID/DERMOID (see page 333).

> Note: large aneurysms or granulomas (TB, sarcoid) may simulate a sellar/suprasellar tumour on CT scan or MRI. If in doubt, perform CTA or MRA prior to operative exploration.

PINEAL REGION TUMOURS

Pineal region tumours are relatively uncommon.
They consists of a variety of different
pathological types and as a result of the direct
anatomical relationship with the third ventricle
include tumours arising at this site. Less than 20%
actually originate from 'pineal' cells.

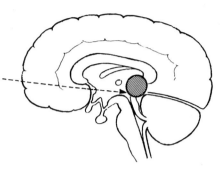

PATHOLOGICAL TYPES

Germ cell tumours: *Germinoma* is the commonest pineal region tumour of germ cell origin.
It is malignant in nature and adheres firmly to surrounding tissues and cells may spread to
the floor and anterior wall of the third ventricle. *Teratomas* are usually well differentiated,
occurring predominantly in males, and formed from various cell types – muscle, bone,
cartilage, dermis. Tumour consistency depends on the predominant cell type. In most the
tumour margin is well defined, but malignant, poorly differentiated forms occasionally occur.

Other germ cell tumours include the highly malignant *yolk sac tumour*, *choriocarcinoma* and
embryonal carcinoma.

Pineocytoma: well differentiated, slowly growing tumour ⎱ rare tumours of true
Pineoblastoma: poorly differentiated, highly malignant tumour ⎰ 'pineal' origin.
Glial cell tumours – **astrocytoma** – arising from cells within the pineal gland, or from
　　　　　　　　　　　　　　　　adjacent brain.
　　　　　　　　　　– **ependymoma** – arising from cells lining the third ventricle.
Meningioma ⎫
Dermoid 　⎬ rarely occur in the pineal region.
Epidermoid ⎭

CLINICAL FEATURES Develop due to:

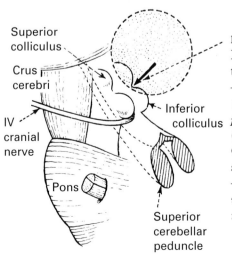

Superior
colliculus
Crus
cerebri
IV
cranial
nerve
Pons
Inferior
colliculus
Superior
cerebellar
peduncle

LOCAL MASS EFFECT
Pressure on the
tectal region (midbrain)
– PARINAUD'S *syndrome*
(impaired upward gaze,
pupillary abnormalities)
(page 155).
Compression of the
aqueduct of Sylvius
– *obstructive hydrocephalus*
with signs and symptoms of
raised intracranial pressure.

EFFECTS FROM
SPREAD THROUGH
THE THIRD
VENTRICLE
e.g. germinoma
– *hypothalamic damage,*
diabetes insipidus,
hypo/hyperphagia,
precocious puberty,
hypopituitarism.
– *optic chiasmal*
involvement with
visual field defects.

345

PINEAL REGION TUMOURS

INVESTIGATIONS

CT scan shows a mass projecting into the posterior aspect of the third ventricle with associated dilatation of the third and lateral ventricles.

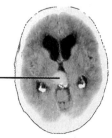

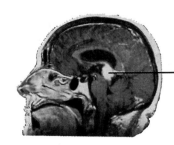

T1 weighted MRI with gadolinium

Sagittal MRI clarifies the exact tumour relationship to the third ventricle.

Pineal region tumour (pineocytoma)

Pineocytomas – may appear calcified.
Teratomas – may contain mixed densities from fat to calcification.

Tumour markers – Serum/CSF human chorionic gonadotrophin – ↑ in choriocarcinoma
(and slight ↑ in some germinomas)
– Serum/CSF alpha fetoprotein – ↑ in yolk sac tumours

CSF cytology: Malignant pineal region tumours can metastasise through CSF and *cytology* is important in planning treatment.

MANAGEMENT

Hydrocephalus often requires urgent treatment with a *ventriculoperitoneal shunt* or 3rd ventriculostomy. Large tumours may obstruct the foramen of Munro, making *bilateral* ventricular drainage necessary.

If biopsy, either via an endoscope or by stereotaxy, confirms a germinoma, or if serum/CSF markers are significantly raised suggesting choriocarcinoma or a yolk sac tumour, then *radiotherapy ± chemotherapy* is the treatment of choice.

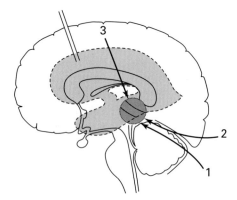

Routes of direct approach
1 – Infratentorial supracerebellar
2 – Suboccipital transtentorial
[3 – Transventricular]

Teratomas, pineocytomas, dermoid or epidermoid cysts and meningiomas require *direct operative exploration* and excision, usually via either the supracerebellar or the transtentorial approach as shown. Pineoblastomas, certain pineocytomas and ependymomas require a combination of *excision + radiotherapy. Chemotherapy* may be added for the more malignant tumours.

When imaging shows disseminated tumour or when CSF cytology is positive, the entire craniospinal axis should be irradiated.

Outcome depends on tumour type. For germinomas and resectable tumours, the outlook is excellent and long-term survival is the rule.

TUMOURS OF THE VENTRICULAR SYSTEM

EPENDYMOMA

Intracranial ependymomas originate from cells lining the ventricular cavities. The majority arise in the 4th ventricle and in this site occur predominantly in children. Most are low grade (grade II), but an anaplastic form (grade III) exists and in about 10% tumour cells seed throughout CSF pathways.

In the *4th ventricle*, ependymomas present with cerebellar signs or, more commonly, with signs and symptoms of raised intracranial pressure from CSF obstruction. *Vomiting* is often an early feature from direct brain stem involvement.

CT scanning shows an isodense mass, with or without calcification, lying within the 4th ventricle and usually enhancing with contrast. *MRI* more clearly delineates the anatomical relationships.

Management

The aim is complete operative removal, although infiltration of the floor of the 4th ventricle may prevent this. Most clinicians advise radiotherapy postoperatively, but its value is limited in the low grade tumours. CSF metastases are treated by total neuraxis irradiation.

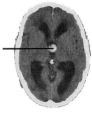

4th ventricle ependymoma

Prognosis

Despite relatively slow growth, results are often disappointing with 5-year survival ranging from 20–50%. Poor prognostic factors include incomplete resection and age < 2 years.

CHOROID PLEXUS PAPILLOMA

Rare, benign tumour with a granular surface and a gritty texture.
They develop from the choroid plexus – in the *4th ventricle – adults*,
　　　　　　　　　　　　　　　　　　　 – in the *lateral ventricle – children*.
Malignant forms occasionally occur in children.
Most patients present with hydrocephalus, either due to obstruction or to excessive CSF secretion from the tumour.
CT scanning shows a hyperdense mass within the ventricular system.
Operative removal gives good results.

COLLOID CYST OF THE THIRD VENTRICLE

A benign cyst, containing a mucoid fluid may arise from embryological remnants in the roof of the third ventricle. When of sufficient size (about 2 cm) it occludes CSF drainage from both lateral ventricles through the foramen of Munro.

Clinical features: Many patients exhibit no symptoms. In others, symptoms occur intermittently, possibly due to a ball-valve effect – headaches, episodes of loss of consciousness or even sudden death.
CT scan shows a small round mass of increased density, lying level with the foramen of Munro, causing lateral ventricular dilatation. The cyst wall will enhance following contrast on MRI.
When *symptomatic*, operative removal through a transcallosal or transventricular approach carries relatively little risk. These cysts can be drained through a stereotactically placed needle or an endoscope, but with this treatment, recurrence almost inevitably occurs.
In *asymptomatic* patients, the risk of sudden death is so small (4 deaths in 1800 patients in 5 years) operative treatment is rarely justified.

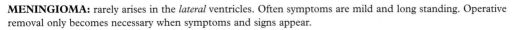

MENINGIOMA: rarely arises in the *lateral* ventricles. Often symptoms are mild and long standing. Operative removal only becomes necessary when symptoms and signs appear.

GERMINOMA
TERATOMA } see Pineal region tumours, page 345.

TUMOURS OF THE ORBIT

The orbital cavity is bounded –

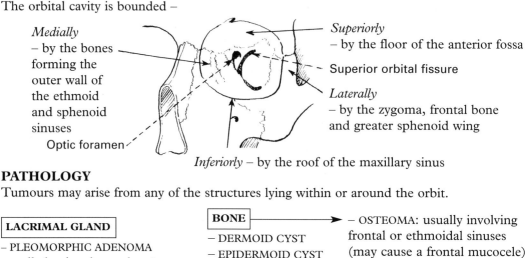

Medially
– by the bones forming the outer wall of the ethmoid and sphenoid sinuses

Optic foramen

Superiorly
– by the floor of the anterior fossa

Superior orbital fissure

Laterally
– by the zygoma, frontal bone and greater sphenoid wing

Inferiorly – by the roof of the maxillary sinus

PATHOLOGY

Tumours may arise from any of the structures lying within or around the orbit.

LACRIMAL GLAND

– PLEOMORPHIC ADENOMA usually benign, but unless excision is complete recurrences occur
– CARCINOMA

LYMPHOID TISSUE

– LYMPHOMA: developing primarily within the orbit, or secondarily to generalised disease

RETINA

– RETINOBLASTOMA: highly malignant tumour of childhood
– MELANOMA

OPTIC NERVE

– GLIOMA (pilocytic astrocytoma): very slow growth (see page 344)
– NEUROFIBROMA/ SCHWANNOMA

BONE
– DERMOID CYST
– EPIDERMOID CYST

– OSTEOMA: usually involving frontal or ethmoidal sinuses (may cause a frontal mucocele)

PARANASAL SINUSES NASOPHARYNX

– CARCINOMA: often invades the medial wall of the orbit early in the course of the disease

OPTIC NERVE SHEATH

– MENINGIOMA: often extends intracranially through the optic foramen (see page 344)

CONNECTIVE TISSUE

– RHABDOMYO-SARCOMA: malignant childhood tumour with rapid growth and local spread

BLOOD BORNE METASTASIS

Adults e.g.
– BREAST Ca.
– BRONCHIAL Ca.
Children
– NEUROBLASTOMA
– EWING'S SARCOMA
– LEUKAEMIA

NON-NEOPLASTIC ORBITAL LESIONS

– CAVERNOUS HAEMANGIOMA/LYMPHANGIOMA: common benign lesions in adults
– ORBITAL GRANULOMA (PSEUDOTUMOUR) } (see over)
– DYSTHYROID EXOPHTHALMOS
– WEGENER'S GRANULOMATOSIS
– SARCOIDOSIS
– HISTIOCYTOSIS X

N.B. CAROTID-CAVERNOUS FISTULA presents with a pulsatile exophthalmos.

TUMOURS OF THE ORBIT

CLINICAL SYMPTOMS AND SIGNS

Orbital pain: prominent in rapidly growing malignant tumours, but also a characteristic feature of orbital granuloma and carotid-cavernous fistula.

Proptosis: forward displacement of the globe is a common feature, progressing gradually and painlessly over months or years (benign tumours) or rapidly (malignant lesions).

Lid swelling: may be pronounced in orbital granuloma, dysthyroid exophthalmos or carotid-cavernous fistula.

Palpation: may reveal a mass causing globe or lid distortion – especially with lacrimal gland tumours or with a mucocele. *Pulsation* indicates a vascular lesion – carotid-cavernous fistula or arteriovenous malformation – listen for a bruit.

Eye movements: often limited for mechanical reasons, but if marked, may result from a dysthyroid ophthalmoplegia or from III, IV or VI nerve lesions in the orbital fissure (e.g. Tolosa Hunt syndrome) or cavernous sinus.

Visual acuity: may diminish due to direct involvement of the optic nerve or retina, or indirectly from occlusion of vascular structures.

INVESTIGATIONS

CT scan with a fast helical scanner is the investigation of choice. It will demonstrate the exact relationship of the lesion to the surrounding bone and will show the presence of any intracranial extension.

Axial view showing an optic nerve glioma. Coronal views are of value in assessing the size of the optic nerve and extraocular muscles and the floor and roof of the orbit

MRI may provide more information in some patients, but eye movements tend to cause artefacts.

MANAGEMENT

BENIGN tumours: require excision, but if visual loss would inevitably result, the clinician may adopt a conservative approach.

MALIGNANT tumours: require biopsy plus radiotherapy. Lymphomas may also benefit from chemotherapy. Occasionally localised lesions (e.g. carcinoma of the lacrimal gland) require radical resection.

Operative approach

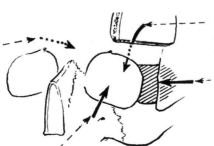

Frontal transcranial: for tumours with intracranial extension or lying posterior and medial to the optic nerve

Contralateral frontal transcranial: for tumours lying inferomedially to the optic nerve

Lateral: for tumours lying superior, lateral or inferior to the optic nerve

Transconjunctival: for tumours lying in the anterior intraconal compartment

349

NON-NEOPLASTIC ORBITAL LESIONS

ORBITAL GRANULOMA (pseudotumour)

Sudden onset of *orbital pain* with *lid oedema, proptosis* and *chemosis* due to a diffuse granulomatous infiltrate of lymphocytes and plasma cells involving multiple structures within the orbit.

This condition usually occurs in middle age and seldom occurs bilaterally. CT scanning or MRI shows a diffuse orbital lesion, although one structure may be predominantly involved, e.g. optic nerve, extraocular muscles or the lacrimal gland. If diagnostic doubt remains, a biopsy is required. Most patients show a dramatic response to high dose *steroid therapy*. If symptoms persist, the lesion should respond well to radiotherapy.

DYSTHYROID EXOPHTHALMOS

The thyrotoxic patient with bilateral exophthalmos presents no diagnostic difficulty, but dysthyroid exophthalmos, with marked lid oedema, lid retraction and ophthalmoplegia *may occur unilaterally* without evidence of thyroid disease.

Coronal CT scanning establishes the diagnosis by demonstrating enlargement of the extraocular muscles – primarily the medial and inferior recti. MRI shows a similar appearance.

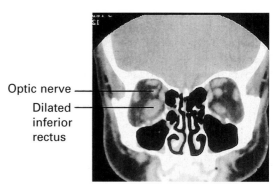

Optic nerve

Dilated inferior rectus

Circulating thyroid hormone levels are often normal. Thyroid releasing hormone stimulation or thyroid suppression tests may support the diagnosis.

Management
Steroids should help. A few patients require orbital decompression in an attempt to prevent corneal ulceration, papilloedema and blindness.

TUMOURS OF THE SKULL BASE

MALIGNANT

CARCINOMA

Carcinoma of the nasopharynx, paranasal sinuses or ear may extend intracranially either by direct erosion or through the skull foramina. It frequently penetrates the dura (in contrast to metastatic carcinoma of the spine) and may involve almost any cranial nerve. Symptoms of nasopharyngeal or sinus disease are often associated with facial pain and numbness. Spread to the CSF pathways leads to *carcinomatous meningitis* and may cause multiple cranial nerve palsies. *Skull X-rays, CT scan* and *MRI scan* will demonstrate a lesion involving the skull base. CT scanning most clearly shows the bone involvement. *Treatment* is usually restricted to retropharyngeal biopsy plus radiotherapy.

CHORDOMA

Rare tumours of notochordal cell rests arising predominantly in the sphenoido-occipital (clivus) and sacrococcygeal regions. Although growth begins in the midline, they often expand asymmetrically into the intracranial cavity. Chordomas may present at any age, but the incidence peaks in the 4th decade. They are locally invasive and rarely metastasise.

Clinical: most patients develop nasal obstruction. Cranial nerve palsies usually follow and depend on the exact tumour site.

Skull X-ray shows a soft tissue mass with an osteolytic lesion of the sphenoid, basi-occiput or petrous apex.

CT scan confirms the presence of a partly calcified mass causing marked bone destruction and extending into the nasopharyngeal space.

MRI scan more clearly demonstrates the structural relationships.

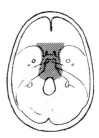

Chordoma – sites of intracranial lesion

Management: the tumour site prevents complete removal. Usually extensive debulking (sometimes through the transoral route) is combined with radiotherapy. Most patients die within 10 years of the initial presentation.

BENIGN

GLOMUS JUGULARE TUMOUR (syn: chemodectoma, paraganglioma)

Rare tumour arising from chemoreceptor cells in the jugular bulb or from similar cells in the middle ear mucosa. This tumour extensively erodes the jugular foramen and petrous bone; many patients present with cranial nerve palsies, especially IX–XII. Chemodectomas occasionally arise at other sites and metastasis may occur.

X-ray and *CT scan* demonstrate an osteolytic lesion expanding the jugular foramen.

MRI shows the anatomical relationships.

Angiography reveals a vascular tumour, usually only filling from the external carotid artery, but occasionally from vertebral branches.

Management: tumour vascularity makes excision difficult. Selective embolisation may considerably reduce the operative risks or provide an alternative treatment. The value of radiotherapy is uncertain.

OSTEOMA

Rare tumours, usually occurring in the frontal sinus and eroding into the orbit, nasal cavity or anterior fossa. If sinus drainage becomes obstructed, a *mucocele* develops, often with infected contents. These lesions require excision, either through an ethmoidal approach or through a frontal craniotomy.

INTRACRANIAL ABSCESS

The advent of antibiotics and improved treatment of ear and sinus infection has led to a reduction in intracranial abscess formation but the incidence still lies at 2–3 patients per million per year.

Pus may accumulate in:
– the extradural space
EXTRADURAL ABSCESS
– the subdural space
SUBDURAL EMPYEMA
– the brain parenchyma
CEREBRAL ABSCESS

CEREBRAL ABSCESS

Source of infection

Haematogenous spread
– Subacute bacterial endocarditis
– Congenital heart disease (especially right to left shunt)
– Bronchiectasis or pulmonary abscess

Chronic otitis media/mastoiditis

Compound depressed fracture

Frontal sinusitis

Basal fracture

Infected dental caries

Local spread
direct penetration of the dura
indirect — extension of an infected thrombus
embolic spread along a vein
Abscess *site* depends on the source, e.g. frontal sinusitis
→ frontal lobes
mastoiditis → temporal lobe
or cerebellum

Organisms: Improved aerobic and anaerobic culture techniques now reveal the responsible organism in over 80% of patients. These depend on the source –

Middle ear – *Strep. milleri, Bacteroides fragilis, E. coli* } often
          Proteus, Strep. pneumoniae. } mixed
Sinus   – *Strep. pneumoniae, Strep. milleri.*
Blood   – *Strep. pneumoniae, Strep. milleri, Staph. aureus.*
Accidental or surgical trauma – *Staph. aureus.*
Immunocompromised patients – *Toxoplasma, Aspergillus, Candida, Nocardia* (see page 510)
                      – *Listeria* (microabscesses)

Pathogenesis

Infection source
Local   Haematogenous

Small vessel occlusion or surface thrombophlebitis may precede parenchymal involvement (bacteria appear to favour ischaemic brain)

↓

Parenchymal bacterial invasion

↓

Polymorphonuclear infiltrate and impaired vascular permeability

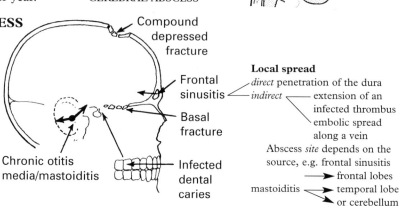

Risk of rupture into adjacent ventricle

'Mass' + surrounding oedema → *raised ICP*

Extension to cortical surface → *purulent meningitis*

ABSCESS

'Daughter' loculi may form

Mature capsule forms with central zone of necrotic tissue, inflammatory cells and necrotic debris.

↑

→ Zone of granulation tissue 'CEREBRITIS' → Thin capsule of fibroblasts and reticular fibres form

INTRACRANIAL ABSCESS

CEREBRAL ABSCESS (*cont'd*)

Clinical effects

Symptoms and signs usually develop over 2–3 weeks and progress. Occasionally the onset is more gradual, but features may develop acutely in the immunocompromised patient. Clinical features arise from:

– Toxicity – *pyrexia, malaise* (although systemic signs often absent).

– Raised intracranial pressure – *headache, vomiting* → *deterioration of conscious level.*

– Focal damage – *hemiparesis, dysphasia, ataxia, nystagmus*
  – *epilepsy* – partial or generalised, occurring in over 30%

– Infection source – *tenderness over mastoid* or *sinuses, discharging ear.*
  bacterial endocarditis – *cardiac murmurs, petechiae, splenomegaly.*

– Neck stiffness due to coexistent meningitis or tonsillar herniation occurs in 25%.

N.B. Beware attributing patient's deteriorating clinical state to the primary condition, e.g. otitis media, thus delaying essential investigations.

Investigations

X-rays of the sinuses and mastoids: opacities indicate infection.

CT scan: in the stage of 'cerebritis' the CT scan may appear normal or only show an area of low density. As the abscess progresses, a characteristic appearance emerges:

CT scan with i.v. contrast

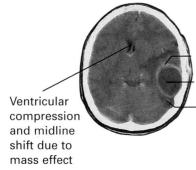

Marked 'ring' enhancement
– usually spherical
Central area of low density

Surrounding area of
low density = oedema

Ventricular
compression
and midline
shift due to
mass effect

N.B. Always administer
i.v. contrast to patients
with suspected
intracranial infection to
avoid overlooking small
abscesses.

CT scan may also reveal opacification
of the mastoids or sinuses.

If abscesses occur at multiple sites, suspect a haematogenous source.

MRI: will more readily detect the 'cerebritic' stage, but does not distinguish infection from other pathologies.

Lumbar puncture is contraindicated in the presence of a suspected mass lesion, but if CSF is obtained inadvertently, this will show ↑ protein e.g. 1 g/l, ↑ white cell count (several hundred/ml) – polymorphs or lymphocytes. The Gram stain is occasionally positive.

Peripheral blood – may show ↑ ESR, leucocytosis. Blood culture is positive in 10%.

INTRACRANIAL ABSCESS

CEREBRAL ABSCESS (*cont'd*)

Management:

1. Antibiotics

Commence i.v. antibiotics on establishing the diagnosis (prior to determining the responsible organism and its sensitivities). Antibiotics are selected on an empirical basis depending on the likely source of the infection and their ability to cross the blood–brain barrier and to achieve therapeutic concentrations in intracranial pus.

Use combined therapy: (note adult doses indicated)

      – CEFTRIAXONE   i.v. 3–4 g/day
      – METRONIDAZOLE   i.v. 500 mg tds

        for a *middle ear source*
        + AMOXICILLIN   i.v. 2 g 4 hourly

        if *endocarditis* or *congenital heart disease*
        + BENZYLPENICILLIN i.v. 1.8–2.4 g 6 hourly

If a *penetrating trauma source*

       – FLUCLOXACILLIN   i.v. 2 g 4 hourly
       ± GENTAMICIN   i.v. 5 mg/kg/day (+ monitor levels)

In immunocompromised patients – see page 510.

Later determination of the organism and its sensitivities permits alteration to more specific drugs. Intravenous antibiotics should continue for 2–3 weeks followed by oral medication for a further 3–4 weeks.

2. Abscess drainage

Various methods exist:

Primary excision of the whole abscess including the capsule (standard treatment of cerebellar abscess)

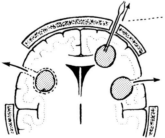

Burrhole aspiration of pus, guided by ultrasound or frameless stereotaxy, with repeated aspiration if required.

Evacuation of the abscess contents under direct vision, leaving the capsule remnants.

Burr hole aspiration is simple and relatively safe. Persistent reaccumulation of pus despite repeated aspiration requires secondary excision. Primary excision removes the abscess in a single procedure, but carries the risk of damage to surrounding brain tissue. Open evacuation of the abscess contents requires a craniotomy, but minimises damage to surrounding brain.

INTRACRANIAL ABSCESS

CEREBRAL ABSCESS

Management: *(cont'd)*

3. Treatment of the infection site

Mastoiditis or sinusitis requires prompt operative treatment, otherwise this acts as a persistent source of infection.

Steroids help reduce associated oedema but they may also reduce antibiotic penetration and impede formation of the abscess capsule. Their value in management remains controversial.

Conservative management: In some situations the risks of operative intervention outweigh its benefits. In those patients, treatment depends on i.v. antibiotics.
Indications: – small deep abscesses, e.g. thalamic (although stereotactic aspiration may help).
  – multiple abscesses.
  – early 'cerebritic' stage.

Prognosis

The use of CT scanning in the diagnosis and management of intracranial abscesses and the recognition and treatment of pathogenic anaerobic organisms have led to a reduction in the mortality rate from 40% to 10%. In survivors, focal deficits usually improve dramatically with time. Persistent seizures occur in 50%.

SUBDURAL EMPYEMA

Subdural empyema occurs far less frequently than intracerebral abscess formation. Infection usually spreads from infected sinuses or mastoids, but may arise from any of the aforementioned sources. The responsible organism is usually *Strep. pneumoniae, Strep. milleri* or *Staph. aureus*. Clinical features match those of intracerebral abscess but since rapid extension occurs across the subdural space, overwhelming symptoms often develop suddenly. Seizures occur in 70% at onset.

CT scan shows a low density extracerebral collection with mass effect, often with enhancement on the cortical surface; occasionally isodense lesions make identification difficult.

Management: Intravenous antibiotic treatment is combined with evacuation of pus either through multiple burr holes or a craniotomy flap. Despite active treatment, the mortality rate still runs at approximately 20%.

GRANULOMA

TUBERCULOMA

Although tuberculomas still constitute an important cause of mass lesions in underdeveloped countries (20% in India), they are now rare in Britain. The lesions may be single or multiple. They often lie in the cerebellum, especially in children.

Clinical features are those of any intracranial mass; alternatively tuberculoma may present in conjunction with tuberculous meningitis.

CT scan clearly demonstrates an enhancing lesion – but this often resembles astrocytoma or metastasis; tuberculomas have no distinguishing features. MRI is even more sensitive and may show additional lesions.

Other investigations: ESR, chest X-ray often fail to confirm the diagnosis. A Mantoux (PPD) test is usually positive but a negative test does not eliminate the diagnosis.

Management: When tuberculoma is suspected, a trial of antituberculous therapy is worthwhile. Follow up CT scans should show a reduction in the lesion size. Other patients require an exploratory operation and biopsy followed by long-term drug treatment.

SARCOIDOSIS

Sarcoidosis is a multisystem disease process of unknown cause whose pathogenesis involves formation of an inflammatory lesion known as a granuloma. Nervous system involvement occurs in 8% and may dominate the presentation.

When sarcoid infiltrates the central nervous system it usually involves the meninges. In some patients mass lesions may arise from the dura, but more commonly signs and symptoms relate to an adhesive arachnoiditis involving the skull base, cranial nerves and pituitary stalk. Mass lesions may occasionally arise within the brain and spinal cord without obvious meningeal involvement.

Investigation: MRI (T1 weighted) shows either a hyperintense mass or multiple periventricular foci. The use of gadolinium and FLAIR (fluid-attenuated inversion recovery) increases the sensitivity of MRI. A definitive diagnosis is based on clinical and radiological evidence of multisystem disease confirmed by characteristic histology.

The diagnosis is often elusive and suggested by clinical presentation supported by some of the following.
– elevated serum and CSF angiotensin converting enzyme (ACE),
– elevated serum immunoglobulins,
– elevated serum calcium,
– elevated CSF cell count (monocytes), IgG, Ig index, and presence of oligoclonal bands.

Management: Immunosuppression with corticosteroids is usually indicated and long-term therapy required. In exacerbation, intravenous pulsed methylprednisolone is used. Success in resistant cases is reported with each of the following – azathioprine, cyclophosphamide, methotrexate, cyclosporin or irradiation.

MOVEMENT DISORDERS – EXTRAPYRAMIDAL SYSTEM

The control of voluntary movement is effected by the interaction of the pyramidal, cerebellar and extrapyramidal systems interconnecting with each other as well as projecting to the anterior horn region or cranial nerve motor nuclei.

The extrapyramidal system consists of paired subcortical masses or nuclei of grey matter **basal ganglia.**

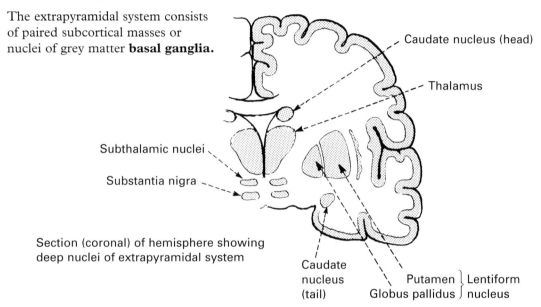

Section (coronal) of hemisphere showing deep nuclei of extrapyramidal system

The caudate nucleus and putamen are collectively referred to as the STRIATUM.

Interconnections of the deep nuclei

The connections between components of the extrapyramidal system and other parts of the brain are complex. However, certain simple observations can be made:

(A) The thalamus plays a vital role in projecting information from the basal ganglia to the motor cortex and back

(B) The cortex projects through the striatum to other basal ganglia

(C) The final common pathway for basal ganglia motor function is the corticospinal or pyramidal tract

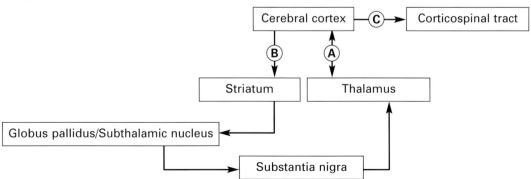

MOVEMENT DISORDERS – EXTRAPYRAMIDAL SYSTEM

NEUROPHARMACOLOGY

The observation that drugs such as reserpine and phenothiazines regularly produce extrapyramidal syndromes has clarified the neurochemical basis of movement disorders and delineated the role of neurotransmitters.

Neurotransmitter substances
are synthesised and stored presynaptically. When released by an appropriate stimulus they cross the synaptic gap and combine with specific receptors of the postsynaptic cell,

e.g. – acetylcholine – serotonin
  – dopamine – glutamate
  – γ-aminobutyric acid

Neuromodulator substances
diminish or enhance the effects of neurotransmitters in the basal ganglia,

e.g. – substance P
  – encephalin
  – cholecystokinin
  – somatostatin.

Acetylcholine
– Synthesised by small striatal cells
– Greatest concentration in striatum
– Excitatory effect.

Dopamine
– Synthesised by cells of substantia nigra (pars compacta) and nigral projections in striatum.
– Greatest concentration in substantia nigra.
– Inhibiting effect.

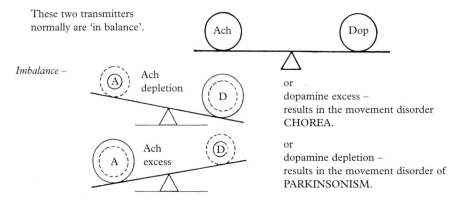

These two transmitters normally are 'in balance'.

Imbalance –

Ach depletion

or
dopamine excess –
results in the movement disorder
CHOREA.

Ach excess

or
dopamine depletion –
results in the movement disorder of
PARKINSONISM.

γ-Aminobutyric acid (GABA) is synthesised from glutamate in the striatum and globus pallidus. It has inhibitory actions and deficiency is associated with Huntington's chorea.

Drugs may produce movement disorders by interfering with neurotransmission in the following ways:

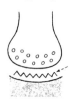

1. – By reducing transmitter presynaptically e.g. tetrabenazine reduces dopamine.

2. – By blocking the receptor site postsynaptically e.g. phenothiazines block dopamine receptors.

Both reduce effective dopamine and create a relative excess of acetylcholine

Parkinsonism

MOVEMENT DISORDERS – EXTRAPYRAMIDAL DISEASES

CLINICAL FEATURES
The effects of disease of the extrapyramidal system on movement can be regarded as *negative* (hypokinetic) and *positive* (hyperkinetic).

Negative features
Bradykinesia: - a loss or slowness of voluntary movement.

A major feature of Parkinson's disease and produces:
– reduced facial expression (mask-like)
– reduced blinking
– reduced adjustments of posture when seated.
When agitated the patient will move swiftly – 'kinesia paradoxica'.

Postural disturbance: most commonly seen in Parkinson's disease.
Flexion of limbs and trunk is associated with a failure to make quick postural or 'righting' adjustments to correct imbalance. The patient falls whilst turning or if pushed.

Positive features

Involuntary movements:
– tremor
– chorea (irregular, repetitive, jerking movements).
– athetosis (irregular, repetitive, writhing movements).
– dystonia (slow, sustained, abnormal movement).
– ballismus (explosive, violent movement).
– myoclonus (shock-like jerks).
Chorea and athetosis may merge into one another – choreoathetosis.

Rigidity

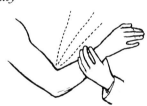

Stiffness felt by the examiner when passively moving a limb. This 'resistance' is present to the same degree throughout the full range of movement, affecting flexor and extensor muscle groups equally and is described as PLASTIC or LEAD PIPE rigidity. When tremor is superimposed upon rigidity it produces a COGWHEELING quality.

In Parkinson's disease both positive features, e.g. tremor, and negative features, e.g. bradykinesia, occur.

In Huntington's chorea positive features, e.g. chorea, predominate.

PARKINSON'S DISEASE

Described by James Parkinson (1817) in 'An essay on the shaking palsy'.
Recognised as an extrapyramidal disorder by Kinnier Wilson (1912).
Annual incidence: 20 per 100 000. Prevalence: 190 per 100 000.
Sex incidence: male:female – 3:2
Age of onset: 50 years upwards. Incidence peaks in mid-70s then declines.
Familial incidence occurs in 5%.

AETIOLOGY

The cause(s) of Parkinson's disease is unknown. Gene mutations have been identified in young onset and familial cases (synuclein & parkin) but epidemiological studies suggest environmental factors are the dominant cause in most (i.e. smoking/herbicide exposure).

The observation that 1-methyl-4-phenyl-1,2,3,6-tetrahydropyridine (MPTP), a meperidine analogue derived during illicit drug production, produces Parkinson's disease in humans and animals has resulted in increased interest in the role of toxins and an animal model for developing new treatments.

Parkinsonian features may be present in many disorders and are not always treatment (L Dopa) responsive. These disorders usually share features of slowness and rigidity (akinetic rigid syndromes).

Parkinson's disease	**Mimics**	– Multiple system atrophy (MSA)
		– Progressive supranuclear palsy (PSP)
		– Corticobasal ganglionic degeneration (CBD)
		– Diffuse Lewy body disease (DLBD)
Secondary Parkinsonism		
– Drug induced (dopamine receptor blockers-antipsychotics/antiemetics)		
– Post traumatic (pugilist's encephalopathy)		
– Vascular disease (small vessel multi-infarct state)		
– Infectious (post encephalitic/prion disease/HIV)		
– Miscellaneous: hydrocephalus/parathyroid/paraneoplastic		

PATHOLOGY of idiopathic Parkinson's disease

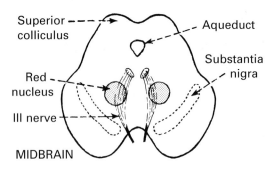

The substantia nigra contains pigmented cells (neuromelanin) which give it a characteristic 'black' appearance (macroscopic). These cells are lost in Parkinson's disease and the substantia nigra becomes pale.
Remaining cells contain atypical eosinophilic inclusions in the cytoplasm – *Lewy bodies* – although these are not specific to Parkinson's disease. Lewy bodies may be found in the cerebral cortex especially when dementia is present (diffuse Lewy body disease).
Changes are seen in other basal nuclei – striatum and globus pallidus.

Radiolabelled ligand studies have identified two dopamine receptors on striatal cell membranes – D_1 – D_2 receptors.

PARKINSON'S DISEASE

CLINICAL FEATURES

Initial symptoms are vague, the patient often complains of aches and pains.

A coarse TREMOR at a rate of 4–7 Hz usually develops early in the disease. It begins unilaterally in the upper limbs and eventually spreads to all four limbs. The tremor is often *'pill rolling'*, the thumb moving rhythmically backwards and forwards on the palm of the hand. It occurs at rest, improves with movement and disappears during sleep.

RIGIDITY is detected by examination. It predominates in the flexor muscles of the neck, trunk and limbs and results in the typical *'flexed posture'*.

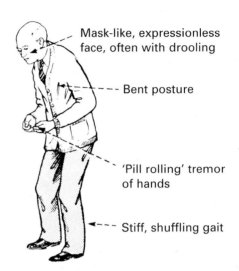

Mask-like, expressionless face, often with drooling

Bent posture

'Pill rolling' tremor of hands

Stiff, shuffling gait

BRADYKINESIA: This slowness or paucity of movement affects facial muscles of expression (mask-like appearance) as well as muscles of mastication, speech, voluntary swallowing and muscles of the trunk and limbs. Dysarthria, dysphagia and a slow deliberate gait with little associated movement (e.g. arm swinging) result.

Tremor, rigidity and bradykinesia deteriorate simultaneously, affecting every aspect of the patient's life:

Handwriting reduces in size.

The gait becomes shuffling and festinant (small rapid steps to 'keep up with' the centre of gravity) and the posture more flexed.

Rising from a chair becomes laborious with progressive difficulty in initiating lower limb movement from a stationary position.

Eye movements may be affected with loss of ocular convergence and upward gaze.

Excessive sweating and greasy skin (seborrhoea) can be troublesome.

Depression, drug-induced confusional states and dementia occur in 30% of patients.

Occasionally autonomic features occur – postural hypotension.

Time of onset is mid–late fifties, juvenile presentation does occur. Such cases are atypical with rigidity more evident than tremor.

Postencephalitic Parkinson's disease (encephalitis lethargica), now rarely encountered, is characterised by an earlier age of onset and oculogyric crises (acute ocular deviation).

PARKINSON'S DISEASE

DIAGNOSIS

The diagnosis of PD in the early stages is difficult. Post-mortem data from the London Brain Bank shows this to be incorrect in 25% of those diagnosed in life.

New tremor in middle age causes particular difficulty – senile/essential & metabolic tremor is generally absent at rest and worsened by voluntary movement.

The diagnostic use of a L-dopa or dopamine agonist (apomorphine) challenge has declined due to concerns that it may increase the risk of subsequent drug induced dyskinesia.

Functional imaging (SPECT & PET) should improve diagnostic accuracy and ensure that persons with conditions unresponsive to treatments (PD mimics) are not unnecessarily exposed to them.

<table>
<tr><td colspan="2" align="center">D2 Receptor SPECT</td><td colspan="2" align="center">FP-CIT SPECT</td></tr>
<tr><td>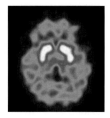</td><td>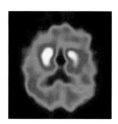</td><td>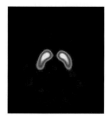</td><td>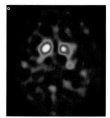</td></tr>
<tr><td align="center">Normal or PD</td><td align="center">Abnormal. PD mimics (reduced uptake)</td><td align="center">Normal</td><td align="center">Abnormal. PD & PD mimics (reduced uptake in tail of caudate)</td></tr>
</table>

The ligand I-IBZM demonstrates the degree of D2 receptor binding. This is normal in PD but reduced in its mimics (MSA/PSP).

The ligand FP-CIT demonstrates the integrity of the presynaptic dopamine terminals. These are normal in essential tremor and reduced in PD and its mimics (MSA/PSP).

PARKINSON'S DISEASE

TREATMENT is symptomatic and does not halt the pathological process though neuroprotective treatments are under trial. It aims at restoring the dopamine/balance:

Levodopa/Dopamine agonists

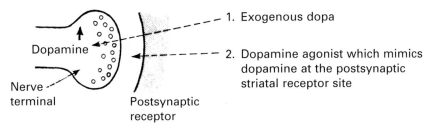

1. Exogenous dopa

2. Dopamine agonist which mimics dopamine at the postsynaptic striatal receptor site

Exogenous dopa

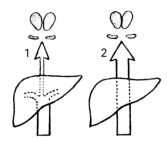

Given as 1 – levodopa, or 2 – levodopa + decarboxylase inhibitor, which prevents peripheral breakdown in the liver allowing a higher concentration of dopa to reach the blood–brain barrier; also the peripheral side effects (nausea, vomiting, hypotension) are diminished.

Central side effects: confusion, depression, dyskinetic movements and following long-term treatment – *'On/Off'* phenomenon (see later).

Controlled-release or long acting preparations produce constant plasma levels and a more even clinical response.

Exogenous dopa improves bradykinesia, rigidity and, to a lesser extent, tremor, but in 20% the response is poor. 'Good' responders often develop central side effects later – especially the 'on/off' phenomenon.

Dopamine agonists: Now used earlier in disease management, they act directly on the dopamine receptor independent of degenerating dopaminergic neurons, have a longer half-life than levodopa providing a more sustained striatal stimulation and do not undergo oxidative metabolism and generate harmful free radicals (neuroprotective). Several agonists are available (*pergolide, pramipexole, ropinirole* and *cabergoline*) each with different receptor affinity and pharmokinetics but with little proven advantage over one another. Apomorphine is a D1 & D2 receptor agonist given by continuous infusion or intermittent injection and is effective in shortening periods of prolonged immobility (freezing).

Side effects: postural hypotension, hallucinations & psychosis, sedation and agonist specific complications (erythromelalgia/pulmonary fibrosis).

COMT inhibitors: (Tolcapone/entacapone) reduce the metabolism of levodopa and are used as adjunctive treatments.

PARKINSON'S DISEASE

TREATMENT (*cont'd*)

Selegiline: the enzymes monoamine oxidase (MAO) A and B play a key role in the breakdown of dopamine. This drug is an MAO-B inhibitor. Its usage results in increased dopamine levels. A randomised study has suggested a neuroprotective as well as symptomatic effect.

Amantidine, an antiviral drug, may help rigidity. The mode of action is not known.

Advances in drug treatment in recent years have reduced the need for **stereotactic surgery** (see page 380), but in patients with intractable tremor this is still of benefit. A stereotactic lesion is made in the globus pallidus or ventrolateral nucleus of the thalamus (contralateral to the tremor). Pallidotomy relieves contralateral dyskinesia.

Human fetal and medullary transplantation: experimental evidence shows that transplantation to the striatum of tissue capable of synthesising and releasing dopamine reverses the motor symptoms of Parkinson's disease. This treatment remains experimental.

Regime of treatment (Drug therapy becomes more complex as disease progresses)

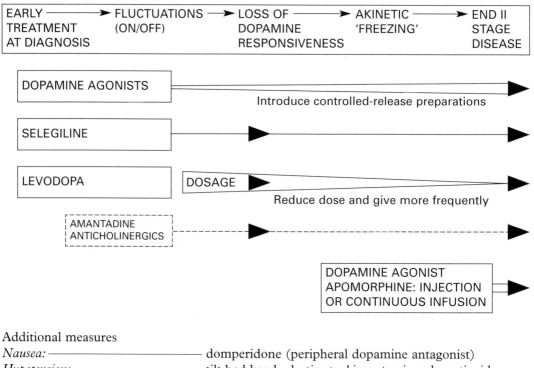

Additional measures

Nausea:	domperidone (peripheral dopamine antagonist)
Hypotension:	tilt bed head, elastic stockings + mineralocorticoid
Peak dose dyskinesia:	lower levodopa dose
End dose dyskinesia:	add dopamine agonist
Nocturnal pain/immobility:	add controlled-release levodopa at night
Confusion/aggravated dementia:	add clozapine (cortical dopamine antagonist)
	if no help reduce levodopa and/or dopamine agonist

CHOREA

An involuntary, irregular, jerking movement affecting limb and axial muscle groups. These movements are suppressed with difficulty and are incorporated into voluntary gestures resulting in a 'semipurposeful' appearance, e.g. crossing and uncrossing of legs.

Causes of chorea

Hereditary: – Huntington's disease
          – Benign chorea

Drugs: – Antiparkinsonian drugs
      – oral contraceptives

Toxins: – alcohol
       – carbon monoxide poisoning

Infections: – Sydenham's chorea
         – encephalitis

Metabolic: – Hyperthyroidism
         – Hypocalcaemia

Immunological: – Systemic lupus erythematosus
             – Polyarteritis nodosa

Miscellaneous: – Chorea gravidarum
             – Polycythaemia rubra vera

HUNTINGTON'S DISEASE

Huntington disease (HD) is inherited as an autosomal dominant disease that gives rise to progressive, selective (localized) neural cell death associated with choreic movements and dementia. The disease is associated with increases in the length of a CAG triplet repeat present in a gene called 'huntingtin' located on chromosome 4p16.3.

Huntington disease has a frequency of 4 to 7 per 100000 persons.

Pathology: Neuronal loss in the striatum is associated with a reduction in projections to other basal ganglia structures. In addition, cells of the deep layers of the frontal and parietal cortex are lost (corticostriatal projections). The neurochemical basis of this disorder involves deficiency of gamma aminobutyric acid (GABA) and acetylcholine with reduced activity of enzymes glutamic acid decarboxylase (GAD) and choline acetyltransferase (CAT).

Symptoms and signs: The classic signs of Huntington disease are progressive chorea, rigidity, and dementia. Typically, there is a prodromal phase of mild psychotic and behavioural symptoms, which precedes frank chorea by up to 10 years.

Chorea – may be the initial symptom. This progressess from mere fidgetiness to gross involuntary movements which interrupt voluntary movement and make feeding and walking impossible.

Dementia – this is of a subcortical type (see page 124).

Behavioural disturbance – personality change, affective disorders and psychosis occur.

Hypotonicity often accompanies fidgety, choreiform movements.

Primitive reflexes – grasp, pout and palmomental – are usually elicited. Eye movements are disturbed with impersistence of gaze.

Diagnosis: Distinguish from benign hereditary chorea in which intellect is preserved. Exclude senile chorea by older age of onset and absence of dementia. MRI shows an increase in the T2 signal in the caudate nucleus. Positron-emission tomography (PET scanning) demonstrates loss of uptake of glucose in the caudate nuclei. Genetic testing is diagnostic.

Prediction of disease: Identifying the CAG repeat provides a reliable method of detecting the disease. Presymptomatic testing is now available in many centres. These tests raise ethical issues but also the possibility of neuroprotective therapy.

Treatment: Phenothiazines, haloperidol or tetrabenazine, may control the movements in the preliminary stages. SSRIs help affective disturbance.

CHOREA

SYDENHAM'S CHOREA

Rare in an age of antibiotic therapy, this condition (also known as St Vitus' dance) followed *streptococcus pneumoniae* infection. Unlike arthritis and carditis, symptoms developed weeks or months after primary infection. Movements are diffuse and often associated with florid behavioural changes.

Pathology: Necrotising arteritis in thalamus, caudate nucleus and putamen.
Diagnosis is confirmed by elevated ESR and ASO (antistreptolysin) titre.
Treatment: Sedation, phenothiazines.
The condition may become recurrent – during pregnancy, intercurrent infection.

CHOREA GRAVIDARUM

Acute onset in pregnancy, usually the first trimester or whilst on oral contraceptive.

Restricted to face or generalised. Perhaps caused by reactivation of Sydenham's chorea. Oestrogens act at dopamine receptors.
Pathology: Unknown.
Treatment: Haloperidol.

SENILE CHOREA

Begins in late middle age unaccompanied by family history or behavioural change. Some patients do have caudate or putaminal atrophy and occasionally test positive for Huntington's disease.

DYSTONIA

Dystonia manifests as a sustained abnormal
posture produced by contraction
of large trunk and limb muscles,
e.g. sustained head retraction ...

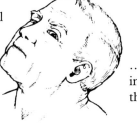

... or sustained
inversion of
the foot.

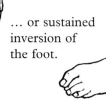

Dystonias may be:
   generalised – idiopathic torsion dystonia,
   or *partial* (focal), e.g. spasmodic torticollis.

The precise neuropathological basis of dystonia is uncertain.

Most *primary* inherited dystonias are caused by mutations in the DYT 1 gene. *Secondary* dystonia occurs as a symptom of sporadic (e.g. Progressive supranuclear palsy) and hereditary degenerative disease (e.g. Wilson's disease), metabolic disorders (e.g. homocysteinuria) or miscellaneous conditions (e.g. drug induced, arteriovenous malformations).

IDIOPATHIC TORSION DYSTONIA
(DYSTONIA MUSCULORUM DEFORMANS)

The first gene identified for idiopathic torsion dystonia, DYT 1, is located on 9q34. The disorder is inherited as an autosomal dominant with reduced penetrance. It is responsible for early-onset generalized dystonia in Ashkenazi Jews.
Initially, a flexion deformity of leg develops when walking.
Movements then become generalised but ultimately constant. Despite eventual gross contortion the postures disappear during sleep.
Diagnosis is made on clinical grounds and by exclusion of other disorders. – EMG studies show inappropriate co-contraction of antagonistic muscle groups.
Pathology: No known pathological substrate.
Treatment: levodopa or carbamezapine are of benefit in some patients; anticholinergics help in others. A small proportion are dramatically dopa-responsive. Pallidal stimulation may benefit (see page 381).

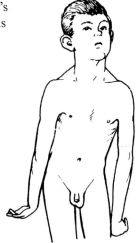

DYSTONIAS – FOCAL AND SEGMENTAL IDIOPATHIC

SPASMODIC TORTICOLLIS (Wry neck)

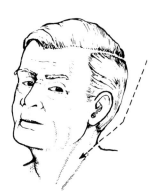

Unilateral deviation of the head.

Aetiology is unknown. Vestibular abnormalities occur on testing, but it is uncertain whether these cause torticollis or result from the abnormal head posture. Familial spasmodic torticollis may be a restricted form of dystonia musculorum.

Dystonic contraction of the *left* sternomastoid produces head turning to the *right*.

Pressure of the index finger on the right side of the chin may turn the head back to the neutral position (geste antagoniste).

Turning of the head is specially noticeable when the patient is walking.

Eventually hypertrophy of the sternomastoid occurs.

Pathology: unknown. **Diagnosis** is based on clinical findings.

Treatment: anticholinergics and phenothiazines produce some benefit in 50% of patients. Injection of *Botulinum* toxin into the sternomastoid muscle gives variable symptomatic relief though requires regular repetition.

Prognosis: Remission occurs in 20% of patients. Dystonia may spread into other muscle groups. In the long term, psychological disturbance often occurs.

DOPAMINE RESPONSIVE DYSTONIA (DRD)

This disorder presents in childhood and generally involves the legs only. Falls are frequent and the response to levodopa is maintained over many years. DRD may be the result of a developmental reduction in the number of dopaminergic nerve endings in the striatum and maps to the same region of 14q as does the gene for the enzyme GTP cyclohydrolase 1 (GCH1) implicated in a hyperphenylalaninaemia.

PROGRESSIVE SUPRANUCLEAR PALSY (PSP)

A condition characterised by gaze palsies, extrapyramidal features, axial dystonia (truncal dystonia) and progressive pseudobulbar palsy. Onset in the 5th to 6th decade. Prominent parkinsonian features can lead to misdiagnosis.

Aetiology: unknown.

Pathology: Neuronal loss is evident in periaqueductal grey matter, brain stem, nuclei, subthalamic nuclei and the superior colliculi. Neurofibrillary tangles as seen in Alzheimer's disease are found.

Signs: Downward eye movement is initially impaired followed by all other voluntary eye movement. Lid retraction is common. Pseudobulbar signs develop (see page 552).
The head then hyperextends (dystonia) and rigidity ensues in the limbs.

Treatment: Levodopa and anticholinergics give disappointing results.

The course is relentless with death in 2–5 years.

WRITER'S CRAMP

Muscles of the hand and forearm tighten on attempting to write and pain may occur in the forearm muscles. Previously regarded as an 'occupational neurosis' but now classified as a partial dystonia.

May be a precursor of Parkinson's disease.

Treatment: Benzodiazepines and anticholinergics are of limited value.

OROMANDIBULAR DYSTONIA

Constant involuntary prolonged tight eye closure (blepharospasm) is associated with dystonia of mouth, tongue or jaw muscles (jaw clenching and tongue protrusion). Response to treatment is poor though phenothiazines should be tried. Section of the nerves to orbicularis oculi muscles will relieve blepharospasm. *Botulinum* toxin injection is also effective.

DRUG INDUCED DYSTONIA

Acute adoption of abnormal dystonic posture – usually head and neck or oculogyric crisis (upward deviation of eyes) – caused by phenothiazines, e.g. haloperidol, metoclopramide.

Anticholinergics, e.g. benzotropine for 24–48 hours helps symptoms settle.

OTHER MOVEMENT DISORDERS

HEMIBALLISMUS

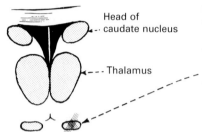

Head of caudate nucleus

Thalamus

This is a movement disorder characterised by unilateral, violent flinging of the limbs. This involuntary movement is occasionally severe enough to throw the patient off balance or even from his bed.

The anatomical basis is a lesion of the *subthalamic nuclei* or its connections contralateral to the abnormal movement. It usually results from vascular disease (posterior cerebral artery territory), but occasionally occurs in multiple sclerosis.

Drug treatment is ineffective. The condition often settles spontaneously.

ATHETOSIS

Athetosis presents in childhood and appears as a slow writhing movement disorder with a rate of movement between that of chorea and dystonia. It usually involves the digits, hands and face on each side.

These abnormal movements may result from:
– Hypoxic neonatal brain damage,
– Kernicterus,
– Lipid storage diseases.

Response to anticholinergics is variable and occasionally dramatic.

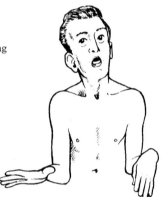

TARDIVE DYSKINESIA

This is a consequence of long-term treatment with neuroleptic drugs – phenothiazines, butyrophenones – and results from the development of drug-induced supersensitive dopamine receptors.

Involuntary movements in the face, mouth and tongue (orofacial dyskinesia) as well as limb movements of a *choreothetoid nature* occur.

This movement disorder may commence even after stopping the responsible drug and can persist indefinitely.

Prevention
Incidence may be reduced by:
1. Drug 'holidays' (periods of rest from causal drug).
2. Early recognition and drug withdrawal.

The practice of increasing the dose of the offending drug when movements occur should be avoided. This will improve movements initially, but they will 'break through' later.

Treatment
Discontinue neuroleptic. If not possible, continue on lowest possible dose. Drugs which increase acetylcholine (anti-cholinesterases), reduce catecholamine release (lithium), or deplete dopamine (reserpine) are variably effective.

TICS

Abrupt jerky movements affecting head, neck and trunk. Tics can be voluntarily suppressed and often take the form of winking, grimacing, shoulder shrugging, sniffing and throat clearing.

Gilles de la Tourette syndrome is characterised by motor and vocal tics, copropraxia (making obscene gestures), coprolalia (obscene utterances) and obsessive behaviour. Onset is in childhood, males are more often affected and the condition may be inherited. However results of a systematic genome screen were negative. A population study showed that 3% of all children and that up to 25% of children requiring special education may have mild to moderate Tourette's syndrome.

The dopaminergic systems in the basal ganglia appear involved, dopamine D2 receptor antagonists improving and dopamimetic agents worsening symptoms.

OTHER MOVEMENT DISORDERS

MALIGNANT NEUROLEPTIC SYNDROME

A rare condition associated with prescribing dopamine antagonist and long-acting depot neuroleptic preparations. Drowsiness, fever, tremor and rigidity occur suddenly. Muscle necrosis (rhabdomyolysis) results in myoglobinuria and occasionally renal failure. Early identification and treatment with dopamine receptor agonist (bromocriptine) and muscle relaxants (sodium dantrolene) may be life saving.

SEROTONIN SYNDROME

SSRIs can cause dystonia and occasionally low-grade fever, confusion, autonomic disturbance, restlessness and rigidity. Early recognition and drug withdrawal is vital for good outcome.

WILSON'S DISEASE (hepatolenticular degeneration)

An autosomal recessive disorder characterised by the build-up of intracellular copper with hepatic and neurological consequences.

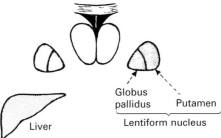

Pathology

Cavitation and neuronal loss occurs within the putamen and the globus pallidus.

The liver shows the appearances of coarse cirrhosis. Copper accumulates in all organs, especially in Descemet's membrane in the eye, nail beds and kidney.

Biochemistry

There is deficiency of α_2 globulin – Ceruloplasmin – which normally binds 98% of copper in the plasma and transfers copper to enzyme (cytochrome oxidase). This results in an increase in loosely bound copper/albumin, and deposition occurs in all organs. Urinary copper is increased.

Clinical features

There are two clinical forms:

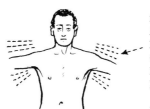

1. *Acute*
Bradykinesia
Behavioural change
Involuntary movements
Liver involvement common

Untreated: death in 2 years
from hepatic and renal failure

2. *Chronic*
Marked proximal 'wing beating' tremor
Dysarthria, dystonia and rigidity
Choreoathetoid movements
Psychosis, behavioural disorders and dementia
Liver involvement less severe

Untreated: death in 10 years

The deposition of copper in Descemet's membrane produces the golden brown *Kayser-Fleischer* ring, which when seen by naked eye or slit-lamp is diagnostic.

Diagnosis

Should be considered in any patient with unusual hepatic and/or neurological features.

Supported by biochemical evidence of abnormal copper metabolism:
– Low ceruloplasmin (less than 20 mg/dl)
– Elevated unbound serum copper
– High urinary copper excretion
– Liver biopsy and copper metabolism tests with radioactive ^{64}Cu.
– MRI (T2) shows thalamic and putaminal hyperintensity.

In families, biochemical tests will identify low ceruloplasmin in carries and in presymptomatic patients. Over 20 mutations in copper transporting ATPase have been identified. Diagnostic genetic testing is not available.

Treatment

Low copper diet and a chelating agent, e.g. penicillamine 1–1.5 g daily. Side effects such as anaphylaxis, skin rash, bone marrow suppression and glomerulonephritis are common in which case trientine is an effective alternative.

Therapy is necessary for the rest of the patient's life. Adequate treatment is compatible with normal life expectancy. Kayser-Fleischer rings will disappear with time.

HYDROCEPHALUS

DEFINITION
Hydrocephalus is an increase in cerebrospinal fluid (CSF) volume, usually resulting from impaired absorption, rarely from excessive secretion.
This definition excludes ventricular expansion secondary to brain shrinkage from a diffuse atrophic process (hydrocephalus ex vacuo).

CSF FORMATION AND ABSORPTION

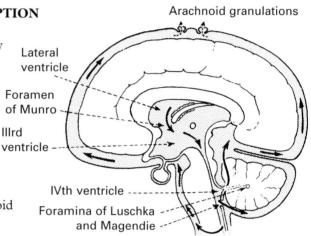

CSF forms at a rate of 500 ml/day (0.35 ml/min), secreted predominantly by the choroid plexus of the lateral, third and fourth ventricles.
CSF flows in a caudal direction through the ventricular system and exits through the foramina of Luschka and Magendie into the subarachnoid space. After passing through the tentorial hiatus and over the hemispheric convexity, absorption occurs through the arachnoid granulations into the venous system.

CLASSIFICATION
'Obstructive' hydrocephalus – obstruction of CSF flow *within* the ventricular system.
'Communicating' hydrocephalus – obstruction to CSF flow *outwith* the ventricular system i.e. ventricular CSF 'communicates' with the subarachnoid space.

CAUSES OF HYDROCEPHALUS

Obstructive

Acquired – Acquired aqueduct stenosis (adhesions following infection or haemorrhage)
– Supratentorial masses causing tentorial herniation
– Intraventricular haematoma
– Tumours – ventricular, e.g. colloid cyst
– pineal region
– posterior fossa
– Abscesses/granuloma
– Arachnoid cysts

Congenital – Aqueduct stenosis or forking
– Dandy-Walker syndrome (atresia of foramina of Magendie and Luschka)
– Chiari malformation
– Vein of Galen aneurysm

Communicating
Thickening of the leptomeninges and/or involvement of the arachnoid granulations
– infection (pyogenic, TB, fungal)
– subarachnoid haemorrhage
– spontaneous
– trauma
– postoperative
– carcinomatous meningitis
Increased CSF viscosity, e.g. high protein content
Excessive CSF production – choroid plexus papilloma (rare)

HYDROCEPHALUS

PATHOLOGICAL EFFECTS

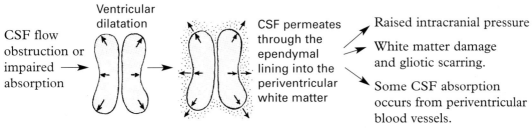

CSF flow obstruction or impaired → absorption

Ventricular dilatation

CSF permeates through the ependymal lining into the periventricular white matter

Raised intracranial pressure

White matter damage and gliotic scarring.

Some CSF absorption occurs from periventricular blood vessels.

In the infant, prior to suture fusion, head expansion and massive ventricular dilatation may occur, often leaving only a thin rim of cerebral 'mantle'. Untreated, death may result, but in many cases the hydrocephalus 'arrests'; although the ventricles remain dilated, intracranial pressure (ICP) returns to normal and CSF absorption appears to balance production. When hydrocephalus arrests, normal developmental patterns resume, although pre-existing mental or physical damage may leave a permanent handicap. In these patients, the rapid return of further pressure symptoms following a minor injury or infection suggests that the CSF dynamics remain in an unstable state.

CLINICAL FEATURES

Infants and young children

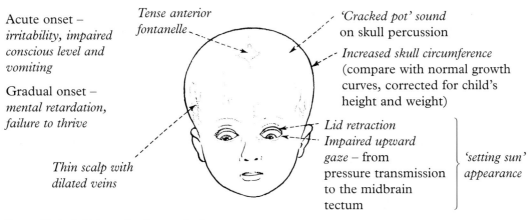

Acute onset – *irritability, impaired conscious level and vomiting*

Gradual onset – *mental retardation, failure to thrive*

Tense anterior fontanelle

Thin scalp with dilated veins

'Cracked pot' sound on skull percussion

Increased skull circumference (compare with normal growth curves, corrected for child's height and weight)

Lid retraction
Impaired upward gaze – from pressure transmission to the midbrain tectum

'setting sun' appearance

Juvenile/adult type hydrocephalus

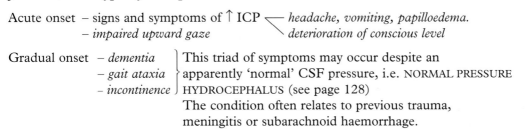

Acute onset – signs and symptoms of ↑ ICP — *headache, vomiting, papilloedema.*
– *impaired upward gaze* — *deterioration of conscious level*

Gradual onset – *dementia*
– *gait ataxia*
– *incontinence*
This triad of symptoms may occur despite an apparently 'normal' CSF pressure, i.e. NORMAL PRESSURE HYDROCEPHALUS (see page 128)
The condition often relates to previous trauma, meningitis or subarachnoid haemorrhage.

HYDROCEPHALUS

INVESTIGATIONS

Skull X-ray
Note: – skull size and suture width.
  – evidence of chronic raised pressure – erosion of the posterior clinoids.
  – associated defects – platybasia, basilar invagination.

CT scan
The *pattern of ventricular enlargement* helps determine the cause, i.e.

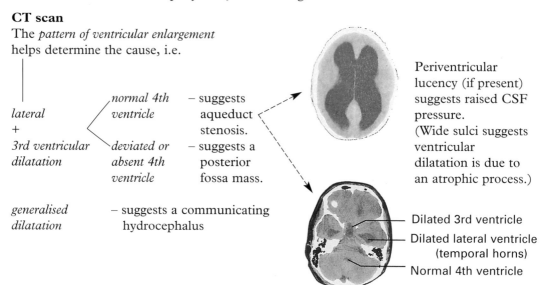

lateral
+
3rd ventricular dilatation

normal 4th ventricle – suggests aqueduct stenosis.

deviated or absent 4th ventricle – suggests a posterior fossa mass.

generalised dilatation – suggests a communicating hydrocephalus

Periventricular lucency (if present) suggests raised CSF pressure.
(Wide sulci suggests ventricular dilatation is due to an atrophic process.)

Dilated 3rd ventricle

Dilated lateral ventricle (temporal horns)

Normal 4th ventricle

Ultrasonography through the anterior fontanelle, usefully demonstrates ventricular enlargement in infants but provides less precise information than CT scanning.

MRI shows similar ventricular expansion, but may more clearly demonstrate periventricular lucency or a neoplastic cause of the obstruction.

ICP monitoring: used to investigate patients with suspected normal pressure hydrocephalus and designed to predict the likelihood of a beneficial response to shunting (see page 129).

Developmental assessment and psychometric analysis detect impaired cerebral function and provide a baseline for future comparison.

MANAGEMENT

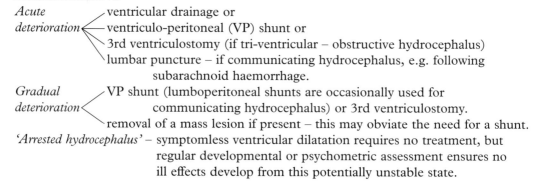

Acute deterioration
  ventricular drainage or
  ventriculo-peritoneal (VP) shunt or
  3rd ventriculostomy (if tri-ventricular – obstructive hydrocephalus)
  lumbar puncture – if communicating hydrocephalus, e.g. following subarachnoid haemorrhage.

Gradual deterioration
  VP shunt (lumboperitoneal shunts are occasionally used for communicating hydrocephalus) or 3rd ventriculostomy.
  removal of a mass lesion if present – this may obviate the need for a shunt.

'Arrested hydrocephalus' – symptomless ventricular dilatation requires no treatment, but regular developmental or psychometric assessment ensures no ill effects develop from this potentially unstable state.

HYDROCEPHALUS

Shunt techniques

A *reservoir* permits CSF aspiration for analysis.
A *valve* is incorporated in the system, with either

– fixed opening pressure
e.g. Heyer-Schulte, Hakim
– variable opening pressure (flow regulated) e.g. Orbis sigma, Delta
– programmable e.g. Medos, Sophy.

Valve opening pressures range from 5–150 mmH$_2$O
[*Lumboperitoneal shunt*
– catheter inserted into the lumbar theca either directly at open operation or percutaneously through a Tuohy needle. The distal end is sited in the peritoneal cavity.]

A *ventricular catheter* is inserted through the occipital (or frontal) horn. The tip lies at the level of the foramen of Munro.

Ventriculoatrial shunt – distal catheter inserted through the internal jugular vein to the right atrium (T6/7 level on chest X-ray).

Silastic tubing tunnelled subcutaneously.

Ventriculoperitoneal shunt – distal catheter inserted into the peritoneal cavity. In children, redundant coils permit growth without revision.

Complications of shunting

Infection: results in meningitis, peritonitis or inflammation extending along the subcutaneous channel. In patients with a V-A shunt, bacteraemia may lead to shunt 'nephritis'. *Staphylococcus epidermidis* or *aureus* are usually involved, with infants at particular risk. Prophylactic antibiotics may minimise the risk of infection, but, when established, eradication usually requires shunt removal.

Subdural haematoma: ventricular collapse pulls the cortical surface from the dura and leaves a subdural CSF collection or tears bridging veins causing subdural haemorrhage. The risk may be reduced with a variable pressure or programmable valve.

Shunt obstruction: blockage of the shunt system with choroid plexus, debris, omentum or blood clot results in intermittent or persistent recurrence of symptoms. Demonstration of an increase in ventricular size compared to a previous baseline CT scan confirms shunt malfunction. Over a third require revision within 1 year and 80% within 10 years.

Low pressure state: following shunting, some patients develop headache and vomiting on sitting or standing. This low pressure state usually resolves with a high fluid intake and gradual mobilisation. If not, insertion of an antisyphon device or conversion to a high pressure valve is required.

Third ventriculostomy: Suitable for patients with tri-ventricular hydrocephalus e.g. obstructive hydrocephalus caused by aquaduct stenosis or a pineal or posterior fossa tumour occluding the posterior end of the 3rd ventricle/aqueduct. By using a flexible or rigid endoscope introduced through a frontal burrhole, a fistula is created in the floor of the 3rd ventricle. This provides an alternative method of treatment, which if successful, avoids the above problems of shunt insertion. About $\frac{2}{3}$ of patients obtain permanent benefit.

Prognosis: Provided treatment precedes irreversible brain damage, results are good with most children attaining normal IQs. Repeated complications, however, particularly prevalent in infancy and in young children carry a significant morbidity.

BENIGN INTRACRANIAL HYPERTENSION

Benign intracranial hypertension (pseudotumour cerebri) is characterised by increased intracranial pressure *without* evidence of an intracranial space-occupying lesion, obstruction to CSF pathways, infection, or hypertensive encephalopathy.

Diagnosis is especially dependent on excluding –
VENOUS OUTFLOW OBSTRUCTION TO CSF ABSORPTION

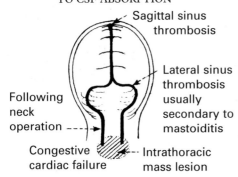

Sagittal sinus thrombosis

Lateral sinus thrombosis usually secondary to mastoiditis

Following neck operation

Congestive cardiac failure

Intrathoracic mass lesion

Where this has been ruled out the cause is obscure but a variety of factors are associated –
DIET – obesity.
 – hyper/hypovitaminosis A.
ENDOCRINE – pregnancy, menarche, menstrual irregularities, Addison's disease.
HAEMATOLOGICAL – iron deficiency anaemia.
 – polycythaemia vera.
DRUGS – oral contraceptives.
 – steroid withdrawal.
 – tetracycline (minocycline)
 – nalidixic acid.
Various mechanisms have been postulated.

– BRAIN SWELLING	Different studies support different mechanisms. The link with obesity suggests an underlying endocrine basis, but, except in Addison's disease, endocrine assessment has failed to reveal abnormalities.
– ↓CSF ABSORPTION	
– ↑CSF SECRETION	

CLINICAL FEATURES

Age: any age, but usually in 3rd and 4th decades.
Sex: female > male

Symptoms	Signs
Headache	Obesity
Visual obscurations	
Impaired visual acuity	← Papilloedema
Diplopia	VI nerve palsy

In women the condition is often ⟶ associated with – recent weight gain, fluid retention, menstrual dysfunction, the first trimester of pregnancy and the postpartum period.

Investigations
CT/MRI brain and orbit (ventricles usually small)
MRV/Venography (to exclude sinus thrombosis)
Visual field charting (enlarged blind spot & peripheral constriction)
Lumbar puncture (measure pressure)

TREATMENT
indicated when:
1. Severe intractable headache
2. Evidence of progressive decrease in visual acuity or visual field loss (severity of papilloedema doesn't predict visual loss)

– Discontinue causative medication if known
– Weight loss
– Acetazolamide (a carbonic anhydrase inhibitor)
– Systemic steroids

If these measures fail, consider – Repeated LPs
 – Optic nerve decompression
 – Lumboperitoneal shunt

PROGNOSIS
Generally a self limiting process especially in pregnancy

CHIARI MALFORMATION

Although the names of two authors (Arnold and Chiari) were originally linked to the description of malformations at the medullary-spinal junction, Chiari must take most credit for providing a detailed description of this condition.

TYPE I

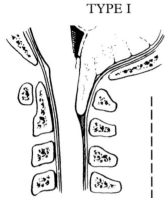

TYPE II

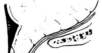

Medulla

TYPE III

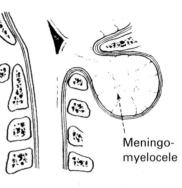

Meningo-myelocele

TYPE I

The cerebellar *tonsils* lie below the level of the foramen magnum (cerebellar ectopia). This may not produce symptoms

Associated conditions

(in symptomatic patients):

Spinal

Syringomyelia ⎱
Hydromyelia ⎰ (50%)

Cranial

Hydrocephalus (10%) (occurs less often than Chiari originally described)

TYPE II

Part of the cerebellar *vermis*, medulla and 4th ventricle extend through the foramen magnum, often to the midcervical region. The lower cranial nerves are stretched and the cervical nerve roots run horizontally or in an upward direction.

Spinal

Syringomyelia ⎱
Hydromyelia ⎰ (90%)

Spina bifida – meningomyelocele, diastomatomyelia

Cervical fusion (Klippel-Feil)

Cranial

Hydrocephalus (85%)
Aqueduct stenosis and forking
Small posterior fossa
Basilar impression
Fusion of both thalami
Fusion of the superior and inferior colliculi
Microgyria
Hypoplastic tentorium cerebelli and falx
Skull lacuniae – vault thinned or defective

Others

Developmental anomalies of the cardiovascular, gastrointestinal and genitourinary systems in 10%

TYPE III

Part of the cerebellum and medulla lie within a cervico-occipital meningomyelocele.

[TYPE IV
Cerebellar hypoplasia – best considered as a separate entity.]

CHIARI MALFORMATION

PATHOGENESIS

Several hypotheses have been proposed to explain the pathological findings of these malformations. Gardner suggested that downward pressure from *hydrocephalus* played an important role in displacing the posterior fossa structures and, when associated with a patent central canal, explained the high incidence of syringomyelia (page 397). Others supposed that *traction* from a tethered spinal cord (dysraphism), or a *CSF leak* through a myelocele into the amniotic sac in fetal life resulted in caudal displacement of the posterior fossa structures. Of these theories, none provides an entirely satisfactory explanation; a more realistic view attributes the hindbrain deformity to *maldevelopment* during early fetal life. This would explain the presence of other developmental anomalies.

CLINICAL PRESENTATION

Depends on age

INFANCY
{ Severe type II (or III) deformities present with *respiratory difficulties* and *lower cranial nerve palsies*. Death may result from *aspiration pneumonia* or *apnoeic attacks*, or from complications of associated malformations, e.g. *spina bifida*. In milder forms, *nystagmus* (horizontal), *retrocollis* (neck extension) and *spasticity* predominate.

CHILDHOOD
{ With increasing age, *gait ataxia* may become evident. Features of an associated syringomyelia – *dissociated sensory loss* and *spastic quadraparesis* often contribute to the clinical problems.

ADULT
{ Only patients with a type I or a mild type II deformity present in adult life –
Occipital headaches are induced by coughing or straining

Nystagmus – downbeat		rotatory	} may result from
(on looking	or	(on lateral	medullary compression
down)		gaze)	or from an associated syringomyelia (see page 397).

Ataxia
Spastic quadraparesis
Progression may eventually lead to severe bulbar symptoms – *lower cranial nerve palsies, respiratory difficulties.*

INVESTIGATIONS

Magnetic resonance imaging (MRI) is the investigation of choice. T1 weighted sagittal and axial scans most clearly demonstrate cerebellar ectopia and the presence or absence of an associated syringomyelia.

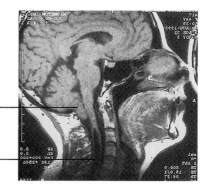

Chiari malformation
(with associated syringomyelia)

CHIARI MALFORMATION

Investigation (*cont'd*)

Straight X-rays
- *Skull:* note the presence of platybasia, basilar impression or lacunae (vault defects).
- *Cervical spine:* note increased canal width or fusion of vertebrae (especially C2,3) – Klippel-Feil syndrome.
- *Lumbosacral spine:* note any associated spina bifida.

Myelography (if MRI unavailable)

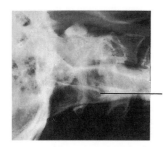

CT scan: difficult to interpret at the cervico-medullary junction, but shows soft tissue filling the spinal canal at this level.

Contrast run up to the foramen magnum with the patient in the supine position outlines a posteriorly situated filling defect.

MANAGEMENT (see also syringomyelia, page 397)

In patients with hydrocephalus and signs and symptoms of raised intracranial pressure. → *Ventriculoperitoneal or atrial shunt* may significantly improve signs and symptoms attributed to the Chiari malformation.

In patients with other symptoms and signs → *Posterior fossa decompression* – by removing the posterior rim of the foramen magnum and the arch of the atlas. For more severe cases, the dura is opened and a graft is inserted. Attempts at freeing tonsillar adhesions should be resisted. An apnoea monitor in the initial postoperative period helps detect potentially fatal apnoea, especially during sleep. In some instances, patients with minimal symptoms or with no evidence of progression may warrant a conservative approach.

PROGNOSIS

Patients with mild symptoms and signs often respond well to operation, but those with long-standing neurological deficits rarely improve. Treatment should aim at preventing further progression.

Further deterioration eventually occurs in one-third, despite operative measures.

SYRINGOBULBIA

Extension of a syringomyelic cavity upwards into the medulla may produce signs and symptoms which are difficult to distinguish from those of medullary compression in the Arnold-Chiari syndrome:

– difficulty in swallowing, dysphonia, dysarthria, vertigo, facial pain
– nystagmus, palatal and vocal cord weakness, occasional facial and tongue weakness.

DANDY-WALKER SYNDROME

This rare developmental anomaly comprises:

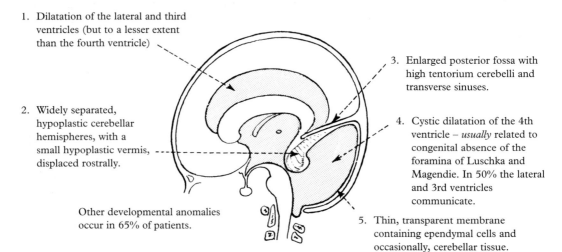

1. Dilatation of the lateral and third ventricles (but to a lesser extent than the fourth ventricle)

2. Widely separated, hypoplastic cerebellar hemispheres, with a small hypoplastic vermis, displaced rostrally.

   Other developmental anomalies occur in 65% of patients.

3. Enlarged posterior fossa with high tentorium cerebelli and transverse sinuses.

4. Cystic dilatation of the 4th ventricle – *usually* related to congenital absence of the foramina of Luschka and Magendie. In 50% the lateral and 3rd ventricles communicate.

5. Thin, transparent membrane containing ependymal cells and occasionally, cerebellar tissue.

CLINICAL PRESENTATION
Infancy: Symptoms and signs of hydrocephalus (page 371) combined with a prominent occiput.
Childhood: Signs of cerebellar dysfunction with or without signs of hydrocephalus.

INVESTIGATIONS
Skull X-ray: Usually shows elevation of the transverse sinuses and occipital bulging, confirming the presence of an enlarged posterior fossa.

CT scan:

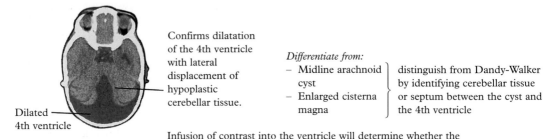

Confirms dilatation of the 4th ventricle with lateral displacement of hypoplastic cerebellar tissue.

Dilated 4th ventricle

Differentiate from:
– Midline arachnoid cyst
– Enlarged cisterna magna
} distinguish from Dandy-Walker by identifying cerebellar tissue or septum between the cyst and the 4th ventricle

Infusion of contrast into the ventricle will determine whether the 4th ventricle communicates with the rest of the ventricular system.

MANAGEMENT
When the dilated 4th ventricle communicates with the rest of the ventricular system, a cystoperitoneal shunt suffices and helps maintain a patent aqueduct. When a 'two-compartment' hydrocephalus exists, both the encysted 4th ventricle and the other ventricles require drainage (i.e. with a cysto-peritoneal and a ventriculo-peritoneal shunt).

Excision of the cyst membrane ('marsupialising' the 4th ventricle) is no longer thought to normalize CSF flow.

PROGNOSIS
Marked neurological impairment prior to treatment carries a poor outlook. In less impaired patients, the prognosis relates more to the presence of other developmental anomalies.

CRANIOSYNOSTOSIS

In normal childhood development, the cranial sutures allow skull enlargement as the brain grows. *Premature fusion of one or more sutures* results in restricted growth of bone alongside the suture and excessive compensatory growth at the non-united joints. The effect depends on the site and number of sutures involved. Sagittal synostosis is the most frequently occurring deformity.

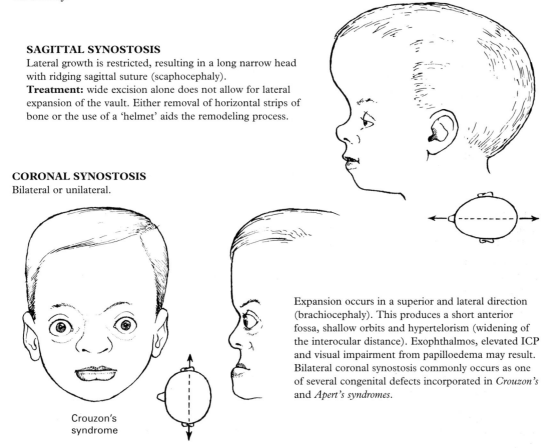

SAGITTAL SYNOSTOSIS
Lateral growth is restricted, resulting in a long narrow head with ridging sagittal suture (scaphocephaly).
Treatment: wide excision alone does not allow for lateral expansion of the vault. Either removal of horizontal strips of bone or the use of a 'helmet' aids the remodeling process.

CORONAL SYNOSTOSIS
Bilateral or unilateral.

Expansion occurs in a superior and lateral direction (brachiocephaly). This produces a short anterior fossa, shallow orbits and hypertelorism (widening of the interocular distance). Exophthalmos, elevated ICP and visual impairment from papilloedema may result. Bilateral coronal synostosis commonly occurs as one of several congenital defects incorporated in *Crouzon's* and *Apert's syndromes*.

Crouzon's syndrome

Involvement of several sutures (oxycephaly) results in skull expansion towards the vertex, the line of least resistance.

PANSYNOSTOSIS (all sutures affected) results in failure of skull growth with a symmetrical abnormally small head and raised intracranial pressure. ICP monitoring or a progressive reduction in normal circumferential growth distinguishes pansynostosis from microcephaly due to inadequate brain development.

Treatment of coronal, metopic and pansynostosis involves extensive craniofacial surgery correcting both cranial and orbital deformities.

Indication for operative treatment is primarily cosmetic when only one suture is involved, but with involvement of two or more sutures operation is also aimed at prevention of visual and cerebral damage from raised ICP.

Posterior plagiocephaly (flattening of the back of the head)

An increasing number of infants present with this condition. This is rarely due to a true lambdoid synostosis but it is thought to be an acquired 'locked suture syndrome' with secondary fusion following posterior moulding. Very few of those who develop a progressive skull deformity require surgical treatment.

STEREOTACTIC SURGERY

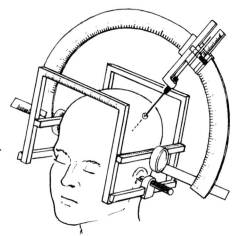

Stereotactic techniques developed initially for lesion making, enable accurate placement of a cannula or electrode at a predetermined target site within the brain with the least risk.

Many different stereotactic frames have been developed, e.g. Leksell, Todd-Wells, Guiot. These, combined with radiological landmarks (usually ventriculography) and a brain atlas, provide anatomical localisation to within ± 1mm. Since some functional variability occurs at each anatomical site, electrode localisation is also based on the recorded neuronal activity and on the effects of electrical stimulation.

CT/MRI STEREOTACTIC SYSTEM

CT and MRI compatible stereotactic systems allow cannula insertion to any point selected on the image. They are all based on the concept of identifiable external reference (fiducial) markers, e.g. Codman-Robert-Wells (CRW) system:

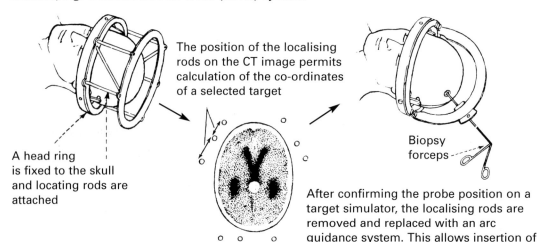

The position of the localising rods on the CT image permits calculation of the co-ordinates of a selected target

A head ring is fixed to the skull and locating rods are attached

Biopsy forceps

After confirming the probe position on a target simulator, the localising rods are removed and replaced with an arc guidance system. This allows insertion of the probe or biopsy forceps, to the target position from any desired direction.

CT/MRI stereosurgery provides the optimal method for the biopsy or aspiration of *small, deeply situated tumours* or *abscesses*. Many now use stereotactic biopsy, for larger tumours. It carries lower risk than handheld biopsy and allows selection of specific areas within the tumour. Functional stereotaxy e.g. thalamotomy, pallidotomy, still requires electrical stimulation for the final localisation.

When combined with craniotomy it permits direct macroscopic examination of a lesion and may aid localisation, e.g. a small arteriovenous malformation. The improved resolution now available with CT/MRI scanning has led to sufficient anatomical localisation for accurate lesion making, obviating the need for ventriculography.

STEREOTACTIC SURGERY

METHODS OF LESION MAKING

Heat   – radiofrequency current delivered through a fine electrode ⎱ lesion size
Cooling   – with a cryogenic probe   ⎰ determined by
Radiation – implantation of radioactive seed, e.g. yttrium^{90} temperature
             – focused beam from cobalt^{60} rods (sited on a specially   change and
                 adapted Leksell frame) or from a linear accelerator.   duration.

USES OF STEREOTACTIC SURGERY

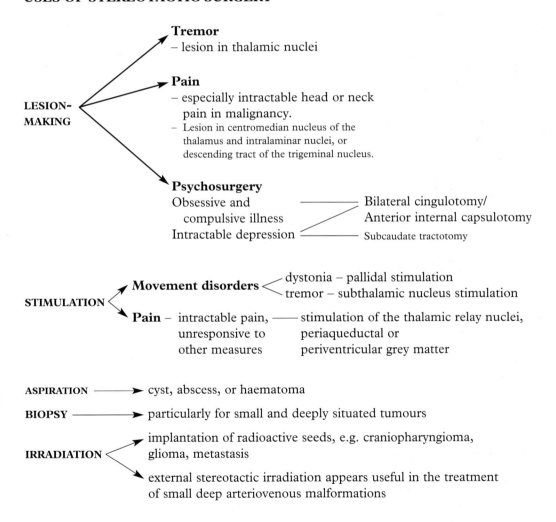

LESION-MAKING

Tremor
– lesion in thalamic nuclei

Pain
– especially intractable head or neck
   pain in malignancy.
– Lesion in centromedian nucleus of the
   thalamus and intralaminar nuclei, or
   descending tract of the trigeminal nucleus.

Psychosurgery
Obsessive and   Bilateral cingulotomy/
   compulsive illness   Anterior internal capsulotomy
Intractable depression   Subcaudate tractotomy

STIMULATION

Movement disorders ⎱ dystonia – pallidal stimulation
                               ⎰ tremor – subthalamic nucleus stimulation

Pain – intractable pain, —— stimulation of the thalamic relay nuclei,
        unresponsive to   periaqueductal or
        other measures   periventricular grey matter

ASPIRATION ——▶ cyst, abscess, or haematoma

BIOPSY ——▶ particularly for small and deeply situated tumours

IRRADIATION ⎱ implantation of radioactive seeds, e.g. craniopharyngioma,
                    glioma, metastasis
                   ⎰ external stereotactic irradiation appears useful in the treatment
                    of small deep arteriovenous malformations

IMAGE GUIDED 'FRAMELESS' STEREOTAXY

Although craniotomy with conventional stereotaxy is feasible, in practice the cumbersome frame, combined with the aiming device, tend to obstruct the operating field. The need for a simultaneous CT or MRI with the head ring and locating rods in place leads to a further inconvenience.

The combination of modern imaging, elaborate computer software and a locating device now permit the surgeon to determine how the tip of a pointer outwith or within the skull, directly relates to a two or even three dimensional CT or MR image.

The accuracy of the technique depends on the quality of the digitised image and on the methods used to *register* the patient's head to the image. The registration of recognisable skin points (e.g. nasion, inner canthus, ears) on the patient to the CT/MR image provides an accuracy of 2–3 mm and this is sufficient for most purposes.

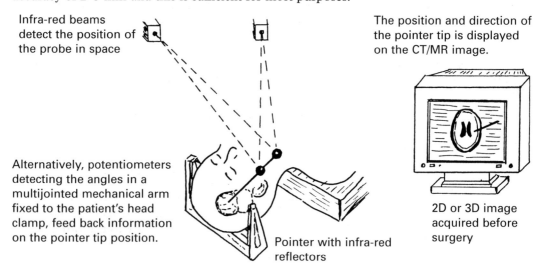

Infra-red beams detect the position of the probe in space

The position and direction of the pointer tip is displayed on the CT/MR image.

Alternatively, potentiometers detecting the angles in a multijointed mechanical arm fixed to the patient's head clamp, feed back information on the pointer tip position.

Pointer with infra-red reflectors

2D or 3D image acquired before surgery

Uses of 'frameless' stereotaxy

Aids accurate positioning of burrholes and bone flap, and the planning of the safest approach to the lesion.

TUMOURS
– biopsy
– resection: locates, then identifies the tumour margins and the position of important adjacent structures
– brachytherapy (see page 310)
EPILEPSY
– defining the extent of resected tissue e.g. amygdalohippocampectomy
– placement of depth electrodes

ARTERIOVENOUS MALFORMATION
– localisation of lesion and the feeding vessels

ABSCESS
– aspiration

ORBIT
– location of intraorbital lesion

Framed stereotactic methods are still required for functional procedures, most of which require a local anaesthetic and patient cooperation. Head movement prevents accurate registration.

PSYCHOSURGERY

In 1935, observation of behavioural changes in chimpanzees following bilateral ablation of the frontal association area, led to the introduction of lesion-making for psychiatric disease (Moniz). The operation of *prefrontal leucotomy* was perfected and used on patients with a wide variety of problems. In Britain, between 1940 and 1955, neurosurgeons performed over 10 000 operations. It became evident that patients with affective problems – depression, anxiety and obsessive compulsive disorder – showed better results than those with schizophrenia.

As a consequence of the introduction of *chlorpromazine* in the 1950s, and the operative complications and results – perhaps limited by poor case selection, prefrontal leucotomy fell into disrepute. The need for a surgical procedure persisted, however, in those patients where drugs had little effect. Despite pharmacological improvements, some patients developed chronically disabling conditions requiring continual hospital care; in others with acute depressive illness, the suicide rate was high.

Stereotactic surgery provided a method of lesion-making which was low risk and this is now generally accepted as a suitable treatment in *selected patients where drug treatment has failed*. Issues of 'informed consent' for such procedures in the mentally ill are often ethically difficult.

INDICATIONS FOR STEREOTACTIC SURGERY AND LESION SITE

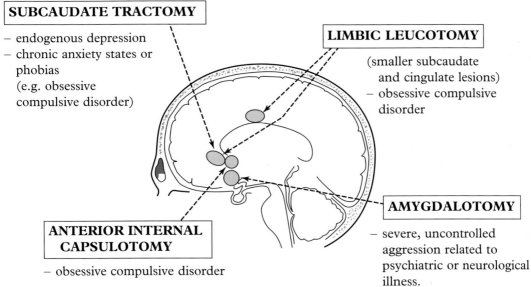

SUBCAUDATE TRACTOMY

– endogenous depression
– chronic anxiety states or phobias
  (e.g. obsessive compulsive disorder)

LIMBIC LEUCOTOMY

(smaller subcaudate and cingulate lesions)
– obsessive compulsive disorder

AMYGDALOTOMY

– severe, uncontrolled aggression related to psychiatric or neurological illness.

ANTERIOR INTERNAL CAPSULOTOMY

– obsessive compulsive disorder

Results

Depression/anxiety states – up to two-thirds benefit from subcaudate tractotomy.
Obsessional neurosis   – 80% improve following limbic leucotomy.

LOCALISED NEUROLOGICAL DISEASE AND ITS MANAGEMENT

B. SPINAL CORD AND ROOTS

SPINAL CORD AND ROOTS

Disorders localised to the spinal cord or nerve roots are detailed below, but note that many diffuse neurological disease processes also affect the cord (see Section V, e.g. multiple sclerosis, Friedreich's ataxia).

SPINAL CORD AND ROOT COMPRESSION

As the spinal canal is a rigidly enclosed cavity, an expanding disease process will eventually cause cord and/or root compression.

Causes

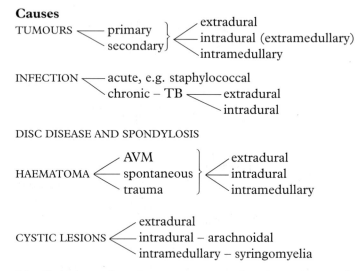

TUMOURS —— primary ⎱ — extradural
secondary ⎰ — intradural (extramedullary)
— intramedullary

INFECTION —— acute, e.g. staphylococcal
chronic – TB —— extradural
intradural

DISC DISEASE AND SPONDYLOSIS

HAEMATOMA —— AVM ⎱ — extradural
spontaneous ⎰ — intradural
trauma — intramedullary

CYSTIC LESIONS —— extradural
intradural – arachnoidal
intramedullary – syringomyelia

Manifestations of cord or root compression depend upon the following:

Site of lesion within the spinal canal:
an expanding lesion outside the cord produces signs and symptoms from root and segmental damage.

ROOT – lower motor neuron (l.m.n.) and sensory impairment appropriate to the distribution of the damaged root.

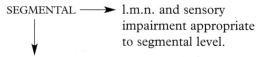

SEGMENTAL ———▶ l.m.n. and sensory impairment appropriate to segmental level.

Interruption of ascending sensory and descending motor tracts produces sensory impairment and an upper motor neuron (u.m.n.) deficit below the level of the lesion.

Lesions within the cord (intramedullary) produce only segmental signs and symptoms.

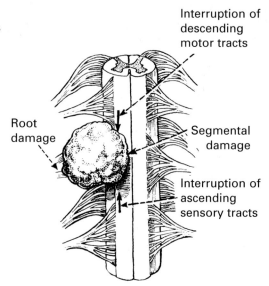

Interruption of descending motor tracts

Root damage

Segmental damage

Interruption of ascending sensory tracts

SPINAL CORD AND ROOT COMPRESSION

Level of the lesion: a lesion above the L1 vertebral body may damage both the cord and its roots. Below this, only roots are damaged.

Vascular involvement: whether neuronal damage results from mechanical stretching or is secondary to arterial ischaemia or venous obstruction remains uncertain. On occasions, clinical findings indicate cord damage well beyond the level of the compressive lesion; this implies a distant ischaemic effect due to blood vessel compression at the lesion site.

Speed of onset: speed of compression affects the clinical picture. Despite producing upper motor neuron damage, a rapidly progressive cord lesion often produces a 'flaccid paralysis' with loss of reflexes and absent plantar responses. This state is akin to 'spinal shock' seen following trauma. Several days or weeks may elapse before tone returns accompanied by the expected 'upper motor neuron' signs.

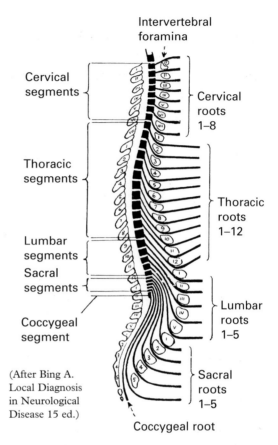

(After Bing A. Local Diagnosis in Neurological Disease 15 ed.)

Clinical features

These depend on the site and level of the compressive lesion.

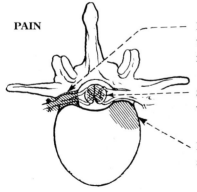

PAIN

ROOT – severe, sharp, shooting, burning pain radiating into the cutaneous distribution or muscle group supplied by the root; aggravated by movement, straining or coughing.

SEGMENTAL – continuous, deep aching pain radiating into whole leg or one half of body; not affected by movement.

BONE – continuous, dull pain and tenderness over the affected area; may or may not be aggravated by movement.

SPINAL CORD AND ROOT COMPRESSION – NEUROLOGICAL EFFECTS

LATERAL COMPRESSIVE LESION

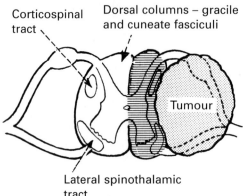

Corticospinal tract

Dorsal columns – gracile and cuneate fasciculi

Tumour

Lateral spinothalamic tract

Root/segmental damage

MUSCLE WEAKNESS in groups supplied by the involved root and segment with LOWER MOTOR NEURON (l.m.n.) signs: – wasting; – loss of tone; – fasciculation; – diminished or absent reflexes. N.B. motor deficit is seldom detected with root lesions above C5 and from T2 to L1.

SENSORY DEFECT of all modalities or hyperaesthesia in area supplied by the root, but overlap from adjacent roots may prevent detection.

Long tract – signs and symptoms
Partial (Unilateral) cord lesion
(Brown-Séquard syndrome)

MOTOR DEFICIT – dragging of the leg. In high cervical lesions weakness of finger movements is noted on the side of the lesion.

UPPER MOTOR NEURON (u.m.n.) signs (maximal on side of lesion):
– weakness in a 'pyramidal' distribution, i.e. arms – extensors predominantly affected; legs – flexors predominantly affected.
– increased tone, clonus; – increased reflexes;
– extensor plantar response.

SENSORY DEFICIT – numbness may occur on the same side as the lesion and a burning dysaesthesia on the opposite side.
– joint position sense and accurate touch localisation (two point discrimination) impaired on side of lesion.
– Pinprick and temperature sensation impaired on opposite side.

BROWN SÉQUARD SYNDROME

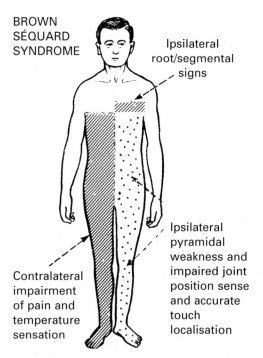

Ipsilateral root/segmental signs

Ipsilateral pyramidal weakness and impaired joint position sense and accurate touch localisation

Contralateral impairment of pain and temperature sensation

In practice, cord damage is seldom restricted to one side. Usually a mixed picture occurs, with an asymmetric distribution of signs and symptoms.
Damage to sympathetic pathways in the T1 root or cervical cord causes an ipsilateral *Horner's syndrome* (page 143).

BLADDER symptoms are infrequent and only occur when cord damage is bilateral. Precipitancy or difficulty in starting micturition may precede retention.

SPINAL CORD AND ROOT COMPRESSION – NEUROLOGICAL EFFECTS

LATERAL COMPRESSIVE LESION (*cont'd*)

Long tract damage – complete cord lesion

MOTOR DEFICIT: the speed of cord compression affects the clinical picture. Slowly growing lesions present with difficulty in walking; the legs may 'jump' at night. Examination reveals u.m.n. signs often with an asymmetric distribution. Rapidly progressive lesions produce 'spinal shock' – the limbs are flaccid, power and reflexes diminished or absent and plantar responses are absent or extensor.

SENSORY DEFICIT: involves all modalities and occurs up to the level of the lesion.

BLADDER: patient first notices difficulty in initiating micturition. Retention follows, associated with incontinence as automatic emptying occurs. *Constipation* is only noticed after a few days. Some patients develop *priapism* (painful erection).

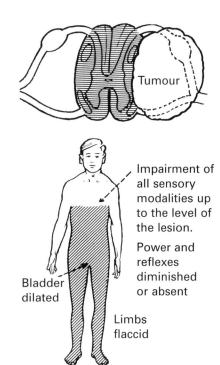

Tumour

Impairment of all sensory modalities up to the level of the lesion.

Power and reflexes diminished or absent

Bladder dilated

Limbs flaccid

CENTRAL CORD LESION

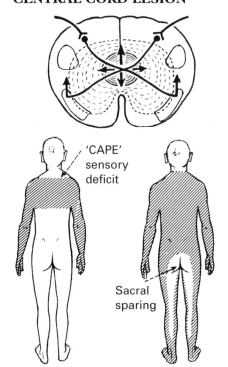

'CAPE' sensory deficit

Sacral sparing

Segmental damage: A central lesion initially damages the second sensory neuron crossing to the lateral spinothalamic tract; pain and temperature sensations are impaired in the distribution of the involved segment. As the lesion expands, anterior horn cells are also involved and a l.m.n. weakness occurs.

Long tract effects: further lesion expansion damages the spinothalamic tract and corticospinal tracts, the most medially situated fibres being involved first. With lesion in the cervical region, the sensory deficit to pain and temperature extends downwards in a 'CAPE'-like distribution. As the sacral fibres lie peripherally in the lateral spinothalamic tract, SACRAL SPARING can occur, even with a large lesion. Involvement of the corticospinal tracts produces u.m.n. signs and symptoms in the limbs below the level of the lesion. The bladder is usually involved late.

In the cervical cord, sympathetic involvement may produce a unilateral or bilateral *Horner's syndrome.*

SPINAL CORD AND ROOT COMPRESSION – NEUROLOGICAL EFFECTS

LOWER CORD (CONUS) CAUDA EQUINA LESIONS

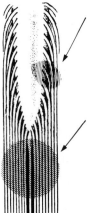

Root or segmental lesions may involve the upper part of the cauda equina and produce root/segmental and long tract signs as described on the previous page, e.g. an expanding proximal L4 root lesion causes weakness and wasting of the foot dorsiflexors, sensory deficit over the inner calf, an increased ankle jerk and an extensor plantar response. Bladder involvement tends to occur late.

The lower sacral roots are involved early, producing loss of motor and sensory bladder control with detrusor paralysis. Overflow incontinence ensues. Impotence and faecal incontinence may be noted. A l.m.n. weakness is found in the muscles supplied by the sacral roots (foot plantarflexors and evertors), the ankle jerks are absent or impaired and a sensory deficit occurs over the 'saddle' area.

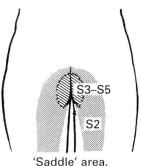

'Saddle' area.

VERTEBRAL COLUMN

If a spinal cord or root lesion is suspected look for:
– *Scoliosis, loss of lordosis* or *limitation of straight leg raising* } – suggests root irritation
– *Paravertebral swelling*
– *Tenderness* on bone percussion } – suggests malignant disease or infection
– *Restricted spinal mobility* – suggests bone, disc or root involvement
– *Sacral dimple or tuft of hair* – suggests spina bifida occulta/dermoid.

SPINAL CORD AND ROOT COMPRESSION – INVESTIGATIONS

STRAIGHT X-RAY On the ANTERO-POSTERIOR views look for:

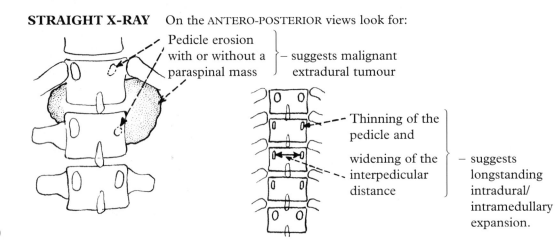

Pedicle erosion with or without a paraspinal mass } – suggests malignant extradural tumour

Thinning of the pedicle and

widening of the interpedicular distance } – suggests longstanding intradural/ intramedullary expansion.

SPINAL CORD AND ROOT COMPRESSION – INVESTIGATIONS

STRAIGHT X-RAY (*cont'd*)

On the LATERAL view

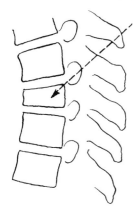

Collapse of the vertebral body suggests malignant infiltration or osteoporosis
(If the disc space is destroyed, infection is more likely)

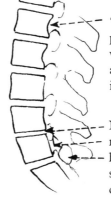

'Scalloping' of the posterior surface of the vertebral body indicates a longstanding intradural lesion

Narrow disc space, narrow canal and hypertrophic facet joints support a diagnosis of disc disease or lumbar spinal stenosis (but not diagnostic)

On OBLIQUE views

Expansion of the intervertebral foramina suggests neurofibroma

Narrowing from osteophytic encroachment indicates possible root compression (but often seen in asymptomatic elderly patients)

MRI

This is now the investigation of choice for spinal disease, whether this lies within or outwith the dura or the spinal cord. Clinical examination and straight X-rays may suggest the level of the lesion and guide the level of examination. If this fails to detect a lesion, then further imaging must cover the whole length of the cord since occasionally the site of compression lies many segments higher than the clinical signs indicate. The examination must involve both T1 and T2 weighted images, the former often repeated with gadolinium enhancement. *Sagittal* or *coronal views* are of value in outlining a section of the spinal cord or the cervical medullary junction. On displaying an abnormality at a particular site, *axial views* at selected levels may provide additional information. MRI differentiates a syrinx (page 397) or a cystic swelling within the spinal cord from a solid intramedullary tumour (page 396).

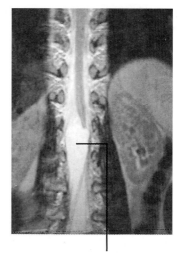

Coronal T2 weighted MRI showing an intradural, extramedullary lesion (ependymoma)

391

SPINAL CORD AND ROOT COMPRESSION – INVESTIGATIONS

MYELOGRAPHY

If MRI is unavailable or contraindicated e.g. pacemaker, myelography is used to screen the spinal cord and the cauda equina. This will identify the level of a compressive lesion and indicate its probable site i.e. intradural, extradural.

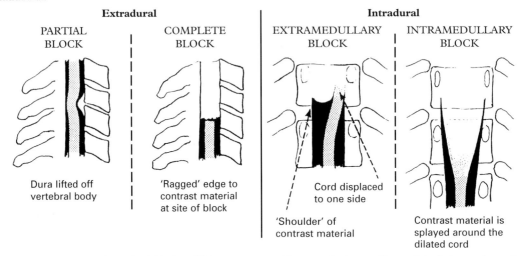

Extradural

PARTIAL BLOCK

Dura lifted off vertebral body

COMPLETE BLOCK

'Ragged' edge to contrast material at site of block

Intradural

EXTRAMEDULLARY BLOCK

Cord displaced to one side

'Shoulder' of contrast material

INTRAMEDULLARY BLOCK

Contrast material is splayed around the dilated cord

Even with an apparent 'complete' block, sufficient contrast medium may be 'coaxed' beyond the lesion to determine its upper extent. If not, a cervical puncture may be necessary.

Lesions in the lumbar and sacral regions require a *'radiculogram'*, outlining the lumbosacral roots.

CT SCAN/CT MYELOGRAPHY

It is impractical to use this as a screening investigation for cord compression, but if the level of interest is known, CT scanning provides useful additional information.

Vertebral body eroded by tumour

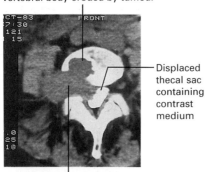

Displaced thecal sac containing contrast medium

Neurofibroma

Plain CT with axial cuts will clearly demonstrate bone erosion, osteophytic outgrowth and thickened facet joints causing narrowing of the spinal canal or intervertebral foramen. Axial cuts will also demonstrate disc herniation, the relationship of vertebral bone destruction to a paraspinal mass (e.g. metastatic tumour) and the extraspinal extent of an intraspinal lesion (e.g. neurofibroma).

CT myelography with axial cuts (CT performed either 6–12 hours after routine myelography or immediately after intrathecal injection of just a few ml of contrast) demonstrates clearly the degree of spinal cord or nerve root compression.

If cord compression is suspect then lumbar puncture and CSF analysis should await imaging.

CSF protein: often increased, especially below a complete block.

CSF cell count: a marked leucocyte count suggests an infective cause – abscess or tuberculosis.

CSF cytology may reveal tumour cells

CSF ANALYSIS

This is of limited value in cord compression. Abnormalities frequently occur, but *lumbar puncture may precipitate neurological deterioration*, presumably due to the creation of a pressure gradient.

SPINAL CORD AND ROOT COMPRESSION

TUMOURS

Incidence: The table shows the number of patients with histologically confirmed tumours admitted to the Institute of Neurological Sciences, Glasgow, over a 5-year period (population 2.7 millions). Tumour types differ in adults and children and are considered separately.

Adults		**Children**		
EXTRADURAL (**78%**)		EXTRADURAL (**78%**)		
Metastasis	118	Metastasis	1	
Myeloma	19	Lymphoma	1	
Neurofibroma	15			
Lymphoma	14			
Others	7			
INTRADURAL (**18%**)		INTRADURAL (**64%**)		
Meningioma	22	Dermoid/epidermoid	6	
Schwannoma	13	Others	1	
Others	4			(Table adapted from Adams, Graham and Doyle: Brain Biopsy, 1982)
INTRAMEDULLARY (**4%**)		INTRAMEDULLARY (**18%**)		
Astrocytoma	8	Astrocytoma	2	
Others	1			

Pathology: The pathological features of spinal tumours match those of their intracranial counterparts (see page 300).

METASTATIC TUMOUR

Occurs in 5% of all cancer patients and accounts for 50% of adult acute myelopathies.

Primary site: Usually breast, lung, prostate or kidney.

Metastatic site: Thoracic vertebrae most often involved, but metastasis may occur at any site and may be multiple.

Clinical features: Bone pain and tenderness are common features usually preceding limb and autonomic dysfunction.

Investigations: Plain radiology may be diagnostic as osteolytic lesions or vertebral collapse are present in most cases. MRI will identify extradural compression and help exclude or confirm multiple level disease.

Management

In earlier years, numerous patients with spinal cord compression were subjected to a 'decompressive' laminectomy followed by radiotherapy. Since metastatic tumour usually involves the vertebral body and pedicles, removal of the spinous processes and the lamina served only to increase instability. Not surprisingly results were extremely poor.

Most now feel that *radiotherapy* is the appropriate initial treatment, once the diagnosis is established, unless known radioresistance or a rapidly deteriorating neurological condition enforces the need for *surgical decompression*. Major operative procedures are inappropriate in the elderly, in patients with paraplegia and in patients with a dismal prognosis from their primary tumour (e.g. small cell bronchial carcinoma). In such patients, if medication fails to control pain, a palliative course of radiotherapy may help.

Aims of surgical treatment
— To establish a histological diagnosis if not already known
— To decompress the spinal cord yet maintain stability of vertebral column
— To produce stability if instability causes excessive pain

393

SPINAL CORD AND ROOT COMPRESSION

Techniques

Biopsy – needle biopsy of a paraspinous mass or trochar biopsy of infiltrated bone

Surgical decompression

> FOR TUMOUR INVOLVING THE VERTEBRAL BODY OR THE PEDICLE–

ANTERIOR TRANSTHORACIC DECOMPRESSION: Provides excellent exposure of the vertebral bodies, but requires the more extensive procedure of a thoracotomy. Usually reserved for patients with the best outcome e.g. breast carcinoma.

> FOR TUMOUR LYING POSTERIOR TO THE CORD OR ONLY INVOLVING THE LAMINA AND SPINOUS PROCESSES –

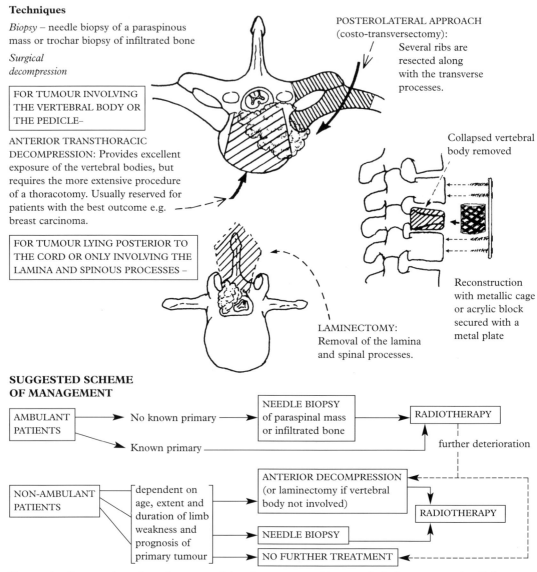

POSTEROLATERAL APPROACH (costo-transversectomy):
Several ribs are resected along with the transverse processes.

Collapsed vertebral body removed

Reconstruction with metallic cage or acrylic block secured with a metal plate

LAMINECTOMY:
Removal of the lamina and spinal processes.

SUGGESTED SCHEME OF MANAGEMENT

AMBULANT PATIENTS → No known primary → NEEDLE BIOPSY of paraspinal mass or infiltrated bone → RADIOTHERAPY

→ Known primary →

further deterioration

NON-AMBULANT PATIENTS → dependent on age, extent and duration of limb weakness and prognosis of primary tumour →

ANTERIOR DECOMPRESSION (or laminectomy if vertebral body not involved)

NEEDLE BIOPSY

NO FURTHER TREATMENT

RADIOTHERAPY

Prognosis: Outcome depends on the nature of the primary tumour. Mean survival after surgery and radiotherapy ranges from 6 months for lung carcinoma to 45 months for prostatic and thyroid carcinoma.

MYELOMA

This malignant condition usually affects older age groups. It is often multifocal, involving the vertebral bodies, pelvis, ribs and skull, but solitary tumours may occur ('plasmacytoma'). Spinal cord compression occurs in 15% of patients with myeloma and rarely without vertebral body involvement due to intradural deposits. If suspect, look for characteristic changes in the plasma immunoglobulins and for Bence-Jones protein in the urine. An isotope bone scan may be less informative than a radiological skeletal survey. Bone marrow shows infiltration of plasma cells. Serum calcium levels may be high.

Management is as for metastatic tumour with additional chemotherapy. The prognosis is variable but patients may survive many years with a solitary plasmacytoma.

SPINAL CORD AND ROOT COMPRESSION

MENINGIOMA

Spinal meningiomas tend to occur in elderly patients and are more common in females than in males. They usually arise in the thoracic region and are almost always intradural. Slow growth often permits considerable cord flattening to occur before symptoms become evident. *MRI* or *CT myelography* will identity the lesion.

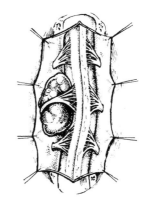

The operative aim is complete removal. Results are usually good, but if the tumour arises anteriorly to the cord, excision of the dural origin is difficult, if not impossible, and recurrence may result.

SCHWANNOMA/NEUROFIBROMA

Schwannomas are slowly growing benign tumours occurring at any level and arising from the posterior nerve roots. They lie either entirely within the spinal canal or 'dumbbell' through the intervertebral foramen, on occasions presenting as a mass in the thorax or posterior abdominal wall.

Neurofibromas are identical apart from their microscopic appearance (page 301) and their association with multiple neurofibromatosis (Von Recklinghausen's disease NF1 – see page 557) – look for café au lait patches in the skin.

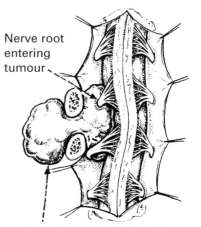

Nerve root entering tumour

Neurofibroma 'dumbbelling' through intervertebral foramen

Schwannomas tend to occur in the 30–60 age group. Typically they present with root pain. Root signs and/or signs of cord compression may follow.

MRI or *CT myelography* identifies an intradural/extramedullary lesion. Oblique X-rays may show foraminal enlargement; CT scan will delineate any extraspinal extension (see page 392). Complete operative removal is feasible but the nerve root of origin is inevitably sacrificed. Overlap from adjacent nerve roots usually minimises any resultant neurological deficit.

SPINAL CORD AND ROOT COMPRESSION

INTRAMEDULLARY TUMOURS

Intrinsic tumours of the spinal cord occur infrequently. In the Glasgow series (Table, page 393) almost all were slowly growing *astrocytomas* (grades I and II) although other series report an equal incidence of *ependymomas*. Cystic cavities may lie within the tumour or at the upper or lower pole. Benign lesions include haemangioblastoma, lipoma, epidermoid, tuberculoma and cavernous angioma.

Clinical features

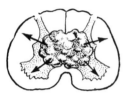

The onset is usually gradual. Segmental pain is common. Interruption of the decussating fibres of the lateral spinothalamic tract causes loss of pain and temperature sensation at the level of the involved segments.

Tumour expansion and involvement of the anterior horn cells produces a lower motor neuron weakness of the corresponding muscle groups; corticospinal tract involvement produces an upper motor neuron weakness below the level of the lesion. The sensory deficit spreads downwards bilaterally, the sacral region being the last to become involved.

Investigations

Straight X-rays occasionally show widening of the interpedicular distance or 'scalloping' of the vertebral bodies. MRI shows widening of the cord and differentiates solid tumour from syringomyelia. It also identifies the extent of the lesion and any associated cysts.

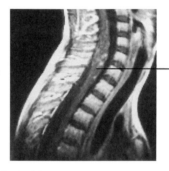

TI weighted sagittal MRI showing intramedullary lesion

Management

When an intrinsic cord tumour is suspected, an exploratory laminectomy is required. An attempt is made to obtain a diagnosis either through a longitudinal midline cord incision or by needle biopsy. Cystic cavities within a tumour or an associated syringomyelia may benefit from aspiration. With some ependymomas and benign lesions, a plane of cleavage is evident and partial or even total removal is possible. Attempted removal of low grade astrocytomas carries less encouraging results and operation is contraindicated in malignant tumours. After tumour biopsy or removal, radiotherapy is often administered, but its value is uncertain.

EPENDYMOMA OF THE CAUDA EQUINA

Over 50% of spinal ependymomas occur around the cauda equina and present with a central cauda equina syndrome (page 390). Operative removal combined with radiotherapy usually gives good long-term results, although metastatic seeding occasionally occurs through the CSF.

SPINAL CYSTIC LESIONS

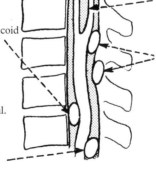

Enterogenous cysts: cysts with a mucoid content are occasionally found lying ventral or dorsal to the cord. They are often associated with vertebral malformation or other congenital abnormality, and are thought to arise from remnants of the neurenteric canal.

Epidermoid/dermoid cysts: may be of developmental origin or may follow implantation from a preceding lumbar puncture procedure.

Intramedullary cystic lesion: syringomyelia (see over) or cystic cavitation within a glioma.

Arachnoid cysts: arachnoid pouches are found incidentally. Myelography has shown that these may communicate with CSF or seal off producing cysts. They occur predominantly in the thoracic region and sometimes cause cord compression. Children with extradural arachnoid cysts frequently develop kyphosis; the causal relationship remains unknown. In ankylosing spondylitis lumbosacral cysts produce a cauda equina syndrome.

SPINAL CORD AND ROOT COMPRESSION

SYRINGOMYELIA

Syringomyelia is the acquired development of a cavity (syrinx) within the central spinal cord. The lower cervical segments are usually affected, but extension may occur upwards into the brain stem (syringobulbia, see page 377) or downwards as far as the filum terminale.

The cavitation appears to develop in association with obstruction:
– around the foramen magnum in conjunction with the *Chiari malformation.*
– secondarily to *trauma* or *arachnoiditis.*

The syrinx may obliterate the central canal leaving clumps of ependymal cells in the wall. In contrast HYDROMYELIA is the congenital persistence and widening of the central canal.

Syringomyelia should be distinguished from cystic intramedullary tumours, although both pathologies may coexist.

Pathogenesis

The exact cause of this condition remains uncertain but theories abound. In 1965, Gardner proposed the *'hydrodynamic theory'*, suggesting that the craniovertebral anomaly may impair CSF outflow from the 4th ventricle to the cisterna magna. This in turn was believed to result in transmission of a CSF arterial pulse wave through a patent central canal, dilating the canal below the level of compression. This theory, however, does not explain the occurrence of syringomyelia in patients with non-patent central canals. It now seems likely that the normal free flow of CSF around the foramen magnum during the cardiac cycle becomes obstructed in patients with the Chiari malformation. In these patients downward movement of the tonsils occurs with each systole causing high CSF pressure waves which force CSF into the cord substance via the Virchow-Robin spaces (extension of the subarachnoid space around the blood vessels that penetrate the cord). This model does not require a patent central canal.

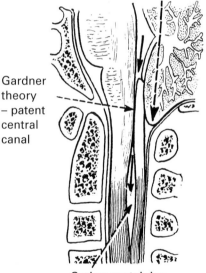

Type I Chiari malformation with cerebellar tonsils impacted in the foramen magnum.

Gardner theory – patent central canal

Syrinx containing fluid identical to CSF

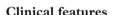

Clinical features

– *Dissociated sensory loss* (i.e. loss of pain and temperature sensation with retention of other senses) occurring in a cape-like distribution. Painless burns are a classic sign.
– *Wasting and weakness of the small muscles of the hand and winging of the scapula* from anterior horn cell involvement. *Scoliosis* often results.
– *Long tract signs* follow.
– *Brain stem signs* may appear, either from syringobulbia or an associated Chiari malformation.
– *Hydrocephalus* occurs in 25% but is usually asymptomatic.

397

SPINAL CORD AND ROOT COMPRESSION

SYRINGOMYELIA (*cont'd*)

Investigations

MRI is the investigation of choice (see page 376). This will demonstrate the syrinx with any associated Chiari malformation and exclude intramedullary tumour.

If MRI is unavailable – MYELOGRAPHY demonstrates widening of the spinal cord. With coexisting Chiari malformations, screening in the *supine* position will show the cerebellar tonsils descending below the foramen magnum.

Historically introduction of air into the CSF space – AIR MYELOGRAPHY – was used to 'collapse' the dilated segment thereby excluding an intrinsic cord tumour. A CT scan, six hours after injection of intrathecal contrast, may show uptake within the syrinx, but beware of misinterpreting normal contrast uptake within spinal cord tissue. Puncture of the syrinx is occasionally possible and subsequent injection of contrast shows its exact extent.

Management

The natural history is variable and operative techniques only of limited benefit. The approach depends on progression of symptoms and the presence or absence of an associated Chiari malformation.

If Chiari malformation is present – *decompression* by removing the posterior rim of the foramen magnum and posterior arch of the atlas and widening the dura with a patch, improves symptoms in most patients and should halt progression. This operation relieves the obstructed foramen magnum and alters the hydrodynamics of the syrinx. If deterioration continues, or if no associated Chiari malformation exists –

Syringostomy:

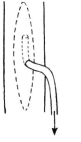

To CSF space
or peritoneum

The syrinx is drained via a silastic tube into the surrounding CSF space.

Alternatively, a syringoperitoneal shunt is performed. Some patients benefit from this procedure but in others, progressive deterioration continues.

Syringomyelia remains a difficult condition to treat. Draining the syrinx into the CSF space by syringostomy may not significantly alter the haemodynamics. Syringoperitoneal shunt may seem to be the most logical approach. Despite all efforts, about one-third of patients suffer progressive deterioration.

SPINAL CORD AND ROOT COMPRESSION

SPINAL INFECTION

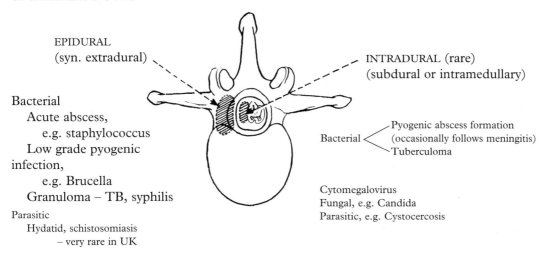

EPIDURAL
(syn. extradural)

INTRADURAL (rare)
(subdural or intramedullary)

Bacterial
  Acute abscess,
    e.g. staphylococcus
  Low grade pyogenic
infection,
    e.g. Brucella
  Granuloma – TB, syphilis
Parasitic
  Hydatid, schistosomiasis
    – very rare in UK

Bacterial ⟨ Pyogenic abscess formation
(occasionally follows meningitis)
Tuberculoma

Cytomegalovirus
Fungal, e.g. Candida
Parasitic, e.g. Cystocercosis

ACUTE EPIDURAL ABSCESS
Tend to occur in debilitated patients – diabetes, malignancy, liver or renal failure, intravenous drug abuse and alcoholism.

Organism: *Staphylococcus aureus* is the most common agent (90% of cases).

Spread: Haematogenous, e.g. from a boil or furuncle, or direct from vertebral osteomyelitis.

Site: Usually thoracic, but may affect any level and be extensive. Cord damage occurs either from direct compression or secondary to a thrombophlebitis and venous infarction.

Clinical features: Develops over several days mimicking a rapidly progressive extradural tumour or haematoma with bilateral leg weakness, a sensory level and urinary retention, but distinguishing features are:
  – very severe pain and tenderness over the involved site.
  – toxaemia: pyrexia, malaise, increased pulse rate.
  – rigidity of neck and spinal column, with marked resistance to flexion.

As the abscess extends upwards, the sensory level may rise.

Investigations: *Straight X-ray* may or may not show an associated osteitis or discitis.
An *MRI* or *myelogram* confirms the site of the extradural lesion.
CSF examination, if performed shows an increased white cell count, usually polymorphonuclear, but may be normal
A *leucocytosis* is usually present in the peripheral blood and the ESR raised.
Blood cultures are often positive.

Management: Urgent decompressive laminectomy and abscess drainage combined with intravenous antibiotic therapy over some weeks provide the best chance of recovery of function. In the cervical spine, anterior collections may be drained through the disc space.

SPINAL CORD AND ROOT COMPRESSION

SPINAL TUBERCULOSIS (Pott's disease of the spine)

In developing countries, spinal TB is mostly a disease of childhood or adolescence. In Britain it usually affects the middle aged and is particularly prevalent in immigrant populations and in the immunocompromised. The incidence is now increasing, probably due to the development of antibiotic resistance.

The lower thoracic spine is commonly involved and the disease initially affects the intravertebral disc and spreads to adjacent vertebral bodies.

Clinical features:

The classic systemic features of weight loss, night fever and cachexia are often absent.

Pain occurs over the affected area and is made worse by weight bearing.

Symptoms and signs of cord compression occur in approximately 20% of cases.

The onset may be gradual as pus, caseous material or granulation tissue accumulate, or sudden as vertebral bodies collapse and a kyphosis develops.

STRAIGHT X-RAYS are characteristic.

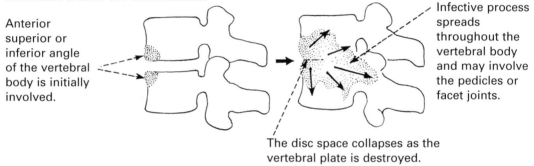

Anterior superior or inferior angle of the vertebral body is initially involved.

Infective process spreads throughout the vertebral body and may involve the pedicles or facet joints.

The disc space collapses as the vertebral plate is destroyed.

MRI with gadolinium shows an epidural mass with paraspinal soft tissue swelling.

Management:

Every effort is made to establish the diagnosis. A *needle biopsy* is often sufficient, but occasionally an exploratory operation (costotransversectomy) is required. Long-term *antituberculous therapy* is commenced.

If signs of cord compression develop, decompression is necessary.

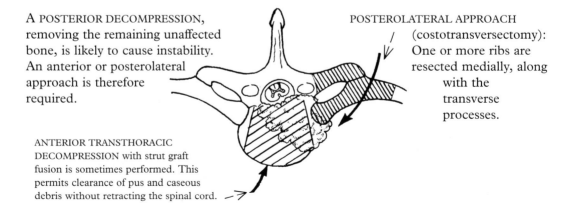

A POSTERIOR DECOMPRESSION, removing the remaining unaffected bone, is likely to cause instability. An anterior or posterolateral approach is therefore required.

POSTEROLATERAL APPROACH (costotransversectomy): One or more ribs are resected medially, along with the transverse processes.

ANTERIOR TRANSTHORACIC DECOMPRESSION with strut graft fusion is sometimes performed. This permits clearance of pus and caseous debris without retracting the spinal cord.

DISC PROLAPSE AND SPONDYLOSIS

Intervertebral discs act as shock absorbers for the bony spine.

A tough outer layer – the annulus fibrosis surrounds a softer central nucleus pulposus.

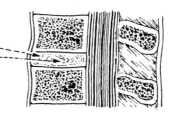

Discs degenerate with age, the fluid within the nucleus pulposus gradually drying out. Disc collapse produces excessive strain on the facet joints, i.e. the superior and inferior articulatory processes of each vertebral body, and leads to degeneration and hypertrophy.

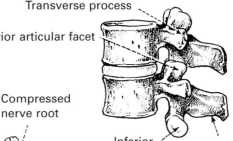

Transverse process

Superior articular facet

Inferior articular facet

Spinous process

LUMBAR DISC PROLAPSE

An *acute disc prolapse* occurs when the soft nucleus herniates through a tear in the annulus and may result from a single or repeated traumatic incidents. Herniation usually occurs posterolaterally and compresses adjacent nerve roots, but may occasionally occur centrally, compressing the cauda equina.

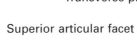

Facet joint

Compressed nerve root

Posterolateral disc protrusion

A 'free fragment' of the nucleus pulposus may extrude and lie above or below the level of the disc space.

Associated hypertrophy of degenerated facet joints is often a further source of back and leg pain and is an important cause of root compression.

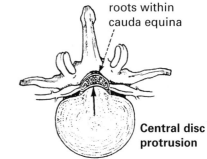

Compressed roots within cauda equina

Central disc protrusion

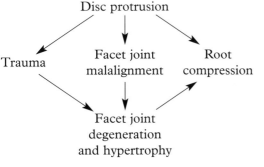

Disc protrusion

Trauma

Facet joint malalignment

Root compression

Facet joint degeneration and hypertrophy

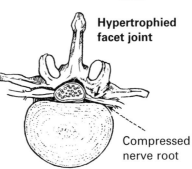

Hypertrophied facet joint

Compressed nerve root

LUMBAR DISC PROLAPSE

A *congenitally narrowed spinal canal* increases susceptibility to the development of nerve root compression. Here the spinal canal diameter is considerably diminished and minor disc protrusion or mild joint hypertrophy may more readily compress the nerve root.

Posterolateral disc herniations usually compress the nerve root exiting through the foramen below the affected level, e.g. an L3/4 disc lesion will compress the L4 nerve root, but large disc protrusions or a free fragment may compress any adjacent root.

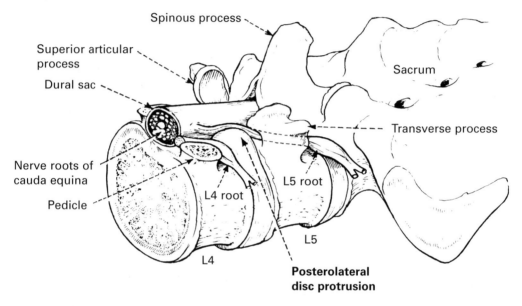

Lumbar disc lesions may occur at any level but L4/5 and L5/S1 are the commonest sites (95%).

CLINICAL FEATURES
Posterolateral disc protrusion

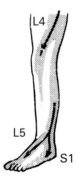

Injury: A history of falling, or lifting heavy weights often precedes the onset of symptoms.

Leg pain: Root irritation or compression produces pain in the distribution of the affected root and this should extend below the mid-calf. Coughing, sneezing or straining aggravates the leg pain which is usually more severe than any associated backache. If compression causes severe root damage the leg pain may disappear as neurological signs develop.

Paraesthesia: Numbness or tingling occurs in the distribution of the affected root.

LUMBAR DISC PROLAPSE

CLINICAL FEATURES (*cont'd*)

'MECHANICAL' SIGNS: Spinal movements are restricted, scoliosis is often present and is related to spasm of the erector spinae muscles, and the normal lumbar lordosis is lost.

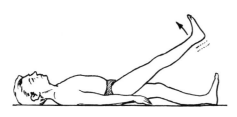

Straight leg raising: L5 and S1 root compression causes limitation to less than 60° from the horizontal and produces pain down the back of the leg.

Dorsiflexion of the foot while the leg is elevated aggravates the pain. Elevation of the 'good' leg may produce pain in the other leg.

(If in doubt about the veracity of a restricted straight leg raising deficit, sit the patient up on the examination couch with the legs straight. This is equivalent to 90° straight leg raising.)

Reverse leg raising (femoral stretch)

Tests for irritation of higher nerve roots (L4 and above)

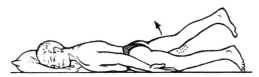

NEUROLOGICAL DEFICIT: Depends on the predominant root involved:

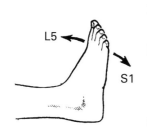

L4 – Quadriceps wasting and weakness; sensory impairment over medial calf; impaired knee jerk.

L5 – Wasting and weakness of dorsiflexors of foot, extensor digitorum longus and extensor hallucis longus; wasting of extensor digitorum brevis; sensory impairment over lateral calf and dorsum of foot.

S1 – Wasting and weakness of plantar flexors; sensory impairment over lateral aspect of foot and sole; impaired ankle jerk.

Root signs cannot reliably localise the level of disc protrusion due to variability of the anatomical distribution.

Central disc protrusion

Symptoms and signs of central disc protrusion are usually bilateral, although one side is often worse than the other.

Leg pain: Extends bilaterally down the back of the thighs. Pain may disappear with the onset of paralysis.

Paraesthesia: Occurs in the same distribution.

Sphincter paralysis: Loss of bladder and urethral sensation with intermittent or complete retention of urine occurs in most patients. Anal sensation is usually impaired and accompanies constipation.

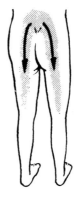

LUMBAR DISC PROLAPSE

Central disc protrusion (*cont'd*)

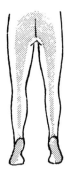

Severe pain associated with lateral disc protrusion may inhibit micturition. In this instance, strong analgesia should allow normal micturition; the presence of normal perineal sensation excludes root compression as the cause of the retention.

Sensory loss: Extends over all or part of the sacral area ('saddle' anaesthesia) and confirms a neurogenic cause for the sphincter disturbance.

Motor loss: Usually presents as foot drop with complete loss of power in the dorsiflexors and plantarflexors of both feet.

Reflex loss: The ankle jerks are usually absent on each side.

INVESTIGATION

Straight X-ray of lumbosacral spine is of limited benefit in the investigation of lumbar disc disease – it may show loss of a disc space or an associated spondylolisthesis (see p. 406). Straight X-rays are *important in excluding other pathology* such as metastatic carcinoma.

CT scanning of lowest three spaces will detect a disc protrusion and demonstrate the extent of root compression. CT scanning also clearly shows hypertrophy of the facet joints and the diameter of the spinal canal (see page 402).

NB *A patient with characteristic 'root' pain in whom CT scanning is negative requires an MRI to exclude a lesion involving the conus medullaris.*

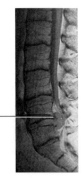

MRI is now the investigation of first choice. Sagittal views combined with axial views at the appropriate level will demonstrate disc disease and exclude a lesion at the conus.

T1 weighted sagittal MRI.

Radiculography shows a filling defect in the theca obliterating or displacing the nerve root sleeve at the disc level. A *CT radiculogram* may demonstrate nerve root displacement more clearly than MRI.

LUMBAR DISC PROLAPSE

Management

(a) Posterolateral disc protrusion

CONSERVATIVE: Most bouts of leg pain settle spontaneously by taking simple measures:
- *Analgesics*
- *Avoiding heavy lifting and bending.* Picking up objects from the floor
  should be performed by bending the knees and keeping the back straight
- Using an *orthopaedic mattress* or hard board under the mattress
- *Bed rest*, but *only* if pain prevents any movement
- *Traction* may help, but pain can return when traction is removed.

INDICATIONS FOR OPERATION
- Severe *unremitting leg pain* despite
  conservative measures.
- *Recurrent attacks* of leg pain,
  especially when causing repeated
  time loss from work.
- The development of a *neurological deficit.*

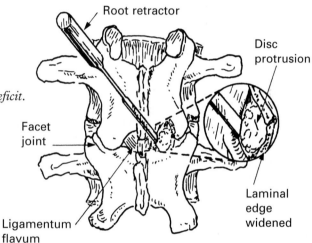

TECHNIQUE: Fenestration usually provides good access. Retraction of the root and dural sac exposes the disc protrusion and allows removal with rongeurs. Any protuberance from the facet joint causing root pressure or narrowing of the root canal is also removed. '**Microdiscectomy**' with an operating microscope allows disc removal through a smaller skin and muscle incision and may reduce the period of hospital care.

RESULTS: Over 80% of patients obtain good results after operation. The remainder may have recurrent problems due to a further disc protrusion at the same or another level. Root damage occurs in <1%.

After disc operation, patients are advised to avoid heavy lifting, preferably for an indefinite period. Persistance in a heavy manual job may lead to further trouble.

In general, patients with clear-cut indications for operation do well, whereas those with dubious clinical or radiographic signs tend to have a high incidence of residual or recurrent problems.

(b) Central disc protrusion

Compression of the cauda equina from a central disc usually requires urgent treatment, particularly if signs and symptoms have developed within 48 hours. The chance of recovery appears to depend on the extent of nerve root damage at the time of the decompression. If severe, e.g. painless urinary retention with overflow incontinence, outcome is poor and the timing of surgery may not influence the results. Recovery of function may continue for up to two years, but results are often disappointing. Although most regain bladder control, few have completely normal function and in many, disordered sexual function persists. In contrast to posterolateral protrusions, large central discs may require a one or two level laminectomy to minimise the risk of further root damage.

LUMBAR SPINAL STENOSIS

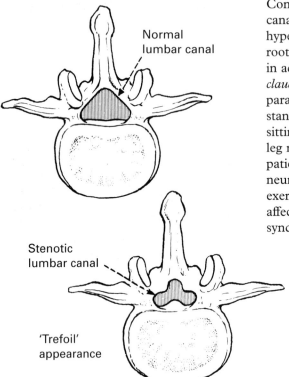

Normal
lumbar canal

Stenotic
lumbar canal

'Trefoil'
appearance

Congenital narrowing of the lumbar spinal canal, or secondary narrowing due to hypertrophic facet joints, may predispose to root compression from a herniated disc, but in addition may produce '*neurogenic claudication*'. Symptoms of root pain, paraesthesia or weakness develop after standing or walking and may be relieved by sitting, bending over or lying down. Straight leg raising is seldom impaired, in contrast to patients with disc protrusion. Objective neurological findings may only appear after exercise. In some patients this condition only affects one side – the 'unilateral facet syndrome'.

Plain X-rays may show thickened joints, but CT scanning, MRI or radiculography is required to establish the diagnosis.

Treatment: A wide laminectomy with root decompression usually produces good results with complete relief of symptoms.

SPONDYLOLISTHESIS

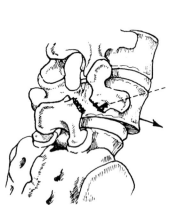

Spondylolisthesis is a forward shift of one vertebral body on another. Slip occurs due to degenerative disease of the facet joints (commonly at L4/L5) or to a developmental break or elongation of the L5 pars intraarticularis causing an L5/S1 spondylolisthesis.

L4

L5

Spondylolisthesis is often symptomless but the resultant narrowing in canal width may accentuate symptoms of root compression from disc protrusion or joint hypertrophy.

Treatment: usually conservative, but if signs of root compression are present, then decompression of the root canal is necessary. Occasionally fusion is required, especially if back pain predominates.

THORACIC DISC PROLAPSE

This occurs rarely (0.2% of all disc lesions) due to the relative rigidity of the thoracic spine.

PRESENTATION

– Root pain and/or
– Progressive or fluctuating paraparesis (may lead to mistaken diagnosis).

As vascular involvement may produce damage above the level of compression, sensory findings may be misleading.

INVESTIGATION

MRI is the investigation of choice and should clearly demonstrate the disc herniation and the extent of the associated cord compression.

CT myelography will clearly demonstrate the lesion if MRI is unavailable.

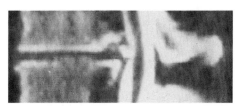

Sagittal reconstruction of CT myelogram showing cord compression from a T11/12 disc protrusion.

MANAGEMENT

Root pain – may settle with bed rest.

In the presence of cord compression or unremitting root pain, either a *posterolateral* or an *anterior transthoracic approach* is used to remove the disc. (A posterior approach – laminectomy – carries an unacceptably high risk of paraplegia.)

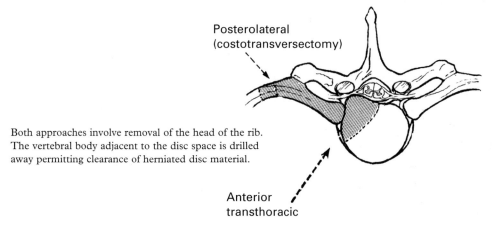

Posterolateral
(costotransversectomy)

Both approaches involve removal of the head of the rib.
The vertebral body adjacent to the disc space is drilled
away permitting clearance of herniated disc material.

Anterior
transthoracic

407

CERVICAL SPONDYLOSIS

The mobile cervical spine is particularly subject to osteoarthritic change and this occurs in more than half the population over 50 years of age; of these approximately 20% develop symptoms. Relatively few require operative treatment.

PATHOGENESIS

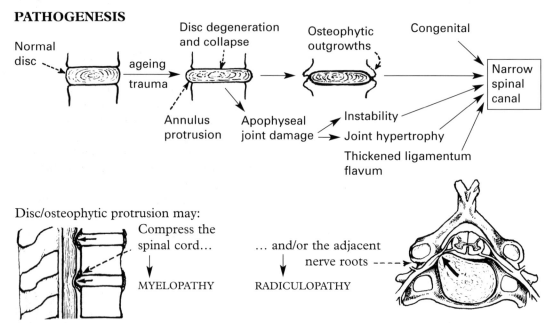

Disc/osteophytic protrusion may:

Compress the spinal cord...

MYELOPATHY

... and/or the adjacent nerve roots

RADICULOPATHY

Resultant damage to the spinal cord may arise from direct pressure or may follow vascular impairment. The onset is usually gradual. Trauma may or may not predispose to the development of symptoms.

CLINICAL FEATURES

Radiculopathy

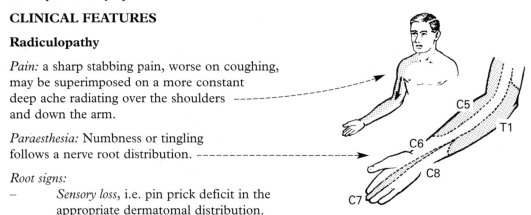

Pain: a sharp stabbing pain, worse on coughing, may be superimposed on a more constant deep ache radiating over the shoulders and down the arm.

Paraesthesia: Numbness or tingling follows a nerve root distribution.

Root signs:
- *Sensory loss,* i.e. pin prick deficit in the appropriate dermatomal distribution.
- *Muscle (l.m.n.) weakness* and wasting in appropriate muscle groups, e.g. C5, C6 . . . biceps, deltoid: C7 . . . triceps.
- *Reflex impairment/loss,* e.g. C5, 6 . . . biceps, supinator jerk: C7 . . . triceps jerk.
- *Trophic change:* In long-standing root compression, skin becomes dry, scaly, inelastic, blue and cold.

CERVICAL SPONDYLOSIS

CLINICAL FEATURES (*cont'd*)

Myelopathy

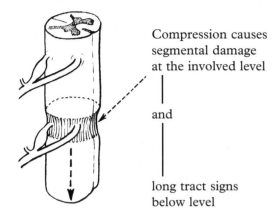

Compression causes segmental damage at the involved level

and

long tract signs below level

Arms: l.m.n. signs and symptoms, as above, at the level of the lesion
and/or
u.m.n. signs and symptoms below the level of the lesion

e.g. C5 lesion $\left\{\begin{array}{l}\text{deltoid and biceps}\\\text{weakness, wasting:}\\\text{diminished biceps jerk:}\\\text{increased finger jerks.}\end{array}\right.$

Legs: u.m.n. signs and symptoms, i.e. difficulty in walking due to stiffness; 'pyramidal' distribution weakness, increased tone, clonus and extensor plantar responses; sensory symptoms and signs are variable and less prominent.
Sphincter disturbance is seldom a prominent early feature.

N.B. Involved segments may extend above or below the level of compression if the vascular supply is also impaired.

INVESTIGATION

Plain X-ray of cervical spine

Look for:
– congenital narrowing of canal, loss of lordosis.
– disc space narrowing and osteophyte protrusion
   (foraminal encroachment is best seen in oblique views).
– subluxation. Flexion/extension views may be required.

MRI: the investigation of first choice. *Sagittal views* clearly demonstrate cord compression at the level of the disc space. Any hyperintensity within the cord on T2 weighting reflects cord damage and may correlate with the severity of the myelopathy and outcome. *Axial views* show cord compression and the degree of foraminal narrowing.

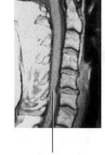

T1 weighted MR showing a C5/6 spondylotic bar

Myelography, particularly when combined with **CT scanning**, shows in detail the degree of spinal cord and nerve root compression from osteophytic outgrowth.

MANAGEMENT

Conservative
– Analgesics
– Cervical collar
– Traction

Symptoms of radiculopathy, whether acute or chronic, usually respond to these conservative measures plus reassurance. Progression of a disabling neurological deficit however demands surgical intervention. The clinician may adopt a conservative approach when a myelopathy is mild, but undue delay in operation may reduce the chance of recovery.

CERVICAL SPONDYLOSIS

MANAGEMENT (*cont'd*)

Indications for operation

1. Progressive neurological deficit – myelopathy or radiculopathy.
2. Intractable pain, when this fails to respond to conservative measures. This is rarely the sole indication for operation and usually applies to acute disc protrusion (see below) rather than chronic radiculopathy.

Operative techniques

1. *Anterior decompression and fusion*
   A core of bone and disc is drilled out allowing removal of the osteophytic projection. Although not essential, some combine this with a bone graft from the iliac crest.

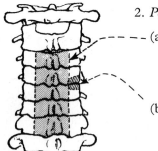

Bone and disc drilled away.

Osteophytes removed with curettes.

Bone graft fuses bodies

Suitable for root or cord compression from an anterior protrusion at one level, although two and even three levels may be decompressed by this method.

2. *Posterior approach*

    (a) *Laminectomy:* a wide decompression, usually from C3–C7, is carried out. Only suitable for multilevel cord compression especially when superimposed on a congenitally narrow spinal canal.

    (b) *Foraminotomy:* the nerve root at one or more levels may be decompressed by drilling away overlying bone.

Results
Operative results vary widely in different series and probably depend on patient selection. Some improvement occurs in 50–80% of patients. Operation should be aimed at preventing progression rather than curing all symptoms.

CERVICAL DISC PROLAPSE
In contrast to cervical spondylosis, cervical 'soft disc' protrusion is uncommon. This tends to occur acutely in younger patients and may be related to a specific incident such as a sudden twist or injury to the neck. The protrusion usually occurs posterolaterally at the C5/C6 or C6/C7 level causing a radiculopathy rather than a myelopathy. Sagittal and axial MRI (or CT myelography) will clearly outline the disc protrusion.

T2 weighted axis MRI showing disc protrusion

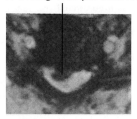

Operative removal through an anterior approach may be required for intractable pain or neurological deficit and gives good results.

410

SPINAL TRAUMA

Approximately 2 per 100 000 of the population per year sustain a spinal injury. Of these, 50% involve the cervical region.

At impact, *spinal cord damage* may or may not accompany the *bony or ligamentous damage*. After impact, stability at the level of injury plays a crucial part in further management. Injudicious movement of a patient with an unstable lesion may precipitate spinal cord injury or aggravate any pre-existing damage.

MECHANISMS OF INJURY

The mechanism of injury helps determine the degree of stability:

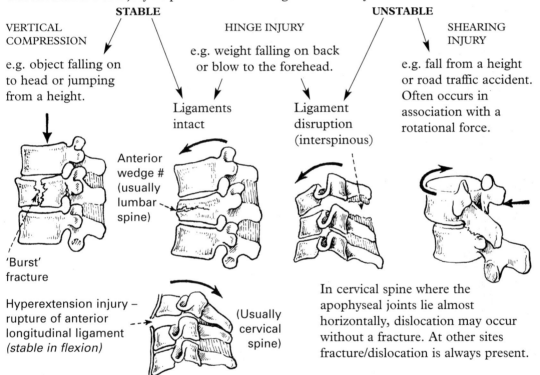

STABLE

VERTICAL COMPRESSION

e.g. object falling on to head or jumping from a height.

'Burst' fracture

HINGE INJURY

e.g. weight falling on back or blow to the forehead.

Ligaments intact

Anterior wedge # (usually lumbar spine)

Hyperextension injury – rupture of anterior longitudinal ligament *(stable in flexion)*

(Usually cervical spine)

Ligament disruption (interspinous)

UNSTABLE

SHEARING INJURY

e.g. fall from a height or road traffic accident. Often occurs in association with a rotational force.

In cervical spine where the apophyseal joints lie almost horizontally, dislocation may occur without a fracture. At other sites fracture/dislocation is always present.

Initial assessment

The *possibility of spinal injury must be considered* at the scene of the accident and all movements and transportation of the patient undertaken with extreme caution especially when comatose. Most spinal injuries occur in conscious patients who complain of *pain, numbness* or *difficulty with limb movements*.

Examination may reveal *tenderness over the spinous processes, paraspinal swelling* or *a gap between the spinous processes*, indicating rupture of an interspinous ligament.

Neurogenic paradoxical ventilation (indrawing of the chest on inspiration due to absent intercostal function) may occur with cervical cord damage.

Bilateral absence of limb reflexes in flaccid limbs, unresponsive to painful stimuli, indicates spinal cord damage (unless death is imminent from severe head injury.)

Painless urinary retention or *priapism* may also occur.

411

SPINAL TRAUMA – INVESTIGATIONS

STRAIGHT X-RAYS

LATERAL VIEW

In the *cervical spine:*
– note evidence of *soft tissue swelling* between the pharynx and the vertebrae.

– ensure *C6 and C7* are included in the film. If not, repeat with gentle downward arm traction, or do a CT scan.

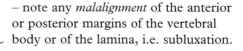

– note any *malalignment* of the anterior or posterior margins of the vertebral body or of the lamina, i.e. subluxation.

– note any undue *widening of the interspinous distance or of the disc space.*

– note *damage to the vertebral body, apophyseal joints, lamina or spinous process,* e.g. anterior wedge collapse, 'burst' fracture.

In the upper thoracic spine only **Tomography** may satisfactorily demonstrate the lateral view.

ANTERO-POSTERIOR VIEW
– note the *alignment* of the spinous processes and the *width of the apophyseal joints* and look for *vertical* fracture lines.

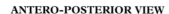

ANTERO-POSTERIOR 'OPEN MOUTH' VIEW
– may be required to demonstrate a *fracture of the odontoid peg.*

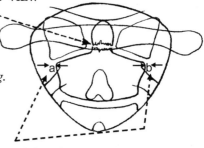

In fractures of C1, if the lateral masses project beyond C2 > 7 mm (i.e. a + b), the transverse ligament is likely to be disrupted indicating an unstable injury (Rule of Spence).

If doubt remains – take **OBLIQUE VIEWS** to demonstrate the intervertebral foramina.

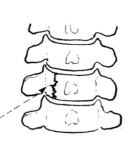

CERVICAL
SPINE

Disruption of the foraminal outline suggests malalignment

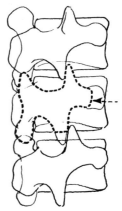

In the LUMBAR spine look for the normal '*scotty dog*' appearance – if misshapen, suggests a fracture/ dislocation.

If in doubt about cervical stability, take **FLEXION/ EXTENSION VIEWS,** but only with expert supervision.

SPINAL TRAUMA – INVESTIGATIONS/MANAGEMENT

CT SCANNING

CT may demonstrate more extensive fracturing than suspected on plain X-rays and aids identification of regions not clearly shown.

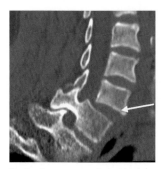

Sagittal reconstruction showing dislocation of the cervico-thoracic junction

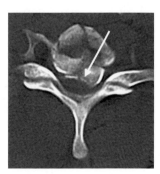

Axial views showing a burst fracture of the vertebral body with retropulsed fragments compromising the spinal canal

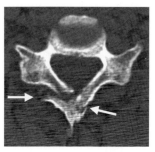

Axial views demonstrating fractures of the lamina and spinal process

MRI may provide additional information of soft disc prolapse or haematoma within the spinal canal, but seldom influences management.

MANAGEMENT

Management depends on the site and stability of the lesion, but basic principles apply.

1. An *unstable* lesion risks further damage to the spinal cord and roots and requires either
   – *operative fixation* or
   – *immobilisation*, e.g. skull traction, Halo or plaster jacket.

2. There is no evidence that 'decompressing' the cord lesion (either anteriorly or posteriorly) improves the neurological outcome, but –

3. If a patient with normal cord function or with an incomplete cord lesion (i.e. with some residual function) *progressively deteriorates*, then *operative decompression* is required.

Many additional therapies and techniques (e.g. steroids, cord cooling, hyperbaric oxygen) have been employed with the aim of improving neurological outcome. Although initial trials with METHYLPREDNISOLONE suggested benefit when given within 8 hours of injury, concern has been raised about the methodological techniques applied. Its use may be associated with an increased incidence of infective complications and its value in improving functional outcome remains unproven.

SPINAL TRAUMA – MANAGEMENT

Management of injury at specific sites

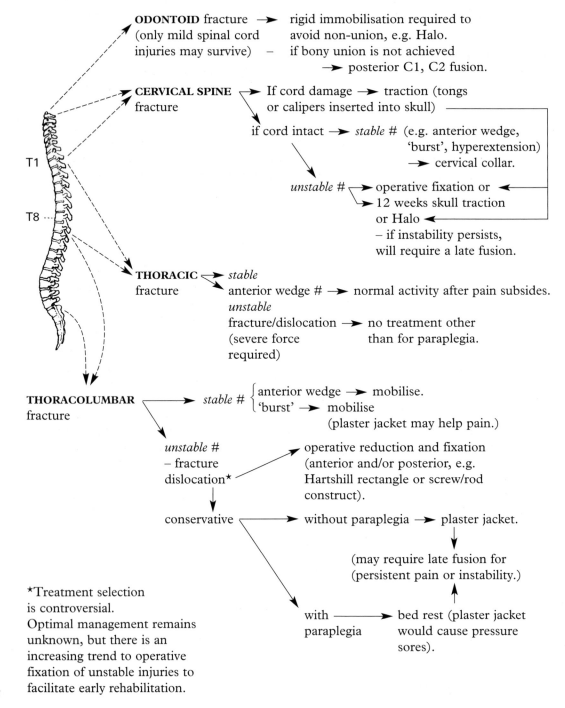

ODONTOID fracture → rigid immobilisation required to
(only mild spinal cord   avoid non-union, e.g. Halo.
injuries may survive) – if bony union is not achieved
                              → posterior C1, C2 fusion.

CERVICAL SPINE → If cord damage → traction (tongs
fracture   or calipers inserted into skull)

if cord intact → *stable* # (e.g. anterior wedge,
                              'burst', hyperextension)
                              → cervical collar.

unstable # → operative fixation or ←
            → 12 weeks skull traction
            or Halo ←
            – if instability persists,
            will require a late fusion.

THORACIC → *stable*
fracture   anterior wedge # → normal activity after pain subsides.
              unstable
              fracture/dislocation → no treatment other
              (severe force   than for paraplegia.
              required)

THORACOLUMBAR ——→ *stable* # { anterior wedge → mobilise.
fracture   'burst' → mobilise
                                          (plaster jacket may help pain.)

unstable #   operative reduction and fixation
– fracture   (anterior and/or posterior, e.g.
dislocation*   Hartshill rectangle or screw/rod
                                construct).

conservative ——→ without paraplegia → plaster jacket.

                              (may require late fusion for
                              (persistent pain or instability.)

with ——→ bed rest (plaster jacket
paraplegia   would cause pressure
              sores).

*Treatment selection
is controversial.
Optimal management remains
unknown, but there is an
increasing trend to operative
fixation of unstable injuries to
facilitate early rehabilitation.

SPINAL TRAUMA – MANAGEMENT

Management of the paraplegic patient

After spinal cord injury, transfer to a spinal injury centre with medical and nursing staff skilled in the management of the paraplegic patient provides optimal daily care and rehabilitation.

Important features include:

1. *Skin care* – requires meticulous attention. Two-hourly turning should prevent pressure sores. Attempt to avoid contact with bony prominences or creases in the bed sheets. Air or water beds or a sheepskin may help.

2. *Urinary tract* – long-term catheter drainage or intermittent self-catheterisation is required. Infection requires prompt treatment. Eventually, training may permit automatic reflex function (in cord lesions) or micturition by abdominal compression (in root lesions). In some, urodynamic studies may indicate possible benefit from bladder neck resection.

3. *Limbs* – intensive physiotherapy helps prevent flexion contractures (in cord injury) and plays an essential role in rehabilitation.

OUTCOME FOLLOWING SPINAL CORD OR ROOT INJURY

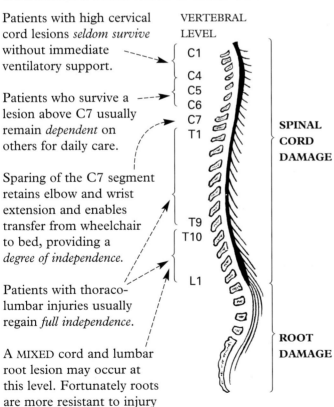

VERTEBRAL LEVEL

Patients with high cervical cord lesions *seldom survive* without immediate ventilatory support.

Patients who survive a lesion above C7 usually remain *dependent* on others for daily care.

Sparing of the C7 segment retains elbow and wrist extension and enables transfer from wheelchair to bed, providing a *degree of independence.*

Patients with thoraco-lumbar injuries usually regain *full independence.*

A MIXED cord and lumbar root lesion may occur at this level. Fortunately roots are more resistant to injury – '*root escape*' – and the outlook is more favourable.

SPINAL CORD DAMAGE

'COMPLETE': if no sign of motor or sensory function within 24 hours, then recovery will not occur. (The early return of anal and penile reflexes is not necessarily a good sign.) After a few days or weeks, tone returns to the flaccid limbs and reflexes become brisk. Flexor spasms may follow with the risk of contractures. A reflex bladder develops with automatic emptying.

'INCOMPLETE': any retention of motor or sensory function indicates an incomplete lesion with the potential for recovery.

ROOT DAMAGE

Recovery may theoretically occur as the roots regenerate, perhaps only after many months delay. The limbs remain flaccid throughout.

415

VASCULAR DISEASES OF THE SPINAL CORD

Blood supply to the spinal cord is complex; the main vessels are the anterior and posterior spinal arteries.

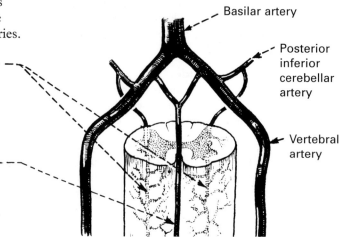

Basilar artery

Posterior inferior cerebellar artery

Vertebral artery

The posterior spinal arteries: usually arise from the posterior inferior cerebellar arteries and form a plexus on the posterior surface of the spinal cord.

The anterior spinal artery: branches from each vertebral artery unite to form a single vessel lying in the median fissure of the spinal cord.

Vertebral artery

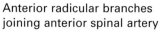

Both anterior and posterior spinal arteries run the length of the spinal cord and receive anastomotic vessels.

The plexus of the posterior spinal artery is joined by approximately 12 *unpaired* radicular feeding arteries. This rich collateral circulation protects the posterior part of the spinal cord from vascular disease.

The anterior spinal artery has a much less efficient collateral supply and is thus more vulnerable to the effects of vascular disease. It is joined by 7–10 *unpaired* radicular branches, usually from the left side.

Cervical arteries arise from vertebral and subclavian vessels, form plexuses and supply the cervical and upper thoracic cord.

Intercostal artery branches supply the midthoracic cord.

Anterior spinal artery is at its narrowest at T8. This level of the spinal cord is liable to damage during hypertension – watershed area.

Artery of Adamkiewicz, the largest radicular artery, supplies the low thoracic and lumbar cord. It usually arises at T9–L2 level and is on the left side in 70% of the population.

Sacral arteries arise from the hypogastric artery and supply the sacral cord and cauda equina.

Anterior radicular branches joining anterior spinal artery

VASCULAR DISEASES OF THE SPINAL CORD

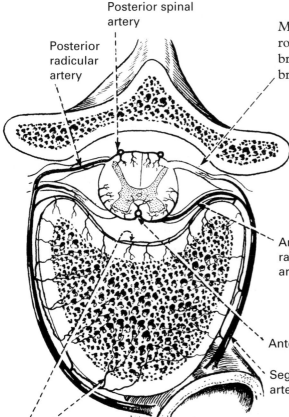

Posterior spinal artery territory
– Posterior one-third of spinal cord.
– Dorsal column.

Virtually no anastomotic communication.

Anterior spinal artery territory
Penetrating branches – anterior and part of
posterior grey matter.
Circumferential branches – anterior white matter.
– Anterior two-thirds of spinal cord.

Posterior spinal artery

Posterior radicular artery

Most radicular vessels only supply the root. On average 12 posterior radicular branches and 8 anterior radicular branches supply the spinal cord.

Atherosclerosis of spinal arteries is rare. When infarction occurs in the anterior spinal artery territory it is often a consequence of disease in the vessels of origin of the segmental arteries, i.e. atheroma or dissection of the aorta.

Anterior radicular artery

Anterior spinal artery

Segmental artery

Aorta

Section through spinal cord in thoracic region.

Rich anastomotic network occurs between each segmental artery through the vertebral body and across the extradural space

417

VASCULAR DISEASES OF THE SPINAL CORD

SPINAL CORD INFARCTION

Anterior spinal artery syndrome

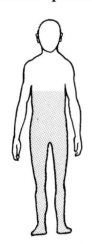

The level at which infarction occurs determines symptoms and signs. Characteristic features include:
– Radicular pain at onset
– Sudden para/quadraplegia
– Flaccid limbs ——$\xrightarrow{\text{days}}$ spastic
– Areflexia ——$\xrightarrow{\text{days}}$ hyper-reflexia and extensor plantar responses
– Sensory loss to pain and temperature up to the level of cord damage
– Preserved vibration and joint position sensation (dorsal columns supplied by the posterior spinal arteries)
– Urinary retention

When only penetrating branches are involved, long tract damage may be selective and sensory loss may be minor.

Spinal cord ischaemia due to aortic atheroma evolves slowly and preferentially affects anterior horn cells.

A pure conus syndrome (page 390) occasionally occurs.

Investigative approach
– *Exclude* other causes of acute para/quadriplegia – cord compression, Guillain Barré syndrome – by appropriate imaging or neurophysiology
– *Confirm* spinal ischaemia by MRI (T2 weighted imaging showing hyperintense signal changes)
– *Explore* possible sources of spinal ischaemia

Small vessel diseases
    diabetes – random or fasting blood glucose
    vasculitis – see pages 263–265
    neurosyphilis – CSF VDRL, FTA and TPI tests (see page 494)
    endarteritis secondary to – CSF meningeal infection or granulomatous disease

aortic (large) vessel diseases
    atheromatous – vascular risk factor e.g. cholesterol
    embolic – echocardiography, blood cultures
    thrombotic – coagulation screen
    dissection/aneurysm – transoesophageal echo (TOE) angiography
    hypotension – ECG, cardiac enzymes

Treatment is symptomatic and the outcome variable.

Posterior spinal artery syndrome
This is rare as white matter structures are less vulnerable to ischaemia. The dorsal columns are damaged and ischaemia may extend into the posterior horns.

Clinical features: – Loss of tendon reflexes/motor weakness
                  – Loss of joint position sense.

Venous infarction
A rapid 'total' cord syndrome with poor outcome often associated with pelvic sepsis.

VASCULAR DISEASES OF THE SPINAL CORD

SPINAL ARTERIOVENOUS MALFORMATION (Angiomatous malformation)

Arterio-venous malformations (AVMs) are congenital abnormalities of blood vessels rather than neoplastic growths. Arteries communicating directly with veins bypass the capillary network which has failed to develop, creating a 'shunt'. The AVM appears as a mass of convoluted dilated vessels.

Site

Cervical: uncommon site (~15%)
Arises from the anterior spinal artery and usually lies within the cord substance (intramedullary).

Upper thoracic: (20%)

Thoracolumbar: this is the commonest site (~ 65%). Most are *dural arterio-venous fistula* where the branches of the radicular artery drain directly into the dural venous plexus; in others the radicular artery drains into the dorsal spinal venous plexus.

Intramedullary lesions at this site are less common.

Spinal AVMs may present clinically at any age in either sex, but dural lesions are most common in males between 40–70 years of age.

Clinical features

SUDDEN ONSET (10–15%)

Due to – subarachnoid haemorrhage: headache, neck stiffness, back and leg pain
    – extradural haematoma
    – subdural haematoma   } signs of acute cord damage.
    – intramedullary haematoma (haematomyelia)

GRADUAL ONSET (85–90%)

Probably due to ↑ *venous pressure* but other factors may play a part:
– venous thrombosis
– 'steal' phenomenon
– venous bulk
– arachnoiditis (if previous bleed).

Progressive deterioration of all spinal modalities simulating cord compression. Pain is common. With thoracolumbar lesions a mixed u.m.n./l.m.n. weakness in the legs is typical. Intramedullary AVMs may cause fluctuating signs and symptoms and may mimic intermittent claudication.

A bruit may be heard overlying a spinal AVM and occasionally midline cutaneous lesions – haemangiomas, naevi or angiolipomas – are found. (Note that cutaneous angiomas are not uncommon and do not necessarily imply an underlying lesion.)

VASCULAR DISEASES OF THE SPINAL CORD

Investigation

MRI will demonstrate abnormal signal from the lesion or from draining veins. *Myelography* will also demonstrate abnormal draining veins. *Selective angiography* is required to delineate arterial feeders.

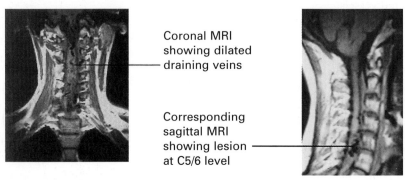

Coronal MRI showing dilated draining veins

Corresponding sagittal MRI showing lesion at C5/6 level

Management

Untreated, 50% of patients with gradual onset of symptoms would be unable to walk within 3 years. Treatment should prevent progression and may well improve a gait or bladder disturbance. Delay may result in irreversible cord damage.

Techniques: *Embolisation* – may successfully obliterate dural AVMs, particularly when fed by one or two dural arteries
– may aid subsequent operative treatment
– or may produce symptomatic improvement in inoperable lesions.

        Surgery – It is important to identify and divide the feeding vessel and excise the shunt. Total excision of all the dilated veins is unnecessary and hazardous. Operative risk for most dural A-V fistula is low and excision provides an alternative to embolisation. In contrast, when an AVM lies within the cord substance and/or ventral to the cord, operative risks are high. Staged pre-operative embolisation may help, but in some, a conservative approach may be appropriate.

Spinal Epidural and Subdural Haematomas: These may present with a rapid onset of paraplegia. Epidural or less commonly, subdural haematoma may occur due to rupture of a spinal AVM, after minor trauma or lumbar puncture, or spontaneously in patients with a bleeding disorder, liver disease or on anticoagulant therapy. MRI (or myelography) clearly demonstrates the lesion. Urgent decompression is required after correcting any coagulation deficit, without waiting for spinal angiography. Pathological examination of the haematoma may reveal angiomatous tissue; in other patients, there is no evident cause.

SPINAL DYSRAPHISM

SPINAL DYSRAPHISM: This term encompasses all defects (open or closed) associated with a failure of closure of the posterior neural arch.

Embryology

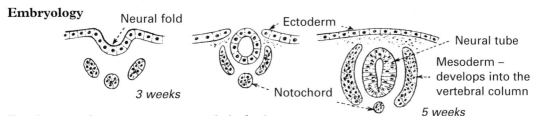

Developmental errors may occur early in fetal life and lead to a variety of spinal defects:

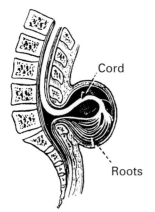
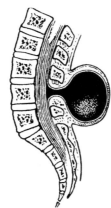
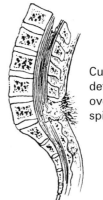

MYELOMENINGOCELE
The spinal cord and roots protrude through the bony defect and lie within a cystic cavity, lined with meninges and/or skin. In most patients, the meningeal covering ruptures and the spinal cord and roots lie exposed to the air – myelodysplasia. CSF may leak from the open lesion.

MENINGOCELE
Cystic CSF filled cavity – lined with meninges but devoid of neural tissue. The cavity communicates with the spinal canal through the bone defect (usually lumbosacral). Meningoceles occur far less frequently than myelomeningocele; they are rarely associated with other congenital anomalies.

SPINA BIFIDA OCCULTA
A bony deficit – present in 5–10% of the population and not clinically significant. Those who also have a lumbosacral cutaneous abnormality however (*tuft of hair, dimple, sinus or 'port wine' stain*) have a high incidence of related underlying defects:
– *diastomatomyelia*
– *lipoma*
– *dermoid cyst*.
These defects may cause symptoms of pain or neurological impairment after many years.

Site: 80% occur in the lumbosacral region.
Incidence: 2/1000 births in the UK, but geographical variation exists (0.2/1000 in Japan) and the incidence is declining. A familial incidence increases the risk (5% if a sibling is affected). Both genetic factors and teratogens, e.g. sodium valproate, have a role. Folic acid before and during pregnancy provides some protection.
Associated abnormalities: *Hydrocephalus, Chiari type II,* aqueduct forking.

421

SPINAL DYSRAPHISM

Clinical assessment

Myelomeningocele: This lesion should be carefully examined for the presence of neural elements. Transillumination of the sac may help. Observation of movement in the limbs and in specific muscle groups, occurring spontaneously and in response to pain applied both above and below the level of the lesion, helps determine the degree and level of neurological damage. Also note the presence of a dilated bladder and a patulous anal sphincter. Look for any associated congenital anomalies, e.g. hydrocephalus, scoliosis, foot deformities.

Meningocele: Patients with this lesion seldom show any neurological deficit.

Investigations

Ultrasound or *MRI* may detect neural elements extending into the sac.

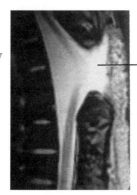

MRI showing a thoracic myelomeningocele with spinal cord extending through the deficit.

Management

Myelomeningocele: Advances in both orthopaedic and urological procedures have considerably improved the long-term management of the associated disabilities in most patients. Active treatment, however, in patients with gross hydrocephalus, complete paraplegia and other multiple anomalies as well as the spinal dysraphism, may merely prolong a painful existence. In these patients, many adopt a thoughtful conservative approach.

Immediate treatment requires closure and replacement of the neural tissues into the spinal canal to prevent infection. If necessary, this initial step provides more time to consider the wisdom of embarking on further active management.

Meningocele: In the presence of a CSF leak, urgent excision is performed; otherwise this is deferred, perhaps indefinitely if the lesion is small.

Spina bifida occulta: Treatment may not be required, although patients with a cutaneous abnormality or with neurological signs, should undergo ultrasound or MRI to exclude an intraspinal anomaly.

Antenatal diagnosis

Screening the maternal serum/amniotic fluid for alpha-fetoprotein and acetylcholinesterase, fetal ultrasonography and contrast enhanced amniography in high risk patients (e.g. with an affected sibling) provides an effective method of detecting neural tube defects. This gives the parents the possibility of therapeutic abortion and in the long term may reduce the incidence of this condition.

SPINAL DYSRAPHISM

TETHERED CORD: in some patients the conus medullaries lies well below its normal level (L1), *'tethered'* by the filum terminale. Since vertebral growth proceeds more rapidly than growth of the spinal cord, tethering may produce progressive back pain or neurological impairment as the cord is stretched.

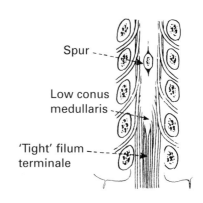

Spur

Low conus
medullaris

'Tight' filum
terminale

DIASTOMATOMYELIA: A congenital splitting of part of the spinal cord by a *bony, fibrous or cartilaginous* spur. This usually lies at the upper lumbar region and extends directly across the spinal canal in an antero-posterior direction. The split cord does not always reunite distal to the spur (diplomyelia).

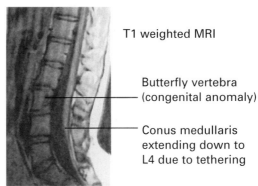

T1 weighted MRI

Butterfly vertebra
(congenital anomaly)

Conus medullaris
extending down to
L4 due to tethering

Investigation: MRI is the investigation of choice in spinal dysraphism, but straight X-ray may reveal associated congenital abnormalities: spina bifida occulta, fused or hemivertebrae. CT scanning may help demonstrate the presence of a bony spur.

Management: Although some recommend prophylactic division of the tethered filum terminale in the absence of neurological impairment, most reserve operative treatment for those who present with a neurological deficit, especially if there is evidence of progression, or prior to correction of any spinal deformity. In contrast, prophylactic removal of the spur in patients with diastomatomyelia is usually performed, even in the absence of neurological impairment.

LIPOMENINGOCELE

Lipomas may occur in association with spinal dysraphism and range from purely intraspinal lesions to very large masses extending along with neural tissues through the bony defect. All are adherent to the conus and closely related to the lumbosacral roots, preventing complete removal and increasing operative hazards.

CONGENITAL DERMAL SINUS TRACT/DERMOID CYST

This congenital defect results from a failure of separation of neuronal from epithelial ectoderm and may occur with other midline fusion defects, e.g. diastomatomyelia and a tethered cord. A tiny sinus in the lumbosacral region may represent the opening of a blind ending duct or may extend into the spinal canal. Dermoid cysts arise at any point along the sinus tract and often lie adjacent to the conus.

Clinical presentation varies from repeated attacks of unexplained meningitis to neurological deficits arising from the presence of an intraspinal mass. Treatment involves excision of the whole tract and any associated cyst (after treating any meningitic infection).

LOCALISED NEUROLOGICAL DISEASE AND ITS MANAGEMENT

C. PERIPHERAL NERVE AND MUSCLE

THE POLYNEUROPATHIES – FUNCTIONAL ANATOMY

The function of the peripheral nervous system is to carry impulses to and from the central nervous system. These impulses regulate motor, sensory and autonomic activities.

The peripheral nervous system is comprised of structures that lie outside the pial membrane of the brainstem and spinal cord and can be divided into cranial, spinal and autonomic components.

STRUCTURE OF THE NERVE CELL AND AXON

Each axon represents an elongation of the nerve cell – lying within the central nervous system, e.g. anterior horn cell, or in an outlying ganglion, e.g. dorsal root ganglion. The cell body maintains the viability of the axon, being the centre of all cellular metabolic activity.

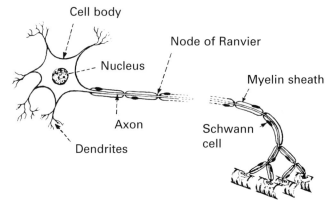

Many axons are surrounded by an insulation of myelin, which is enveloped by the Schwann cell membrane. Myelin is a protein–lipid complex. The membrane of the Schwann cell 'spirals' around the axon resulting in the formation of a multilayered myelin sheath.

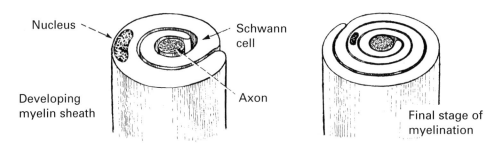

All axons have a cellular sheath – Schwann cell – but not all axons are myelinated.

Schwann cells with associated myelin are 250–1000 µm in length and separated from each other by the node of Ranvier. The axon is bare at this node and, during conduction, impulses jump from one node to the next – *saltatory* conduction. The rate of conduction in myelinated nerves is markedly increased in comparison with unmyelinated fibres. Myelin thus facilitates fast conduction. In unmyelinated fibres conduction depends upon the diameter of the nerve fibre, this determining the rate of longitudinal current flow.

THE POLYNEUROPATHIES – FUNCTIONAL ANATOMY

SPINAL PERIPHERAL NERVOUS SYSTEM

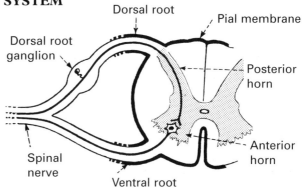

Entry to and exit from the central nervous system is achieved by paired spinal nerve roots (30 in all).

These dorsal and ventral roots lie in the spinal subarachnoid space and come together at the intervertebral foramen to form the spinal nerve.

The dorsal roots contains sensory fibres, arising from specialised sensory receptors in the periphery.

The dorsal root ganglia are collections of sensory cell bodies with axons extending peripherally as well as a central process which passes into the spinal cord in the region of the posterior horn of grey matter and makes appropriate central connections.

Sensation can be divided into:
- *Pain and temperature*
- *Simple touch*
- *Discriminatory sensation* – proprioception, vibration.

These different forms of sensation are carried from the periphery by axons with specific characteristics. The central connections and pathways vary also (see page 198).

The anterior horns of the spinal cord contain cell bodies whose axons pass to the periphery to innervate skeletal muscle – the alpha motor neurons. Smaller cell bodies also project into the anterior root and innervate the intrafusal muscle fibres of muscle spindles – the gamma motor neurons.

Each alpha motor neuron through its peripheral ramifications will innervate a number of muscle fibres. The number of fibres innervated from a single cell varies from less than 20 in the eye muscles to more than 1000 in the large limb muscles (innervation ratio). The alpha motor neuron with its complement of muscle fibres is termed the *motor unit*.

PERIPHERAL NERVES

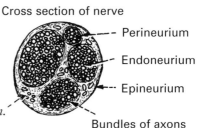

Cross section of nerve

Peripheral nerves are composed of many axons bound together by connective tissue. A 'mixed' nerve contains motor, sensory and autonomic axons.

The blood supply to these bundles is by means of small nutrient vessels within the epineurium – the *vasa nervorum.*

427

THE POLYNEUROPATHIES – FUNCTIONAL ANATOMY

PERIPHERAL NERVES (cont'd)
Nerve fibre type
Axons within the peripheral nerve vary structurally. This is related to function. Three distinct fibre types can be distinguished:

TYPE A   2–20 µm in diameter.
              Myelinated.
  Function: Motor and sensory (vibration, proprioception).
              Conduction velocity: 10–70 metres/second.

TYPE B   3 µm diameter.
              Thinly myelinated.
  Function: Mainly preganglionic autonomic, some pain and temperature.
              Conduction velocity: 7–5 metres/second.

TYPE C   <1 µm diameter.
              Unmyelinated.
  Function: Sensory – pain and temperature.
              Conduction velocity: <2 metres/second.

The structure of the spinal peripheral nervous system has been considered but the arrangement is also important. Spinal nerves, after emerging from the intervertebral foramen pass into the brachial plexus to supply the upper limbs and the lumbosacral plexus to supply the lower limbs.

The thoracic nerves supply skeletal muscles and subserve sensation of the thorax and abdomen.

The Autonomic Nervous System is described on page 455.

PATTERNS OF INJURY

Damage may occur to: axon, myelin sheath, cell body, supporting connective tissue and nutrient blood supply to nerves. Three basic pathological processes occur.

WALLERIAN DEGENERATION

Degeneration of axon distally following its interruption

SEGMENTAL DEMYELINATION

DISTAL AXONAL DEGENERATION

Distal to injury the axon disintegrates and the myelin breaks up into globules.

Approximation of nerve ends result in regeneration. The basement membrane of the Schwann cell survives and acts as a skeleton along which the axon regrows.

Scattered destruction of the myelin sheath occurs without axonal damage.

The primary lesion affects the Schwann cell. Prognosis for recovery is good because the muscle is not denervated.

Damage to the cell body or to the axon will affect the viability of the axon which will 'die back' from the periphery. Loss of the myelin sheath occurs as a secondary event.

Recovery is slow because the axon must regenerate. When the cell body is destroyed reinnervation of muscle can only occur from surrounding nerves.

THE POLYNEUROPATHIES – SYMPTOMS

Sensory

Negative phenomena – loss of sensation.

Disease of *large myelinated fibres* produces loss of touch and joint position perception.

Patients complain of difficulty in discriminating textures. Their hands and feet feel like cotton wool. Gait is unsteady, especially when in darkness where vision cannot compensate for loss of joint position sensation (proprioception).

Disease of *small unmyelinated fibres* produces loss of pain and temperature appreciation as a consequence of which painless burns/trauma result. Damage to joints without pain results in a 'neuropathic' joint (Charcot's joint) in which traumatic deformity is totally painless.

Positive phenomena

Disease of *large myelinated fibres* produces paraesthesia – a 'pins and needles' sensation with a peripheral distal distribution.

Disease of *small unmyelinated fibres* produces painful positive phenomena:

International Association for the Study of Pain (IASP) definitions has clarified the following.
- analgesia   absent sensitivity to a painful stimulus
- hyperalgesia   increased sensitivity to a painful stimulus
- hypoalgesia   reduced sensitivity to painful stimulus
- hyperaesthesia increased sensitivity to any stimulus
- hypoaesthesia   reduced sensitivity to any stimulus
- hyperpathia   increased sensitivity with increasing threshold to repetitive stimulation
- allodynia   pain provoked by a non-painful stimulus

Complex regional pain syndromes (CRPS) were previously termed 'reflex sympathetic dystrophy' and 'causalgia'. These may follow a simple soft tissue injury (CRPS-1) or injury to a large peripheral nerve (CRPS-2). Allodynia and hyperalgesia are associated with local changes in temperature and skin appearance (oedema and discoloration). The pain has a burning, shooting quality. Motor manifestations (weakness or involuntary movements) are common and the pathophysiologic mechanism unknown.

Motor
The patient notices weakness:
- When distal, e.g. difficulty in clearing the kerb when walking
- When proximal, e.g. difficulty in climbing stairs or combing hair
- Cramps may be troublesome
- Twitching of muscles (fasciculation) may be felt.

THE POLYNEUROPATHIES – SIGNS

SENSORY EXAMINATION

All modalities are tested
Light touch ⎫
Two point discrimination ⎬ Functions of large myelinated sensory fibres.
Vibration sensation ⎪
Joint position perception ⎭

Temperature perception ⎫ Functions of small unmyelinated
Pain perception. ⎭ and thinly myelinated sensory fibres.

Initially the area of total sensory loss is defined. The test object, e.g. a pin, should be moved from anaesthetic to normal area; it is more accurate to state when an object is felt rather than when it disappears.

In polyneuropathies, sensory loss is symmetrical and follows a characteristic stocking and glove distribution. --------→

Examination of gait is important; with joint position impairment, sensory ataxia is evident. Romberg's test is positive (see page 189). Neuropathic burns/ulcers or joints may be present.

Trophic changes
  – Cold blue extremities.
  – Cutaneous hair loss.
  – Brittle finger/toe nails occasionally occur.

The AXON REFLEX can be used to 'place' lesions in the sensory pathway.

Normally:
  the skin is scratched – local vasoconstriction (white reaction) ⎫ due to local
      next – local oedema (red reaction) ⎭ histamine release.
  and finally – surrounding vasodilation or flare, dependent on antidromic impulses from the dorsal root ganglion along an intact sensory neuron.

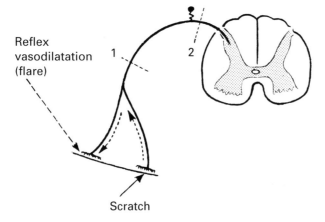

Reflex vasodilatation (flare)

1

2

Scratch

1. A distal sensory lesion will result in an absent flare response.
2. A proximal root lesion will not impair the response.

THE POLYNEUROPATHIES – SIGNS

MOTOR EXAMINATION

Muscle wasting. Evident in axonal but absent in demyelinating neuropathies. Oedema of immobile limbs may mask wasting. The 1st dorsal interosseus muscle in the upper limbs and extensor digitorum brevis in the lower limbs are muscles that commonly first show wasting in the neuropathies, but examine all muscle groups. Look for *fasciculations* – irregular twitches of groups of muscle fibres due to diseased anterior horn cells, these may be induced by exercise or muscle percussion.

Muscle weakness. The degree of weakness is 'scored' using the MRC (Medical Research Council) scale.

Score 0   – No contraction
Score 1   – Flicker
Score 2   – Active movement/gravity eliminated
Score 3   – Active movement against gravity
Score 4   – Active movement against gravity and resistance
Score 5   – Normal power

Weakness is proportional to the number of affected motor neurons. It develops suddenly or slowly and is generally symmetrical, usually starting distally in the lower limbs and spreading to upper limbs in a similar manner before ascending into proximal muscle groups. This pattern of progression is supposedly due to the 'dying back' of axons towards their nerve cells – the longest being the most vulnerable.

Some neuropathies, e.g. Guillain Barré, chronic inflammatory demyelinating polyneuropathy, may affect proximal muscle groups first.

In severe neuropathies, truncal and respiratory muscle involvement occurs. Respiratory muscle weakness may result in death.

Tendon reflexes

The tendon reflex depends on:
- stretch of the muscle spindle (1),
- activation of spindle afferent fibres (2),
- monosynaptic projections to the alpha motoneurons (3)

The gamma motoneuron fibres, projecting to the spindle (4) 'modulate' activity in the reflex loop.

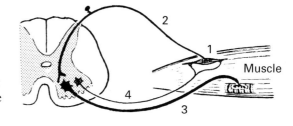

Reflexes commonly tested:

Deltoid	– C5,6 – Circumflex nerve		Triceps	– C6,7,8 – Radial nerve	
Biceps	– C5,6 – Musculocutaneous nerve		Knee	– L2,3,4 – Femoral nerve	
Supinator	– C6,7 – Radial nerve		Ankle	– S1,2 – Sciatic nerve	

The tendon reflexes are lost when any component of the reflex response is affected by disease. Reflexes are lost early in peripheral neuropathies when power and muscle bulk appear normal. Distal reflexes are generally lost before proximal ones.

THE POLYNEUROPATHIES – CLASSIFICATION

There are several approaches to classification:

    by MODE OF ONSET – acute, subacute, chronic

    by FUNCTIONAL DISTURBANCE – motor, sensory, autonomic, mixed

    by PATHOLOGICAL PROCESS – axonal, demyelinating

    by CAUSATION – e.g. infections; carcinomatous, diabetic, inflammatory, vascular

    by DISTRIBUTION – e.g. symmetrical, asymmetrical; proximal, distal.

Clinically it is of most value to classify the neuropathies according to mode of onset. The following table is for reference. Certain neuropathies will be dealt with separately (see pages 436–441).

	CAUSE	FUNCTIONAL DISTURBANCE	PATHOLOGY
ACUTE A few days– 4 weeks	**Inflammatory** —— (Postinfectious Guillain-Barré	Predominantly motor Distal or proximal Autonomic disturbance	Demyelinative with perivascular lymphocytic infiltration
	Diphtheria ———	Cranial nerve onset Mixed motor/sensory	Demyelinative. No inflammatory infiltration.
	Porphyria ———	Motor (may begin in arm). Autonomic disturbance Minimal sensory loss.	Axonal
SUBACUTE Develop over weeks	**Drug-induced** Isoniazid Metronidazole Dapsone Nitrofurantoin Cisplatin Vincristine etc.	Usually mild sensory motor disturbance Dapsone – pure motor involvement	Axonal degeneration
	Intramuscular injection	Localised neuropathies	
	Environmental **toxins** Solvents Lead Acrylamide Carbon disulphide Hexocarbons Organophosphates	— Occasionally acute Usually sensory, motor disturbance; severity related to dose Lead – severe, predominantly motor with arms involved first	Lead – axonal degeneration with segmental demyelination. Other heavy metals and solvents produce axonal degeneration
	Nutritional ——— Deficiency B complex (includes alcoholic neuropathy)	Sensory disturbance with 'burning feet' and other painful dysaesthesiae Motor component may be present and severe Autonomic disturbance is common but mild	Axonal degeneration with segmental demyelination. (Demyelination is minimal in alcoholic neuropathy)
	Substance abuse – Solvents Heroin	Sensory (facial numbness), motor disturbance Peripheral nerve lesion and plexopathies	Axonal degeneration

THE POLYNEUROPATHIES – CLASSIFICATION

	CAUSE	FUNCTIONAL DISTURBANCE	PATHOLOGY
CHRONIC Develop over months, years	**Malignant disease** – (Paraneoplastic)	Sensory or sensory/motor Chronic though sometimes subacute	Normally axonal Anti-neuronal antibodies (anti-Hu)
	Paraproteinaemias – e.g. Monoclonal gammopathies (IgG, IgA, IgM)	Sensory/motor disturbance	Axonal or demyelinative degeneration
	Connective tissue **disorders** Rheumatoid arthritis	In rheumatoid arthritis multiple mononeuropathy is common Motor/sensory disturbance is rare	Occlusion of nutrient blood vessels to nerves (vasa nervorum)
	Systemic lupus erythematosus	Systemic lupus erythematosus – mild motor/sensory disturbance	
	Polyarteritis nodosa Sclerodema	Polyarteritis nodosa usually produces multiple mononeuropathy	
	Amyloid disease Primary, familial or secondary	Motor/sensory disturbance with autonomic involvement Also may develop 'entrapment' neuropathies	Thickened nerves with amyloid deposition as well as small fibre axonal degeneration
	Metabolic disorders – Uraemia Hyperthyroidism	Uraemic neuropathy is sensory/motor in type. Hypothyroidism produces mild sensory/motor disturbance.	Axonal degeneration
	Diabetes	Diabetic neuropathy takes many forms	
	Chronic **inflammatory** **demyelinating** **polyneuropathy (CIDP)**	Sensory, motor disturbance	Demyelination
	Hereditary **neuropathies** Refsum's disease	A phytanic acid storage disorder. Onset in first decade and slowly progressive. A severe sensorimotor neuropathy with associated cerebellar ataxia, ichthyosis, pigmentary retinal degeneration, deafness and cardiac abnormalities. Elevated serum phytanate	Schwann cell hyperplasia – hypertrophic neuropathy
	Hereditary motor and sensory neuropathy (HMSN)	See page 441	

INVESTIGATION OF NEUROPATHY

Despite extensive investigation, the cause of chronic neuropathy cannot be identified in 30% of such cases.

The following conditions require exclusion before a chronic neuropathy is classified as idiopathic or of unknown aetiology: diabetes, uraemia, deficiency states, connective tissue disorders, paraproteinaemias, underlying malignancy, drugs and toxins. Hereditary disease can sometimes be excluded by clinical examination and genetic analysis of relatives.

The cause of acute or subacute neuropathy can usually be defined. Here, CSF examination may prove a useful diagnostic investigation, e.g. Guillain-Barré syndrome.

SPECIAL INVESTIGATIONS

1. Nerve conduction studies

An electrical stimulus is applied at points along a nerve (20–100 V for 0.05–0.1 ms) and the evoked muscle response recorded. By applying a stimulus at various points along a nerve and recording the latency between stimulus and muscle response the motor conduction velocity of a particular nerve may be measured.

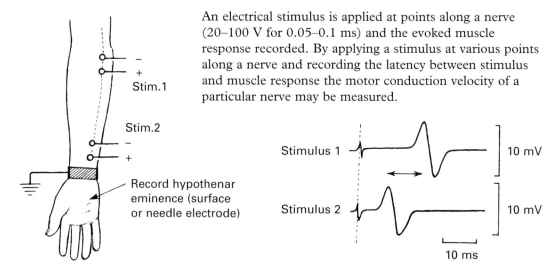

$$\text{Conduction velocity} = \frac{\text{Distance between two stimuli}}{\text{Difference in conduction time between the two sites}}$$

Motor conduction velocity can be measured in most motor peripheral nerves from the brachial plexus in the upper limbs and sciatic and femoral outlets in the lower limbs.

These studies not only aid in the diagnosis of generalised neuropathies but also in entrapments, e.g. ulnar nerve at elbow or median nerve at wrist (carpal tunnel syndrome).

INVESTIGATION OF NEUROPATHY

Sensory conduction can also be measured:

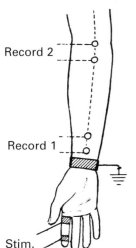

Record 2

Record 1

Stim.

The index finger is stimulated and the evoked sensory potential recorded at wrist and elbow. Measurements enable calculation to be made of the latencies and conduction velocity. Note the considerable difference in amplitude between sensory and motor evoked potentials.

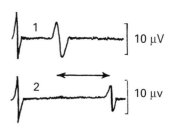

1   10 µV

2   10 µv

$$\text{Conduction velocity} = \frac{\text{Distance between two recording sites}}{\text{Difference in latency between the two evoked responses}}$$

GENERAL OBSERVATIONS

Amplitude of response – a function of the number of axons which respond to stimulation.

Latency of response – a function of the speed at which the largest fibres in a nerve will conduct.

Axonal degeneration → *reduced amplitude or absence of response* to stimulation with mild slowing of conduction velocity.

Demyelinative disorders → marked *slowing of conduction velocity (30% at least reduced) with progressive reduction of amplitude.*

Localised compression of nerve → slowing of conduction in region of block, e.g. over the elbow when ulnar nerve is compressed at that site. Conduction block, distant from entrapment sites may suggest multifocal motor neuropathy (see page 440).

2. Electromyography

A fine needle is inserted into the muscle and the recorded activity displayed on an oscilloscope. Electromyography is primarily of value in muscle disease but can also give indirect evidence of a neuropathic process. The presence of denervation in paraspinal muscles indicates proximal nerve root disease.

If chronic denervation has occurred, reinnervation may be present with long duration high amplitude motor unit potentials.

Also, with voluntary efforts, poor recruitment of motor units is seen on the oscilloscope screen.

The concentric needle has at its centre an insulated wire and potential differences between the centre and outer casing are measured

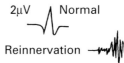

2µV   Normal

Reinnervation

Long duration, high amplitude, polyphasia

3. Nerve biopsy

A biopsy is most likely to aid diagnosis in asymmetric multiple mononeuropathies (vasculitis, amyloidosis, sarcoidosis etc). The sural nerve is usually chosen, provided its sensory conduction is abnormal.

435

THE POLYNEUROPATHIES – SPECIFIC TYPES

ACUTE INFLAMMATORY POSTINFECTIOUS POLYNEUROPATHY (GUILLAIN-BARRÉ SYNDROME)

Incidence: 2 per 100 000 population per year. Characteristically it occurs 1–3 weeks after a viral or other infection or immunisation.

Aetiology/pathology

The condition may follow viral infection, e.g. varicella-zoster, mumps and *cytomegalovirus*. It is also associated with *Mycoplasma, Campylobacter,* infections, immunisations with both live and dead vaccines, antitoxins, trauma, surgery and, rarely, malignant disease and immunodeficiency.

Both antibody and cell-mediated reactions to peripheral nerve myelin are involved. Some patients produce antibodies to myelin glycoproteins or gangliosides, others develop a T cell-mediated assault on myelin basic protein.

Segmental demyelination results with secondary axonal damage if the process is severe. Perivascular infiltration with lymphocytes occurs within peripheral nerves and nerve roots. Lymphocytes and macrophages release cytotoxic substances (cytokines) which damage Schwann cell/myelin.

When axon damage and nerve cell death occur, regeneration cannot take place.

Clinical features

Sensory symptoms predominate at the beginning with paraesthesia of the feet, then hands. Pain, especially back pain, is an occasional initial symptom. Weakness next develops – this may be generalised, proximal in distribution or commence distally and ascend. Tendon reflexes are absent or depressed. In severe cases, respiratory and bulbar involvement occurs. Weakness is maximal three weeks after the onset. Tracheostomy/ventilation is required in 20% of cases. Facial weakness is present to some extent in 50% of cases. Papilloedema may occur when CSF protein is markedly elevated (blocked arachnoid villi?). Autonomic involvement – tachycardia, fluctuating blood pressure, retention of urine – develops in some cases.

Variants are common (20% of cases).
– acute motor axonal neuropathy (AMAN)
– acute motor, sensory axonal neuropathy (AMSAN)

Investigations

CSF protein is elevated in most patients but often not until the second or third week of illness. Cells are usually absent but in 20% up to 50 cells/mm^3 may be found.

Nerve conduction studies
When carried out early in the illness, these may be normal. Findings of multifocal demyelination soon develops with slowing of motor conduction, conduction block and prolonged distal motor latencies.

Ancillary investigations
Performed to identify any precipitating infection: e.g. viral and bacterial studies. Electrolytes are checked for inappropriate secretion of antidiuretic hormone and immune complex glomerulonephritis.

THE POLYNEUROPATHIES – SPECIFIC TYPES

ACUTE INFLAMMATORY POSTINFECTIOUS POLYNEUROPATHY (*cont'd*)

Diagnosis is based on clinical history supported by CSF and neurophysiological investigation and exclusion of acute spinal cord disease, porphyria and myasthenia gravis.

Treatment

Supportive care in HDU/ITU with prevention of respiratory and autonomic complications provides the best chance of a favourable outcome. Signs of impending respiratory failure – forced vital capacity (FVC) below 18 ml/kg, arterial $PaCO_2$ > 6.5 kPa and PaO_2 < 8 kPa on oxygen – indicate elective intubation for ventilation. When respiratory assistance is likely to exceed 2 weeks, tracheotomy should be performed.

Subcutaneous low molecular weight heparin with support stockings must be given where the degree of immobility makes thromboembolism a possible complication.

Both plasma exchange (PE) and intravenous immune globulin (IVIG), 0.4 g/kg – are equally effective at speeding recovery and improving outcome. IVIG is the preferred treatment because of ease of administration but is not without side effects (flu-like symptoms, vasomotor instability, congestive cardiac failure, thrombotic complications – strokes and myocardial ischaemia, transient renal failure and anaphylaxis)

Treatment is generally given to those who can no longer walk and is deferred in milder cases.

Steroids are no longer justified, two trials showing no benefit.

Outcome

Mortality – 2%. Of those progressing to respiratory failure, 20% are left severely disabled and 10% moderately disabled. In milder cases the outcome is excellent. Recurrence – 3%.

Miller Fisher variant of Guillain-Barré

The Miller Fisher syndrome consists of ophthalmoplegia, areflexia and ataxia without significant limb weakness. Serum IgG antibodies to a specific ganglioside are characteristic. Management is that of Guillain-Barré.

THE POLYNEUROPATHIES – SPECIFIC TYPES

CHRONIC INFLAMMATORY DEMYELINATING POLYNEUROPATHY (CIDP)

Similar to Guillain-Barré but with a progressive or fluctuating course over weeks or months and rarely involving cranial nerves or respiratory function.

Pathology: Segmental demyelination with remyelination (onion bulb formation) and sparse mononuclear inflammatory change.

Prevalence – 3% of all neuropathies

Incidence – 5 per million

Age of onset: mean 35 yrs (fluctuating course – younger, progressive – older)

Diagnosis: Electrophysiology – conduction velocity < 70% of normal
– conduction block (outwith entrapment sites)
– prolonged distal latencies

Distinguish from – hereditary neuropathy (HSMN type 1 page 441)
– paraprotein and lymphoma associated neuropathy (page 440)
– multifocal motor neuropathy with conduction block (page 440)
– HIV neuropathy (page 512)

Treatment

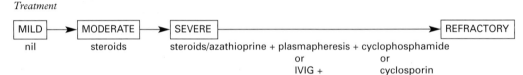

MILD → MODERATE → SEVERE → REFRACTORY

nil   steroids   steroids/azathioprine + plasmapheresis + cyclophosphamide
or   or
IVIG +   cyclosporin

About two thirds of patients respond to steroids, PE or IVIG. In moderate/ severe cases steroids should be used initially (cost and ease of use) followed, if response unsatisfactory, by IVIG and finally PE. Despite little evidence, immunosuppressive drugs (azathioprine, cyclophosphamide or cyclosporin) are deployed in resistant cases.

Outcome with treatment – 30% symptom free – 45% mild disability – 25% severe disability

DIABETIC NEUROPATHY

This condition is uncommon in childhood and increases with age.

Peripheral nerve damage is related to poor control of diabetes. This is more common in insulin-dependent patients. Damage results from either metabolic disturbance with sorbitol and fructose accumulation in axons and Schwann cells or an occlusion of the nutrient vessels supplying nerves (vasa vasorum). The frequent occurrence of neuropathy with other vascular complications – retinopathy and nephropathy – suggests that the latter is the more usual mechanism. Neurological complications correlate with levels of glycosylated haemoglobin A1C, an indicator of the long-term control of hyperglycaemia.

THE POLYNEUROPATHIES – SPECIFIC TYPES

DIABETIC NEUROPATHY *(cont'd)*

Classification

Polyneuropathy

Asymmetrical neuropathy

Present in 30% of all diabetics, but only 10% are symptomatic. Distal weakness and sensory loss is usual. Two forms of sensory neuropathy occur – large fibre, causing ataxia and small fibre causing a painful anaesthesia.

Autonomic neuropathy

In most patients with peripheral neuropathy, some degree of autonomic disturbance is present. Occasionally this predominates:
– pupil abnormalities
– loss of sweating
– orthostatic hypotension
– resting tachycardia
– gastroparesis and diarrhoea
– hypotonic dilated bladder
– impotence.

Diabetic amyotrophy – Much less common than polyneuropathy. Pain and weakness rapidly develop. The anterior thigh is preferentially affected with wasting of the quadriceps, loss of the knee jerk and minimal sensory loss. The condition is due to anterior spinal root or plexus disease. Imaging the lumbar roots and plexus excludes other causes. Functional recovery is good.

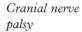

Cranial nerve palsy

An oculomotor palsy, usually without pain, may occur with pupillary sparing, which helps to differentiate from an aneurysmal cause. The 6th and 7th cranial nerves may also be involved in diabetes. Complete recovery is the rule.

Treatment

Improved control of diabetes is essential.

Carbamazepine, gabapentin, antidepressants or α-adrenergic blockers, e.g. phenoxybenzene, help control pain.

Drugs which reduce aldose reductase and halt accumulation of sorbitol and fructose in nerves are being evaluated.

Management of autonomic neuropathy – see page 457.

Asymmetrical neuropathies usually spontaneously recover, whereas prognosis for symmetric neuropathies is less certain.

THE POLYNEUROPATHIES – SPECIFIC TYPES

CARCINOMATOUS POLYNEUROPATHY

Sensory or mixed 'sensorimotor' neuropathy is often associated with malignant disease, particularly small cell carcinoma of the lung. Neuropathy may also occur with Hodgkin's disease and lymphomas. The neuropathy is characterised by the presence of antibodies (anti Hu) that are detected in serum. Such antibodies not only recognise antigen in tumours but also bind to peripheral nervous system neurones.

Pathology

The sensory type is characterised by degeneration and inflammatory changes in the dorsal root ganglion. The ventral roots and peripheral nerve motor fibres are spared. In the sensorimotor type, degeneration of the dorsal root ganglion is less marked and axonal and demyelinative changes affect motor and sensory fibres equally.

Clinical features

Symptoms and signs may predate the appearance of causal malignant disease by months or even years.

Sensory neuropathy: Progressive sensory loss often commencing in upper limbs is associated with paraesthesia, unpleasant 'burning' dysaesthesia and sensory ataxia.

Sensorimotor neuropathy: The onset is gradual with distal sensory loss and mild motor weakness. Occasionally a more acute, severe neuropathy resembling Guillain-Barré syndrome occurs.

Detection and treatment of the underlying malignancy may lead to recovery of the neuropathy. Alternatively the use of immunosuppressive agents, plasma exchange or intravenous gammaglobulin (IVIG) may help.

MULTIFOCAL MOTOR NEUROPATHY WITH CONDUCTION BLOCK

This presents with asymmetric lower motor neuron weakness and may be mistaken for motor neuron disease. Neurophysiological investigation shows 'conduction block' at sites distant from possible entrapment. Antibodies to gangliosides (Anti GM1) are found in serum. Immunosuppressive treatment (cyclophosphamide) or intravenous immunoglobulin (IVIG) when indicated, result in clinical improvement.

NEUROPATHIES ASSOCIATED WITH PARAPROTEINS

Approximately 10% of patients with late onset chronic peripheral neuropathy have a circulating monoclonal paraprotein in the serum. If myeloma, lymphoma, amyloidosis and Waldenström's macroglobinaemia are excluded, the condition is referred to as a 'monoclonal gammopathy of uncertain significance' (MGUS). IgM is reactive, in 50% of cases, against myelin associated glycoprotein. IgA and IgB are not. Neuropathies may be axonal, demyelinating or mixed and show a variable response to immunotherapy.

PORPHYRIA

Acute intermittent porphyria is an autosomal dominant disorder in which symptoms of abdominal pain, psychosis, convulsions and peripheral neuropathy occur.

The metabolic fault occurs in the liver. An increased production of porphobilinogen is reflected by its increased urinary excretion. δ-amino laevulic acid, a porphyrin precursor, is also increased.

Clinical features

The onset is acute and predominantly motor with upper limb and occasional cranial nerve involvement. Respiratory failure occurs in severe cases. Autonomic involvement with tachycardia, blood pressure changes, abdominal pain and vomiting often develop. The neuropathy must be distinguished from Guillain-Barré.

Clinical course is variable. Spontaneous recovery occurs over several weeks. Respiratory failure will require ventilation and carries a poor prognosis. During an attack, a high carbohydrate diet and prevention and treatment of electrolyte disturbances are essential. Chelating agents (EDTA or Penicillamine) are used in severe cases. Recurrent attacks may be anticipated. Certain drugs may precipitate these attacks and must be avoided, e.g. sulphonamides, barbiturates, phenytoin, griseofulvin.

THE POLYNEUROPATHIES – SPECIFIC TYPES
– INHERITED NEUROPATHIES

HEREDITARY MOTOR SENSORY NEUROPATHY (HMSN) (Charcot–Marie–Tooth)

A heterogeneous group of disorders with a prevalence of 1:2500 – the largest category of genetic neurological disease. The characteristic appearance is that of distal wasting, the lower limbs having an 'inverted wine bottle' appearance.

Classification	Clinical features	Pathology	Neuro-physiology	Inheritance	
HMSN type I	Age of onset < 30 yrs. Wasting and weakness of intrinsic foot muscles, peroneal and tibial groups. Distal upper limb involvement. Pes cavus/hammer toes – 75%. Palpable peripheral nerves – 25%. Associated ataxia and tremor – 10%.	Demyelination with thickened 'onion bulb' areas of remyelination.	Motor conduction velocities slowed < 38 m/sec in common peroneal nerve.	*Autosomal dominant* 70% of cases are due to duplication of 17p 11.2 in PMP (peripheral myelin protein) 22 gene. X linked cases result from point mutations in the Connexin 32 gene.	
HMSN type II	Age of onset > 30 yrs. Wasting and weakness as type I. Foot deformities absent. Peripheral nerves not palpable.	Axonal loss.	Motor conduction velocities normal or marginally slowed.	*Autosomal dominant –* mechanism and gene locus unknown.	
HMSN type III (Dejerine–Sottas disease)	Age of onset: childhood. Wasting and weakness may be proximal. Peripheral nerves and spinal roots thickened. CSF protein elevated.	Demyelination with 'onion bulb' formation.	Motor conduction velocities profoundly slowed – 5–10 m/sec	*Autosomal recessive –* point mutation chromosome 1 or 17 or sporadic	

Complex forms of HMSN occur and the above classification is by no means complete. Several pedigrees show additional features such as – optic atrophy, retinopathy, deafness, ataxia, spasticity and cardiomyopathy. Such 'extra' features complicate a simple classification. Treatment is symptomatic with provision of appropriate footwear, splints or orthopaedic procedures to maintain mobility. In adult onset disease, the rate of progression is exceedingly slow. The demonstration of genetic markers and the application of nerve conduction studies allows early and correct diagnosis in those at risk. Nerve biopsy is of no diagnostic value.

Other rare forms of hereditary neuropathy

- *Hereditary sensory and autonomic neuropathies*
  - Autosomal recessive
    Childhood onset
    Characterised by insensitivity to pain and disordered sweating
- *Hereditary neuropathy with liability to pressure palsies (HNPP)*
  - Autosomal dominant (deletion in PMP 22 gene)
    Adult onset
    Characterised by recurrent entrapment neuropathies
    e.g. carpal tunnel syndrome
- *Hereditary neuropathy with spinocerebellar degeneration*
  - e.g. Friedreich's ataxia (pages 548–549)
- *Hereditary neuropathy with metabolic defect*
  - e.g. Familial amyloid neuropathy – mutation of transthyretin gene
    Porphyria – abnormality of hepatic haem biosynthesis
    Refsum's disease – abnormality of phytanic acid metabolism.

PLEXUS SYNDROMES AND MONONEUROPATHIES

Disease of a single peripheral or cranial nerve is termed *mononeuropathy*. When many single nerves are damaged one by one, this is described as *mononeuritis multiplex*. Damage to the brachial or lumbosacral plexus may produce widespread limb weakness which does not conform to the distribution of any one peripheral nerve. A knowledge of the anatomy and muscle innervation of the plexuses and peripheral nerves is essential to localise the site of the lesion and thus deduce the possible causes.

Certain systemic illnesses are associated with the development of mononeuropathy or mononeuritis multiplex:
  – diabetes mellitus
  – sarcoidosis
  – vasculitis
  – leprosy (worldwide commonest cause)

Entrapment mononeuropathies result from damage to a nerve where it passes through a tight space such as the median nerve under the flexor retinaculum of the wrist. These are often related to conditions such as acromegaly, myxoedema and pregnancy, in which soft tissue swelling occurs. A familial tendency to entrapment neuropathy has been described.

Cranial nerve mononeuropathies have been dealt with separately.

BRACHIAL PLEXUS
The plexus lies in the posterior triangle of the neck between the muscles scalenius anterior and scalenius medius.

At the root of the neck the plexus lies behind the clavicle.

The plexus itself gives off several important motor branches:

1. Nerve to rhomboids

2. Long thoracic nerve
   – to serratus ant.

3. Pectoral nerves – to pectoralis major

4. Suprascapular nerve
   – to supraspinatus
   infraspinatus

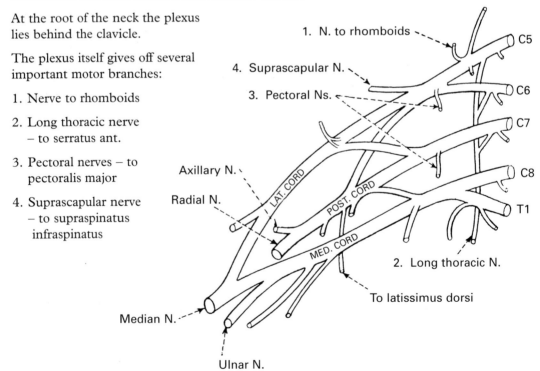

1. N. to rhomboids — C5
4. Suprascapular N.
3. Pectoral Ns. — C6
C7
Axillary N.
Radial N.
LAT. CORD
POST. CORD
MED. CORD
C8
T1
2. Long thoracic N.
To latissimus dorsi
Median N.
Ulnar N.

BRACHIAL PLEXUS SYNDROMES

UPPER PLEXUS LESION (C5C6)

Traction on the arm at birth (Erb-Duchenne paralysis) or falling
on the shoulder may damage the upper part (C5C6) of the plexus.

Deltoid
Supraspinatus } paralysed.
Infraspinatus

Biceps
Brachialis } elbow flexors – also paralysed.

Adductors of shoulder – mildly affected.

When damage to C5C6 is more proximal, nerve to rhomboids and long thoracic nerve may
be affected.

POSTERIOR CORD LESION (C5C6C7C8)

Deltoid
Extensors of elbow (triceps)
Extensors of wrist (extensor carpi radialis longus } paralysed
    and brevis, extensor carpi ulnaris)
Extensors of fingers (extensor digitorum)

LOWER PLEXUS LESION (C8T1)

Forced abduction of the arm at birth (Klumpke's paralysis) or trauma may produce damage
to the lower plexus. This results in paralysis of the intrinsic hand muscles producing a claw
hand, C8T1 sensory loss and a Horner's syndrome (page 143) if the T1 root is involved.

N.B. A combined ulnar and median nerve lesion will produce a similar picture in the hand
but with involvement also of flexor carpi ulnaris and pronator teres.

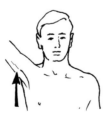

TOTAL BRACHIAL LESION

This results in complete flaccid paralysis and anaesthesia of the arm.

The presence of a Horner's syndrome indicates proximal T1 nerve root involvement.

N.B. When trauma is the cause of brachial paralysis, early referral to a specialist unit with
experience in the surgical repair of plexus injuries is advised.

BRACHIAL PLEXUS SYNDROMES

THORACIC OUTLET SYNDROME

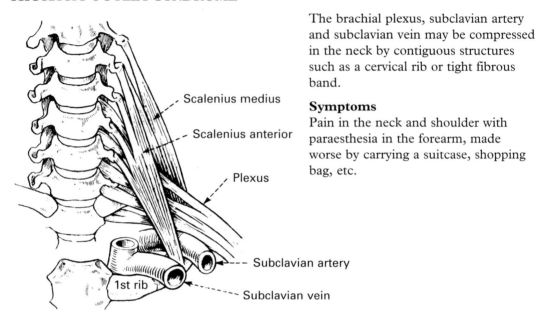

Scalenius medius

Scalenius anterior

Plexus

Subclavian artery

1st rib

Subclavian vein

The brachial plexus, subclavian artery and subclavian vein may be compressed in the neck by contiguous structures such as a cervical rib or tight fibrous band.

Symptoms

Pain in the neck and shoulder with paraesthesia in the forearm, made worse by carrying a suitcase, shopping bag, etc.

Signs

Sensory loss in a T1 distribution.
Wasting and weakness of thenar and occasionally interosseous muscles.
Signs of vascular compression:
– Unilateral Raynaud's phenomenon.
– Pallor of limb on elevation.
– Brittle trophic finger nails.
– Loss of radial pulse in arm on abduction and external rotation at
  the shoulder or on bracing the shoulders – ADSON's sign.
– Subclavian venous thrombosis may occur, especially after excessive usage of arm.

Investigation

Coronal MRI is the definitive investigation.
Plain radiology of the thoracic outlet may reveal a cervical rib or prolonged transverse process. Nerve conduction/electromyography will distinguish this from other peripheral nerve lesions. Arteriography or venography is occasionally necessary if there are obvious vascular problems.

Treatment

In middle-aged people with poor posture and no evidence of abnormality on plain radiology, neck and postural exercises are helpful.

In younger patients with clinical and electrophysiological changes supporting the radiological abnormalities, exploration and removal of a fibrous band or rib may afford relief.

BRACHIAL PLEXUS SYNDROMES

Ensure orthopaedic mimics, rotator cuff injury or shoulder joint contractures, are considered prior to assessment.

BRACHIAL NEURITIS (Neuralgic amyotrophy)

Brachial neuritis is a relatively common disorder sometimes associated with:
- Viral infection (infectious mononucleosis, cytomegalovirus)
- Vaccination (tetanus toxoid, influenza) — Probable variant of Guillain-Barré
- Strenuous exercise

In most cases it develops without any evident precipitating cause.

Clinical features

- Acute onset with preceding shoulder pain.
- Weakness is usually proximal, though the whole arm may be affected.
- Occasionally both arms are affected simultaneously.
- Sensory findings are minor (loss over the outer aspect of the shoulder) and occur in 50%.
- Reflex loss occurs.
- Wasting is apparent after 3–6 weeks.
- Recurrent episodes can occur, especially in the presence of a family history.

Differential diagnosis

A painful weak arm. *Consider:*
- Cervical spondylosis.
- Cervical disc lesion.
- Brachialgia due to local bursitis.
- Polymyalgia rheumatica.

Investigation

CSF may show a mild protein rise and a pleocytosis.
Nerve conduction studies will show slowing in affected nerves after 7–10 days.

Treatment

Narcotic analgesics may be required if pain is extreme. Corticosteriods are normally given though the value of immunotherapy is uncertain. By 2 yrs – 75% have fully recovered. Brachial neuritis may be familial. Recurrent attacks occur in Hereditary Neuropathy with liability to Pressure Palsies – HNPP (Page 441). Autosomal dominant forms of Hereditary Neuralgic Amyotrophy (HNA), both acute and chronic are described, some linked to chromosome 17q.

PANCOAST's TUMOUR

Involvement of the plexus by apical lung tumour (usually squamous cell carcinoma). The lower cervical and upper thoracic roots are involved.

Clinical features

- Severe pain around the shoulder and down the inside of the arm.
- Weak wasted hand muscles.
- Sensory loss (C8T1).
- Horner's syndrome (invasion of sympathetic chain and stellate ganglion).
- Rarely medial extension can involve the recurrent laryngeal nerve (hoarseness & bovine cough).

RADIATION PLEXOPATHY

Now infrequently seen after irradiation of axillary nodes in breast Ca. Onset usually 2–4 yrs after exposure to high radiation dose (>44–50 Gy). Thickening of the vascular endothelium causes ischaemia of the plexus. Symptoms start with paraesthesia in the hand and progress slowly to involve all lower plexus structures with wasting, weakness, reflex & sensory loss.

UPPER LIMB MONONEUROPATHIES

LONG THORACIC NERVE (C5C6C7)
Supplies: Serratus anterior muscle

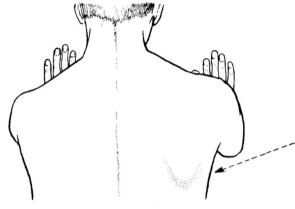

Damaged by:
- Carrying heavy objects
- Strapping the shoulder
- Limited brachial neuritis
- Diabetes mellitus

Results in:
Winging of the scapula when arms are stretched in front

SUPRASCAPULAR NERVE (C5C6)
Supplies: Supraspinatus and infraspinatus muscles.

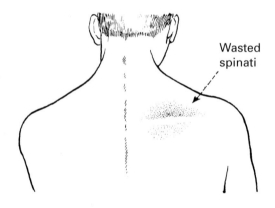

Wasted spinati

Damaged by:
- [as for Long thoracic nerve (above)]

Results in:
- Weakness of abduction of arm (supraspinatus)
- Weakness of external rotation of arm (infraspinatus).

AXILLARY NERVE (posterior cord) (C5C6)
Supplies: Deltoid and teres minor muscles.

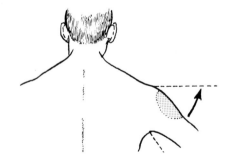

Damaged by:
- Shoulder dislocation.
- Limited brachial neuritis.

Results in:
- Weakness of abduction of shoulder between 15–90° and sensory loss over the outer aspect of the shoulder.

UPPER LIMB MONONEUROPATHIES

MUSCULOCUTANEOUS NERVE (Lateral cord) (C5C6)

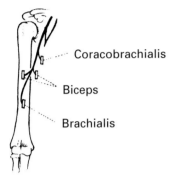

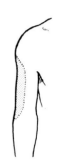

Sensory supply: Lateral border of the arm.

Damaged by:
- Fracture of the humerus.
- Systemic causes.

Results in:
- Weakness of elbow flexion and forearm supination with characteristic sensory loss and absent biceps reflex.

Coracobrachialis

Biceps

Brachialis

RADIAL NERVE (Posterior cord) (C6C7C8)

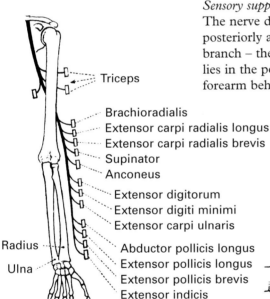

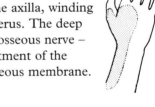

Sensory supply: Dorsum of hand.
The nerve descends from the axilla, winding posteriorly around the humerus. The deep branch – the posterior interosseous nerve – lies in the posterior compartment of the forearm behind the interosseous membrane.

Triceps

Brachioradialis
Extensor carpi radialis longus
Extensor carpi radialis brevis
Supinator
Anconeus

Extensor digitorum
Extensor digiti minimi
Extensor carpi ulnaris

Radius
Ulna

Abductor pollicis longus
Extensor pollicis longus
Extensor pollicis brevis
Extensor indicis

Damaged by:
- Fractures of the humerus.
- Prolonged pressure (Saturday night palsy).
- Intramuscular injection.
- Lipoma, fibroma or neuroma.
- Systemic causes.

Results in:
- Weakness and wasting of muscles supplied, characterised by wrist drop with flexed fingers (weak extensors). Sensory loss on dorsum of hand and forearm. Loss of triceps reflex (when lesion lies in the axilla) and supinator reflex.

The *posterior interosseous branch* of the radial nerve can be compressed at its point of entry into the supinator muscle. The clinical picture is similar to a radial nerve palsy, only brachioradialis and wrist extensors are spared. Examination shows weakness of finger extension with little or no wrist drop.

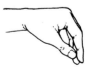

UPPER LIMB MONONEUROPATHIES

MEDIAN NERVE (Lateral and medial cords) (C7C8)

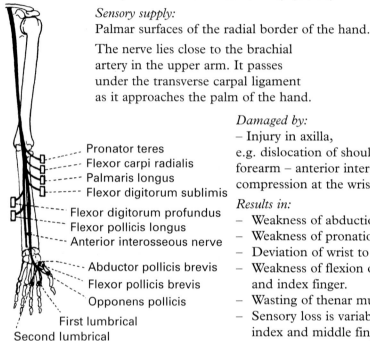

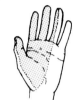

Sensory supply:
Palmar surfaces of the radial border of the hand.

The nerve lies close to the brachial artery in the upper arm. It passes under the transverse carpal ligament as it approaches the palm of the hand.

Pronator teres
Flexor carpi radialis
Palmaris longus
Flexor digitorum sublimis

Flexor digitorum profundus
Flexor pollicis longus
Anterior interosseous nerve

Abductor pollicis brevis
Flexor pollicis brevis
Opponens pollicis

First lumbrical
Second lumbrical

Damaged by:
– Injury in axilla,
e.g. dislocation of shoulder, compression in the forearm – anterior interosseous branch, compression at the wrist (carpal tunnel syndrome).

Results in:
– Weakness of abduction and apposition of thumb.
– Weakness of pronation of the forearm.
– Deviation of wrist to ulnar side on wrist flexion.
– Weakness of flexion of distal phalanx of thumb and index finger.
– Wasting of thenar muscles is evident.
– Sensory loss is variable but most marked on index and middle fingers

Carpal tunnel syndrome

The most common entrapment neuropathy, more frequent in women, results from median nerve entrapment under the transverse carpal ligament at the wrist.

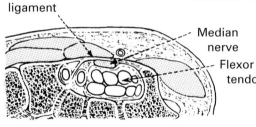

Transverse carpal ligament

Median nerve

Flexor tendons

Causes: – Connective tissue thickening, e.g.
– Rheumatoid arthritis
– Acromegaly
– Hypothyroidism.
– Infiltration of ligament, e.g. amyloid disease.
– Fluid retention, e.g. in pregnancy, weight gain.

Symptoms:
Pain, especially at night, and paraesthesia, eased by shaking the hand or dangling it out of the bed.
Objective findings may follow with cutaneous sensory loss and wasting and weakness of thenar muscles (abductor and opponens pollicis). Percussion on the nerve at the wrist produces heightened paraesthesia (Tinel's sign).
Nerve conduction studies are helpful in confirming diagnosis by showing slowing of conduction over the wrist.
Treatment: of the cause, weight loss and diuretics. Surgical division of the transverse ligament if symptoms fail to improve produces excellent results (90% symptom free).

UPPER LIMB MONONEUROPATHIES

ULNAR NERVE (Medial cord) (C7C8)

Sensory supply:
Both palmar and dorsal surfaces of the ulnar border of the hand.

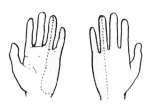

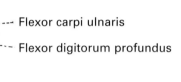

– Flexor carpi ulnaris

– Flexor digitorum profundus

– Adductor pollicis

– 1st dorsal interosseous

Flexor
Opponens } digiti minimi
Abductor

In the upper arm the nerve is closely related to the brachial artery and the median nerve, and passes behind the medial epicondyle of the humerus into the forearm.

In the hand, close to the hamate bone, it divides into deep and superficial branches.

Damaged by:
– Injury at elbow, e.g. dislocation.
– Entrapment at elbow or distal to the medial epicondyle.
– Pressure on the nerve in the palm of the hand damages the deep branch resulting in wasting and weakness without sensory loss.

Results in:
– Weakness and wasting of muscles supplied, with a characteristic posture of the hand – *ulnar claw hand* – as well as sensory loss. The level of the lesion dictates the extent of the motor paralysis. Nerve conduction studies are helpful in confirming entrapment at the elbow.

Surgical transposition may be necessary in such cases.

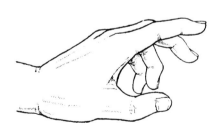

LUMBOSACRAL PLEXUS

LUMBAR PLEXUS

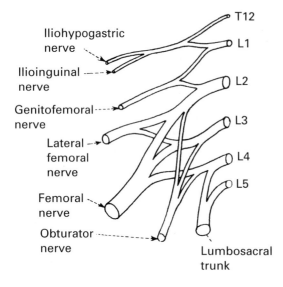

Iliohypogastric nerve

Ilioinguinal nerve

Genitofemoral nerve

Lateral femoral nerve

Femoral nerve

Obturator nerve

T12
L1
L2
L3
L4
L5

Lumbosacral trunk

The plexus is located in the psoas muscle. The important branches are the femoral and obturator nerves.

The femoral nerve (L2L3L4) emerges from the lateral border of the psoas muscle and leaves the abdomen laterally below the inguinal ligament with the femoral artery.

The obturator nerve (L2L3L4)

SACRAL PLEXUS

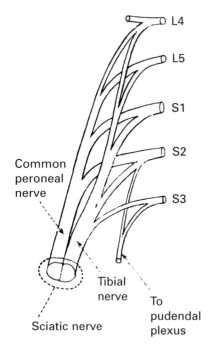

L4
L5
S1
S2
S3

Common peroneal nerve

Tibial nerve

Sciatic nerve

To pudendal plexus

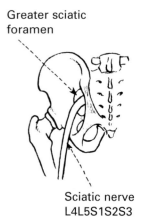

Greater sciatic foramen

Sciatic nerve L4L5S1S2S3

The plexus is located on the posterior wall of the pelvis. The five roots of the plexus divide into anterior and posterior divisions. The L4L5S1S2 divisions form the common peroneal nerve.

The L4L5S1S2S3 anterior divisions form the tibial nerve. Both these nerves fuse to form the sciatic nerve.

The posterior divisions S2S3 pass to the pudendal plexus.

The common peroneal and tibial nerves (sciatic nerve) leave the pelvis by the greater sciatic foramen. In the popliteal fossa the sciatic nerve splits into its constituent nerves.

LUMBOSACRAL PLEXUS SYNDROMES

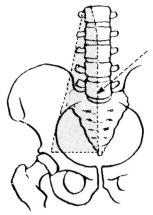

The proximity of the plexus to important abdominal and pelvic structures renders it liable to damage from disease of these structures.

Trauma following surgery, e.g. hysterectomy, lumbar sympathectomy or during labour. Compression from an abdominal mass, e.g. aortic aneurysm. Infiltration from pelvic tumour. Radiotherapy.

Symptoms may be unilateral or bilateral, depending upon causation. Weakness, sensory loss and reflex changes are dictated by the location and extent of plexus damage. Pain of a severe burning quality may be present; it may be worsened by coughing, sneezing, etc.

In general:

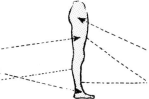

Lower plexus lesions produce:
Weakness of posterior thigh (hamstring) and foot muscles with posterior leg sensory loss.

Upper plexus lesions produce:
Weakness of hip flexion and adduction with anterior leg sensory loss.

The lumbosacral plexus may be affected in the same way as the brachial plexus in brachial neuritis – lumbosacral neuritis – the association with infection, etc., being similar. Recovery is usually good. Recurrent and familial cases occur. Plexus lesions also occur in *diabetes mellitus* and *vasculitis*. In both, the symptoms and signs may be bilateral. Investigate with CT/MR and neurophysiology.

LOWER LIMB MONONEUROPATHIES

FEMORAL NERVE (L1L2L3)

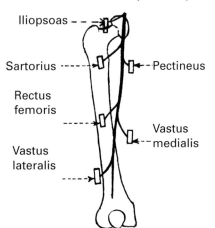

Iliopsoas
Sartorius
Rectus femoris
Vastus lateralis
Pectineus
Vastus medialis

Damaged by:
- Fractures of the upper femur
- Congenital dislocation of the hip, hip surgery
- Neoplastic infiltration
- Psoas muscle abscess
- Haematoma into iliopsoas muscle (haemophilia, anticoagulants)
- Systemic causes of mononeuropathy, e.g. diabetes.

Results in:
- Weakness of hip flexion
- Weakness of knee extension with wasting of thigh muscles
- Sensory loss over the anterior and medial aspects of the thigh
- The knee jerk is lost.

451

LOWER LIMB MONONEUROPATHIES

OBTURATOR NERVE (L2L3L4)

Damaged by: – Same process as the femoral nerve.
– During labour and occasionally as a consequence of compression by hernia in the obturator canal.

Results in: – Weakness of hip external rotation and adduction.
– The patient may complain of inability to cross the affected leg on the other.
– Sensory loss is confined to the innermost aspect of the thigh.
– The adductor reflex is absent (adductor response to striking the medial epicondyle).

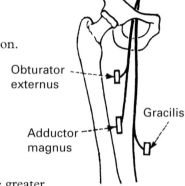

SCIATIC NERVE (L4L5S1S2)

The nerve descends between the ischial tuberosity and the greater trochanter of the femur. In the thigh it innervates the hamstring muscles (semitendinosus, semimembranosus and biceps).

Damaged by: – Congenital or traumatic hip dislocation.
– Penetrating injuries.
– Accidental damage from 'misplaced' intramuscular injection.
– Entrapment at sciatic notch.
– Systemic causes of mononeuropathy

Results in: – Weakness of hamstring muscles with loss of knee flexion.
– Distal foot and leg muscles are also affected.
– Sensory loss involves the outer aspect of the leg.
– The ankle reflex is absent.

COMMON PERONEAL NERVE (L4L5)

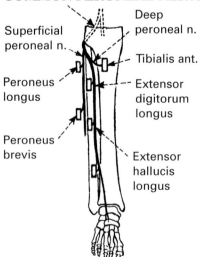

The nerve arises from the division of the sciatic nerve in the popliteal fossa. It bears a close relationship with the head of the fibula as it winds anteriorly. It divides into superficial and deep branches as well as giving off a purely sensory branch which, with sensory twigs from the tibial nerve, forms the sural nerve, mediating sensation from the dorsum and lateral aspect of the foot.

Damaged by: – Trauma to the head of the fibula; pressure here from kneeling, crossing legs.
– Systemic causes of mononeuropathy, e.g. diabetes.

Results in: Weakness of dorsiflexion and eversion of the foot. The patient walks with a 'foot drop'. Sensory loss involves the dorsum and outer aspect of the foot. Partial common peroneal nerve palsies are common with very selective muscle weakness.

LOWER LIMB MONONEUROPATHIES

POSTERIOR TIBIAL NERVE (S1S2)

This nerve also arises from the division of the sciatic nerve in the popliteal fossa and descends behind the tibia, terminating in the medial and lateral plantar nerves which innervate the small muscles of the foot. The sensory branch contributes to the *sural nerve*.

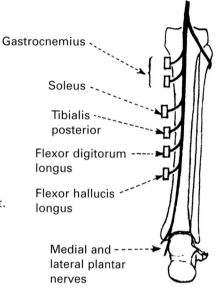

Damaged by:
Trauma in the popliteal fossa.
- Fracture of the tibia.
- Systemic causes of mononeuropathy.

Results in:
- Weakness of plantar flexion and inversion of the foot.
- The patient cannot stand on toes.
- Sensory loss involves the sole of the foot.
- The ankle reflex is lost.

Tarsal tunnel syndrome

The posterior tibial nerve may be entrapped below the medial malleolus. This produces a burning pain in the sole of the foot. Weakness of toe flexion and atrophy of small muscles of the foot occur in advanced cases. A prolonged sensory conduction velocity confirms the diagnosis. Surgical decompression is often required.

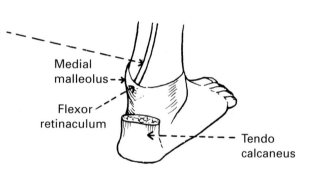

PLANTAR AND SMALL INTERDIGITAL NERVES

Compression of these nerves at the sole of the foot produces localised burning pain. Involvement of inter-digital nerves produces pain and analgesia in adjacent halves of neighbouring toes.

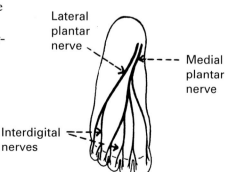

AUTONOMIC NERVOUS SYSTEM

The autonomic nervous system maintains the visceral and homeostatic functions essential to life. It is divided into SYMPATHETIC and PARASYMPATHETIC components and contains both motor (efferent) and sensory (afferent) pathways.

Both sympathetic and parasympathetic systems are regulated by the *limbic system*, *hypothalamus* and *reticular formation*. Fibres from these structures descend to synapse with preganglionic neurons in the intermediolateral column T1–T12 (sympathetic) and in the III, VII, IX and X cranial nerve nuclei and S2–S4 segments of the cord (parasympathetic).

PARASYMPATHETIC OUTFLOW

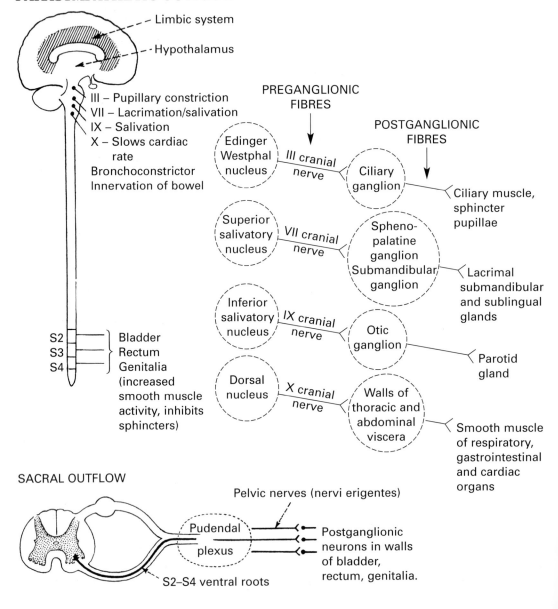

AUTONOMIC NERVOUS SYSTEM

SYMPATHETIC OUTFLOW

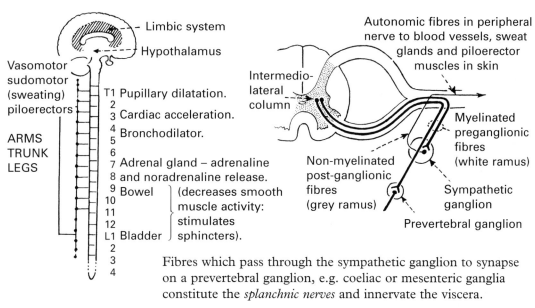

- Limbic system
- Hypothalamus

Vasomotor
sudomotor
(sweating)
piloerectors

ARMS
TRUNK
LEGS

T1 Pupillary dilatation.
2
3 Cardiac acceleration.
4 Bronchodilator.
5
6
7 Adrenal gland – adrenaline
8 and noradrenaline release.
9 Bowel ⎫ (decreases smooth
10 ⎪ muscle activity:
11 ⎬
12 ⎪ stimulates
L1 Bladder ⎭ sphincters).
2
3
4

Autonomic fibres in peripheral
nerve to blood vessels, sweat
glands and piloerector
muscles in skin

Intermedio-
lateral
column

Myelinated
preganglionic
fibres
(white ramus)

Non-myelinated
post-ganglionic
fibres
(grey ramus)

Sympathetic
ganglion

Prevertebral ganglion

Fibres which pass through the sympathetic ganglion to synapse
on a prevertebral ganglion, e.g. coeliac or mesenteric ganglia
constitute the *splanchnic nerves* and innervate the viscera.

AFFERENT AUTONOMIC NERVOUS SYSTEM

Sympathetic

Terminate in spinal cord in intermediate zone of grey matter – in relation to preganglionic
neurons.
Function: Important in the appreciation of visceral pain.

Parasympathetic

Afferent fibres from the mouth and pharynx, and respiratory, cardiac and gastrointestinal
systems, travelling in the VII, IX and X cranial nerves, terminate in the nucleus of tractus
solitarius.
Function: Important in maintaining visceral reflexes.
The sacral afferents end in the S2–S4 region in relation to preganglionic neurons.

NEUROTRANSMITTER SUBSTANCES

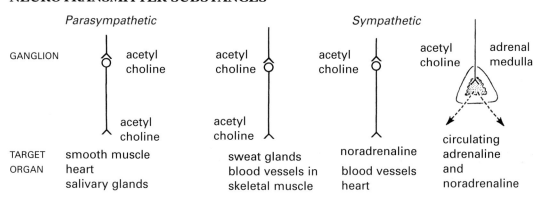

Parasympathetic

Sympathetic

GANGLION

acetyl
choline

acetyl
choline

acetyl
choline

acetyl
choline

adrenal
medulla

acetyl
choline

acetyl
choline

noradrenaline

circulating
adrenaline
and
noradrenaline

TARGET
ORGAN

smooth muscle
heart
salivary glands

sweat glands
blood vessels in
skeletal muscle

blood vessels
heart

455

TESTS OF AUTONOMIC FUNCTION

BLOOD PRESSURE CONTROL

1. Maintenance of blood pressure with alteration in posture – is normally dependent upon reflex baroreceptor function. A fall in BP occurs with efferent or afferent lesions – postural (orthostatic) hypotension.
2. Exposure to cold induces vasoconstriction and a rise in BP – cold pressor test. Stress will produce a similar pressor response, e.g. ask patient to do mental arithmetic.
   Both central and peripheral lesions affect these tests.
3. Valsalva manoeuvre:
   The patient exhales against a closed glottis, increases intrathoracic pressure and thus reduces venous return and systemic BP. The heart rate accelerates to maintain BP. On opening the glottis, venous return increases and an overshoot of BP with cardiac slowing occurs. An impaired response occurs with afferent or efferent autonomic lesions.
4. Noradrenaline infusion test:
   A postganglionic sympathetic lesion results in 'supersensitivity' of denervated smooth muscle to adrenaline, with a marked rise in BP following infusion.

HEART RATE

1. Massage of the carotid sinus should stimulate the baroreceptors, increase vagal parasympathetic discharge and slow the heart rate. Either efferent or afferent lesions abolish this response.
2. Atropine test:
   Intravenous atropine 'blocks' vagal action and with intact sympathetic innervation results in an increase in heart rate.

SWEATING

A rise in body temperature causes increased sweating, detectable on the skin surface with starch-iodide paper. Any lesion from the central to the postganglionic sympathetic system impairs sweating.

SKIN TEMPERATURE

Skin temperature is a function of the sympathetic supply to blood vessels. With pre- or postganglionic lesions the skin becomes warm and red. With chronic postganglionic lesions the skin may become cold and blue (denervation hypersensitivity) compare the temperature of various regions.

PUPILLARY FUNCTION

Check the response to light and accommodation.
Pharmacological tests are important:
1. Atropine – blocks parasympathetic system – dilates pupil.
2. Cocaine – stimulates adrenergic receptors – dilates pupil.

In highly specialised units detailed neurophysiology (e.g. thermal threshold measurements) and plasma concentrations of neurotransmitters and hormones at rest and in response to baroreceptor stimulation are employed to characterize the site and selectivity of the autonomic lesion.

AUTONOMIC NERVOUS SYSTEM – SPECIFIC DISEASES

Symptoms of autonomic dysfunction occur in many common conditions which affect both the parasympathetic and sympathetic pathways e.g. cerebrovascular disease.

The following are less common disorders which primarily may affect the autonomic nervous system –

IDIOPATHIC ORTHOSTATIC HYPOTENSION

Two types of this condition are recognised:
1. Due to degeneration of sympathetic postganglionic neurons.
2. Due to degeneration of sympathetic preganglionic neurons of the intermediolateral column T1–T12 – SHY-DRAGER SYNDROME.

In the latter disorder, features of extrapyramidal system involvement are also found.

Both disorders are characterised by: postural hypotension: anhidrosis (absent sweating): impotence: sphincter disturbance: pupillary abnormalities.

The disorders may be separated pharmacologically; the postganglionic disorders shows hypersensitivity (denervation hypersensitivity) to noradrenaline infusion.

Treatment

Drugs such as fludrocortisone increase blood volume and may prevent postural hypotension.

DIABETIC AUTONOMIC NEUROPATHY

Symptoms of autonomic dysfunction are common in long-standing insulin-dependent diabetics:

Impotence/retrograde ejaculation.

Bladder dysfunction – decreased detrusor muscle action – resulting in increased residual volume.

Nocturnal diarrhoea.

GI dysfunction – vomiting from gastroparesis.

Orthostatic hypotension.

These problems arise from damage to both sympathetic and parasympathetic postganglionic neurons.

Treatment

Improve diabetic control and treat symptoms e.g. fludrocortisone for BP control.

POST-INFECTIOUS POLYNEUROPATHY – Guillain-Barré syndrome (see previous chapter). Autonomic involvement occurs commonly in this disorder and may present major problems in patient management. The lesion may involve the afferent or efferent limbs of the cardiovascular reflexes (baroreceptor reflexes) resulting in postural hypotension, episodes of hypertension and cardiac dysrhythmias.

Occasionally the postinfectious neuropathy is purely autonomic.

HEREDITARY SENSORY & AUTONOMIC NEUROPATHY (HSAN)

This group of rare, generally recessively inherited disorders are characterised by insensitivity to pain, anhidrosis (absence of sweating), orthostatic hypotension and unexplained fevers from birth. Riley-Day syndrome is typical of these though its gene mutation is confined to Ashkenazi Jewish families.

PRIMARY AMYLOIDOSIS

Autonomic involvement with orthostatic hypotension, impotence, diarrhoea and bladder involvement may accompany sensorimotor neuropathy in the primary and hereditary forms. Amyloid infiltration affects autonomic ganglia.

ADIE'S SYNDROME

A tonic pupil (page 142) associated with areflexia and occasionally widespread autonomic dysfunction, e.g. segmental hypohidrosis (absent sweating) and diarrhoea.

AUTONOMIC DYSFUNCTION IN QUADRIPLEGIA (autonomic dysreflexia)

A high cervical lesion which completely severs the spinal cord, e.g. traumatic cervical fracture/dislocation will isolate all but the cranial parasympathetic outflow. As a result, disturbed autonomic function is inevitable but variable.

Autonomic reflexes are retained – Passive movement or tactile stimulation of limbs may result in blood pressure rise, bradycardia, sweating, reflex penile erection (priapism).

AUTONOMIC NERVOUS SYSTEM – BLADDER INNERVATION

Efferent innervation

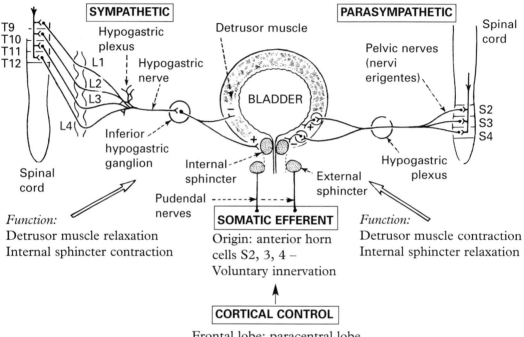

SYMPATHETIC

T9, T10, T11, T12

Hypogastric plexus

L1, L2, L3, L4

Hypogastric nerve

Inferior hypogastric ganglion

Spinal cord

Detrusor muscle

BLADDER

Internal sphincter

Pudendal nerves

External sphincter

PARASYMPATHETIC

Spinal cord

Pelvic nerves (nervi erigentes)

S2, S3, S4

Hypogastric plexus

Function:
Detrusor muscle relaxation
Internal sphincter contraction

SOMATIC EFFERENT

Origin: anterior horn cells S2, 3, 4 – Voluntary innervation

Function:
Detrusor muscle contraction
Internal sphincter relaxation

CORTICAL CONTROL

Frontal lobe: paracentral lobe
– initiates micturition
– inhibits micturition

Afferent innervation

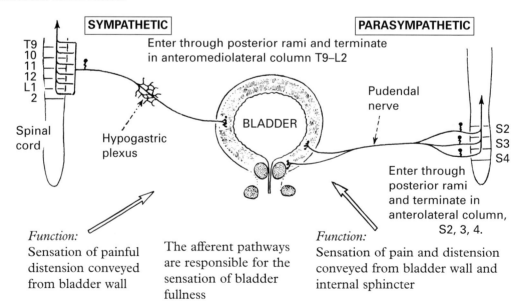

SYMPATHETIC

T9, 10, 11, 12, L1, 2

Spinal cord

Hypogastric plexus

Enter through posterior rami and terminate in anteromediolateral column T9–L2

BLADDER

Pudendal nerve

PARASYMPATHETIC

S2, S3, S4

Enter through posterior rami and terminate in anterolateral column, S2, 3, 4.

Function:
Sensation of painful distension conveyed from bladder wall

The afferent pathways are responsible for the sensation of bladder fullness

Function:
Sensation of pain and distension conveyed from bladder wall and internal sphincter

MICTURITION

PROCESS OF MICTURITION

1. Cortical centre – removal of conscious inhibition of micturition.
2. Voiding – wave-like detrusor muscle contractions with relaxation of internal and external sphincters.
3. Voiding completed – detrusor muscle relaxation
   contraction of internal sphincter
   contraction of external sphincter.
4. Voiding may be voluntarily interrupted before complete bladder emptying by forced voluntary contraction of the external sphincter.

DISORDERS OF MICTURITION

Complete or partial spinal cord lesion

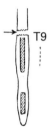 isolates segmental innervation from cortical control

Retention develops

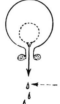

Increase in the intravesical pressure eventually overcomes internal sphincter integrity and 'dribbling overflow incontinence' results.

After some days or weeks a REFLEX BLADDER develops – *automatic emptying may be induced by abdominal tapping*. This voiding is often inadequate due to reflex contractions of the external sphincter before bladder emptying (autonomic dysnergia). High residual volumes result.

Lesions of the cauda equina

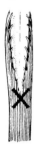 Result in a parasympathetic denervated bladder which enlarges – flaccid neurogenic bladder – again with 'overflow incontinence'

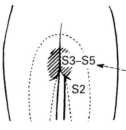

Sensation is lost in the sacral dermatomes. Anal tone is diminished and the anal reflex absent.

After weeks or months, abdominal compression combined with a Valsalva manoeuvre can induce efficient bladder emptying.

Urinary and, less commonly, associated faecal incontinence occurs in women following traumatic childbirth with injury to the innervation of striated pelvic floor musculature.

BOWEL AND SEXUAL FUNCTION

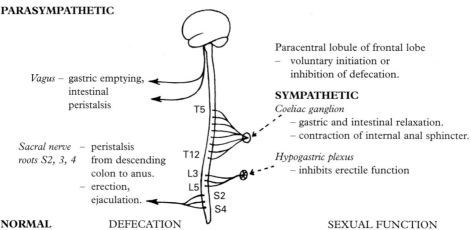

PARASYMPATHETIC

Vagus – gastric emptying, intestinal peristalsis

Sacral nerve – peristalsis
roots S2, 3, 4 from descending colon to anus.
– erection, ejaculation.

T5
T12
L3
L5
S2
S4

Paracentral lobule of frontal lobe
– voluntary initiation or inhibition of defecation.

SYMPATHETIC
Coeliac ganglion
– gastric and intestinal relaxation.
– contraction of internal anal sphincter.

Hypogastric plexus
– inhibits erectile function

NORMAL PROCESS	**DEFECATION**

DEFECATION
1. Faeces arrive at rectosigmoid junction:
   – cortical awareness of urge to defecate
   – release of sympathetic tone.
2. Relaxation of pelvic floor muscles and internal anal sphincter. Lowering of anorectum.
3. Voluntary opening of external anal sphincter.
4. Parasympathetic peristalsis and Valsalva manoeuvre empty the rectum.

SEXUAL FUNCTION
Parasympathetic:
– penile/clitoral erection.
   Reflex – in response to tactile stimulation of erogenous zones.
   Psychogenic – sexual thoughts or visual erotic stimulation – orgasm, ejaculation
Sympathetic:
– mainly anti-erectile action.

COMPLETE OR PARTIAL CORD LESION

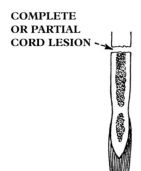

Bowel atony for up to 1 week. → Faecal retention with impaction and faecal fluid overflow (spurious diarrhoea).
Impaired/absent external sphincter tone becomes spastic after days or weeks.
→ *Regular bowel emptying reflexly in response to digital stimulation or suppositories achieves continence.*

♂ Prolonged reflex erection (priapism) may occur for 2–3 days, then:
– Erections and ejaculation lost for weeks or months, then:
– Reflex erections (only tactile) appear but reflex ejaculation seldom returns.
Fertility is impaired or lost

♀ Vaginal sensation and lubrication are lost. Fertility is retained.

CONUS LESION

→ Mixed upper and lower neuron pattern

Loss of genital sensation.
Loss of reflex erections and ejaculation (psychogenic erection may be retained).
Male infertile; female fertility retained.
Male erection may be achieved by cavernosal blockade using intracavernosal injection of papaverine HCl.

CAUDA EQUINA LESION

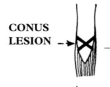

Flaccid external sphincter. Faecal retention with impaction and faecal fluid overflow.
Regular clearance of constipated stool by manual evacuation or Valsalva manoeuvre achieves continence.

DISEASES OF SKELETAL (VOLUNTARY) MUSCLE

Normal skeletal muscle morphology

A skeletal muscle is composed of a large number of muscle fibres separated by connective tissue (endomysium) and arranged in bundles (fasciculi) in which the individual fibres are parallel to each other. Each fasciculus has a connective tissue sheath (perimysium) and the muscle itself is composed of a number of fasciculi bound together and surrounded by a connective tissue sheath (epimysium).

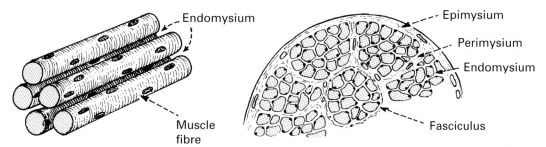

The three envelopes (sheaths) are made up of connective tissue richly endowed with blood vessels and fat cells (lipocytes).

The muscle fibre

This is a large multinucleated cell
with an outer membrane – SARCOLEMMA
and a cytoplasm – SARCOPLASM
within which lie the MYOFIBRILS

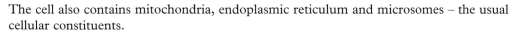

Each muscle fibre has its own endplate approximately half way along its length.

The cell also contains mitochondria, endoplasmic reticulum and microsomes – the usual cellular constituents.

Fats, glycogen, enzymes and myoglobin lie within the sarcoplasm and related structures.

The **MYOFIBRILS** are the contractile components of muscle.

Each myofibril is 1 μ in diameter and contains filaments of *myosin* and *actin* interdigitating with each other between each Z line. When muscle contracts or relaxes these filaments slide over each other producing shortening and lengthening of the muscle fibre. The striated appearance of skeletal muscle is a consequence of differing concentrations of actin and myosin. These resultant bands are designated as shown.

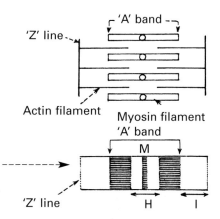

MUSCLE MORPHOLOGY AND FUNCTION

Fibre type

It is possible to distinguish two main types of muscle fibre on pathological and physiological study: Type I: Slow twitch, fatigue resistant.
Type II: Fast twitch, fatigue dependent.

Characteristics:	**Type I**	**Type II**
	ATPase stain: Light	ATPase stain: Dark
	Oxidative metabolism	Glycolytic metabolism
	Abundant mitochondria	High glucogen content

The muscle fibre type is influenced by its innervation that further determines its pattern of use; all muscle fibres innervated by a single motor neuron (the motor unit) have identical physiological and pathological parameters. The distribution of muscle fibre types differ in specific muscles within the body according to function – the muscles of the erector spinae are rich in oxidative, fatigue resistant fibres while the converse is true in triceps.

Neuromuscular junction

Each muscle fibre receives a nerve branch from the motor cell body in the anterior horn of the spinal cord or cranial nerve motor nuclei.

When a nerve fibre reaches the muscle it loses its myelin sheath and its neurilemma then merges with the sarcolemma under which the axon spreads out to form the motor endplate. The axon fibre with its endings and muscle fibres it supplies is called the MOTOR UNIT. The number of muscle fibres in a motor unit varies: in the eye muscles it is small (5–10), whereas in the limb muscles the number is large (in the gastrocnemius about 1800). Each motor unit contains only one type of muscle fibre, i.e. type I or type II. The neuromuscular junction is the point at which neuromuscular transmission is effected. The motor endplate is separate from the sarcoplasm by the synaptic cleft.

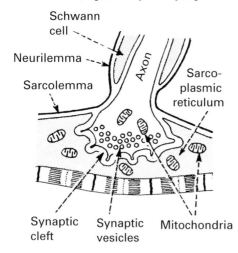

Schwann cell
Neurilemma
Sarcolemma
Axon
Sarco-plasmic reticulum

Synaptic cleft   Synaptic vesicles   Mitochondria

Physiology
Muscle contraction results from the following:
1) A depolarisation wave arrives at the axon terminus and opens voltage sensitive Ca^{2+} channels
2) Ca^{2+} entry triggers fusion of synaptic vesicles with the axon membrane which then release acetylcholine into the synaptic cleft
3) Acetylcholine attaches to end-plate receptors with Na^+ entry into muscle. Post synaptic depolarisation initiates an action potential that spreads along the sarcolemmal membrane.
4) Release of Ca^{2+} from the sarcoplasmic reticulum and the interaction of actin and myosin result in muscle contraction.

The enzyme cholinesterase, found in high concentration at motor endplates, destroys acetylcholine so that normally a single nerve impulse only gives rise to a single muscle contraction.

MUSCLE MORPHOLOGY AND FUNCTION

Biochemistry

Muscle contraction requires adenosine triphosphate (ATP). This may be generated either by carbohydrate breakdown (glycogenolysis and glycolysis,) or lipid breakdown (beta-oxidation). These non-oxygen requiring processes produce only a limited amount of ATP but also generate Acetyl- Co-A which, in the presence of oxygen, is further metabolised through the Krebs cycle within the mitochondria. This process yields even greater quantities of ATP.

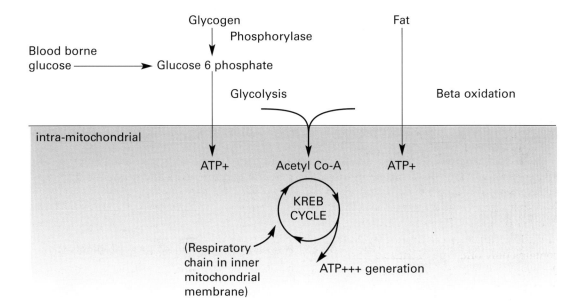

The biochemical pathways yielding energy from the Krebs cycle reactions are dependent on proteins coded for by both the nuclear and mitochondrial genome. Mitochondrial DNA (mtDNA) is present in many copies per mitochondrion, with many mitochondria per cell. The usual state is that all an individual's mtDNA has the same sequence – homoplasmy – but in the mitochondrial disorders mutations are frequently present in only a proportion of the mtDNA – heteroplasmy. The distribution of these populations is not homogeneous across tissues and these features make the diagnosis of disorders associated with abnormalities of mtDNA difficult when the mutation may not be detected in blood but may be present in varying amounts in muscle or other affected tissues (see page 478).

MUSCLE DISEASE – HISTORY, EXAMINATION AND INVESTIGATIONS

History taking

This must include

- *A family history* paying particular attention to additional features that can be associated with muscle disease (e.g. deafness if a mitochondrial disorder is suspected or diabetes and cataracts with Myotonic Dystrophy).
- *Age at onset.* Parents describe delay in early motor milestones or a history of poor athletic abilities. Old photographs show long-standing facial weakness or ptosis.
- *A full drug and alcohol history.*
- *Terminology.* Patients should be given the opportunity to expand on terms such as 'weakness', 'cramp' or 'fatigue'. These are often used to describe symptoms distinct from their strict medical definitions.
- *Pattern of weakness.* Proximal weakness will produce difficulty in descending stairs or rising from a low chair or drying hair. Distal weakness causes difficulty with latch keys, ascending stairs and scuffing toes.
- *Pain and cramp.* Their relationship to exercise should be noted. In disorders of glycolysis a cramp develops in the exercising muscle after a minute or so whereas in Carnitine-palmityl transferase deficiency cramp and rhabdomyolysis follows some hours later.
- *Fatiguability.* This occurs in neuromuscular transmission disorders and mitochondrial disease.

Examination

This must assess

- *Walking* – here a waddling or foot drop gait is noted or other neurological problems such as Parkinsonism identified.
- *The distribution of weakness and wasting* will distinguish proximal, distal and generalised myopathies. Involvement of anatomically adjacent muscles is a feature of the muscular dystrophies. The face must be carefully examined for minor bilateral facial weakness; mild ptosis and limitation of extraocular movements. Muscle weakness should be graded using a standard scale (Medical Research Council scale – page 431).
- *The presence of pseudohypertrophy and contractures* (easily missed at hips, ankles and elbows) should be noted.

Investigations

- *Creatine kinase (CK):* this sarcoplasmic enzyme is released from the damaged muscle membrane. High levels are associated with Muscular Dystrophies and Rhabdomyolysis but normal values do not exclude milder muscle disease (benign recessive dystrophies, mitochondrial and some metabolic disorders).
- *Neurophysiology:* may differentiate neurogenic from myopathic weakness and provide evidence of muscle membrane damage (e.g. inflammatory myopathies), but normal studies do not exclude muscle disease.
- *Muscle biopsy:* Routine staining of frozen material identifies some disorders but immunohistochemical analysis and appropriate mutation studies are needed for the diagnosis of others (e.g. Muscular Dystrophies). The choice between needle and open biopsy is difficult – the former is simpler but no less painful; the latter may be preferable to avoid sampling error.

INHERITED MUSCLE DISORDERS

The muscular dystrophies (MD) are genetically determined progressive disorders of muscle characterised by cycles of muscle fibre necrosis, regeneration, eventual fibrosis and replacement with fatty tissue. Originally defined and described on patterns of weakness (e.g. Facio-scapulo-humeral muscular dystrophy) they are now defined on the basis of known gene loci and protein product. This is not yet possible in all dystrophies but a continuing reclassification is taking place. Many disorders are associated with abnormalities in the dystrophin associated glycoprotein complex. Congenital myopathies are associated with morphological muscle abnormalities without necrosis and with a more benign prognosis. The metabolic myopathies present with pain, weakness or fatigue.

Xp2.1 DYSTROPHIES (DUCHENNE & BECKER MUSCULAR DYSTROPHY)

The gene for dystrophin is located at Xp2.1. Point mutations and deletions affecting the terminal domains are more often associated with the severe clinical phenotype of Duchenne, while deletions within the central rod domain are associated with the milder Becker Dystrophy.

DUCHENNE DYSTROPHY

Clinical features

Duchenne MD has an incidence of 1:3500 male births. It is characterised by delayed early motor development usually noted between ages 1 and 3 years, followed by scoliosis, contractures and eventual loss of ambulation at around 12 years of age. Pseudohypertrophy of muscle, in particular the calf, is a characteristic (occurring in 80%) but not a pathognomonic feature.

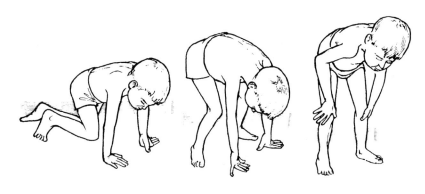

The child cannot climb stairs or rise from a low chair and when attempting to rise from the ground will 'climb up him' – Gower's sign (not diagnostic of the condition, but indicative of pelvic muscle weakness).

465

INHERITED MUSCLE DISORDERS

Investigation

Gene testing on serum may establish the diagnosis. The Dystrophin gene is large and many protocols only screen a part of it. A 'negative test' therefore does not rule it out and muscle biopsy with immunological testing is necessary. This demonstrates the absence of dystrophin. Female carriers can be detected by PCR.

Creatine kinase (CK) – substantially elevated (several thousand times). The enzyme is raised at birth and elevated in female carriers (in earlier times this formed the basis for counselling).

Electrocardiogram – 80% show conduction disorders, tall precordial R waves and deep left precordial Q waves. Echocardiography should be repeated occasionally to detect developing cardiomyopathy.

Electromyography – shows severe myopathic change.

Life expectancy has risen from late teens to late 20s or early 30s with the use of surgery to correct scoliosis, active control of contractures and non-invasive ventilation. Death occurs from respiratory insufficiency and infection or is 'sudden' and presumed to be related to cardiac disease. Long term care of affected individuals should be co-ordinated with anticipation rather than reaction to the evolution of disease.

BECKER DYSTROPHY

Abnormalities within the dystrophin gene may be associated with a spectrum of presentations from Duchenne to the milder condition described by Becker. Becker MD is rarer than Duchenne MD – incidence 1:35 000, presenting at a later age usually with limb-girdle involvement and pseudohypertrophy. These later milder presentations may also occur in some female carriers of the mutation. Cardiac involvement may be symptomatic in up to 10% of affected individuals and female carriers and is not related to the mutation or the severity of limb muscle disease.

The diagnosis is established in up to 80% of cases with serum DNA analysis. In the rest a combination of immunohistochemical demonstration of the relative absence of dystrophin, elevated CK, the clinical pattern and pedigree analysis make the diagnosis.

MUSCULAR DYSTROPHIES

DYSTROPHIES WITH PARTICULAR PATTERNS OF WEAKNESS

Facioscapulohumeral (FSH)

An autosomal dominant disorder, variable in severity and associated with a contraction of a series of 3.3 kB repeats at locus 4q35. Incidence 1–2:100 000. The mechanism by which this mutation causes disease is not known.

The clinical features include
- Facial weakness (which may be mild or asymmetrical)
- Periscapular weakness producing winging of the scapula and rising up of the scapulae on attempted abduction
- Weakness of the humeral muscles
- A predominantly proximal lower limb pattern of weakness giving a dromedary or camel-backed gait

Pseudohypertrophy is not a feature.

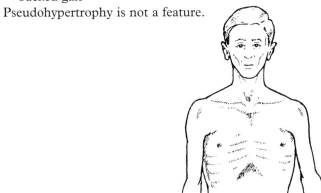

Severity is variable, ranging from severe childhood forms to later onset disease that may be asymptomatic. CK levels may only be raised to 1.5–2 upper limit or normal. EMG and muscle biopsy will show myopathic abnormalities but have no specific features; although secondary inflammatory change on biopsy may lead to an erroneous diagnosis of Polymyositis. Cardiac involvement is not a feature. High frequency sensorineural hearing loss and exudative retinal telangiectases complicate some early onset cases (Coat's syndrome). Prognosis is dependent on the degree of respiratory muscle involvement. Some may benefit from ventilatory support.

Scapuloperoneal

A dominant or recessive disorder that involves proximal upper and distal lower limb muscles. Onset is in adulthood with foot drop followed by weakness in scapular deltoid, triceps and biceps muscle groups. Differentiation from spinal muscular atrophy and inflammatory muscle disease is difficult.

Distal

Distal weakness due to primary dystrophies is rare with the exception of Myotonic Dystrophy. Both autosomal dominant and recessive patterns are described and may involve upper or lower limb muscles at onset. Some are associated with vacuolation of muscle fibres.

MUSCULAR DYSTROPHIES

DYSTROPHIES WITH PARTICULAR PATTERNS OF WEAKNESS (*cont'd*)

Emery Dreifuss

Rare but important because of its cardiac complications. Both X-linked and dominant forms reported (the dominant form is now classified as LGMD type 2). Contractures of the spine produce an appearance of hyperextension. Contractures of elbows and ankles occur early. Weakness may be in a scapuloperoneal distribution. Life threatening cardiac condition defects are virtually universal and ventricular tachyarrythmias occur in a proportion. Patients will require pacing and some have implanted defibrillators. Respiratory muscle weakness may occur.

Oculopharyngeal

This is another very rare pattern of weakness associated with a small GCG trinucleotide expansion in the PABP2 gene on chromosome 14. Inheritance is autosomal dominant. Occurs with a mean age of onset of 50 years with a combination of ptosis, ophthalmoparesis and dysphagia. Limb weakness may occur. Muscle biopsy shows rimmed vacuoles and filamentous intranuclear inclusions.

Limb girdle syndromes and limb girdle muscular dystrophy (LGMD)

Slowly progressing proximal weakness is a common presentation of both primary and secondary myopathies. A large number of proteins with differing functions produce a similar LGMD phenotype. Recessive forms are more common than dominant ones. The differential diagnosis of limb girdle distribution weakness is wide (see table).

CATEGORIES	EXAMPLES	SUGGESTIVE FEATURES
Non-dystrophic genetic myopathies	Desmin myopathy, congenital structural myopathies (nemaline etc.)	Early onset, presence of contractures, often very thin muscles yet only mild weakness
Metabolic myopathies	Acid Maltase deficiency, McArdles disease, mitochondrial disorders	Pain, variability, exercise intolerance
Endocrine	Hypo- and hyperthyroidism, osteomalacic myopathy, Cushing's syndrome	Diffuse pattern of weakness, endocrine features may not be prominent
Toxic/metabolic	Steroid therapy, alcohol, statins	Should be apparent from history
Inflammatory	Polymyositis	See discussion below
Limb Girdle Muscular Dystrophy (LGMD)	At least 3 dominant and 9 recessive forms. Precise diagnosis requires specialised investigation	Symmetry, focal involvement of individual muscles, cardiac conduction defects, contractures from early stages

MUSCULAR DYSTROPHIES

MYOTONIC DYSTROPHY (MyD)

Myotonic Dystrophy is an autosomal dominant multisystem disorder caused by an unstable trinucleotide repeat expansion in a non-coding sequence at position 19q13.3. This expansion is thought to be pathogenic because of indirect effects on adjacent gene(s). It may present at any age with an incidence of 5 per 100 000.

Whilst neuromuscular features may not be prominent, the condition is usually characterised by the presence of MYOTONIA – failure of immediate muscle relaxation after contraction has ceased.

It can be demonstrated by:

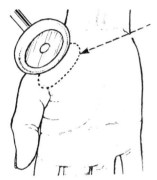

1. Striking a muscle with the tendon hammer and watching the resultant 'dimple' persist for a while before filling up.

2. Asking the patient to grip an object then suddenly release it. The slow relaxation and opening of the hand grip will make the object appear 'stuck' to the fingers.

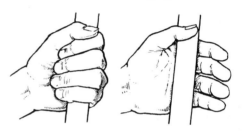

Clinical features

The facial appearance is typical:

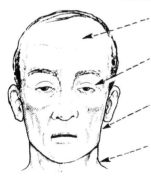

Frontal baldness
Myopathic face with ptosis
Jaw hanging and wasting of muscles of mastication resulting in hollowing of temporal fossae and cheeks
Wasting of neck and shoulder girdle muscles also is evident

In the limbs – weakness and wasting are distal though the hands are spared until late.

– Cataracts
– Disorders of smooth muscle; gut motility disorders, constipation, poor bladder emptying.
– Cardiac disease; dilated cardiomyopathy and atrio-ventricular block requiring cardiac pacing
– Respiratory failure; due to intercostals and diaphragmatic weakness, impaired swallowing with risk of aspiration and central sleep apnoea (many patients benefit from nocturnal respiratory support).
– Diabetes; due to insulin resistance
– Testicular atrophy and subfertility

MUSCULAR DYSTROPHIES

MYOTONIC DYSTROPHY (MyD) (cont'd)

Diagnosis

In classic adult-onset cases, clinical diagnosis is straightforward with demonstration of progressive distal and bulbar dystrophy in the presence of myotonia, with frontal balding, and cataracts. Clinical diagnosis can be more difficult in mild cases, where cataracts may be the only manifestation. Direct analysis, by Southern blotting on peripheral leucocytes, of the size of the CTG repeat permits DNA diagnosis. Normal individuals have 5 to 37 CTG repeats, whereas patients have 50 to several thousand CTG repeats.

The importance of recognition of the disorder lies in the management of complications and genetic advice. The gene defect instability (number of repeats) between generations accounts for the wide clinical variability (phenotype) of MyD. Females are at risk of delivering a severely affected child who, due to respiratory failure, may not survive the neonatal period. Occasionally persons first present, either spontaneously or following anaesthesia, with unexpected respiratory failure or sudden death.

When molecular tests are negative but clinical features suggestive two rare alternative disorders are considered –

1. DYSTROPHIA MYOTONICA 2 (MyD 2)

Genetically distinct form of myotonic dystrophy. Affected family members show remarkable clinical similarity to classic MyD (myotonia, proximal and distal limb weakness, frontal balding, cataracts, and cardiac arrhythmias). Disease locus maps to a 10 cM region of 3q.

2. PROXIMAL MYOTONIC MYOPATHY (PROMM)

This dominant disorder presents with myotonia in 30s–40s and mild proximal weakness in the fifth to seventh decades of life. Muscle biopsy demonstrates a non-specific mild myopathy with hypertrophy of type 2 fibres. Cataracts identical to those found in MyD occur in 15 to 30% of patients. Cardiac symptoms (arrhythmias) are infrequent. The gene causing PROMM is also located on 3q, suggesting that PROMM and MyD 2 are either allelic disorders or caused by closely linked genes.

DYSTROPHIES: GENERAL PRINCIPLES

It may not be possible to diagnose or exclude a specific type of dystrophy but practical issues apply to all:
– *Genetics*. The implications for the family of differing modes of inheritance are clear. Help should be sought from a clinical geneticist to discuss these even if no molecular diagnosis has been reached but an inherited disorder suspected. Isolated cases of LGMD may represent a new dominant mutation and its phenotype is extremely variable. Both patients and their partners should be made aware of such issues.
– *Cardiac disease*. This is critically important in the Emery-Dreifuss syndrome where life-threatening conduction defects are inevitable but also occur in Xp2.1 related dystrophies and Polymyositis. In the absence of a proven diagnosis, ECGs should be performed at 12 monthly intervals and echocardiography also if symptoms suggestive of cardiac failure develop.
– *Respiratory failure* related to diaphragmatic weakness, a prominent feature of Xp2.1, MD, LGMD, other forms of MD and inflammatory muscle disease. Late deterioration in some of the congenital myopathies may also lead to sleep disordered breathing. It is important to be aware of this, as non-invasive nocturnal ventilatory support is frequently beneficial to such patients.

INFLAMMATORY MYOPATHY

Primary inflammatory myopathies are clinically, pathologically and therapeutically distinct entities. Inflammatory changes are probably due to an immune mediated process rather than directly pathogenic. These are acquired as opposed to the inherited dystrophies and are classified as follows:

Polymyositis —— Childhood form
⟍ Adult form

Dermatomyositis

Inclusion body myositis

Inflammatory myopathy associated with malignant disease

Inflammatory myopathy associated with collagen vascular disorders – e.g. lupus erythematosus, systemic sclerosis, rheumatoid arthritis.

Infective – *Viral* e.g. coxsackie, echo. *Parasitic*, e.g. cysticercosis, trichinosis, taenia solium, toxoplasma, toxocara.

Sarcoid myopathy – some with this multi-system disease have granulomas in skeletal muscle.

POLYMYOSITIS/DERMATOMYOSITIS

There are two principal forms of inflammatory myopathy – polymyositis and dermatomyositis – which are separated clinically by the dermatological findings in the latter. All age groups are affected. Annual incidence is 8 per 100 000. These disorders are sporadic though familial cases are described.

An autoimmune basis for these disorders is supported by:
– response to immunosuppressive therapy.
– association with other known immunological disorders, e.g. collagen vascular disorders.
– elevated IgG in blood and presence of circulating autoantibodies, e.g. antinuclear antibody in some cases.
– an increased incidence of certain histocompatibility antigens (HLA antigens) – B_8, DR3.
– the reproduction of a similar disorder in laboratory animals by injection of muscle extract with Freund's adjuvant.

Humoral and cell mediated immune mechanisms seem responsible for these disorders but the trigger factor(s) remain unknown.

INFLAMMATORY MYOPATHY

Clinical presentation
Onset is acute or subacute over a period of several weeks and may follow systemic infection.

Systemic symptoms prevail at onset, e.g. lassitude, and are then followed by muscle weakness. Extensive oedema of skin and subcutaneous tissues is common (especially in the periorbital region).

POLYMYOSITIS

Muscles may be painful and tender in 60% of cases though onset is often painless.

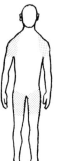

Proximal muscles are first involved and initially weakness may be asymmetrical e.g. one quadriceps only.

Weakness of posterior neck muscles will result in the head 'lolling' forwards.

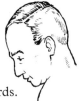

Occasionally weakness may spread into distal limb muscle groups.

Pharyngeal and laryngeal involvement results in dysphagia and dysphonia. Cardiac muscle may also be involved. Respiratory muscle weakness causes respiratory failure (this may be disproportionately severe).

The eye muscles are *not* involved unless there is coexistent myasthenia gravis.

Reflexes are retained (if absent, consider underlying carcinoma with added neuropathy).

Differential diagnosis
Inclusion body myositis.
Acid maltase deficiency
Limb girdle muscular dystrophy (LGMD)
Drug induced, toxic and metabolic myopathies.

DERMATOMYOSITIS

Often more severe and acute
Characterised by skin rash.
Violet discoloration of light exposed skin.

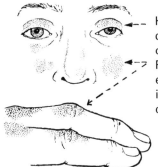

Heliotropic discoloration of eyelids
Raised scaly erythematous rash involving nose and cheeks, shoulders, extensor surfaces of limbs and knuckles

Telangiectasia and tightening of skin are common and small ulcerated vasculitic lesions develop over bony prominences.

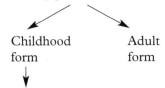

Childhood form   Adult form

Multisystem involvement.
Calcification develops in skin and muscle with extrusion through skin.
Muscle contractures develop – tip-toe gait.
Gastrointestinal ulceration occurs.

The muscle weakness is as in polymyositis but in childhood dermatomyositis may be very severe, involving chewing, swallowing and breathing.

INFLAMMATORY MYOPATHY

INCLUSION BODY MYOSITIS (IBM)

Recognised now as the commonest inflammatory muscle disorder in the middle aged and elderly (women are less commonly affected and more likely to be younger). Unlike the other inflammatory myopathies symmetrical weakness is painless and distal including foot extensors and finger flexors. Most patients have a protracted course unaffected by immunosuppressive therapies. Occasionally it is associated with connective tissue disorders such as Sjögren's syndrome.

Investigations

Diagnosis is supported by the following investigations:

Muscle enzymes
Creatine kinase (CK) is elevated.
Released from necrotic muscle, it is
an indicator of disease activity and severity

Circulating antibodies
e.g. rheumatoid factor, antinuclear
factor. Present in 40%.

Electromyography
Shows a typical myopathic pattern.

Erythrocyte sedimentation rate (ESR)
Elevated in most patients.

Muscle biopsy shows necrosis of muscle fibres with inflammatory cells – lymphocytes, plasma cells, leucocytes.

The distinguishing features of the common inflammatory myopathies and responses to treatment are summarised as follows:

	Dermatomyositis	**Polymyositis**	**Inclusion body myositis**
Clinical features	Proximal weakness	Proximal weakness	Axial and asymmetric distal weakness
Neurophysiology	Myopathic	Myopathic	Mixed neurogenic/ myopathic
Pathology	Necrosis, secondary inflammatory infiltrate, perifascicular atrophy of muscle fibres	Necrosis, inflammatory infiltrate, T cell mediated necrosis; invasion of healthy muscle fibres	Necrosis, inflammatory cell infiltrate. Vacuolation with inclusion bodies and paired helical filaments at EM
Therapy	Steroids, intravenous immunoglobulin	Steroids; usually with azathioprine	None proven to benefit
Associations	Paraneoplastic in adults	Weakly paraneoplastic	Sjögren's etc.

INFLAMMATORY MYOPATHY

OUTCOME OF INFLAMMATORY MYOPATHIES

The natural history of these conditions is uncertain; mortality is low though perhaps only a minority recover completely. Inclusion body myositis is slowly and steadily progressive. Polymyositis and dermatomyositis respond in varying degrees to treatment and eventually become inactive. Safe monitoring of treatments and protection against side effects (e.g. steroid induced bone disease) is critical.

POLYMYOSITIS AND DERMATOMYOSITIS ASSOCIATED WITH MALIGNANT DISEASES

Approximately 10% of adults with inflammatory myopathy have underlying neoplasia usually carcinoma. In dermatomyositis, of those over 40 years of age as many as 60% harbour neoplasia. Neoplasia may present before or after the development of inflammatory myopathy.

POLYMYOSITIS AND DERMATOMYOSITIS ASSOCIATED WITH COLLAGEN VASCULAR DISEASES

Approximately 15% of adults with inflammatory myopathy have symptoms and signs of an associated collagen vascular disorder.

In 5–10% of persons with these disorders (systemic lupus erythematosus etc.), inflammatory myopathy develops at some stage in their illness.

In the 'overlap' syndromes (mixed collagen vascular diseases) muscle involvement is more common.

ENDOCRINE MYOPATHIES

Unlike inflammatory myopathy the weakness in these conditions is more chronic and is unassociated pathologically with inflammation. Serum CK is usually normal and EMG and biopsy (if performed) show non-specific myopathic changes. Correction of the underlying endocrine disturbance results in recovery. Usually the other features of endocrine dysfunction are more problematical and myopathy is of secondary importance.

Pituitary

Acromegaly
Proximal weakness with fatigue. Entrapment neuropathies, e.g. carpal tunnel syndrome may complicate the clinical picture of myopathy. Other features of growth hormone excess are evident.

Parathyroid

Hyperparathyroidism and osteomalacia.
Weakness of a proximal distribution with muscle tenderness occurs in 50% of patients with osteomalacia but is less common in primary hyperparathyroidism. The legs are mainly affected and a waddling gait results. Pathogenesis of hyperparathyroid myopathy is uncertain; hypercalcaemia, Vitamin D deficiency or chronic phosphate deficiency is implicated, tetany results and the CK may be elevated but weakness is uncommon.

Adrenal

Hyperadrenalism and hypoadrenalism
These may both be associated with proximal myopathy. Muscle weakness, fatigue and cramping are frequent in *Addison's disease* with attacks of severe episodic hypokalaemic weakness (periodic paralysis) requiring glucocorticoid and mineral corticoid replacement. Hypokalaemic periodic paralysis is also frequent in *hyperaldosteronism. Cushing's syndrome* and exposure to excessive exogenous glucocorticoids commonly results in insidious proximal weakness. Reduction of steroid dosage results in improvement.

Thyroid

Hyperthyroidism
Weakness occurs in 20% of thyrotoxic patients. Shoulder girdle weakness is more marked than pelvic. Reflexes are brisk, fasciculation and atrophy may be present. *Distinction must be made from motor neuron disease.* There is always clinical evidence of thyrotoxicosis in these patients. Diagnosis is confirmed by thyroid function studies.

Hypothyroidism
Hypothyroidism impairs muscle glycolysis and mitochondrial oxidative capacity. Proximal weakness involves pelvic girdle more than shoulder. Painful cramps and muscle stiffness are common.
Muscle enlargement in limbs and tongue often occur (Hoffman's syndrome). There is always clinical evidence of hypothyroidism in these patients. Diagnosis is confirmed by thyroid function tests and response to thyroid hormone therapy is excellent.

In chronic proximal weakness, careful clinical history taking, examination and appropriate investigation will separate the various endocrine causes.

METABOLIC MYOPATHIES: THE PERIODIC PARALYSES

Periodic paralyses are associated with changes in serum potassium concentrations. The *primary periodic paralyses* are classified into two categories: *hypokalemic* and *hyperkalemic* (or potassium-sensitive). Hypokalemic periodic paralysis shows the clearest relationship between episodic weakness and alterations in potassium. Hyperkalemic periodic paralysis is more accurately a 'potassium sensitive' periodic paralysis as weakness can be provoked by potassium administration, whilst serum potassium may rise only marginally during spontaneous attacks. *Paramyotonia* can be associated with either hypo or hyperkalaemic periodic paralysis.

Importantly episodes of weakness, with alterations in serum potassium, are most commonly *secondary* to drugs (e.g. diuretics and corticosteroids) or disorders such as alcoholism, renal and endocrine disease. (See page 475.)

Hypokalaemic periodic paralysis
Autosomal dominant.
The gene has been mapped on chromosome 1, mutations resulting in upset of the dihydropyridine receptor, a voltage-gated calcium channel.
Onset in second decade.
Precipitated by: exercise, carbohydrate load.
Commences in proximal lower limb muscles and rapidly becomes generalised. Onset usually in morning on wakening.
Attacks last from 4 to 24 hours.
Bulbar muscles/respiration unaffected.
K^+ falls as low as 1.5 meq/l.
Treatment:
Acute – oral KCl.
Prophylactic _ acetazolamide;
   low carbohydrate,
   high K^+ diet.
With age, attacks become progressively less frequent.

Hyperkalaemic periodic paralysis
Autosomal dominant or recessive.
Chromosome 17 location.
Na^+ channel gene defect
Onset in infancy/childhood.
Precipitated by: rest after activity or by cold.
Commences in lower limbs and evolves rapidly.
Attacks are of short duration (less than 60 min).
Myotonia is evident in some patients.
K^+ rises only slightly.
Treatment:
Acute – intravenous calcium gluconate or sodium chloride.
Prophylactic – Acetazolamide is effective prophylaxis .

Paramyotonia congenita
The gene is the same gene that is responsible for the hyperkalaemic form. The mutations that cause the paramyotonia are due to impaired inactivation of skeletal muscle sodium channels.
Onset in infancy.
Precipitated by: rest after exercise, fasting and cooling.
Commences in proximal muscles.
Repetitive muscle contractions produce increasing stiffness.
EMG findings are specific with marked spontaneous activity in limb cooling.
Treatment.
Na^+ channel blockers, Tocainide or Mexiletine.

Normokalaemic periodic paralysis
There are patients with episodic weakness in whom no alteration in serum potassium can be found. Many are sensitive to the administration of oral potassium salts. Treatment is the same as for the hyperkalaemic form but there is no response to acetazolamide. Muscle biopsy in these patients showed occasional vacuoles and prominent tubular aggregates.

Thyrotoxic periodic paralysis
Attacks of paralysis are associated with hypokalaemia and are clinically similar to those of the hypokalaemic form. Mainly occurs in Asians and rarely in non-Asians. The majority of patients experience their first attack in their 30s. There is a marked (20 to 1) male to female predominance.

METABOLIC AND TOXIC MYOPATHIES

Metabolic myopathies

A group of genetically determined biochemical disorders of muscle characterised by myalgia, cramps, weakness and fatigue. These are divided into conditions with *reduced exercise tolerance* and those of *static weakness*. These complex disorders of muscle carbohydrate and lipid metabolism require specialist evaluation. Diagnosis requires detailed muscle staining to demonstrate enzyme loss critical to specific metabolic pathways.

The following disorders are representative but not comprehensive.

McArdle's disease – disorder of carbohydrate metabolism – block in glycolytic pathway (phosphorylase deficiency). Muscle phosphorylase deficiency is a phenotypically heterogeneous autosomal recessive disorder. In some patients phosphorylase is absent whilst in others present but defective. The gene defect localises to chromosome 10.

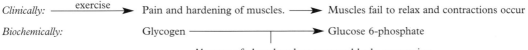

Clinically: ──── exercise ────► Pain and hardening of muscles. ────► Muscles fail to relax and contractions occur

Biochemically: Glycogen ──────────────────────► Glucose 6-phosphate

Absence of phosphorylase enzyme blocks conversion
Myoglobin appears in the urine

Diagnosis: Failure of serum lactate to rise following exercise.
Muscle biopsy – absence of phosphorylase activity with appropriate histochemical staining.
Can be diagnosed from leucocyte DNA.

Treatment with oral fructose may help.

Carnitine palmitoyltransferase deficiency – Carnitine palmitoyltransferase (CPT) enzymes transfer fatty acids across the muscle mitochondrial membrane. CPT 1 attaches and CPT 2 detaches these fatty acids.

Infrequent episodes of myalgia and myoglobinuria following fasting or strenuous exercise. Onset is in adolescence, occasionally in adulthood. Though an autosomal recessive disorder, males are more commonly symptomatic. Neurological examination is normal. Serum CK, EMG and muscle biopsy (including histochemistry) are normal between attacks. Patients are advised to take a low fat/high protein and carbohydrate diet and to avoid prolonged exercise or fasting.

Acid maltase deficiency (ADM) – A lysosomal glycogen storage disease with infantile, childhood, and adult types. The casual gene localises to chromosome 17 with different mutations accounting for ages of onset. Treatment is supportive, genetic counselling essential.

Infantile AMD (Pompe's disease) – progressive muscle weakness, cardiomegaly with congestive heart failure. Death occurs before 1 year. Glycogen accumulates in cardiac, skeletal muscle and in the CNS.

Childhood AMD – slower clinical course, with respiratory muscle weakness developing between 5 and 20 years. Histologically, muscle contains glycogen-filled vacuoles.

Adult AMD – proximal weakness in 3rd or 4th decade mimicking limb-girdle muscular dystrophy or polymyositis. Respiratory muscles are severely affected with risk of death from respiratory failure. Muscle biopsy again shows glycogen-filled vacuoles. Liver, heart and central nervous system are spared.

Carnitine deficiency – Carnitine transports long-chain fatty acids into the mitochondria. Deficiency results in systemic or myopathic features.

Systemic carnitine deficiency – childhood onset weakness with hypoglycaemic encephalopathy, precipitated by fasting and resembling Reye's syndrome (page 504). Serum and muscle carnitine levels are low. Biopsy shows an excessive number of lipid droplets in type 1 fibres. The liver, kidney, and heart contain excessive lipid. Cardiomyopathy is fatal.

Myopathic carnitine deficiency – muscle weakness, exertional myalgias and myoglobinuria. Onset of symptoms is usually in childhood but can be delayed until adulthood. Some cases are complicated by cardiomyopathy. Muscle biopsy shows excessive lipid droplets, especially in type 1 fibres. Muscle and serum carnitine levels are low.

Toxic myopathies

Necrotising myopathy is the pathological consequence of toxic muscle insult characterised by muscle weakness, pain, and tenderness. Investigations – elevated serum CK, myoglobinuria, myopathic motor units and fibrillation on EMG. Muscle biopsy – necrosis and regeneration. Numerous drugs have been incriminated. Examples are: Lovastatin, when combined with other medications such as cyclosporin. Clofibrate in renal failure or hypoalbuminaemia. Epsilon-aminocaproic acid, procainamide, zidovudine (AZT) and phencyclidine. Focal muscle necrosis can be caused by intramuscular injections.

MITOCHONDRIAL DISORDERS

The DNA of the mitochondria (mtDNA) is circular, and while mitochondria themselves reproduce by binary fission, mtDNA replication is controlled by the eukaryotic genome. Mitochondrial disorders are transmitted through the maternal line and not by affected males (mtDNA transmits through the ovum not sperm). The relative proportion of normal to abnormal mtDNA determines the degree of expression (phenotype) for the mutation. As well as muscle involvement, characterised by ragged red muscle fibres on biopsy, many other clinical features are associated with mtDNA mutation syndromes and include:

- Seizures, respiratory insufficiency, weakness and vomiting and failure to thrive in the neonate.
- Developmental delay, ataxia, optic atrophy, progressive external ophthalmoplegia, sensorineural deafness, stroke-like episodes, dementia, exercise intolerance, and short stature.
- Renal failure, diabetes mellitus, cataract and cardiomyopathy.

Certain specific syndromes are recognised though overlap and diversity of phenotype is common.

CPEO (Chronic progressive external ophthalmoplegia)

Adolescence/adult onset of ptosis and ophthalmoplegia (without diplopia) often associated with mild proximal myopathy. When associated with heart block and retinopathy – Kearns Sayre syndrome (KSS).
Differentiate from ocular myasthenia (page 150).
Investigations Large deletion in mt DNA in skeletal muscle biopsy and serum.
Prognosis good with very slow progression. Heart block may require pacing.

MELAS (Mitochondrial encephalopathy, lactic acidosis and stroke-like syndrome)

Adult onset of stroke-like episodes (posterior hemisphere) associated with focal seizures and vascular headache. 'Strokes' are not in vascular territories and are due to failure to utilise substrates rather than to a lack of them.
Differentiate from other causes of 'young' stroke.
Investigations CT/MRT shows posteriorly placed ischaemic changes, elevated lactate in serum and CSF. 'Ragged red' fibres on muscle biopsy and two-point mutation in tRNA Leu gene of mt DNA.
Prognosis is variable. Seizures and headache followed by 'strokes' and eventual dementia.

NARP (Neuropathy, ataxia and retinitis pigmentosa)

Adult onset of sensory/motor neuropathy, ataxia and chronic visual impairment. The rarest mitochondrial syndrome. In some, shares a similar molecular basis as Leigh's syndrome and can demonstrate maternal, autosomal recessive or X linked inheritance.
Differentiate from other causes of ataxic neuropathy e.g. Freidreich's.
Investigations Point mutations mt DNA (ATPase) detected in serum.
Prognosis is uncertain, dementia occurs in time.

MERRF (Myoclonic epilepsy with ragged red fibres)

Adult onset of myoclonus, seizures and ataxia occasionally associated with respiratory failure. Disease expression is variable.
Differentiate from other types of myoclonic epilepsy.
Investigations Elevated lactate i.e. serum and CSF. 'Ragged red' fibres in muscle biopsy and point mutation in tRNA Lys gene of mt DNA in skeletal muscle biopsy and serum.
Prognosis is poor in fully expressed disease – death from seizures or respiratory failure.

LHON (Leber's hereditary optic neuropathy)

Adult subacute onset of loss of central vision, initially unilateral but bilateral in all patients after 1 year. Visual acuity may be reduced to hand movements only due to marked optic atrophy. Male/female ratio: 3:1.
Differentiate from optic neuritis, alcohol/tobacco amblyopia and anterior ischaemic optic neuropathy.
Investigations Several mt DNA mutations have been detected in serum.
Prognosis for visual recovery varies and depends on the specific mutation, as do other accompanying neurological features. In the majority visual loss is irreversible.

Leigh's syndrome

Infant or childhood onset of subacute necrotising encephalomyelopathy characterised by psychomotor retardation, ataxia, optic atrophy and ophthalmoplegia.
Differentiate from other causes of progressive encephalopathy of childhood e.g. inborn errors of metabolism.
Investigations CT/MRI brain stem changes, elevated lactate and pyruvate dehydrogenase complex in CSF and serum and various mutations at Xp 22.1 and mt DNA (ATPase).
Prognosis is poor with early death.

There is no proven therapy for these conditions. Co-morbid conditions such as infection, cardiac involvement and diabetes mellitus should be treated conventionally. Pharmacologic therapies that may bypass biochemical defects are worth using e.g. L. Carnitine, Ubiquinone, riboflavin, thiamine and free radical scavengers (Vits C and E).

MYASTHENIA GRAVIS

Myasthenia gravis is a disorder of neuromuscular transmission characterised by:

– Weakness and fatiguing of some or all muscle groups.
– Weakness worsening on sustained or repeated exertion, or towards the end of the day, relieved by rest.

This condition is a consequence of an autoimmune destruction of the NICOTINIC POSTSYNAPTIC RECEPTORS FOR ACETYLCHOLINE.

Myasthenia gravis is rare, with a prevalence of 5 per 100 000. The increased incidence of autoimmune disorders in patients and first degree relatives and the association of the disease with certain histocompatibility antigens (HLA) – B_7, B_8 and DR_2 – suggests an IMMUNOLOGICAL BASIS.

AETIOLOGY

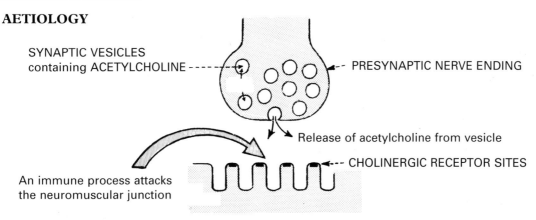

SYNAPTIC VESICLES
containing ACETYLCHOLINE ----- PRESYNAPTIC NERVE ENDING

Release of acetylcholine from vesicle

CHOLINERGIC RECEPTOR SITES

An immune process attacks
the neuromuscular junction

Antibodies bind to the receptor sites resulting in their destruction (complement mediated). These antibodies are referred to as ACETYLCHOLINE RECEPTOR ANTIBODIES (AChR antibodies) and are demonstrated by radioimmunoassay in the serum of 90% of patients.

Human purified IgG (containing AChR antibodies) injected into mice induces myasthenia-like disease in these recipient animals.

In human myasthenia gravis a reduction of acetylcholine receptor sites has been demonstrated in the postsynaptic folds. Reduced receptor synthesis and increased receptor destruction, as well as the blocking of receptor response to acetylcholine, all seem responsible for the disorder.

The rôle of the thymus: Thymic abnormalities occur in 80% of patients. The main function of the thymus is to affect the production of T-cell lymphocytes, which participate in immune responses. Thymus dysfunction is noted in a large number of disorders which may be associated with myasthenia gravis, e.g. systemic lupus erythematosus.

MYASTHENIA GRAVIS – PATHOLOGY

Changes are found in the THYMUS gland and in muscle.

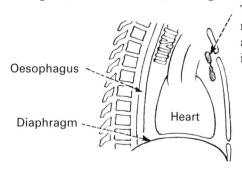

The gland is most active during the induction of normal immune responses in the neonatal period and attains its largest size at puberty after which it involutes.

Oesophagus

Diaphragm

Heart

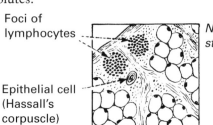

Foci of lymphocytes

Epithelial cell (Hassall's corpuscle)

Normal structure

In myasthenia gravis:
20%: involuted gland

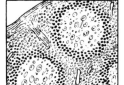

70%: show hyperplasia with lymphoid follicles demonstrating germinal centres

10%: thymoma, and encapsulate tumour of lymphoid and epithelial cells which may be locally invasive but rarely metastasises.

Muscle biopsy may show abnormalities:
– Lymphocytic infiltration associated with small necrotic foci of muscle fibre damage.
– Muscle fibre atrophy (type I and II or type III alone).
– Diffuse muscle necrosis with inflammatory infiltration (when associated with thymoma).

Motor point biopsy may show abnormal motor endplates. Supravital methylene blue staining reveals abnormally long and irregular terminal nerve branching.
Light and electron microscopy show destruction of ACh receptors with simplification of the secondary folds of the postsynaptic surface.

CLINICAL FEATURES
Up to 90% of patients present in early adult life (<40 years of age). Female:male ratio 2:1. The disorder may be selective, involving specific groups of muscles.

Several clinical subdivisions are recognised:
    Class 1 – ocular muscles only – 20%
    Class 2 – Mild generalised weakness
    Class 3 – Moderate generalised and mild to moderate ocular-bulbar weakness ⎫ 80%
    Class 4 – Severe generalised and ocular-bulbar weakness
    Class 5 – Myasthenic crises

Approximately 40% of class I will eventually become widespread. The rest remain purely ocular throughout the illness.
Respiratory muscle involvement accompanies severe illness.

MYASTHENIA GRAVIS – PATHOLOGY

CLINICAL FEATURES (*cont'd*)

Cranial nerve signs and symptoms

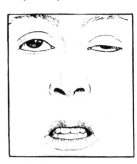 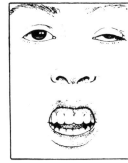

– Ocular involvement produces ptosis and muscle paresis.
– Weakness of jaw muscles allows the mouth to hang open.
– Weakness of facial muscles results in expressionless appearance.

– On smiling, buccinator weakness produces a characteristic smile (myasthenic snarl).

Bulbar involvement may result in: – dysarthric dysphonic speech and dysphagia.
– nasal regurgitation of fluids – nasal quality to speech.

Weakness of 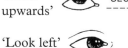 ... and ... in the same patient is characteristic.
eye opening ... (ptosis)   closing ...   (failure to 'bury' eyelashes)

The demonstration of *fatiguing* is important in reaching diagnosis and in monitoring the response to treatment:

'Look upwards'   SECONDS ------> SECONDS ------>   Ptosis becomes apparent and the eye drifts to neutral position

'Look left'   SECS -----> SECS ----->

Ptosis becomes apparent and a dysconjugate drift develops

Fatiguing of other bulbar muscles may be demonstrated by:
– blowing out cheeks against pressure.
– counting as far as possible in one breath, etc.

The tongue occasionally shows the characteristic triple grooved appearance with two lateral and one central furrow.

Limb and trunk signs and symptoms

Weakness of neck muscles may result in lolling of the head. Proximal limb muscles are preferentially affected. Fatigue may be demonstrated by movement against a constant resistance.

Limb reflexes are often hyperactive and fatigue on repeated testing.
Muscle wasting occurs in 15% of cases.
Stress, infection and pregnancy and drugs that alter neuromuscular transmission all exacerbate the weakness

Natural history:
(Before treatment became available)

10% of patients entered a period of remission of long duration.
20% experienced short periods of remission (1 to several months).
30% progressed to death.
The remainder showed varying degrees of disability accentuated by exercise.

481

MYASTHENIA GRAVIS – DIFFERENTIAL DIAGNOSIS

Distinguish from:

– The patient who complains of fatiguing easily – general weakness/debility (e.g. chronic fatigue syndrome) & functional weakness.
– The patient with progressive ophthalmoplegia, e.g. mitochrondrial myopathy, oculopharangeal dystrophy.
– The patient with multiple sclerosis – diplopia, dysarthria and fatigue with a relapsing and remitting course.
– The patient with the Lambert-Eaton myasthenic syndrome (see page 545).

INVESTIGATION

PHARMACOLOGICAL

Anticholinesterase drugs are used to confirm diagnosis.

Tensilon (edrophonium) – short action, 2–4 minutes, given i.v. 2–10 mg slowly, with atropine available to counter muscarinic side effects (nausea and bradycardia). This is positive when noticeable improvement in weakness occurs on objective testing. A control injection of saline is useful, especially when assessing limb weakness only. The Tensilon test may be negative in ocular myasthenia and give a false positive in the Lambert-Eaton syndrome.

SEROLOGICAL

Acetylcholine receptor antibodies are detected in 90% of patients and are virtually specific to this disease. In ocular myasthenia, only 60% show antibodies. Magnitude of titres correlates with disease severity.

Other antibodies e.g. microsomal, colloid, rheumatoid factor, gastric parietal cell antibody – are occasionally found. These reflect the overlap between myasthenia gravis and other autoimmune disorders.

Anti striated muscle antibodies are found in 30% of all patients and in 90% of those with thymoma.

ELECTROPHYSIOLOGICAL

Reduction of the amplitude of the compound muscle action potential evoked by repetitive supramaximal nerve stimulation – 'the decrementing response'.

Various rates of stimulation; even as low as 3/second may produce a decrementing response.

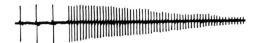

Single fibre electromyography – measure of 'Jitter' – the time interval variability of action potentials from two single muscle fibres of the same motor unit – is a more sensitive index of neuromuscular function and is increased (95% of mild cases are abnormal).

ADDITIONAL

Chest X ray will show a large mediastinal mass but will not exclude a small thymoma. CT of chest should be performed in all newly diagnosed cases.

MYASTHENIA GRAVIS – TREATMENT

In severely ill patients, the first priority is to protect respiration by intubation and, if necessary, ventilation.

Anticholinesterase drugs
This is the longest established form of treatment (1930s).

Anticholinesterase drugs inhibit **cholinesterase**, the enzyme responsible for the breakdown of acetylcholine, allowing enhanced receptor stimulation. As a result, more acetylcholine is available to effect neuromuscular transmission.

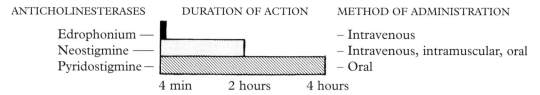

ANTICHOLINESTERASES   DURATION OF ACTION   METHOD OF ADMINISTRATION

Edrophonium —   – Intravenous
Neostigmine —   – Intravenous, intramuscular, oral
Pyridostigmine —   – Oral

4 min   2 hours   4 hours

A muscarinic inhibitor, atropine, may be required to counter side effects (nausea, vomiting, diarrhoea, muscle fasciculations and increasing weakness). Anticholinesterases rarely give complete symptomatic relief and large doses can result in a *cholinergic crisis*

- worsening weakness
- increased sweating, saliva and bronchial secretions
- small pupils (miosis)
- eventual respiratory failure.

Atropine may mask early warning symptoms of this potential life-threatening state.

Steroids
Because this disorder is immune-mediated steroids are a logical choice in generalised and occasionally severe ocular disease. Prednisone 60 mg/day is initially used. Deterioration may briefly occur before improvement. Because of this low-dose regimes are often preferred, increasingly slowly from prednisone 25 mg alternate days. Once a response occurs, dosage is reduced.

Immunosuppressants other than steroids
These drugs (azathioprine and cyclosporine) are considered in patients who do not respond to steroids or who require an unacceptably high steroid maintenance dose.

Thymectomy
There are two indications for this:
1. When thymoma is present
2. When myasthenia is generalised and benefits of surgery outweigh risks.

Trans-sternal is preferred to supra-sternal approach giving better chance of total clearance. Within 5 yrs of surgery 70% of patients are in remission.

MYASTHENIA GRAVIS – TREATMENT

Plasmapheresis

Plasma filtration removes antibodies and other circulating factors and has short term benefit (4–6 weeks). A plasma volume of 1.5–2 litres is exchanged 3–5 times over a 6–8 day period. The technique is expensive and carries risks (hypotension, metabolic disturbance and thrombo-embolism). It is used to stabilise refractory cases and prior to thymectomy in severe disease.

Immunoglobulin (IVIG)

May be used in place of plasmapheresis at a dose of 400 mg per kg intravenously daily for 5 days. Mechanism may act by blocking ACh receptors. A positive response (75% of patients) lasts for 2–3 months. Treatment is expensive and long term effects and complications unknown.

SUMMARY OF TREATMENT

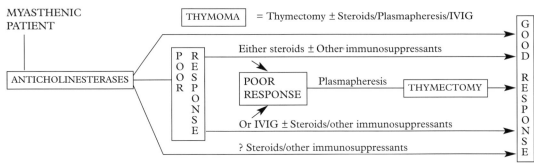

Anticholinesterases should be required throughout the whole illness. When immunological control of the disease is obtained, these drugs may be stopped.

EMERGENCY TREATMENT – MYASTHENIC/CHOLINERGIC CRISES

- Identify and treat precipitating cause, e.g. infection, drug interaction or overdose
- Sit patient at 45°, clear airway, give nasal O_2 and if overt respiratory failure – intubate and ventilate for as long as required.

Myasthenic crisis

- IV neostigmine 8–12 mg/24 hrs
- sc. Atropine 0.5 mg tds
- Prednisolone 100 mg daily
- Consider plasmapheresis or IVIG
- Change IV to oral anticholinesterases when able to swallow

Cholinergic crisis

- Withdraw all anticholinesterases
- Monitor respiratory function (vital capacity)
- Wean from ventilation when appropriate
- Re-introduce oral anti-cholinesterases in low dose and gradually increase

NEONATAL form of myasthenia gravis: this develops in a number of infants of myasthenic mothers.
- Suggested by poor crying/sucking and floppy limbs.
- Presents within 48 hours of birth and may persist until the end of 3rd month.
- Caused by passive transplacental passage of IgG (acetylcholine receptor antibodies).
- Treatment with anticholinesterases is required until spontaneous recovery occurs. Remission occurs following exchange transfusion. This disorder may occur in infants even when their mother has been in remission for many years.

CONGENITAL MYASTHENIAS

These non-immunologic disorders are due to pre, post and mixed synaptic defects. They generally present in infancy though onset can be delayed into adult life. Characteristically fatiguing weakness affects limb (with associated skeletal abnormalities when early age of onset), ocular, bulbar and respiratory muscle groups. AChR antibodies are absent, electrophysiological assessment complex and treatments supportive though some respond to anticholinesterases or 3,4-diaminopyridine.

MULTIFOCAL NEUROLOGICAL DISEASE AND ITS MANAGEMENT

BACTERIAL INFECTIONS – MENINGITIS

ACUTE BACTERIAL MENINGITIS

In most cases the infection causing meningitis arises in the nasopharynx; intravascular invasion (bacteraemia) and penetration of the blood–brain barrier follow mucosal involvement with entry into the CSF. Bacteria may invade the subarachnoid space directly by spread from contiguous structures, e.g. sinuses and fractures. Specific characteristics of the capsule determine whether meninges are breached. Humoral defences against bacteria are absent in the CSF offering little resistance to infection.

Causative organisms

In neonates   – Gram –ve bacilli, e.g. *E. coli, Klebsiella.*
                  Haemophilus influenzae.
In children   – *Haemophilus influenzae.* Pneumococcus (*Strep. pneumoniae*).
                  Meningococcus. (*Neisseria meningitidis*).
In adults   – Pneumococcus. Meningococcus.

Other bacteria – *Listeria monocytogenes, Streptococcus pyogenes* and *Staphylococcus aureus* – are occasionally responsible.
Host factors (congenital or acquired immune deficiency, hyposplenism and alcoholism) predispose to infection, as do environmental factors (overcrowding and poverty).
Infections of mixed aetiology (two or more bacteria) may occur following head injury, mastoiditis or iatrogenically after lumbar puncture.

Pathology

The presence of the blood–brain barrier limits host defence mechanisms and enables multiplication of organisms.

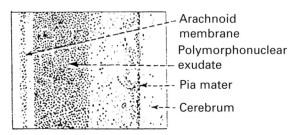

Arachnoid
membrane
Polymorphonuclear
exudate
Pia mater
Cerebrum

A purulent exudate most evident in the basal cisterns extends throughout the subarachnoid space.
The underlying brain, although not invaded by bacteria, becomes congested, oedematous and ischaemic. The integrity of the pia mater normally protects against brain abscess formation.

The cytokines, interleukin, tumour necrosis factor, and prostaglandin E2 are released as part of an acute inflammatory response. They increase vascular permeability, cause a loss of cerebrovascular autoregulation and exacerbate neuronal injury.
The inflammatory exudate may also affect vascular structures crossing the subarachnoid space producing an *arteritis* or *venous thrombophlebitis* with resultant *infarction*. Similarly, cranial nerves may suffer direct damage.
Hydrocephalus can result from CSF obstruction.

Clinical

The classical clinical triad is fever, headache and neck stiffness.

Prodromal features (variable)	*Meningitic symptoms*
A respiratory infection	Severe frontal/occipital headache
otitis media or pneumonia	Stiff neck
associated with muscle pain	Photophobia.

ACUTE BACTERIAL MENINGITIS

Clinical (*cont'd*)

Systemic signs: – High fever. Transient purpuric or petechial skin rash in meningococcal meningitis.

Meningitic signs:
Neck stiffness – gentle flexion of the neck is met with boardlike stiffness

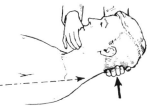

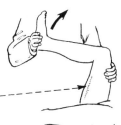

Kernig's sign – stretching the lumbar roots produces pain

Associated neurological signs
– Impaired conscious level
– Focal or generalised seizures are frequent.
– Cranial nerve signs occur in 15% of patients.
– Sensorineural deafness (not due to concurrent otitis media but to direct cochlear involvement) – 20%
– Focal neurological signs – hemiparesis, dysphasia, hemianopia, papilloedema – occur in 10%.

Non-neurological complications

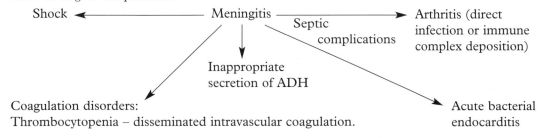

Shock ← Meningitis → Arthritis (direct infection or immune complex deposition)

Septic complications

Inappropriate secretion of ADH

Coagulation disorders:
Thrombocytopenia – disseminated intravascular coagulation.

Acute bacterial endocarditis

Features specific to causative bacteria

Haemophilus meningitis	*Meningococcal meningitis*	*Pneumococcal meningitis*
Generally occurs in small children. Preceding upper respiratory tract infection. Onset abrupt with a brief prodrome.	Often occurs in epidemics where the organism is carried in the nasopharynx. Septicaemia can occur with arthralgia; purpuric skin rash. When overwhelming, confluent haemorrhages appear in the skin due to disseminated intravascular coagulation.	Predominantly an adult disorder. Often associated with debilitation, e.g. alcoholism. May result from pneumonia, middle ear, sinus infection or follow splenectomy. Onset may be explosive, progressing to death within a few hours.
Outcome Generally good Less than 5% mortality.	Gradual onset – good prognosis. Sudden onset with septicaemia – poor outcome. Overall mortality – 10%.	Mortality – 20%. Poor prognostic signs – coma, seizures, increased protein in CSF.

ACUTE BACTERIAL MENINGITIS

Investigations

1. If patient is in coma or has papilloedema or focal neurological signs → exclude an intracranial mass with a *CT scan*. If the patient is deteriorating rapidly, or has a bleeding disorder that cannot be rapidly corrected, take off blood cultures and commence antibiotics (see below) *prior* to scanning.

2. If above signs are absent or CT scan excludes a mass lesion → *confirm diagnosis with a lumbar puncture and identify the organism.*

CSF examination – moderate increase in pressure < 300 mm CSF.

– Gram stain of spun-down sediment.

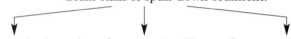

Gram +ve paired cocci	Gram –ve bacilli	Gram –ve intra and extracellular cocci
= pneumococcus	= haemophilus	= meningococcus

– cell count is elevated, 100–10 000 cells/mm^3 (80–90% polymorphonuclear leucocytes).
– glucose is depressed.
– enzyme lactic dehydrogenase is elevated.
– culture CSF

Serological/immunological tests

The latex particle agglutination (LA) test, for the detection of bacteria antigen in CSF, has a sensitivity 80% for haemophilus and pneumococcus and 50% for meningococcus (100% specificity). The polymerase chain reaction (PCR), for the detection of bacteria nucleic acid in CSF, is available for all the suspected organisms. The specificity and sensitivity of PCR is unknown and the delay (3 to 5 days) to process results, makes the test less helpful than the combination of Gram's stain, culture, and the LA test.

Blood cultures

– Organism isolated in 80% of cases of Haemophilus meningitis.
– Pneumococcus and meningococcus in less than 50% of patients.

3. Check serum electrolytes.
   – important in view of the frequency of inappropriate antidiuretic hormone secretion.

4. Detect the source of infection.
   – Chest X-ray – pneumonia   – Skull X-ray – fracture
   – Sinus X-ray – sinusitis   – Petrous views – mastoiditis

Treatment

Once meningitis is suspected, treatment must commence immediately, often before identification of the causative organism. Antibiotics must penetrate CSF, be in appropriate bactericidal dosage and be sensitive to causal organism once identified.

Initial therapy (before organism identification)

Neonates (above 1 month)	– ampicillin, + aminoglycoside and cephalosporin
Children (under 5 years)	– ampicillin, + cephalosporin
Adults	– penicillin G, or cephalosporin
Immunocompromised patient	– ampicillin + cephalosporin

ACUTE BACTERIAL MENINGITIS

Treatment (*cont'd*)

Steroids

A four-day regimen of dexamethasone 10 mg six hourly, starting before or with the first dose of antibiotics, is now recommended in all patients with acute bacterial meningitis. A pivotal study (New England Journal of Medicine 2002; 347:1549) showed a risk reduction of an unfavourable outcome compared with placebo (15 per cent versus 25 per cent). The proportion who died was 7 per cent in the dexamethasone and 15 per cent in the placebo group.

Therapy after organism identification

ORGANISM	ANTIBIOTIC	CHILD mg/kg/day	ADULT	ALTERNATIVE THERAPY
Haemophilus	Chloramphenicol and/or cefotaxime	100 200	2–4 g/day 6–12 g/day	Ampicillin Cefuroxime
Pneumococcus	Benzylpenicillin	180	20 million units	Chloramphenicol Cefotaxime Cefuroxime
Meningococcus	Benzylpenicillin	180	20 million units	Chloramphenicol Cetatamin
E. coli	Cefotaxime	200	6–12 g/day	Ampicillin Gentamicin
Listeria	Ampicillin ± gentamicin	200 5–7	8 g/day (5–7 mg/kg/day)	Chloramphenicol Cotrimoxazole

Duration

Meningococcus ⎱
Haemophilus ⎰ continue for at least 1 week after afebrile.

Pneumococcus – continue for 10–14 days after afebrile

Monitoring

In a deteriorating patient, CT scan will exclude the development of hydrocephalus, abscess or subdural empyema. In suspected sinus thrombosis MR venography may be required.

Remove any source of infection, e.g. mastoidectomy or sinus clearance.

In meningococcal meningitis the risk to household contacts is increased (500–800 x) and chemoprophylaxis should be offered – rifampicin 600 mg b.d. for 48 hours. Vaccines are also available.

Meningitis/CSF shunts

Meningitis infection may follow CSF drainage operations for hydrocephalus. This may occur in the immediate postoperative period or be delayed for weeks or months. Clinical features of raised intracranial pressure may coexist due to shunt blockage. Bacteraemia is inevitable and blood cultures identify the responsible organism – usually *Staphylococcus albus*. The infection seldom resolves with antibiotic therapy alone and shunt removal is usually required.

BACTERIAL INFECTIONS – CNS TUBERCULOSIS

Tuberculosis is an infection caused in man by one of two mycobacteria – *Mycobacterium tuberculosis* and *Mycobacterium bovis*. The disease involves the nervous system in 10% of patients.

MENINGITIS

This is the commonest manifestation of tuberculous infection of the nervous system. *In children*, it usually results from bacteraemia following the initial phase of primary pulmonary tuberculosis.

In adults, it may occur many years after the primary infection.

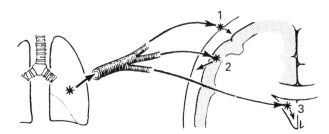

Following bacteraemia, metastatic foci of infection lodge in:
  1. Meninges
  2. Cerebral or spinal tissue
  3. Choroid plexus

Rupture of these encapsulated foci results in spread of infection into the subarachnoid space. In adults, reactivity of metastatic foci may occur spontaneously or result from impaired immunity (e.g. recent measles, alcohol abuse, administration of steroids).

The clinical features of tuberculous meningitis (TBM) result from:
  – Infection.
  – Exudation – which may obstruct the basal cisterns and result in hydrocephalus.
  – Vasculitis – secondary to inflammation around vessels, resulting in infarction of brain and spinal cord.
  The basal meninges are generally most severely affected.

Clinical features

The majority of patients are adults; childhood TBM is now rare. Non-specific prodromal symptoms develop over 2–8 weeks.

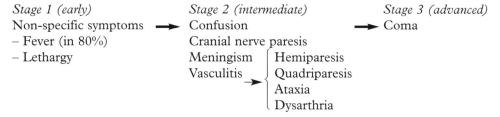

Staging is useful for predicting outcome.

Seizures may occur at the onset. Involuntary movements (chorea, myoclonus) occur in 10%.

Atypically the illness may develop slowly over months presenting with dementia or rapidly like pyogenic (bacterial) meningitis. Occasionally cerebral features prevail rather than signs of meningitis.

Untreated, the illness may progress from phase 1 to death over a 3-week period.
Arachnoiditis inflammatory exudate may result in hydrocephalus/dementia/blindness.

TUBERCULOUS MENINGITIS

Investigations

- *General:* Anaemia, leucocytosis. Hyponatraemia (if inappropriate ADH secretion occurs).

- *Cerebrospinal fluid*
  - Cell count, differential count, cytology (50–4000/mm^3 – predominantly lymphocytes)
  - Glucose, with a simultaneous blood sugar (<50% blood glucose)
  - Protein (>1g/l)
  - Acid-fast stain, Gram stain, appropriate bacteriologic culture and sensitivity, India ink (all causes of lymphocytic meningitis)
  - Cryptococcal antigen, herpes antigen (other causes of lymphocytic meningitis)
  - Culture for *M. tuberculosis* (50–80% positive)
  - Polymerase chain reaction (PCR) to detect Mycobacterium DNA – specificity and sensitivity 100% and 70%.

- *Tuberculin skin test:* Positive in 50% of cases. (Negative if recent steroids or acquired primary infection.)

- *Chest x-ray:* – hilar lymphadenopathy/ infiltrate/cavitations/effusion/scar.

- *CT scan and MRI* – hydrocephalus, basal meningeal thickening, infarcts, oedema, tuberculomas and obliteration of the subarachnoid space.

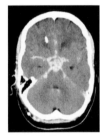

CT scan with i.v. contrast Thickened, enhancing basal meninges

Diagnosis

Diagnosis is based on the clinical presentation with characteristic CSF findings.

DIFFERENTIAL DIAGNOSIS – Viral meningoencephalitis
– Subacute/chronic meningitis (see pages 513, 514).

Treatment

If suspect, commence antituberculous treatment.

Recommended treatment programme:

Normal regime:

Isoniazid (300 mg daily)
Rifampicin (600 mg daily) ——— 2 months ———▸ Isoniazid ———▸ 6 months
Pyrazinamide (15–30 mg/kg daily)   Rifampicin

Drug resistance suspected due to previous antituberculous therapy, e.g.
  - Developing countries
  - History of previous infection.
→ Add a fourth drug – streptomycin (1 g daily) or ethambutal (25 mg/kg daily).

Isoniazid and pyrazinamide penetrate meninges well; other drugs penetrate less well especially when the inflammation begins to settle.

TUBERCULOUS MENINGITIS

Treatment (*cont'd*)

Side effects:
– Isoniazid may produce peripheral neuropathy – protect with pyridoxine 50 mg daily.
– Ethambutol may produce optic atrophy – check colour vision.
– Streptomycin may cause 8th cranial nerve damage (vertigo and deafness).
– Nausea, vomiting, abnormal liver function and skin rashes may occur with all antituberculous drugs.

Evidence concerning the duration of anti-tuberculous treatment is conflicting. Conventionally therapy is given for 6–9 months, although some still recommend it for 24 months.

Intrathecal therapy: Since CSF penetration, especially with streptomycin, is poor, some recommend intrathecal treatment. Streptomycin 50 mg may be given daily or more frequently in seriously ill patients.

When obstructive hydrocephalus occurs, combined intraventricular (through the shunt reservoir or drainage catheter) and lumbar intrathecal treatment injections may be administered.

Steroid therapy: Adjunctive steroids might be of benefit in patients with TBM. A recent Cochrane review suggested publication bias could account for some positive results. No data are available on the use of steroids in HIV positive TBM.

Steroids tend to be given when – conscious level declines
                                – neurological signs progress
                                – spinal block develops (manifesting as paraplegia).

Hydrocephalus
Progressive dilatation of the ventricles impairing conscious level requires CSF drainage – either temporarily with a ventricular catheter (permitting intraventricular drug administration) or permanently with a ventriculoperitoneal/atrial shunt. Surgery may also be considered for co-existent tuberculomas and tuberculous abscesses though these often resolve with drug therapy.

The course of treated tuberculous meningitis
Outcome is influenced by the patient's age, general state of health, timing of initiation of treatment and the development of arachnoiditis and vascular complications.

Treatment in early stages is associated with a 10% mortality, in later stages with a 50% mortality. Of those who survive, neurological sequelae persist in 30% – hemiplegia, hypothalamic/pituitary dysfunction, blindness, deafness, dementia and epilepsy.

With treatment, CSF sugar quickly returns to normal; the cellular reaction gradually diminishes over 3–4 months; the protein level may take a similar time to return to normal.

Tuberculous meningitis in AIDS
Atypical mycobacteria such as *M. avium* and *fortuitum* should be considered. Response to treatment is generally good. TBM tends to occur in the earlier phases of immunodeficiency with CD4 T cell count, at <400 per mm^3.

OTHER FORMS OF CNS TUBERCULOUS INFECTION

TUBERCULOMAS OF THE BRAIN

Tuberculomata may occur in cerebral hemispheres, cerebellum or brain stem with or without tuberculous meningitis, and may produce a space-occupying effect. They consist of caseating granulomas made up of epitheloid cells and macrophages containing mycobacteria. Lesions may be single or multiple. CT and MRI demonstrate lesions but appearances are not pathognomonic. Most resolve over a few weeks with antituberculous therapy.

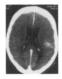

CT scan with i.v. contrast
Enhancing tuberculoma at grey/white matter junction

POTT'S DISEASE

Chronic epidural infection follows tuberculous osteomyelitis of the vertebral bodies. This arises in the lower thoracic region, can extend over several segments and may spread through the intervertebral foramen into pleura, peritoneum or psoas muscle (psoas abscess).

TUBERCULOUS MENINGOMYELITIS

Infection of the leptomeninges results in an exudate that encases the spinal cord and nerve roots. This produces back pain, paraesthesia, lower limb weakness and loss of bowel and bladder control. Imaging may be normal while CSF shows high protein, lymphocytes and rarely acid fast bacilli. This disorder is now more frequent in AIDS patients. Differential diagnosis includes cytomegalovirus, cryptococcus, syphilis and lymphoma. Laminectomy and meningeal biopsy may be required to establish diagnosis. When suspected, empirical theory with antituberculous drugs is appropriate.

Clinical features:

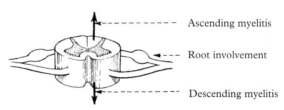

- - - May result from downward spread of intracranial infection

- - - - or direct spread from epidural infection.

*- - - - Occasionally arises from rupture of local metastatic focus; resultant infection is confined to the spinal level.

- - - - - Ascending myelitis

- - - - Root involvement

- - - - - Descending myelitis

Results in – Weakness
       – pyramidal and segmental.
    – Root pain.
    – Sensory loss.
    – Sphincter disturbance.

SPIROCHAETAL INFECTIONS OF THE NERVOUS SYSTEM

SYPHILIS

This infectious disease is caused by the spirochaete *Treponema pallidum*. Entry is by:
  – inoculation through skin or mucous membrane (sexually transmitted) – acquired syphilis.
  – transmission in utero – congenital syphilis.

In the last 30 years, there has been a steady decline in incidence regardless of race and ethnicity. Despite this, it still remains an important health problem in certain geographic areas.

Up to 10% of patients with HIV will test positive for syphilis. All patients with neurosyphilis should be tested for this.

The natural history of infection is divided into:

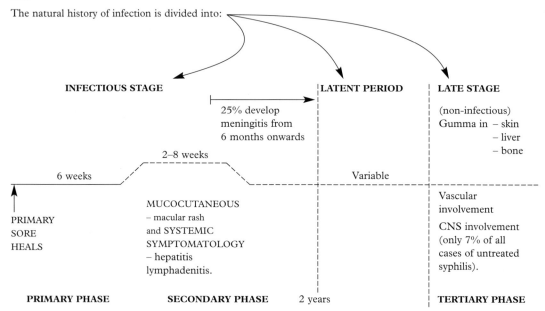

The *chancre* or *primary sore* on skin or mucous membrane represents the local tissue response to inoculation and is the first clinical event in acquired syphilis.
The organism, although present in all lesions, is more easily demonstrated in the primary and secondary phases.
In congenital syphilis fetal involvement can occur even though many years may elapse between the mother's primary infection and conception.
Widespread recognition and efficient treatment of the primary infection have greatly reduced the late or tertiary consequences.
Not all patients untreated in the secondary phase progress to the tertiary phase.
In HIV patients the neurological complications occur earlier and advance more quickly.

Investigations

Spirochaetes can be demonstrated microscopically by dark field examination in primary and secondary phase lesions.

Serological diagnosis depends on detection of antibodies.
1. Non-specific (Reagin) antibodies (IgG and IgM).
   Reagin tests involve complement fixation.
   The Venereal Disease Research Laboratory (VDRL) test is the commonest and when strongly positive indicates active disease (may be negative in HIV).
2. Specific treponemal antibodies (do not differentiate between past and present infection). Fluorescent treponemal antibody absorption (FTA) test and Treponema immobilisation (TPI) test.
3. *Treponema pallidum* DNA can be detected in the CSF of patients by PCR (sensitivity 60%).

SPIROCHAETAL INFECTION – NEUROSYPHILIS

The initial event in neurosyphilis is meningitis. Of all untreated patients 25% develop an acute symptomatic syphilitic meningitis within 2 years of the primary infection.

ACUTE SYPHILITIC MENINGITIS: Three clinical forms are recognised:

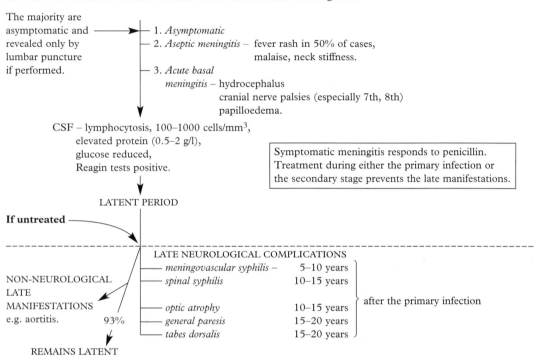

The majority are asymptomatic and revealed only by lumbar puncture if performed.

1. *Asymptomatic*
2. *Aseptic meningitis* – fever rash in 50% of cases, malaise, neck stiffness.
3. *Acute basal meningitis* – hydrocephalus
   cranial nerve palsies (especially 7th, 8th)
   papilloedema.

CSF – lymphocytosis, 100–1000 cells/mm^3,
elevated protein (0.5–2 g/l),
glucose reduced,
Reagin tests positive.

> Symptomatic meningitis responds to penicillin.
> Treatment during either the primary infection or
> the secondary stage prevents the late manifestations.

LATENT PERIOD

If untreated

LATE NEUROLOGICAL COMPLICATIONS

meningovascular syphilis –	5–10 years
spinal syphilis	10–15 years
optic atrophy	10–15 years
general paresis	15–20 years
tabes dorsalis	15–20 years

after the primary infection

NON-NEUROLOGICAL LATE MANIFESTATIONS e.g. aortitis.   93%

REMAINS LATENT

Late neurological complications occur in only 7% of **untreated** cases.
These forms are exceptionally rare and the clinical syndromes mentioned above seldom occur in a 'pure' form.

MENINGOVASCULAR SYPHILIS

'Early' late manifestation resulting in an obliterative endarteritis and periarteritis.

Presents as a 'stroke' in a young person – hemisphere, brain stem or spinal. Granulations around the base of the brain may produce cranial nerve palsies or even hydrocephalus.

CSF – lymphocytes 100/mm^3, protein ↑, gammaglobulin ↑, positive serology. Penicillin arrests progression.

SPINAL SYPHILIS

Chronic meningitis with subpial damage to the spinal cord.
Presents as a progressive paraplegia, occasionally with radicular pain and wasting in upper limbs – ERB's PARAPLEGIA. CSF – as meningovascular syphilis. Penicillin arrests progression.

OCULAR MANIFESTATIONS

Meningitis around optic nerve with subpial necrosis may be the only manifestation of late syphilis.
Presents as a constriction of the visual fields with a progressive pallor of the optic disc:
– if both eyes are affected, the vision is rarely saved.
– if only one eye is involved, treatment with penicillin will save the other.
Neuroretinitis, uveitis and chorioretinitis occur, especially in HIV patients.

SPIROCHAETAL INFECTION – NEUROSYPHILIS

GENERAL PARESIS

Characterised by dementia – with memory impairment, disordered judgement and disturbed affect – manic behaviour, delusions of grandeur (rare).

There are two phases: 1. Pre-paralytic – with progressive dementia.

                      2. Paralytic – when corticospinal and extrapyramidal symptoms and signs develop associated with involuntary movements (myoclonus).

Argyll Robertson pupils may be present (see page 135).

At autopsy, meningeal thickening, brain atrophy and perivascular infiltration with plasma cells and lymphocytes are evident; culture from the cortex may reveal an occasional treponema.

CSF – lymphocytes 50/mm^3, protein $\uparrow$ 0.5–2 g/l, gammaglobulin $\uparrow$.

Reagin tests in CSF positive in the majority.

Treatment in the preparalytic phase will halt progression in 40%.

TABES DORSALIS

Posterior spinal root and posterior column dysfunction –$\rightarrow$ account for symptoms.

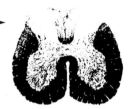

Pupillary abnormality (Argyll Robertson) and optic atrophy occur. Peripheral reflexes are lost and joint position and vibration sensation is impaired. A positive Romberg's test (page 180) indicates a sensory ataxia.

Pain loss results in trophic lesions and occasionally a Charcot joint may develop. – – – – – – – – – – – – – – – – – –$\rightarrow$

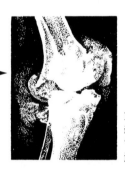

Urinary incontinence, impotence and constipation also occur. 'Lightning pains', visceral crises (abdominal pain/ diarrhoea) and rectal crises (tenesmus) are frequent.

Repeated trauma to an insensitive joint results in 'painless' osteoarthritis and joint destruction.

The CSF is more normal than in general paresis. The Reagin test may be negative in 30 per cent. Treatment may produce some improvement; it will not reverse joint destruction.

SYPHILITIC GUMMA presenting as an intracranial mass is extremely rare.

TREATMENT OF NEUROSYPHILIS

Penicillin G.	2–4 megaunits i.v.	(When patient sensitive to penicillin
or	4-hourly for 10 days.	$\downarrow$
Procaine Penicillin	600 000 units i.m.	erythromycin or
	daily for 15 days.	tetracycline may be given
Benzathine Penicillin	2–4 megaunits i.m. weekly × 3.	orally over 30 days.)

To prevent congenital syphilis penicillin should be given to all neonates and infected mothers during the first 4 months of pregnancy.

The Jarisch-Herxheimer reaction – tachycardia/fever – occurs in one-third of patients within a few hours of commencing treatment; it is believed to be due to endotoxin release from killed organisms. Steroids should counter the reaction, especially in tertiary syphilis.

CSF follow up: CSF is checked initially and at 6 monthly intervals until normal.

Cell count and degree of positivity of VDRL are the best indicators of persistent infection.

Failure of treatment is common in HIV positive patients and more frequent retesting of blood and CSF is necessary.

SPIROCHAETAL INFECTION

LYME DISEASE (NEUROBORRELIOSIS)

Originally described in the community of Old Lyme, this is a disorder, caused by the spirochaete *Borrelia burgdorferi*, characterised by relapsing and remitting arthralgia associated with a characteristic skin rash (*erythema chronicum migrans*) and neurological features. The organism, related to the treponemes, is prevalent throughout Europe and North America and is carried by ixodes ticks.

Clinical features

Only a minority of persons bitten by an infected tick develop the disease. Spirochaetocidal activity in normal serum and the immune response normally provide protection. It rarely occurs in HIV patients.

Stage 1: Spring/summer –
Tick bite → flu-like symptoms, arthralgia and skin rash (erythema chronicum migrans).
Treatment with antibiotics is usually curative.

Untreated and small
number of treated patients.

Stage 2: Several weeks/months later –
Subacute lymphocytic meningitis – both illnesses are often mild, clear
Subacute encephalitis   spontaneously and occasionally are unrecognised.
Cranial nerve involvement – Facial nerve palsy with or without
                                subacute lymphocytic meningitis.
Peripheral neuropathy – Subacute demyelinating and axonal sensory/motor neuropathy
                            associated with severe root pain (radiculitis). – Bannwarth's syndrome.
CSF examination in stage 2: Lymphocytosis   Elevated immunoglobulins.
                             Oligoclonal bands.   Elevated *anti*Burgdorferi antibodies.
                                    An unknown proportion progress.

Stage 3: Several months/years later –
Arthritis
Diffuse CNS involvement – chronic/subacute encephalitis.
                            – focal brain disease.
                            – *psychiatric* disease with fatigue and diffuse muscle pain.

Diagnosis

Antibody tests
   – Immunofluorescence assay (IFA)
   – Enzyme-linked immunoabsorbent assay (ELISA). } in serum and CSF.

In endemic areas up to 5% of the population are positive, although with lower titres than symptomatic patients.

In patients from endemic areas:

with meningitis/CN palsy   diagnosis is definite, but   *PCR* if available gives the definitive answer.
encephalitis/radiculitis   in stage 3 this is often
+ CSF profile   uncertain and blind trials   *MRI* is abnormal in 25% with subcortical
+ positive serology   of therapy are given.   (T2) white matter lesions.

Treatment

Stage 1 – Oral antibiotics: penicillin, erythromycin or tetracycline.
Stage 2 – I.V. penicillin G. 20 million units for 10 days (or ceftriaxone).
Stage 3 – as stage 2.

If symptoms persist – wrong diagnosis with misleading titres, or
                    – immune mediated damage.

Steroids can be used in late stages when symptoms have not responded to antibiotics.

SPIROCHAETAL INFECTION

LEPTOSPIROSIS

Leptospira interrogans is transmitted to man in the infected urine of wild and domestic animal carriers. Subclinical infection commonly occurs in high-risk occupations, e.g. sewer workers. Symptomatic illness is usually mild and only 10% of patients develop jaundice and haemorrhagic complications (Weil's disease).

Clinical features

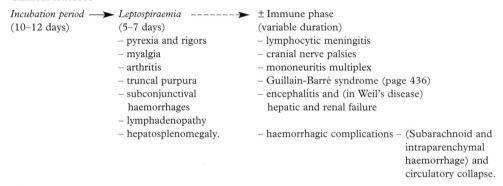

Incubation period ⟶ *Leptospiraemia* ------➤ ± Immune phase
(10–12 days)   (5–7 days)   (variable duration)

            – pyrexia and rigors   – lymphocytic meningitis
            – myalgia   – cranial nerve palsies
            – arthritis   – mononeuritis multiplex
            – truncal purpura   – Guillain-Barré syndrome (page 436)
            – subconjunctival   – encephalitis and (in Weil's disease)
              haemorrhages   hepatic and renal failure
            – lymphadenopathy
            – hepatosplenomegaly.   – haemorrhagic complications – (Subarachnoid and
                                           intraparenchymal
                                           haemorrhage) and
                                           circulatory collapse.

Diagnosis

A combination of abnormal liver and renal function with elevated creatine kinase suggest the diagnosis. Leptospirae can be isolated from blood and CSF (in the immune phase) but diagnosis is usually confirmed by demonstrating agglutinating antibodies (ELISA detected IgM).

Treatment

The disease is usually self limiting and therapy unnecessary. Early treatment in the leptospiraemic phase with Penicillin G 12 million units daily and tetracycline 500 mg four times per day may minimize the immune-mediated complications. Support of hepatic/renal failure and management of haemorrhagic complications may be life-saving.

PARASITIC INFECTIONS OF THE NERVOUS SYSTEM – PROTOZOA

TOXOPLASMOSIS

A world-wide parasitic infection affecting many species, including man.

Organism: An anaerobic intracellular protozoan, *Toxoplasma gondii.*

The majority of infections in man are asymptomatic (30% of the population have specific antibodies indicating previous exposure).

In the host

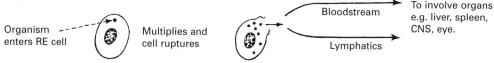

Transmission: Eating uncooked meat or contact with faeces of an infected dog or cat (definitive hosts).

There are two forms of toxoplasmosis:

CONGENITAL – when a previously unaffected woman contracts infection during pregnancy (subclinical infection); transplacental spread results in fetal infection.

Premature delivery occurs in 25%.

Neurological complications:
– hydrocephalus,
– aqueduct stenosis,
– microcephaly.

Non-neurological featues:
– skin rash, jaundice, hepatosplenomegaly, choroidoretinitis.

Skull X-ray shows:
– curvilinear calcification (basal ganglion and periventricular regions).

Varying degrees of organ involvement may occur. The only manifestation may be choroidoretinitis in an otherwise healthy child.

ACQUIRED – symptomatic infection is uncommon and may be associated with underlying systemic disease or immunosuppression (e.g. AIDS).

Fever and fatigue with muscle weakness and lymphadenopathy result. Abnormal lymphocytes in peripheral blood leads to confusion with *infectious mononucleosis.* The neurological features are those of a meningoencephalitis with focal signs and depressed conscious level. Choroidoretinitis occasionally occurs.

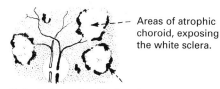

Areas of atrophic choroid, exposing the white sclera.

Retinal pigment epithelium becomes hyperplastic – densely pigmented areas result.

Diagnosis:

Organisms are seldom identified.

IgG antibodies indicate previous exposure, positive IgM and high or rising IgG confirm active infection. Serological tests may be negative in AIDS.

In *acquired infection* CT shows characteristic ring shaped contrast enhancement. MRI is even more sensitive. Brain biopsy is necessary for exclusion of CNS lymphoma and for definitive diagnosis.

N.B. Rubella, cytomegalovirus and herpes simplex can also spread transplacentally and cause jaundice and hepatosplenomegaly. Cytomegalovirus may also produce choroidoretinitis and intracranial calcification.

Treatment

Sulphadiazine and pyrimethamine (Dapaprim) with folinic acid for 6 weeks. In AIDS newer drugs, such as clarithromycin and azithromycin, have also been used with some success. In this patient group recurrence after discontinuation of therapy mandates life long treatment. Give steroids when choroidoretinitis is present.

MALARIA

Plasmodium falciparum, the agent of malignant tertiary malaria, is responsible for *cerebral malaria.* Infected red blood cells adhere to vascular endothelium and block the microcirculation. Endothelial damage produces cerebral oedema. Confusion, focal signs, convulsions and coma occur. Diagnosis depends on demonstrating parasites in peripheral blood. Parenteral anti malaria treatment (chloroquine), exchange transfusion and supportive therapy may be life saving. Overall mortality is 10%. Complete recovery without sequelae is expected in survivors.

VIRAL INFECTIONS

General principles

Invasion of the nervous system may occur as part of a generalised viral infection. Occasionally nervous system involvement is disproportionately severe and symptoms of generalised infection are slight.

Viruses enter the body through the: *respiratory tract,*
gastrointestinal tract,
genitourinary tract or by
inoculation through the skin.

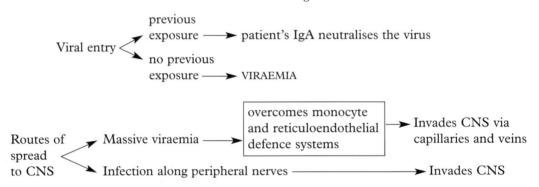

Viral entry
— previous exposure ⟶ patient's IgA neutralises the virus
— no previous exposure ⟶ VIRAEMIA

Routes of spread to CNS
— Massive viraemia ⟶ overcomes monocyte and reticuloendothelial defence systems ⟶ Invades CNS via capillaries and veins
— Infection along peripheral nerves ⟶ Invades CNS

After CNS penetration, the clinical picture depends upon the particular virus and the cells of the nervous system which show a specific susceptibility.

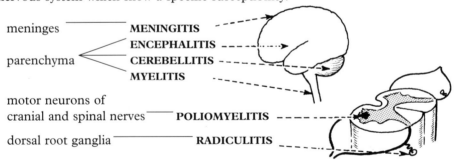

meninges —— **MENINGITIS**

parenchyma
ENCEPHALITIS
CEREBELLITIS
MYELITIS

motor neurons of cranial and spinal nerves —— **POLIOMYELITIS**

dorsal root ganglia —— **RADICULITIS**

Some viruses cause a chronic, progressive infection, others remain dormant for many years within the nervous system before becoming symptomatic.

MENINGITIS

Meningitis is the commonest type of viral infection of the central nervous system. The term *aseptic meningitis* includes viral meningitis as well as other forms of meningitis where routine culture reveals no other organisms.

Common causal viruses —
ENTEROVIRUSES
MUMPS VIRUS
HERPES SIMPLEX (subtype 2)
EPSTEIN-BARR VIRUS (EBV)

Rare causal viruses —
LYMPHOCYTIC CHORIOMENINGITIS
HUMAN IMMUNODEFICIENCY VIRUS (HIV)

VIRAL INFECTIONS – MENINGITIS

Clinical features of acute aseptic meningitis

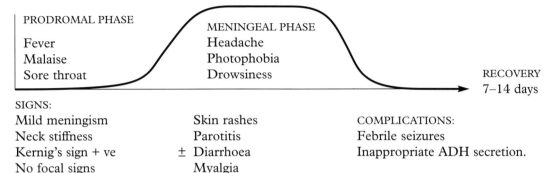

PRODROMAL PHASE

Fever
Malaise
Sore throat

MENINGEAL PHASE

Headache
Photophobia
Drowsiness

RECOVERY
7–14 days

SIGNS:

Mild meningism	Skin rashes	COMPLICATIONS:
Neck stiffness	Parotitis	Febrile seizures
Kernig's sign + ve	± Diarrhoea	Inappropriate ADH secretion.
No focal signs	Myalgia	

Enterovirus infection e.g. Coxsackie or echo viruses – affects children/young adults and occurs seasonally in late summer.
Spread is by the faecal/oral route.

Mumps – affects children/young adults. Winter/spring incidence.

Herpes simplex (type 2) – accounts for 5% of viral meningitis. Develops in 25% of patients with primary genital infection (suspect in sexually active adults). Can cause a recurrent meningitis (Mollaret's meningitis).

Lymphocytic choriomeningitis – affects any age and is a consequence of airborne spread from rodent droppings.

Human Immunodeficiency Virus (HIV) – suspect in high risk groups (page 511). HIV antibodies are often absent and develop 1–3 months later during convalescence.

Investigations
The CSF cell count is elevated (lymphocytes or monocytes) with a normal glucose and protein. PCR detection of viral DNA/RNA in CSF though diagnostic, is rarely thought necessary. Virus may be cultured from throat swabs or stool. Serological tests on serum in acute and convalescent phases are especially valuable in detecting mumps and herpes simplex (type 2).

Differential diagnosis
From other causes of an aseptic meningitis which are usually subacute or chronic in onset:

- *Tuberculous or fungal* meningitis
- *Leptospirosis*
- *Sarcoidosis*
- *Carcinomatous* meningitis
- Partially treated *bacterial* meningitis
- *Parameningeal* chronic infection which evokes a meningeal response, e.g. mastoiditis.

The self-limiting and mild nature of viral meningitis should not lead to confusion with these more serious disorders.

Prognosis is excellent and **treatment** symptomatic.

VIRAL INFECTIONS – PARENCHYMAL

Viruses may act:

> *directly* → acute viral encephalitis or meningoencephalitis,
> or *indirectly via the immune system* → allergic or postinfectious encephalomyelitis and
> postvaccinial encephalomyelitis.

Also, a 'toxic' encephalopathy may develop during the course of a viral illness in which inflammation is not a pathological feature – REYE'S SYDNROME.

ACUTE VIRAL ENCEPHALITIS

Viral infection causes neuronal and glial damage with associated inflammation and oedema.

Viral encephalitis is a worldwide disorder with the highest incidence in the tropics.

Common causal viruses:

World-wide:	Rare forms in specific areas:	
– Mumps	St Louis	– Arthropod-borne – USA
– Herpes simplex	West Nile	– Arthropod-borne – Africa/India
– Varicella zoster	Russian spring/summer	– Arthropod-borne – eastern Europe
– Epstein-Barr		
– Arboviruses		

Encephalitis following childhood infections – measles, varicella, rubella – is presumed to be *postinfectious* and not due to direct viral invasion, though the measles virus has occasionally been isolated from the brain.

Clinical features:

Signs and symptoms:
General: pyrexia, myalgia, etc.
Specific to causative virus, e.g. features of infectious mononucleosis (Epstein–Barr).
Meningeal involvement (slight) → neck stiffness, cellular response in CSF.
Signs and symptoms of parenchymal involvement – focal and/or diffuse.

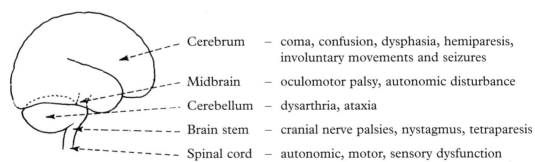

Cerebrum	–	coma, confusion, dysphasia, hemiparesis, involuntary movements and seizures
Midbrain	–	oculomotor palsy, autonomic disturbance
Cerebellum	–	dysarthria, ataxia
Brain stem	–	cranial nerve palsies, nystagmus, tetraparesis
Spinal cord	–	autonomic, motor, sensory dysfunction

In general, the illness lasts for some weeks.

Prognosis is uncertain and depends on the causal virus as do neurological sequelae.

VIRAL INFECTIONS – PARENCHYMAL

Herpes Simplex (HSV) and Varicella-Zoster (UZV) commonly cause disease in humans.

HERPES SIMPLEX ENCEPHALITIS

HSV-1 is the commonest cause of sporadic encephalitis.

One third occur due to primary infection; two thirds have pre-existing antibodies (*reactivation*).

Clinical features

A world-wide disorder occurring during all seasons and affecting all ages.

Incidence: 1/250 000

General symptoms at onset – headache, fever – with evolution over several days to seizures and impaired conscious level.

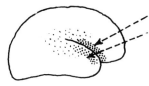 Inferior frontal and temporal lobes are selectively involved and signs and symptoms reflect this – olfactory or gustatory hallucinations, behavioural disturbance, complex partial seizures, dysphasia (dominant hemisphere) and hemiparesis.
Cerebral oedema may result in tentorial herniation.

Investigations

MR imaging: T2 weighted MRI showing temporal and orbitofrontal hyperintensities typical of herpes simplex encephalitis.

CSF examination reveals 5–500 lymphocytes. The protein is mildly elevated and the glucose is normal.

EEG examination shows generalised slowing with bursts of 'periodic' high voltage slow wave complexes over the involved temporal lobe.

MR imaging: T2 weighted MRI showing temporal and orbitofrontal hyperintensities typical of herpes simplex encephalitis

Polymerase chain reaction (PCR) on CSF may be negative in the first 48 hours. The quantity of HSV DNA then increases and, if initially negative and the clinical course is suggestive, the examination should be repeated. Also paired sera and CSF should be sent for HSV antibody (CSF HSV-specific antibody can still be detected up to 30 days).

Brain biopsy seldom required in view of the above new diagnostic techniques.

This shows evidence of a necrotising encephalitis with intranuclear eosinophilic inclusion bodies.

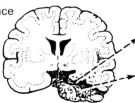

Demonstrate herpes simplex antigen by immunofluorescence.

Isolate virus by culture (positive in 48 hours).

Differential diagnosis

Consider:
– other forms of encephalitis
– cerebral abscess
– brain tumour.

Treatment: Acyclovir inhibits DNA synthesis, is relatively non-toxic and significantly reduces morbidity and mortality. When the diagnosis is considered, treatment must start without delay.

Varicella-Zoster Virus (VZV) encephalitis may complicate chicken pox, or a cutaneous zoster eruption. CSF shows a mild lymphocytosis (<100 cells/mm^3), a slight increase in the protein and a normal glucose. PCR detects VZV DNA. The virus can be grown from CSF and antibodies detected. Treatment with acyclovir or famciclovir is effective. Vasculitis may complicate.

VIRAL INFECTIONS – REYE'S SYNDROME

REYE'S SYNDROME

This rare encephalopathy, associated with fatty changes in the liver and other viscera, is almost exclusively confined to children. It is due to aspirin useage in infection with Influenza A, Influenza B or varicella–zoster viruses.

Incidence

Since 1980 the incidence of this condition has dropped dramatically, in part due to avoidance of salicylates in children.

Pathology

Neurons and glial cells are swollen; the liver, heart and kidney show fatty infiltration.

Pathogenesis

Viral synergism with an environmental factor, e.g. salicylates, may be responsible.
Morphological changes in mitochondria indicate a central role.

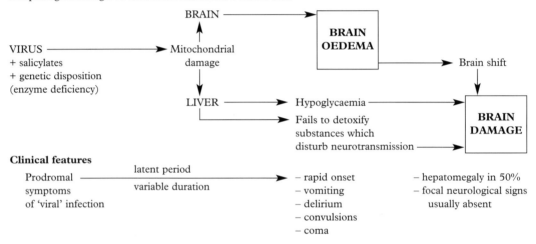

Clinical features

Prodromal — latent period, variable duration →
symptoms
of 'viral' infection

– rapid onset
– vomiting
– delirium
– convulsions
– coma

– hepatomegaly in 50%
– focal neurological signs
  usually absent

Death results from raised intracranial pressure.

Investigations

– Raised liver enzymes (ALT & AST) – Hypoglycaemia (in infants) – Increase in serum fatty acids
– Elevated serum ammonia – Prolonged prothrombin time Aminoaciduria

CT/MRI show appearances of diffuse cerebral oedema

Differential diagnosis

Consider other causes of raised intracranial pressure in childhood, especially
– lead encephalopathy,
– lateral sinus thrombosis, e.g. following mastoiditis.

Treatment

Treatment aims at lowering intracranial pressure with the aid of intracranial pressure monitoring (see page 51). In addition, blood glucose must be maintained and any associated coagulopathy treated. Reduction of ammonia may be achieved by peritoneal dialysis or exchange transfusion.

Prognosis

Early diagnosis and supportive treatment has reduced the mortality from 80% to 30%.

When raised intracranial pressure is present, mortality increases to 50% and a high proprotion of survivors have cognitive disorders.

A condition similar to Reye's syndrome occurs in some children with family history of 'sudden infant death'. A deficiency of medium chain acetyl-CoA dehydrogenase (an enzyme essential for fatty acid metabolism) is found. Carnitine deficiency results as a consequence of 'alternative pathway' fatty acid metabolism. *Siblings of children with Reye's syndrome should be screened for this disorder.*

VIRAL INFECTIONS – CHRONIC DISORDERS

In these disorders the infection results in a chronic progressive neurological condition.
The evidence of a viral etiology is:
Direct – finding of inclusion bodies, demonstration of viral particles or isolation of virus.
Indirect – relationship of onset of symptoms to a preceding viral illness, transmission of illness from one host to the next
N.B. Not all these features are present in any one illness

SUBACUTE SCLEROSING PANENCEPHALITIS (SSPE)
Caused by measles-like paramyxovirus – isolated from brain biopsy.
Less common with the availability of widespread primary measles vaccination.

Clinical features: A world-wide disorder. Incidence: 1 per million per year. Onset: between ages 7–10 years.

Stage 1: Behavioural problem, declining school performance, progression → dementia
Stage 2: Chorioretinitis, myoclonic jerks, seizures, ataxia, dystonia
Stage 3: Lapses into rigid comatose state

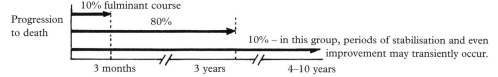

The illness may occur after measles vaccination or following clinical infection at an early age (under 2 years).
Accompanying features of infection, i.e. pyrexia, leucocytosis, are absent.

Investigations

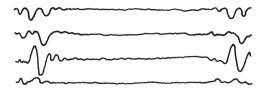

CSF examination shows elevated γ globulin with IgG oligoclonal bands; elevated measles antibodies (75% of total CSF IgG).

Blood examination shows elevated serum measles antibodies.

EEG – shows periodic high voltage slow wave complexes on a low voltage background trace.

Pathology
Changes involve both white and grey matter, especially in the posterior hemispheres. Brain stem, cerebellum and spinal cord are also affected. Oligodendrocytes contain eosinophilic inclusion bodies. Marked gliosis occurs with perivascular lymphocyte and plasma cell cuffing.

Treatment: There is no effective treatment. Since the introduction of measles vaccination there has been a marked reduction of SSPE.

Subacute measles encephalitis may follow measles infection in children on *immunosuppressive drug treatment* or with *hypogammaglobulinaemia.* The clinical course is different however from SSPE and EEG and CSF findings are less specific.

PROGRESSIVE RUBELLA PANENCEPHALITIS
Similar to SSPE with a fatal outcome, caused by rubella virus.
Presents at a later age (10–15 years)
Progressive dementia.
Ataxia. Spasticity. Myoclonus.
Treatment: No effective treatment

CSF shows high γ globulin.
Antibodies elevated in serum and CSF to rubella.
Biopsy does not show inclusion bodies.

PRION DISEASES

Fatal conditions characterised by the accumulation of a modified cell membrane protein – Prion protein or PrP (proteinaceous infectious particle) within the central nervous system.

Clinical features are dependent on site and rate of deposition of PrP. A similar disorder in cattle, bovine spongiform encephalopathy (BSE) may be a source of infection in man.

The Prion theory

Experimental and epidemiological evidence supports transmissibility. Physical properties of the infective agent – heat and radiation resistance and absence of nucleic acid – suggests it is comprised solely of protein. This infectious protein when innoculated modifies normal cell membrane protein which acts as a template for further conversion to abnormal protein. This host-encoded protein accumulates without any inflammatory or immune response. In familial cases a point mutation in the prion gene explains disease susceptibility.

Creutzfeldt-Jakob disease (CJD)

A worldwide disorder with incidence 1:1 000 000. Approximately 90% of cases are sporadic and 10% familial caused by mutations in the prion protein (PRNP) gene on chromosome 20. Age of onset 50–60 years. Non specific symptoms at onset (anxiety and depression) are rapidly followed by myoclonus, ataxia, akinetic rigid state, dementia. Death within 12 months is usual. Iatrogenic disease occurs following corneal or dural grafts, depth electrodes and cadaveric derived human growth hormone treatment.

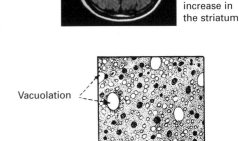

MRI – T2 signal increase in the striatum

Investigation

EEG – 1–2 Hz triphasic sharp waves with periodic complexes
CSF – increase in protein 14–3–3 (a protein kinase inhibitor)

[The combined EEG and CSF findings, where positive, have diagnostic sensitivity/specificity of 97%]

Pathology

– Neuronal degeneration occurs with marked astrocytic proliferation and amyloid plaque formation. Vacuolation of glial cells results in a characteristic spongiform appearance.

Vacuolation

Treatment – supportive.

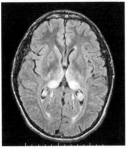

MRI – T2 signal increase in the thalamus (pulvinar sign)

New Variant CJD (vCJD)

Generally affects younger age group. Psychiatric symptoms of depression, anxiety, or withdrawal are common early manifestations. Neurological symptoms appear approximately 6 months later, with paraesthesias an early feature. Eventually sufferers exhibit ataxia, progressive dementia and involuntary movements (myoclonus, chorea, or dystonia).

Only 50% of patients have protein 14–3–3 proteins in CSF. EEG reveals non-specific slowing (the periodic complexes of sporadic CJD are absent).

PRNP gene mutations are found with patients homozygous for methionine at the 129 codon. Neuropathological changes – 'florid' plaques in the cerebral and cerebellar cortex, severe thalamic gliosis, and spongiform change with diffuse accumulation of prion proteins.

Gerstmann Straussler syndrome (GSS)

A similar disorder condition to CJD. Cases are familial and characterised by specific pathology of spongiform changes associated with amyloid plaques containing PrP immunoreactive proteins. Clinical features are nonspecific – ataxia, Parkinsonism, dementia. Death occurs within 5 years of contact.

Kuru

An extensively studied disorder of Papua New Guinea. It is of interest in view of man to man spread from cannibalism.

VIRAL INFECTIONS – MYELITIS AND POLIOMYELITIS

MYELITIS

Acute viral transverse myelitis is rare. It can occur in association with measles, mumps, Epstein-Barr, herpes zoster/simplex, enterovirus infections HIV, HTLV-1 and 2 and smallpox. Fever, back and limb pain precede paralysis, sensory loss and bladder disturbance. Initially paralysed limbs are flaccid, but over 1–2 weeks spasticity and extensor plantar responses develop. Good recovery occurs in 30%. Death from respiratory failure is rare (5%).

Investigations

Myelography when performed is normal. MRI may demonstrate focal cord signal changes. CSF shows elevated protein with a neutrophil or lymphocytic response. Serological tests will occasionally identify the causal virus. Electrophysiology distinguishes from Guillain-Barré syndrome.

Treatment

Supportive; the place of steroids remains unproven.

It is not clear whether the pathological effects (perivenous demyelination) result from direct or delayed (immunological) reactions to the virus.

POLIOMYELITIS

An acute viral infection in which the anterior horn cells of the spinal cord and motor nuclei of the brain stem are selectively involved. A major cause of paralysis and death 30 yrs ago, now rare with the introduction of effective vaccines and improved sanitation.

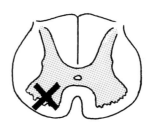

Causative viruses:

The poliovirus is a picornavirus (RNA virus).

Three immunological distinct strains have been isolated. Immunity to one does not result in immunity to the other two.

Coxsackie and echoviruses (also picornaviruses), may produce a clinically identical disorder.

Pathology

Initially – inflammatory meningeal changes, followed by – inflammatory cell infiltration (polymorphs and lymphocytes) around the brain stem nuclei and anterior horn cells. Neurons may undergo necrosis or central chromatolysis.

Microglial proliferation follows.

Mode of spread

Spread by faecal/oral route. Once ingested the virus multiplies in the nasopharynx and gastrointestinal tract.

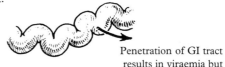

Penetration of GI tract results in viraemia but CNS involvement occurs in only a very small proportion. Most infected patients are asymptomatic. Virus excretion continues in the faeces for as long as three months after the initial infection – carrier state.

Epidemiology

A highly communicable disease which may result in epidemics.

Seasonal incidence – late summer/autumn.

World-wide distribution, although more frequent in northern temperate climates.

Prophylactic vaccination has produced a dramatic reduction in incidence in the last 25 years. In developing countries without a vaccination programme, the disease remains a problem.

Clinical features

Infection may result in:

– Subclinical course + resultant immunity (majority)
– Mild non-specific symptoms of viraemia + resultant immunity
– Meningism without paralysis
  (PREPARALYTIC) + resultant immunity
– Meningism followed by paralysis
  (PARALYTIC) + resultant immunity.

VIRAL INFECTIONS – POLIOMYELITIS

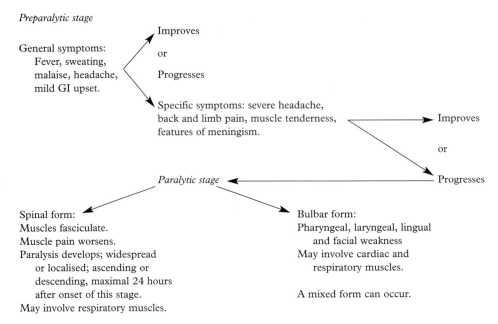

Preparalytic stage

General symptoms:
Fever, sweating,
malaise, headache,
mild GI upset.

Improves

or

Progresses

Specific symptoms: severe headache,
back and limb pain, muscle tenderness,
features of meningism.

Improves

or

Progresses

Paralytic stage

Spinal form:
Muscles fasciculate.
Muscle pain worsens.
Paralysis develops; widespread
or localised; ascending or
descending, maximal 24 hours
after onset of this stage.
May involve respiratory muscles.

Bulbar form:
Pharyngeal, laryngeal, lingual
and facial weakness
May involve cardiac and
respiratory muscles.

A mixed form can occur.

Diagnosis
During the meningeal phase, consider other causes of acute meningitis.
Once the paralytic phase ensues, distinguish from the Guillain-Barré syndrome and transverse myelitis.
The clinical picture + CSF examination (polymorphs and lymphocytes increased; protein elevated with normal glucose) are sufficient to reach the diagnosis.
Poliovirus RNA can be detected in faeces or CSF by PCR.

Prognosis

In epidemics, a mortality of 25% results from respiratory paralysis. Improvement in muscle power usually commences one week after the onset of paralysis and continues for up to a year.

Only a proportion of muscles remain permanently paralysed; in these, fasciculation may persist. In affected limbs, bone growth becomes retarded with shortening as well as thinning.

Treatment
The patient is kept on bed rest and fluid balance carefully maintained.
Respiratory failure may require ventilation.
Avoid the development of deformities in affected limbs with physiotherapy and splinting.

Post-Polio Syndrome
A significant proportion of polio patients develop late sequelae often 30 yrs after initial illness – fatigue, myalgia and progressive muscle atrophy with weakness are characteristic.

Prophylaxis

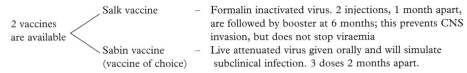

2 vaccines
are available

Salk vaccine

– Formalin inactivated virus. 2 injections, 1 month apart,
are followed by booster at 6 months; this prevents CNS
invasion, but does not stop viraemia

Sabin vaccine
(vaccine of choice)

– Live attenuated virus given orally and will simulate
subclinical infection. 3 doses 2 months apart.

VIRAL INFECTIONS – VARICELLA-ZOSTER INFECTION

Varicella (chickenpox) and herpes zoster (shingles) are different clinical manifestations of infection by the same virus – *Varicella–Zoster*, a DNA human herpes virus.

Conditions caused:
- an acute encephalitis
- viral meningitis
- myelitis

- postinfectious encephalomyelitis
- postinfectious polyneuropathy (Guillain-Barré syndrome).

SHINGLES

This occurs after virus reactivation, dormant after the primary infection (chickenpox).

Pathology: The virus involves the *dorsal root* (sensory) ganglion of the spinal cord or the *cranial nerve* sensory ganglion – trigeminal or geniculate.

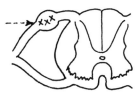

The inflammatory process may spread into the spinal cord and involve posterior and anterior horns. Similarly inflammatory changes may occur in the brain stem.

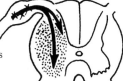

Clinical features

Patients are usually over 50 years of age. Sexes are affected equally. Recurrence is rare. Often occurs in immunocompromised patients e.g. lymphoma. Also associated with spinal/nerve root trauma.

Initial feature:
A vesicular skin rash associated with a burning, painful sensation. Vesicles contain clear fluid and conform to a dermatome distribution. After 1–3 weeks, the vesicles crust over and leave irregular skin depigmentation with scarring.

Motor weakness occurs in 20% due to damage of the anterior horn cell. More widespread spinal (myelitis) or encephalic involvement occurs in the immunodeficient. In these patients extensive cutaneous lesions are common (disseminated zoster).

Cranial nerve ganglia involvement:

– *Trigeminal:* usually ophthalmic division with vesicles above the eye and associated corneal ulceration
       – HERPES ZOSTER OPHTHALMICUS.

– *Geniculate:* vesicles within the external auditory meatus and ear drum. Ipsilateral deafness and facial weakness result. – RAMSAY HUNT SYNDROME.

Diagnosis: Based on clinical features. Virus DNA can be detected in vesicular fluid by PCR.

Treatment

This depends on the severity and location of skin lesions. Mild disease requires symptomatic treatment only. Severe disease, involvement in immunocompromised patients, or ophthalmic vesicles require acyclovir either orally or intravenously.

POST HERPETIC NEURALGIA

This is a condition which occurs in 10% of all patients. The incidence rises with age. A chronic, uncomfortable, burning pain presents in the territory of the involved dermatome. The pathogenesis is unknown.

Treatment with antidepressants, anticonvulsants, e.g. carbamazepine, transcutaneous stimulation (TCS) or sympathetic ganglion block may help, but results are unpredictable.

Varicella and Herpes Zoster CNS involvement

Patients with AIDS and other immunocompromising disorders risk severe, life-threatening CNS involvement – encephalitis, cerebral vasculitis, myelitis or brain stem encephalitis. Herpes Zoster ophthalmicus can be associated, in the middle aged, with delayed major cerebral artery territory infarction. This presents 4–6 weeks after infection. Stroke also occurs as a remote complication of childhood varicella, usually within 12 weeks of clinical chickenpox. These are both due to virus-induced damage to cerebral arteries (vasculitis). The role of anti-viral drugs and steroids is uncertain.

509

OPPORTUNISTIC INFECTIONS

These infections occur in immunocompromised patients. Certain types of immunological deficiency tend to be associated with specific forms of infection.

T cell/macrophage deficiency	*B cell immunoglobulin deficiency*	*Granulocyte deficiency*
Causes: e.g. AIDS	Chronic lymphatic leukaemia	Marrow infiltration
Lymphoreticular tumours	Primary hypogammaglobulinaemia	Aplastic anaemia
Immunosuppressant drugs	Splenectomy	Chemotherapy/ radiotherapy
Organisms:		
Viruses – Cytomegalovirus	Measles	
Herpes simplex/zoster	Enteroviruses	
JC virus		
Bacteria – Listeria	*Streptococcus pneumoniae*	Enterobacteria
Nocardia	*Haemophilus influenzae*	*Staphylococcus aureus*
Mycobacterium, etc.	*Pseudomonas aeruginosa*, etc.	*P. aeruginosa*, etc.
Fungi – Aspergillus		*Aspergillus*
Candida		*Candida*
Mucoraceae		*Mucoraceae*
Parasites – Toxoplasmosis		

CLINICAL SYNDROMES, DIAGNOSIS AND TREATMENT

Clinical Syndrome	Diagnosis		Treatment
CEREBRAL ABSCESS	CT scan	→ Common bacteria	
	Blood culture	→ *Listeria*	→ Ampicillin or erythromycin
	Drainage or	→ *Nocardia*	→ Sulphonamide or cycloserine
	biopsy and culture	→ *Candida*	→ Amphotericin B & 5-fluorocytosine
OTHER INTRA-CRANIAL MASS LESIONS	CT/MR scan	→ *Aspergillus*	→ Surgical removal (if indicated) Amphotericin B & 5-fluorocytosine
	Serum antibodies		
	Biopsy	→ *Toxoplasmosis*	→ Pyrimethamine, sulphadiazine & folinic acid
ENCEPHAL-OPATHY	EEG		
	CT/MR scan	→ *Toxoplasmosis*	→ Pyrimethamine, sulphadiazine & folinic acid
	Serum antibodies	→ Cytomegalovirus	→ Gancyclovir or Foscarnet
	Viral isolation	→ JC virus	→ Cytosine arabinoside
	(biopsy)	(progressive	
	Intracellular	multifocal	
	inclusion bodies	→ encephalopathy)	
CRANIAL NERVE PALSIES	Skull X-ray		
	CT/MR scan	→ *Candida*	→ Amphotericin B & 5-fluorocytosine
	CSF/blood culture	→ *Mucoraceae*	→ Radical sinus and orbital surgery and amphotericin B
	Serum antibodies		
	Nasal swab		
MENINGITIS	CT/MR scan	→ Common bacteria	
	CSF/blood culture	→ *Mycobacterium*	
	Serum antibodies	→ *Cryptococcus*	→ Amphotericin B & 5-fluorocytosine
	Antigen agglutin-ation tests	→ *Listeria*	→ Ampicillin or erythromycin
		→ *Nocardia*	→ Sulphonamide or cycloserine
		→ *Candida*	→ Amphotericin B & 5-fluorocytosin
RETINITIS	Serum antibodies	→ *Toxoplasmosis*	→ Pyrimethamine, sulphadiazine & folinic acid
	Viral isolation	→ Cytomegalovirus	→ Gancyclovir or Foscarnet

ACQUIRED IMMUNODEFICIENCY SYNDROME (AIDS)

Human immunodeficiency virus (HIV-I) has *lymphotropic* (CD4 lymphocytes) and *neurotropic* (microglial) properties. Neurological features develop in 80% of infected individuals manifesting as either direct effects of the HIV virus or infections, tumours and associated vascular disorders due to immunodeficiency. AIDS is the end stage of chronic infection.

Prevalence of AIDS and HIV infection

Certain individuals are 'at risk' of infection:

– homosexual males
– I.V. drug users
} and heterosexual partners

– Babies born to infected individuals
– Recipients of blood products, e.g. haemophiliacs.

The incidence of HIV infection in 'at risk' groups varies considerably.
Sex education, supply of clean needles to addicts, active drug-dependence programmes and specific precautions in the preparation of blood products are necessary to limit its spread.

Current prevalence of HIV – USA 140/million (New York 991/million).

CLINICAL COURSE OF HIV INFECTION

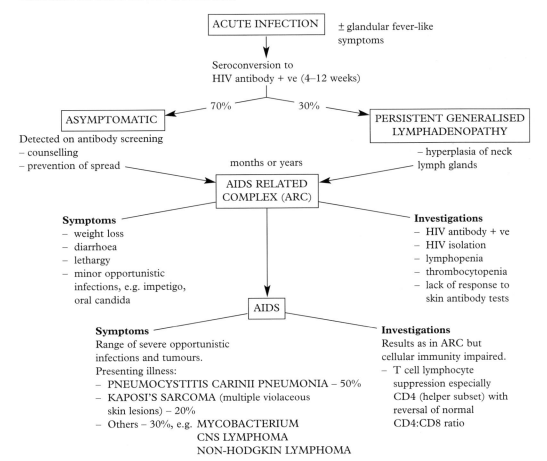

ACUTE INFECTION	± glandular fever-like symptoms

Seroconversion to
HIV antibody + ve (4–12 weeks)

70%   30%

ASYMPTOMATIC

Detected on antibody screening
– counselling
– prevention of spread

PERSISTENT GENERALISED LYMPHADENOPATHY

– hyperplasia of neck lymph glands

months or years

AIDS RELATED COMPLEX (ARC)

Symptoms
– weight loss
– diarrhoea
– lethargy
– minor opportunistic infections, e.g. impetigo, oral candida

Investigations
– HIV antibody + ve
– HIV isolation
– lymphopenia
– thrombocytopenia
– lack of response to skin antibody tests

AIDS

Symptoms
Range of severe opportunistic infections and tumours.
Presenting illness:
– PNEUMOCYSTITIS CARINII PNEUMONIA – 50%
– KAPOSI'S SARCOMA (multiple violaceous skin lesions) – 20%
– Others – 30%, e.g. MYCOBACTERIUM
                 CNS LYMPHOMA
                 NON-HODGKIN LYMPHOMA

Investigations
Results as in ARC but cellular immunity impaired.
– T cell lymphocyte suppression especially CD4 (helper subset) with reversal of normal CD4:CD8 ratio

511

NEUROLOGICAL PRESENTATIONS OF HIV INFECTION

Cerebral tumours
Primary cerebral lymphoma
Metastatic systemic lymphoma —— CT/MR scan
Metastatic Kaposi's sarcoma
Infections
Encephalitis
  Cytomegalovirus
  Herpes zoster/simplex ———— CT/MR scan
  Toxoplasmosis   Antibody tests
  Progressive multifocal   Biopsy
    leukoencephalopathy
Cerebral abscess
  E. coli
  Aspergillus – ———— CT/MR scan
  Candida   Aspiration/culture
  Nocardia   Antibody tests
Meningitis
  HIV-1
  Mycobacterium
  Listeria – ———— CSF exam and culture
  Syphilis   Antibody tests
  Aspergillus

AIDS dementia (in 15%)
Direct HIV infection with
demyelination and perivascular ———— CT/MR scan
inflammatory changes. Intellectual   Psychometry
decline of subcortical type
(page 127).

Retinopathy
Cytomegalovirus ———— Fundal exam.
Toxoplasmosis   Antibody tests

Myelopathy
Acute reversible
Compression –   abscess
              – systemic lymphoma. ——— Spinal CT/MRI
Ascending   – cytomegalovirus   Antibody tests
                herpes zoster/simplex

Vascular disorders
Intracranial haemorrhage
cerebral infarction (septic ——— CT/MR scan
emboli or thrombosis)

Peripheral neuropathy
Herpes zoster radiculopathy
Cauda equina syndrome (cytomegalovirus)   Nerve conduction studies
Acute reversible demyelination   Antibody tests
Chronic demyelination

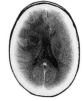

Cerebral
toxoplasmosis

Treatment

Opportunistic infection – treatment of specific infection (see page 510).

> With known HIV + ve patients, invasive procedures such as biopsy are
> often avoided and trials of therapy are administered, e.g. cerebral
> toxoplasmosis – trial of pyrimethamine and sulphadiazine, monitored with
> CT/MRI. If lesions do not resolve → biopsy (? lymphoma).

Highly active antiretroviral therapy (HAART) with effective treatment for infections and neoplastic complications
has significantly improved outcome. Mean survival time for HIV-infected persons currently exceeds 10 years. The
prolonged survival of HIV-infected persons increases their risk of developing PML or CNS lymphoma (these
responding poorly to treatment).

HAART management comprises two nucleoside reverse transcriptase inhibitors (e.g. *zidovudine* and *didanosine*) and
a protease inhibitor (e.g. *ritonavir* or *indinavir*), or a nonnucleoside reverse transcriptase inhibitor (*nevirapine*). This
combination is given to HIV-infected individuals with detectable viral loads or immunologic dysfunction (less than
500 CD4+ cells/mm^3). HAART results in immunological and neurocognitive improvement, even when HIV is
advanced. Treatment aims at reducing the viral load to undetectable levels, PCR having a central role in monitoring
therapy and identifying drug resistance.

SUBACUTE/CHRONIC MENINGITIS

This entity is characterised by symptoms and signs of meningeal irritation which persist and progress over weeks without improvement. Unlike acute meningitis, the onset is insidious; cranial nerve signs and focal deficits such as hemiparesis, dementia and gradual deterioration of conscious level may predominate. Predisposing factors include immunosuppression or immunocompromised host. The outcome depends upon aetiology and the early instigation of appropriate treatment.

Chronic meningitis is associated with certain CSF findings.
- Lymphocytosis + low glucose (relative to serum level)
- Lymphocytosis + normal glucose.

Diagnosis depends upon CSF examination.
Lumbar puncture should be performed in suspicious cases as soon as CT scan has ruled out a mass lesion.

SUBACUTE/CHRONIC MENINGITIS WITH A MARKED REDUCTION IN CSF GLUCOSE

Causes	Diagnosis	Specific features	Treatment
M. tuberculosis	See page 491		
Fungi *Cryptococcus* *Nocardia* *Candida* *Aspergillus*	Diagnosis suggested by chest X-ray – pulmonary infiltrations, CT/MR evidence of meningeal enhancement and associated hydrocephalus CSF abnormalities lymphocytosis, low glucose and high protein with appropriate staining, culture and agglutination/complement-fixation tests.	Clinical features similar to tuberculous meningitis.	Amphotericin B + fluorocytosine or fluconazole
Carcinomatous meningitis – lung/breast/gastrointestinal tract Leukaemia/ lymphoma Glioma Medulloblastoma Melanoma.	Evidence of primary neoplasm. *CT* or *MR* evidence of meningeal enhancement *CSF* Malignant cells seen in fresh centrifuged filtered sample. Tumour markers: – carcinoembryonic antigen (CEA) – β-microglobulin Meningeal biopsy rarely necessary but diagnostic	Back pain/ radicular involvement common. Hydrocephalus in 30%	Consider irradiation followed by intrathecal methotrexate or monoclonal targeting (see page 310). Leukaemia/ lymphoma requires specialist advice

SUBACUTE/CHRONIC MENINGITIS

SUBACUTE/CHRONIC MENINGITIS WITH A MARKED REDUCTION IN CSF GLUCOSE

Causes	Diagnosis	Specific features	Treatment
Parameningeal infections Cerebral abscess Epidural abscess Sinusitis Mastoiditis	Evidence of primary infected source *X-rays* Sinuses, mastoids. *CT/MR* scan – cerebral or cerebellar abscess *CSF* microscopy/culture *Blood* cultures	Prodromal sinus or middle ear infection	Appropriate antibiotic therapy and, if indicated, surgical drainage of loculated parameningeal infection

Bacteria:
 Treponema
 Brucella
 Leptospira
 Listeria
 Borrelia
 Burgdorferi
	CSF
	 Isolate organism (if possible)
	 Serological tests
	 Serum
	 Serological tests
		Treponema – page 495
		   Sexual contact
		 Brucella
		   Contact with
		   infected cattle
		 Leptospira – page 498
		   Contact with
		   contaminated rat,
		   dog or cattle urine
		 Listeria – page 510
		   Contaminated
		   foods
		 Borrelia
		 Burgdorferi – page 497
		   Tick bite
			Appropriate antibiotic

Miscellaneous
Parasites, e.g.
  toxoplasma – see page 499
  Sarcoidosis – see page 356
Behçet's disease
Whipple's disease
Systemic lupus
  erythematosus – see page 263

Chemical
 – leakage from
  epidermoid
  dermoid cyst or
  craniopharyngioma
 – Intrathecal drugs
  and contrast material

Despite extensive investigation, a group of patients with chronic meningitis exists in whom no cause is found.

DEMYELINATING DISEASE

Demyelinating disorders of the central nervous system affect *myelin* and/or *oligodendroglia* with relative sparing of *axons*.

The central nervous system is composed of *neurons* with *neuroectodermal* and *mesodermal* supporting cells.

The neuroectodermal cells comprise:

astrocytes
ependymal cells
oligodendrocytes.

The oligodendrocytes, like Schwann cells in the peripheral nervous system, are responsible for the formation of *myelin* around central nervous system *axons*.

One Schwann cell myelinates one axon but one oligodendrocyte may myelinate several contiguous axons, and the close proximity of cell to axon may not be obvious by light microscopy.

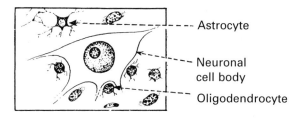

Oligodendrocytes are present in grey matter near neuronal cell bodies and in white matter near axons.

Myelin is composed of *protein* and *lipids*.
Protein accounts for 20% of total content.
The lipid fraction may be divided into:
    cholesterol
    glycophosphatides (lecithins)
    sphingolipids (sphingomyelins).

The laying down of myelin in the central nervous system commences at the fourth month of fetal life in the median longitudinal bundle, then in frontal and parietal lobes at birth. Most of the cerebrum is myelinated by the end of the 2nd year. Myelination continues until the 10th year of life.

Myelin disorders may be classified as diseases in which:

1. Myelin is inherently abnormal or was never properly formed – these disorders generally present in infancy and early childhood and have a biochemical basis, e.g. leukodystrophy.

2. Myelin which was normal when formed breaks down as a consequence of pathological insult, e.g. *multiple sclerosis*.

MULTIPLE SCLEROSIS

Multiple sclerosis (MS) is a common demyelinating disease, normally characterised by focal disturbance of function and a relapsing and remitting course.

The disease occurs most commonly in temperate climates and prevalence differs at various latitudes:

	Latitude (°N)	Rate/100 000 (adjusted)
Orkneys and Shetland	60	309
England (Cornwall).	51	63
Italy (Bari)	41	13

The disease usually occurs in young adults with a peak age incidence of 20–40 years. Slightly more females than males are affected. There is a 3% risk of disease if a sibling or parent is affected.

PATHOLOGY

Scattered lesions with a greyish colour, 1 mm to several cm in size, are present in the white matter of the brain and spinal cord and are referred to as *plaques*. The lesions lie in close relationship to veins (postcapillary venules) – perivenous distribution.

RECENT LESIONS ⟶ LATER ⟶ OLD LESIONS

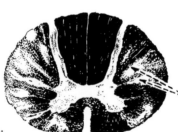

Myelin destruction
Relative axon sparing
Perivenous infiltration with mononuclear cells and lymphocytes. Interstitial oedema is evident in acute lesions.
Breakdown of blood–brain barrier occurs and may be essential for myelin destruction.

Astrocyte proliferation

Relatively acellular and more clearly demarcated. Within these plaques bare axons are surrounded by astrocytes
Axon loss accounts for increasing disability.

Thoracic spinal cord showing established plaques of demyelination

PATHOGENESIS

Immune deficiency has been suggested. This might explain the possible persistence of a latent virus and variations in immune status could be the basis of 'relapses and remissions'. T lymphocytes and macrophages found in plaques may be sensitized to myelin antigens.

Hereditary/genetic factors appear significant. There is an increased familial incidence of multiple sclerosis. This has led to the study of *histocompatibility antigens* (HL-A). An association between A3, B7, B18 and DW2/ DRW2 and multiple sclerosis has been demonstrated. Concordance rate in monozygotic twins is 30% and in dizygotes 5%. Affected women transmit MS to offsping more frequently than affected men suggesting that mitochondrial genes contribute to inheritance.

Viruses may be important in the development of multiple sclerosis, infection perhaps occurring in a genetically/immunologically susceptible host.

Elevated serum and CSF antibody titres have been found to:
– varicella zoster, measles, rubella and herpes simplex during relapse.

Biochemical: No biochemical effect has been demonstrated – myelin appears normal before breakdown and the proposed excess of dietary fats or malabsorption of unsaturated fatty acids is unproven.

MULTIPLE SCLEROSIS

PATHOGENISIS (*cont'd*)

In summary – the causation is probably multifactorial.

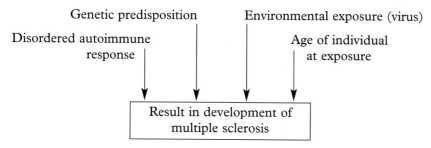

CLINICAL FEATURES

Peak age of onset	– 20–25 years
Childhood onset rare	–2%
Patients presenting >50 years	– 5%
Patients presenting >60 years	– 1%

Multiple sclerosis is usually characterised by:
– Signs and symptoms of widespread white matter disease.
– A relapsing and remitting or progressive course.

Symptoms at onset

1. *Vague symptoms:* lack of energy, headache, depression, aches in limbs – may result in diagnosis of psychoneurosis. These symptoms are eventually associated with:

2. *Precise symptoms:*
(initial symptom of
multiple sclerosis
expressed as a %)

Sensory disturbance	– 40%
Retrobulbar neuritis	– 17%
Limb weakness	– 12%
Diplopia	– 11%
Vertigo	
Ataxia	– 20%
Sphincter disturbance	

Trigeminal neuralgia may be an early symptom of multiple sclerosis, and this should be considered in the young patient with paroxysmal facial pain.

MULTIPLE SCLEROSIS

Sensory symptoms

Numbness and paraesthesia are common and often minor and transient. Paraesthesia is more often due to posterior column demyelination than to spinothalamic tract involvement.

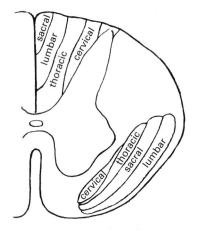

Posterior column lesions result in impaired vibration sensation and joint position sensation. In such cases a limb may be rendered 'useless' by the absence of positional awareness.

Lhermitte's sign: with cervical posterior column involvement sudden neck flexion will evoke a 'shock-like' sensation in the limbs.

Spinothalamic lesions result in dysaesthesia – an unpleasant feeling of burning, coldness or warmth, with associated sensory loss to pain and temperature contralateral to the lesion.

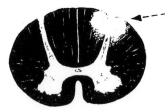

A plaque at the posterior root entry zone will result in loss of *all* sensory modalities in that particular root distribution.

Motor symptoms

Monoparesis and paraparesis are the most common motor symptoms. Hemiparesis and quadriparesis occur less commonly.

Paraparesis is the result of spinal demyelination, usually in the cervical region.

Signs: – Increased tone
      – Hyperactive tendon reflexes, extensor plantar response and absent abdominal reflexes
      – Pyramidal distribution weakness.

N.B. A plaque at the anterior root exit zone may result in lower motor neuron signs (reflex loss and segmental wasting)

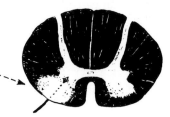

MULTIPLE SCLEROSIS

Loss of vision

Acute optic neuritis (Retrobulbar neuritis): Visual loss associated usually with a central scotoma and recovery over some weeks. This commonly occurs in young adults. The visual loss develops over several days and is often associated with pain on ocular movement (irritation of the dural membrane around the optic nerve). In milder forms, only colour vision is affected. Typically only one eye is affected, although occasionally both eyes simultaneously or consecutively are involved.

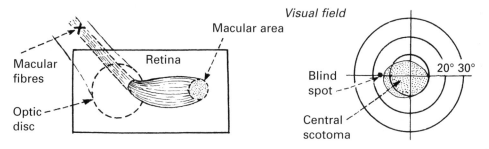

On examination: Disturbance of visual function ranges from a small central scotoma to complete loss. Fundal examination reveals swelling – papillitis – in up to 50% of patients, depending upon the proximity of the plaque to the optic nerve head.

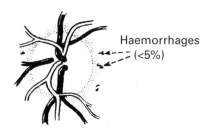

'Sheathing' from an inflammatory exudate around peripheral retinal venules is common. Reduced visual acuity distinguishes papillitis from papilloedema.

Investigation: Visual evoked responses (VERs) show delay. High resolution CT or MRI of the optic nerve excludes tumour. MR confirms the presence of plaque.

Treatment: The optic neuritis study group showed that IV or oral steroids compared with placebo accelerated recovery though at 2 years there was no significant difference in eventual visual function. Oral steroids were associated with a higher risk of recurrent optic neuritis. Intravenous steroids appeared (within the next 2 years) to reduce the risk of subsequent MS.

Outcome: 90% of patients recover most vision, although symptoms may transiently return following a hot bath or physical exercise – Uhthoff's phenomenon. Following recovery the optic disc develops an atrophic appearance with a pale 'punched out' temporal margin.

Subsequent course:
The optic neuritis study group reported 12% of cases had developed clinically definite MS within 2 years (4% with a normal and 30% with an abnormal cranial MRI). Thereafter the risk is 5–6% per annum.

Acute bilateral optic neuritis: less common than unilateral disease and progression to MS not as likely. Occasionally followed by a transverse myelitis (Neuromyelitis optica, page 525). Examination of mitochondrial DNA distinguishes from Leber's hereditary optic neuropathy (page 547).

MULTIPLE SCLEROSIS

Disturbance of ocular movement

Diplopia may result from demyelination affecting the brain stem pathway of the III, IV or VI cranial nerves. Abnormality of eye movements with or without diplopia occurs when supranuclear or internuclear connection are involved. The latter results from a lesion in the medial longitudinal fasciculus – *internuclear ophthalmoplegia* (I.N.O.) – and in young persons is pathognomonic of MS.

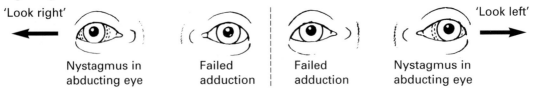

'Look right'			'Look left'
Nystagmus in abducting eye	Failed adduction	Failed adduction	Nystagmus in abducting eye

Nystagmus may be an incidental finding on neurological examination. It is unusual in multiple sclerosis when the eyes are in the primary position, and is commonly seen on lateral gaze. Pupillary *abnormalities* may occur from:

 – sympathetic involvement in the brain stem (Horner's syndrome)
 – III nerve involvement, or
 – II nerve involvement.

The swinging light test is a sensitive test of impaired afferent conduction in the II nerve. Alternating the light from one eye to the other results eventually in 'pupillary escape' – the pupil dilates despite the presence of direct light.

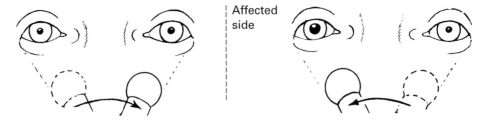

Affected side

OTHER FEATURES

Vestibular symptoms: Vertigo of central type may be a presenting problem or it may develop during the course of the illness. Hearing loss is rare.

Ataxia of gait and limb inco-ordination are frequently present. The gait ataxia may be cerebellar or sensory type (see Romberg's test). Limb inco-ordination, intention tremor and dysarthria indicate cerebellar involvement.

Sphincter disturbance with urgency or precipitancy of micturition and eventual incontinence occurs. Conversely urinary retention in a young person may be the first symptom of disease. On direct questioning, impotence is frequently found.

Mental changes: Mood change – euphoria or depression occur. Cognitive impairment develops in advanced cases. Generalised fatigue is common.

Emotional lability: Uncontrolled outbursts of crying or laughing, result from involvement of pseudobulbar pathways.

Paroxysmal (symptoms occurring momentarily throughout any stage of the disease): paraesthesia, dysarthria, ataxia, pain, e.g. trigeminal neuralgia, photopsia (visual scintillations), epilepsy.

MULTIPLE SCLEROSIS

CLINICAL COURSE

The pattern of illness in individual sufferers cannot be predicted. Several different rates of disease activity and progression have been defined.

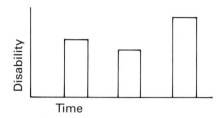

1. *Relapsing and remitting*
Of all patients with MS, 70% pass through this stage. With each attack recovery is virtually complete. This phase of illness may persist for many years. The explanation of why relapses take place is unknown.

2. *Secondary progressive and relapsing/remitting secondary progressive*
After a period of time, relapsing and remitting MS attacks are followed by incomplete recovery and cumulative loss of function and disability. At any one time, the chronic progressive stage accounts for 20% of all sufferers. Converting from relapsing and remitting to secondary progressive occurs on average 6–10 years after the initial symptoms.

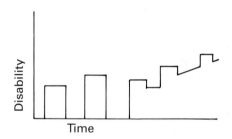

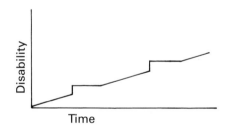

3. *Primary progressive*
This form is common in late onset MS (>45 yrs) and accounts for 15% of all patients. Symptoms and signs are usually spinal and relapses absent in the context of insidious progression.

4. *Benign*
This is defined as low disability (EDSS <3) 10 years after onset. The true incidence of such cases is difficult to define and patients may still progress in time to major disability. Some support for a benign form comes from the occasional incidental autopsy finding of MS.

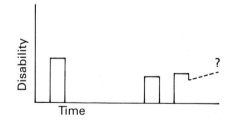

Recognition of different phases of MS is essential in selecting patients for new disease-modifying treatments. The degree of disability can be recorded using specific scales such as the Kurtzke score or the Extended Disability Status Score (EDSS).

[This is a 10 point non-linear scale where 1 = no symptoms or signs, 6 = a walking aid to achieve a short distance, 8 = restricted to bed/wheelchair and 10 = death due to MS].

MULTIPLE SCLEROSIS

INVESTIGATIONS
The development of imaging and laboratory testing has advanced diagnostic accuracy.

Neurophysiological: may detect
a second asymptomatic lesion
(see page 53).

1. *Visual evoked potential (VEP).* In optic
nerve involvement the latency of the large
positive wave (p.102) is delayed beyond
110 msec. The amplitude of the waves
may also be reduced.

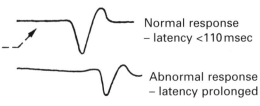

Normal response
– latency <110 msec

Abnormal response
– latency prolonged

2. *Somatosensory evoked response (SSEP)*
may detect central sensory pathway
lesions.

3. *Brain stem auditory evoked potential
(BAEP)* may detect brain stem lesions.

Cerebrospinal fluid examination by lumbar puncture
A mild pleocytosis (25 cells/mm^3), mainly
lymphocytes, is occasionally found. The
total protein may be elevated, although
this rarely exceeds 100 mg/l. An increase
in gammaglobulin occurs in 50–60% of
cases. Electrophoresis of CSF using agar
or acrylamide shows discrete bands which
are not present in serum.

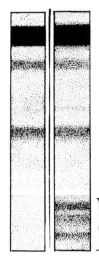

NORMAL

These bands are found in up
to 95% of patients with
established disease and in
50–60% after the first attack.
Oligoclonal bands (OCBs) are
not specific to MS but persist
indefinitely, unlike other
inflammatory neurological
diseases (see following page).

OLIGOCLONAL
BANDS

MRI
This has contributed enormously to the diagnosis and understanding
of MS. Normal white matter appears dark with low signal intensity in
T2 weighted images. Myelin breakdown produces a longer relaxation
time and increased signal on T2. Gliosis produces similar changes.
The presence of white matter abnormalities with a periventricular
distribution is suggestive but not diagnostic of MS. Paramagnetic
contrast (Gadolinium) will show active inflammation. A combination
of MRI and CSF (oligoclonal band) will rule out MS if both are
negative. MR may predict long term outcome – following a single
episode of demyelination (e.g. optic neuritis or transverse myelitis).
Those with cranial MR abnormalities will relapse sooner than those
without. At present MRI does not correlate well with disability, but
newer techniques may be more sensitive measures of disease
progression.

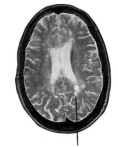

Periventricular lesions,
most evident at frontal
and occipital horns.
Abnormalities are also
seen in the brain stem
and cerebellum. Lesions
of the optic nerves and
spinal cord are more
difficult to detect.

MULTIPLE SCLEROSIS

Diagnostic criteria have been proposed (Poser Committee 1983). These were primarily conceived for research and clinical trials of therapy but are also of use to the clinician.

CLINICALLY DEFINITE ———————— Two attacks of ——— clinical signs or investigative
symptoms   evidence of two lesions.

LABORATORY SUPPORTED DEFINITE ——— | ——————— clinical signs or investigative
evidence of one lesion.
Abnormal CSF (oligoclonal bands).

CLINICALLY PROBABLE ———————— | ——————— clinical signs or investigative
evidence of one lesion.

LABORATORY SUPPORTED PROBABLE ——— ▼ ——————— abnormal CSF (oligoclonal bands).

(Modified from Poser Ann. Neurol. 1985 13:227–231.)

Complex new criteria incorporating MRI findings have been suggested (Ann. Neurol 2001; 50: 121–7).

DIFFERENTIAL DIAGNOSIS

Many conditions mimic multiple sclerosis and unless strict diagnostic criteria are adhered to other treatable disorders will be missed.

Conditions with similar clinical presentations to MS

Inflammatory disorders
- Systemic lupus erythematosus
- Polyarteritis nodosa
- Behçet's disease

Isolated cranial disorders
- AVM
- Meningioma

Granulomatous disorders
- Sarcoidosis
- Wegener's granulomatosis

Miscellaneous disorders
- Spinocerebellar degeneration
- Mitochondrial disorders
- Adrenoleukodystrophy

Isolated spinal cord/foramen magnum disorders
- Extrinsic/intrinsic tumours
- Vitamin B_{12} disease
- Lyme disease
- Acute disseminated encephalomyelitis

Conditions with similar MRI appearances to MS

- Vasculitis
- Sarcoidosis
- Leukodystrophies
- Acute disseminated encephalomyelitis
- Small vessel vascular disease
- Decompression sickness
- Lyme disease
- Chronic inflammatory demyelinating polyneuropathy

Conditions with similar CSF profile to MS (presence of oligoclonal bands)

- HIV infection
- Lyme disease
- Syphilis
- Chronic meningitis
- Neurosarcoidosis
- Subacute sclerosing panencephalitis (SSPE)

MULTIPLE SCLEROSIS – TREATMENT

SYMPTOMATIC

• Spasticity
Drugs that act at spinal or skeletal muscle level
– Baclofen (GABA derivative)
– Dantrolene (direct action on muscle)
– Tizanidine (α_2 adrenergic agonist)
Baclofen can be administered intrathecally (implantable drug delivery system) in severe cases.

• Urinary symptoms
Incomplete bladder emptying – intermittent self-catheterisation
Detrusor instability – anticholinergics (oxybutynin, tolterodine)
                    – Desmopressin spray.

• Bowel symptoms
– lactulose
– loperamide (opiate receptor agonist – increases anal sphincter tone).

• Pain
Analgesics, anticonvulsants, antidepressants, NSAIDs and transcutaneous electrical nerve stimulation (TENS)

• Paroxysmal symptoms
e.g. tonic seizures – anticonvulsants

• Fatigue/Mood change
Amantadine, modafinil and SSRIs.

• Tremor/Ataxia
Betablockers, primidone and in severe cases thalamic ablation or stimulation.

ACUTE RELAPSE
Methylprednisone 3 g i.v. over 3 days followed by oral prednisone taper (40 mg reducing over 3 weeks). Check for infection beforehand, monitor blood glucose and consider an H_2 blocker for ulcer prophylaxis. Methylprednisone can also be given orally.

MODIFY NATURAL HISTORY
No benefit from long-term steroids. Cyclophosphamide, azathioprine, total lymphoid irradiation and plasma exchange – anecdotal evidence of benefit in aggressive illness. Low dose methotrexate of marginal value in primary and secondary progressive disease.

Interferons (1a & 1b) and copolymer 1 These drugs are considered early in disease course, especially when prognosis seems unfavourable (frequent relapses or rapid progression). Effects on MRI progression are impressive but clinical outcomes (in the short term) less so. Treatments are by injection (i.m. or s.c), dose uncertain, costs significant and long-term benefits and hazards unknown. In the UK treatment can only be initiated by neurologists in patients with some retained mobility and continuing relapses. Outcomes are being accessed as part of a national surveillance scheme.

OTHER DEMYELINATING DISEASES

NEUROMYELITIS OPTICA (Devic's disease)

A subacute disorder characterised by simultaneous or consecutive demyelination of the optic nerves and spinal cord. Whether a distinct entity or variant of MS is uncertain. Pathologically demyelination is associated with marked cavitation and necrosis (possibly due to severe oedema confined and compressed by the pia of the optic nerves and spinal cord). Systemic lupus erythematosus, Behçet's disease and sarcoidosis produce a similar picture.

Clinical features

Visual loss is rapid, bilateral and occasionally total.
Spinal cord symptoms follow – hours, days or occasionally weeks later.
Back pain and girdle pain. Paraesthesia in lower limbs.
Paralysis may ascend to involve respiratory muscles.
Urinary retention is common.
Recovery is complete in 60–70% of patients. When recurrent attacks occur, this results in an aggressive course with a high fatality.

Examination

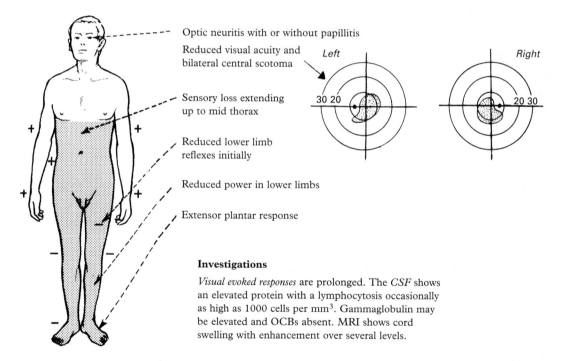

Optic neuritis with or without papillitis

Reduced visual acuity and bilateral central scotoma

Sensory loss extending up to mid thorax

Reduced lower limb reflexes initially

Reduced power in lower limbs

Extensor plantar response

Investigations

Visual evoked responses are prolonged. The *CSF* shows an elevated protein with a lymphocytosis occasionally as high as 1000 cells per mm^3. Gammaglobulin may be elevated and OCBs absent. MRI shows cord swelling with enhancement over several levels.

Treatment

Patients may respond to i.v. methylprednisone or plasma exchange. Supportive treatment is required to minimise complications (DVT/PE, decubiti, contractures). Ventilatory support is sometimes required and may be permanent. Attempts to prevent relapses with immunosuppressive drugs (azathioprine, cyclophosphamide) are disappointing.

TRANSVERSE MYELITIS

This occasionally occurs as the first manifestation of MS but this also occurs with viral infection (e.g. herpes virus), vasculitis and atherosclerotic vascular disease. Only 4% of patients with normal cranial MRI progress to MS. Investigations should exclude other causes of acute spinal cord syndrome – spinal cord compression – by MRI.

OTHER DEMYELINATING DISEASES

ACUTE DISSEMINATED ENCEPHALOMYELITIS (ADEM) (postinfectious encephalomyelitis)

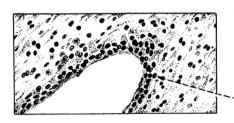

ADEM is an acute immune-mediated demyelinating disorder in which small foci of demyelination with a perivenous distribution are scattered throughout the brain and spinal cord. Lesions are 0.1–1.0 mm in diameter.

Microglial, plasma cell and lymphocyte exudate around venules. Myelin becomes fragmented.

This disorder may follow upper respiratory and gastrointestinal infections (viral), viral exanthems (measles, chickenpox, rubella, etc.) or immunisation with live or killed virus vaccines (influenza, rabies).

Measles is the commonest cause occurring in 1 per 1000 primary infections; next Varicella zoster (chickenpox), 1 per 2000 primary infections.

Clinical features: Within days or weeks of resolution of the viral infection, fever, headache, nausea and vomiting develop. Meningeal symptoms (neck stiffness, photophobia) are then followed by drowsiness and multifocal neurological signs and symptoms – hemisphere brain stem/cerebellar/spinal cord and optic nerve involvement. Myoclonic movements are common.

Predominantly *spinal*, *cerebral* or *cerebellar* forms occur, though usually the picture is mixed. Optic nerve involvement takes the form of optic neuritis. Rarely the peripheral nervous system is involved.

Diagnosis: No diagnosis test.
CSF – 20–200 mononuclear cells.
Total protein and γ globulin raised.
Peripheral blood may be normal or show neutrophilia, lymphocytosis or lymphopenia.

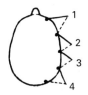

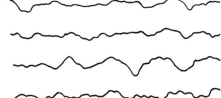

Generalised asynchronous delta activity

The electroencephalogram (EEG) shows diffuse slow wave activity.
CT scan is normal. MRI shows small focal white matter changes, simultaneously enhancing with contrast indicating that all are of the same degree of acuteness (unlike MS).

Diagnosis is straightforward when there is an obvious preceding viral infection or immunisation. When viral infection *immediately* precedes, distinction from acute encephalitis is often impossible.

Separation from acute MS may be difficult. Fever, meningeal signs with elevated CSF protein above 100 mg/ml with cell count greater than 50 per mm^3 suggest ADEM.

Pathology: demyelination is limited to perivascular areas and lesions do not approach the same size as in MS.

Outcome: The illness is typically monophasic.
The mortality rate is 20%.
Full recovery occurs in 50%.
Poor prognosis is associated with an abrupt onset and the degree of deficit.

Treatment: Steroids are used, although no controlled trials have been conducted. Large dosage is recommended during the acute phase. Cyclophosphamide may be used in refractory cases.

OTHER DEMYELINATING DISEASES

ACUTE HAEMORRHAGIC LEUKOENCEPHALITIS

This is a rare demyelinating disease. It is regarded as a very acute form of postinfectious/acute disseminated encephalomyelitis.

Clinical picture: Antecedent viral infection, depression of conscious level and multifocal signs and symptoms. Focal features may suggest a mass lesion or even herpes simplex encephalitis.

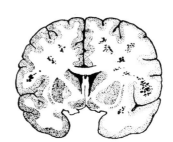

The diagnosis is only really possible at biopsy or autopsy, but elevated CSF pressure, lymphocytosis and erythrocytes in CSF and xanthochromic appearance of fluid are all suggestive.

Pathology: Perivascular polymorph infiltration. Microscopic and macroscopic haemorrhage. Perivascular demyelination and necrotising changes in vessels.

Treatment: Steroids in high dosage should be used though evidence of value in this rare condition is scant.

PROGRESSIVE MULTIFOCAL LEUKOENCEPHALOPATHY

This is a demyelinative disease occurring in association with systemic illness in which cell-mediated and occasionally humoral immunity is depressed, e.g. AIDS (4% of cases), lymphoma, sarcoidosis, systemic lupus erythematosus. The disorder is due to reactivation of previous papovavirus (SV40 or JC virus) infection.

Clinical picture: Features of diffuse process – personality change, hemiparesis, cortical visual loss, seizures, etc. Duration of illness: 3–6 months. Non-remitting and fatal.

Pathology: Demyelination without inflammatory response, especially in subcortical white matter. Electron microscopy – papovavirus in oligodendroglia.

Diagnosis: CT scanning and MR reveal widespread multifocal white matter damage. Definitive diagnosis is made from brain biopsy. Virus can be isolated by inoculation on to glial tissue culture.

Treatment: interferon-alpha and cytosine arabinoside may slow progression.

LEUKODYSTROPHIES

Inborn errors of metabolism may affect the normal development of myelin. These genetic disorders usually present in infancy or childhood but occasionally produce their first manifestations in adult life.

3 specific types are recognised
- Metachromatic leukodystrophy
- Globoid cell leukodystrophy
- Adrenomyeloneuropathy or adrenoleukodystrophy (ADL).

The last condition is sex linked, characterised by adrenal insufficiency and disordered myelin in brain, spinal cord and peripheral nerve. The clinical picture is highly variable and results from a defect in beta oxidation of very long chain fatty acids (VLCFA) which build up in blood and skin fibroblasts. Dietary treatments (Lorenzo's oils) lower these and may slow progression of this fatal disorder. Heterozygote female carriers may become symptomatic with a late onset progressive myelopathy.

NEUROLOGICAL COMPLICATIONS OF DRUGS AND TOXINS

Introduction

Drugs and toxins commonly affect the nervous system. They cause a spectrum of disorders of which most are potentially reversible on withdrawal of the causal agent.

Diagnostic suspicion is especially dependent upon history:
– Availability of drugs.
– Occupational/industrial exposure to toxins.

Drug toxicity may result from:
– The chronic abuse of drugs, e.g. barbiturates, opiates.
– The side effects of drug therapy, e.g. anticonvulsants, steroids.
– The wilful overdosage of drugs, e.g. sedatives, antidepressants.

Toxin exposure may be:
– Accidental: industrial or household poisons, e.g. organophosphates, carbon monoxide, turpentine.
– Wilful: solvent abuse.

History and examination

When acute intoxication is suspected, the following clinical features are supportive.

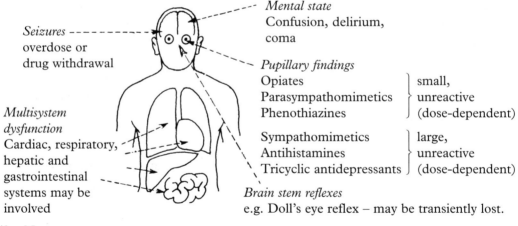

Seizures
overdose or
drug withdrawal

*Multisystem
dysfunction*
Cardiac, respiratory,
hepatic and
gastrointestinal
systems may be
involved

Mental state
Confusion, delirium,
coma

Pupillary findings
Opiates   } small,
Parasympathomimetics } unreactive
Phenothiazines   } (dose-dependent)

Sympathomimetics   } large,
Antihistamines   } unreactive
Tricyclic antidepressants } (dose-dependent)

Brain stem reflexes
e.g. Doll's eye reflex – may be transiently lost.

Also: Note
– Puncture marks in narcotic addicts
– The presence of a snout area rash in solvent abusers

– Rashes in barbiturate poisoning
– Respiration rate in salicylate poisoning
– Skin colour in carbon monoxide poisoning.

Clinical features:

While the neurological picture is generally diffuse, certain pronounced symptoms occur with one drug or toxin and not with another. The following table should act as a guide to diagnosis and alert the clinician to the possible offending substance.

For treatment, the reader is advised to consult an appropriate pharmacology or general medical text.

DRUG-INDUCED NEUROLOGICAL SYNDROMES

HEADACHE

Vasodilators: antihistamines, sympathomimetics, calcium channel blockers, bronchodilators, ergotamine, cocaine
Dopamine agonists
Non-steroidal anti-inflammatories

SEIZURES

Antidepressants, antimicrobials: cycloserine, isoniazid, metronidazole, penicillin
Antineoplastics: vincristine, methotrexate.
Analgesics: pentazocine, fentanyl, opiates
Anaesthetics: ketamine, halothone, althesin
Bronchodilators. Sympathomimetics
Miscellaneous: amphetamine, baclofen, lithium, iodinated contrast media, insulin

CONFUSION/DELIRIUM

Anticholinergics. Anticonvulsants
Antimicrobials: iosiazid, rifampicin
Antineoplastics: vincristine
Dopamine agonists. Tranquillisers
Miscellaneous: cimetidine, ranitidine, lithium

PERIPHERAL NEUROPATHY

Antimicrobials: ethambutol, isoniazid, nitrofurantoin, metronidazole, dapsone
Antineoplastics: cytosine arabinoside, cisplatin, procarbazine, vincristine (and other vinca alkaloids)
Antirheumatics: colchicine, D-penicillamine, gold, indomethacin
Miscellaneous: cimetidine, phenytoin

RETINOPATHY

Antimalarials: chloroquine, mepacrine

VIII NERVE DAMAGE

Aminoglycoside antibiotics: gentamicin, kanamycin, neomycin, streptomycin
Miscellanous: cisplatin, ethycrinic acid, quinine, salicylates

VISUAL DISTURBANCE

Phenothiazines Miscellaneous: ethambutol, indomethacin, tamoxifen

OPTIC NEURITIS

Antimicrobials: chloramphenicol dapsone, isoniazid, streptomycin
Miscellaneous: chlorpropamide

MOVEMENT DISORDERS

Antiemetics: metoclopramide
Butyrophenones: haloperidol, droperidol
Dopamine agonists. Phenothiazines: chlorpromazine, thioridazine
Tricyclic antidepressants

ATAXIA

Anticonvulsants: carbamezepine, phenytoin, primidone
Antineoplastics: cytosine arabinoside, fluoracil
Phenothiazines: sedatives; barbiturates, chloral hydrate. *Tranquillisers:* diazepam

MUSCLE PAIN AND WEAKNESS

Antineoplastics: cytosine arabinoside, methotrexate, thiopeta
Miscellaneous: clofibrate, D-penicillamine, danazol, L-tryptophan.

Drug screen in suspected overdosage
Too often the clinician, when managing drug or toxin overdosage, requests a 'drug screen'. The techniques used in detection, e.g. gas chromatography, thin-layer chromatography and immunological tests, are sophisticated and time-consuming and may require samples of serum, urine or both.
The clinician must 'narrow down the field' from the history and presenting symptoms/signs and discuss with the laboratory the class of drug or toxin he suspects.
A knowledge of the blood level of some drugs, e.g. salicylates, barbiturates, is important in deciding the approach to treatment.

SPECIFIC SYNDROMES OF DRUGS AND TOXINS

NEUROLEPTIC MALIGNANT SYNDROME

A rare life-threatening disorder induced by initiation, increase or reintroduction of neuroleptic drugs (e.g. chlorpromazine, haloperidol). The condition appears to result from acute dopamine receptor blockade and is characterised by *hyperpyrexia, bradykinesia, rigidity, autonomic disturbance, alteration of consciousness* and *high serum muscle enzymes (creatine kinase)*. The causal drug should be withdrawn and the patient cooled. Give dopamine agonists with dantrolene sodium to control bradykinesia and rigidity respectively. Death occurs in 15% from renal failure and/or cardiovascular collapse.

SOLVENT ABUSE

The abuse of volatile solvents is an increasing problem especially in children. The purpose of inhalation is to achieve a state of euphoria. Habituation develops. Commonly used substances are: aerosols, cleaning fluids, nail varnish remover, lighter fluids, 'model' glue. The 'active' components of these are simple carbon-based molecules, e.g. benzene, hexane and toluene.

Symptoms of acute intoxication:
- Euphoria
- Dysarthria, ataxia, diplopia
- Delusions and hallucinations occur, followed by seizures if exposure has been prolonged.
    Death may result:
- Aspiration/asphyxiation
- Cardiac arrhythmias
- Renal or hepatic damage.

Symptoms of chronic abuse;
- Behavioural disturbance.
- Chronic ataxia.
- Sensorimotor peripheral neuropathy.

Treatment of acute intoxication is symptomatic; there are no specific antidotes.
Industrial exposure to hydrocarbons produces similar symptoms.

ORGANOPHOSPHATES

These are widely used as insecticides (sheep dip) and herbicides. They cause symptoms by phosphorylation of the enzyme acetyl cholinesterase. Acute intoxication produces seizures, autonomic disturbance and coma. Chronic exposure results in fatigue, muscle weakness and fasciculation associated with non-specific weight loss and cognitive impairment.

LEAD EXPOSURE

Lead has no biological function. It is present in normal diet as well as in the atmosphere from automobile fumes and in the water supply of old buildings containing lead tanks and piping. Occupation exposure occurs in plumbers, burners and smelters.
Lead excess interferes with *haem* synthesis. This results in the accumulation of 'blocked' metabolites such as aminolevulinic acid (ALA) in serum and urine. It also inhibits oxidative enzymes (e.g. Superoxide dismutase). Anaemia occurs with a characteristic finding in the blood film (basophilic stippling).
Both the peripheral and central nervous systems are affected.

ADULTS
A chronic motor neuropathy with minor sensory symptomatology. Axonal damage predominates.

rarely
Acute encephalopathy

CHILDREN
Peripheral neuropathy is rare.
Encephalopathy is characteristic.
(Lead salts cross blood–brain barrier more easily in children)

Acute fulminating with confusion, impaired conscious level, coma, seizures, papilloedema.

Chronic with fatigue and irritability, headache, apathy.

Treatment

Chelating agents (e.g. calcium disodium edetate – EDTA – or D-penicillamine) and i.v. mannitol in acute encephalopathy with papilloedema.
In acute fulminating encephalopathy the mortality has been reduced to 5%, but neurological sequelae are common.

SPECIFIC SYNDROMES OF DRUGS AND TOXINS

COMPLICATIONS OF RECREATIONAL DRUG ABUSE

The problems of drug abuse are of epidemic proportions. An increasing number of neurological syndromes are recognised.

	Cocaine	Metamphetamine and Ecstasy	Heroin	Phencyclidine
Origin	Alkaloid from leaves of erythroxylon coca plant	Synthetic amphetamines	Alkaloid from poppy – papaver somiferin	Synthetic anaesthetic agent
Clinical use	Pain relief	Anorexia Narcolepsy Depression	Pain relief	Anaesthetic agent
Popular name(s)	'Coke', 'Snow', 'Crack' (potent pica base form)	'Speed' 'Uppers'		'Angel dust'
Method of taking	Oral Intranasal Intravenous	Oral Intravenous 'high speeding'	Oral Smoked Intravenous	Oral Smoked Intranasal
Mode of action	Blocks reuptake of dopamine and noradrenaline and augments neurotransmission (sympathomimetic)	Increases release of dopamine and adrenaline and augments neurotransmission (sympathomimetic)	Acts as opiate receptors located on the surface of neurons	Interference with multiple neurotransmitter function
Moderate dosage	Alertness ↑ Euphoria Blood pressure ↑	Alert ↑ Euphoria Blood pressure ↑	Pupillary constriction Pleasurable abdominal sensation Facial flushing	Alertness ↑ Sweating Blood pressure ↑ Heart rate↑
Excessive dosage	Blood pressure ↑↑ Temperature ↑ Respiration ↓ Cardiac dysrhythmia and sudden death	Blood pressure ↑↑ Temperature ↑ Respiration ↓ Cardiac dysrhythmia and sudden death	Pin-point pupils Respiration ↓ coma	Dysarthria Psychosis Nystagmus Cardiac Ataxia dysrhythmia Vigilant but and sudden unresponsive death
Treatment	Haloperidol (blocks dopamine reuptake) Hypotensive agents Dysrhythmic agents Anticonvulsants	As for cocaine	Naloxone (opiate antagonist) Clonidine or Methadone (for withdrawal symptoms)	Haloperidol (for psychosis)
Neurological complications	Headache Tremor Myoclonus Seizures	Chorea Intracranial haemorrhage (drug-induced vasculitis)	Myelitis Neuropathies and Plexopathies (immune mediated)	Dystonia Athetosis Seizures Rhabdomyolysis

All recreational drugs are associated with increased risk of cerebral or spinal infarction or intracerebral haemorrhage. (Mechanisms are varied – drug-induced hypertension, coagulopathies, foreign body (talc) embolisation and septic emboli from infective endocarditis.)

All intravenous drug abusers are at risk of HIV infection and its complications (page 511)

METABOLIC ENCEPHALOPATHIES

In general terms, the clinical features of metabolic encephalopathy are relatively stereotyped.

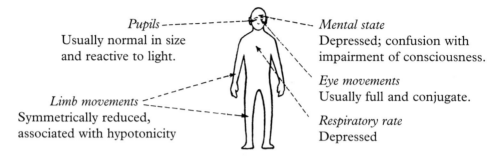

Pupils ------------ *Mental state*
Usually normal in size   Depressed; confusion with
and reactive to light.   impairment of consciousness.

Eye movements
Usually full and conjugate.

Limb movements
Symmetrically reduced,
associated with hypotonicity

Respiratory rate
Depressed

These features are characteristic but exceptions occur in specific encephalopathies –

	Pupils	*Eye movements*
Hypoxia	large-reactive	Hypoxia (severe)

No movement
– conjugate

| Hepatic encephalopathy | small-reactive | Hepatic encephalopathy (severe) |

No movement
– dysconjugate

Limb movements
Hepatic encephalopathy
Non-ketotic
   hyperosmolar coma ⎱ Hemiparesis can occur
Hypoglycaemia
Uraemia

Respiratory rate
Hepatic encephalopathy
increased

Hepatic encephalopathy ⎱
Uraemic encephalopathy ⎰ Involuntary movements
Hypoxia, hypercapnia

Asterixis – a flapping movement noted in the hands when the wrists are hyperextended

Myoclonus – a sudden jerk of muscle groups occasionally resulting in limb movement (page 188).

Beware of the possibility of multiple pathology, e.g. an alcoholic patient with a chronic subdural haematoma may also have liver failure and thiamine deficiency.

CLASSIFICATION AND BIOCHEMICAL EVALUATION

Many metabolic disturbances cause an acquired encephalopathy in adults.

The most frequently encountered are:

– *Hypoxic*	Less commonly:
– *Hypercapnoeic*	– Hyponatraemia. Hypernatraemia.
– *Hypoglycaemic*	– Hypokalaemia. Hyperkalaemia.
– *Hyperglycaemic*	– Hypocalcaemia. Hypercalcaemia.
– *Hepatic*	– Hypothyroidism. Lactic acidosis.
– *Uraemic*	– Addison's disease.

Drugs and toxins producing encephalopathy are dealt with separately (page 529).

Laboratory assessment of suspected metabolic encephalopathy

All patients should have a basic biochemical screen:

– Serum urea and electrolytes.
– Liver function (albumin, globulin, bilirubin, alkaline phosphatase and enzymes) and random blood glucose.
– Blood gases (pH, PO_2 PCO_2).
– Serum ammonia.
– Electroencephalography – slow wave activity (theta or delta) supports the diagnosis of a diffuse dysfunction: hepatic encephalopathy shows a specific triphasic slow wave configuration.
– CT scan – if the above tests are normal or coexisting structural brain disease is suspected.

Calculation of the *anion gap* may be helpful in the diagnosis of encephalopathies, especially *lactic acidosis*. The sum of the anions (Cl^- and HCO_3^-) normally equals the sum of the cations (Na^+ and K^+). An increase in the gap in the absence of ketones, salicylates and uraemia suggests lactic acidosis.

HYPOXIC ENCEPHALOPATHY

Impaired brain oxygenation results from:

– Reduced arterial oxygen pressure – lung disease.
– Reduced haemoglobin to carry oxygen – anaemia or blood loss.
– Reduced flow of blood containing oxygen (ischaemic hypoxia) – due to reduced cardiac output (with reduced cerebral blood flow).
– Biochemical block of cerebral utilisation of oxygen – rare (e.g. cyanide poisoning).

When cerebral arterial PO_2 falls below 35 mmHg (4.5 kPa), anaerobic metabolism takes over; this is not efficient and a further drop in PO_2 will result in neurological dysfunction. The extent of hypoxic damage depends not only upon the duration of hypoxia but also on other factors, e.g. body temperature – hypothermia protects against damage. The irreversibility of hypoxic damage is explained by the 'no flow phenomenon' – after 3–5 minutes the endothelial lining of small vessels swells – even with reversal of hypoxia, flow through these vessels is no longer possible.

SPECIFIC ENCEPHALOPATHIES

HYPOXIC ENCEPHALOPATHY (*cont'd*)

Pathology
As a consequence of high metabolic demand, some areas are more susceptible than others.

Vulnerability to hypoxia

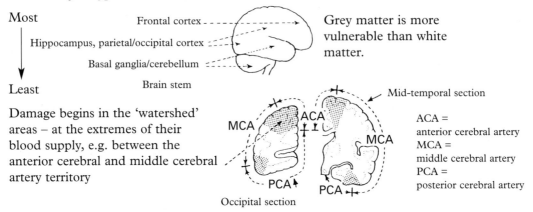

Most

Frontal cortex

Hippocampus, parietal/occipital cortex

Basal ganglia/cerebellum

Brain stem

Least

Grey matter is more vulnerable than white matter.

Damage begins in the 'watershed' areas – at the extremes of their blood supply, e.g. between the anterior cerebral and middle cerebral artery territory

Mid-temporal section

Occipital section

ACA = anterior cerebral artery
MCA = middle cerebral artery
PCA = posterior cerebral artery

Microscopic changes depend upon the delay between the hypoxic event and death.

Immediate:	*At 48 hours:*	*At several days/weeks:*
Scattered petechial haemorrhages.	Cerebral oedema associated with petechial haemorrhage.	Necrosis in cortical grey matter and globus pallidus with associated astrocytic proliferation. The cerebellum and brain stem may also be affected.

Clinical features:
e.g. Severe hypoxia from circulatory arrest

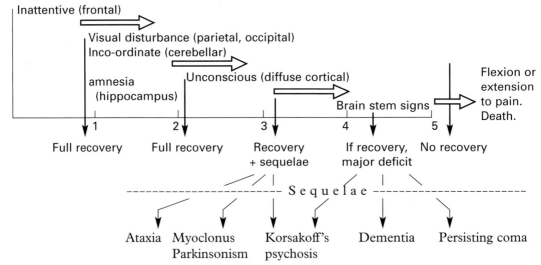

Inattentive (frontal)

Visual disturbance (parietal, occipital)
Inco-ordinate (cerebellar)

amnesia (hippocampus)

Unconscious (diffuse cortical)

Brain stem signs

Flexion or extension to pain. Death.

1 — Full recovery
2 — Full recovery
3 — Recovery + sequelae
4 — If recovery, major deficit
5 — No recovery

— — — — — — — — — — — — — — — — S e q u e l a e — — — — — — — — — — — — — — — —

Ataxia   Myoclonus   Korsakoff's   Dementia   Persisting coma
Parkinsonism   psychosis

Delayed hypoxic encephalopathy refers to the rare occurrence of a full clinical recovery followed after some weeks by a progressive picture → deterioration of conscious level → death. Widespread subcortical demyelination is found at autopsy.

SPECIFIC ENCEPHALOPATHIES

HYPERCAPNIC ENCEPHALOPATHY: the consequence of an elevated arterial carbon dioxide level.

Clinical features:

Headache, confusion, disorientation, involuntary movements.
Papilloedema, depressed limb reflexes, extensor plantar responses.

Diagnosis:

A P_{CO_2} greater than 50 mmHg (6 kPa) with a reduced P_{O_2} is found on arterial blood sampling.

The presence of headache, confusion and papilloedema may suggest intracranial tumour. If hypercapnia has not been diagnosed, such patients inevitably are referred for CT brain scan.

HYPOGLYCAEMIA ENCEPHALOPATHY: the consequence of insufficient glucose reaching the brain and may
result from – overdosage of diabetic treatment
                   – insulin secreting tumour – insulinoma
                   – hepatic disease with reduction of liver glycogen.

Serum glucose levels of 1.5 mmol/l are associated with the onset of encephalopathy. Levels at 0.5 mmol/l are associated with coma.

Pathology:

Changes occur in the cerebral cortex – focal necrosis surrounded by neuronal degeneration. Subcortical grey matter (caudate nucleus) and cerebellum are vulnerable.

Clinical features:

These, as with hypoxia, depend upon the duration and severity of hypoglycaemia.

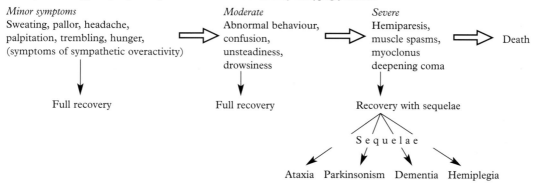

Minor symptoms
Sweating, pallor, headache,
palpitation, trembling, hunger,
(symptoms of sympathetic overactivity)

↓
Full recovery

Moderate
Abnormal behaviour,
confusion,
unsteadiness,
drowsiness

↓
Full recovery

Severe
Hemiparesis,
muscle spasms,
myoclonus
deepening coma

↓
Recovery with sequelae

Sequelae

Ataxia   Parkinsonism   Dementia   Hemiplegia

Death

Repeated mild to moderate episodes may result in a chronic cerebellar ataxia.

Repeated severe attacks may result in a mixed myelopathy/peripheral neuropathy which is distinguished from motor neuron disease by the presence of sensory signs.

HYPERGLYCAEMIC ENCEPHALOPATHY

Two types of encephalopathy develop as a consequence of hyperglycaemia:

Diabetic ketoacidotic coma
Accumulation of acetone and ketone bodies in blood results in acidosis. Hyperventilation ensues with a reduction in P_{CO_2} and HCO_3^-. Osmotic diuresis due to hyperglycaemia results in dehydration.

The neurological presentation is that of confusion, progression to coma and, if untreated, death.

Diabetic hyperosmolar non-ketotic coma

This results from the hyperosmolar effect of severe hyperglycaemia. Reduction of the intracellular compartment results. Involuntary movements, seizures and hemiparesis may occur. Vascular thrombosis is not uncommon. Ketoacidosis is mild or does not occur.

SPECIFIC ENCEPHALOPATHIES

HEPATIC ENCEPHALOPATHY

Neurological signs and symptoms secondary to hepatic dysfunction may arise in:
– acute liver failure.
– chronic liver failure complicated by infection or gastrointestinal haemorrhage.
– chronic liver failure producing characteristic *hepatocerebral degeneration*.

Clinical features:

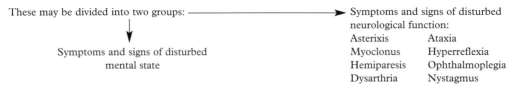

These may be divided into two groups: ⟶ Symptoms and signs of disturbed neurological function:

Asterixis	Ataxia
Myoclonus	Hyperreflexia
Hemiparesis	Ophthalmoplegia
Dysarthria	Nystagmus

Symptoms and signs of disturbed mental state

The encephalopathy is progressive.

Pathology

Neuronal loss with gliosis is noted in the cerebral cortex as well as basal ganglia, cerebellum and brain stem. Astrocytes with irregular and enlarged nuclei are characteristic.

Hepatocerebral degeneration produces varying symptoms and signs. Dementia is associated with dysarthria and ataxia. Primitive reflexes, choreoathetosis, myoclonus, tremor and pyramidal signs may also be present.

Consciousness is *not* impaired.

URAEMIC ENCEPHALOPATHY

Clinical features:

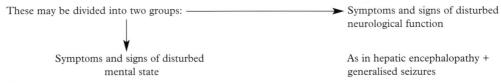

These may be divided into two groups: ⟶ Symptoms and signs of disturbed neurological function

Symptoms and signs of disturbed mental state

As in hepatic encephalopathy + generalised seizures

Pathology:

Uraemia may produce non-specific pathological findings in the nervous system. Peripheral nervous system involvement occurs in chronic renal failure.

Dialysis encephalopathy is encountered in persons on renal dialysis exposed to high aluminium levels in the dialysate. The features are those of dementia, behavioural changes, seizures and myoclonus. The condition progresses unless aluminium levels are controlled.

Specific investigations and treatment of individual metabolic encephalopathies do not come within the scope of this book.

NUTRITIONAL DISORDERS

INTRODUCTION
Nutritional deficiency presents a massive problem in the developing world. In Western countries, alcoholism is the major cause of the neurological syndromes resulting from dietary deficiency with faddism and malabsorption disorders accounting for only a small number.

Vitamins appear important nutrients and certain disorders such as Wernicke Korsakoff syndrome (thiamine) or subacute combined degeneration (vit. B_{12}) are attributed to a single deficiency. Others such as polyneuropathy result from multiple deficiency.

Vitamin deficiency in itself does not always produce symptoms; a dietary excess of carbohydrate seems essential for the development of the neurological features of thiamine deficiency.

As a rule, nutritional disorders of the nervous system present clinically in a symmetrical manner.

WERNICKE KORSAKOFF SYNDROME
This syndrome is comprised of an acute and a chronic phase:

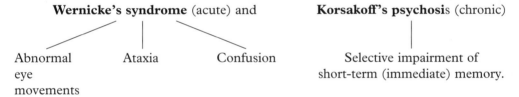

Wernicke's syndrome (acute) and   **Korsakoff's psychosis** (chronic)

| Abnormal eye movements | Ataxia | Confusion | Selective impairment of short-term (immediate) memory. |

Patients often demonstrate additional features of nutritional deficiency – peripheral neuropathy, trophic skin changes and autonomic dysfunction (arrhythmias, postural hypotension and hypothermia). Features of acute alcohol withdrawal often co-exist.

Cause

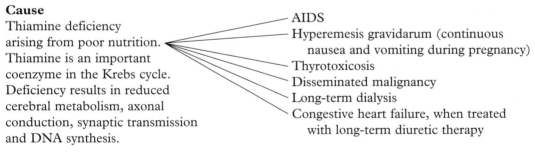

Thiamine deficiency arising from poor nutrition. Thiamine is an important coenzyme in the Krebs cycle. Deficiency results in reduced cerebral metabolism, axonal conduction, synaptic transmission and DNA synthesis.

- AIDS
- Hyperemesis gravidarum (continuous nausea and vomiting during pregnancy)
- Thyrotoxicosis
- Disseminated malignancy
- Long-term dialysis
- Congestive heart failure, when treated with long-term diuretic therapy

N.B. Korsakoff's psychosis may also be caused by head injury, anoxia, epilepsy, encephalitis and vascular diseases.

WERNICKE'S SYNDOME
Diagnosed in 0.1–0.4% of hospital admissions.

Pathology:
Neuronal, axonal and myelin damage occur symmetrically in the mamillary bodies, the walls of the third ventricle, thalamus and periaqueductal grey matter. Secondary vascular proliferation and haemorrhages occur within these lesions.

WERNICKE KORSAKOFF SYNDROME

WERNICKE'S SYNDROME (*cont'd*)

Clinical features: *Acute in onset*

Ocular involvement:

Horizontal and vertical nystagmus is evident. Unilateral or bilateral VI nerve paresis commonly occur. Retinal haemorrhages occur. Pupillary involvement and complete ophthalmoplegia are rare. Polyneuropathy is present in 80% of cases. Vestibular disturbances will occur occasionally and accentuate the ataxia. Autonomic disturbance is common.

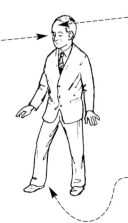

Confusion:
Disorientated and inattentive.
Coma may ensue
Withdrawal symptoms of alcohol:
– agitation, delusions and hallucinations – develop following admission to hospital.
Ataxia – is often the presenting symptom. May be mild or severe with inability to stand.
Lower limb (heel to shin) ataxia is modest.
Upper limbs are spared.

Investigation

- Serum B_1 levels may be low.
- Pyruvate is elevated.
- Transketolase activity is decreased (enzyme in hexose monophosphate shunt).
- MRI may show mamillary body atrophy.

Treatment

Intravenous (i.v.) Pabrinex containing thiamine (B_1), riboflavin (B_2), pyridoxine (B_6), is the only available treatment. Oral treatment is ineffective. Treatment must be given immediately to persons with a suggestive clinical picture and evidence of chronic alcohol use. Those with a history of alcohol abuse requiring IV glucose should be treated prophylactically (thiamine is critical for the metabolism of carbohydrate and levels can be exhausted by a sudden load).

With treatment – Eyes improve – in days, though nystagmus may persist for months.
　　　　　　　 – Ataxia improves – in weeks.
Overall mortality: 15% → coma → death.
Failure to recognise and promptly treat can result in Korsakoff's syndrome or psychosis.

KORSAKOFF'S PSYCHOSIS

Sometimes encountered in traumatic or infective brain disorders, though normally overlaps with Wernicke's syndrome.

Pathology

Lesions are identical in distribution to those of Wernicke's syndrome without haemorrhagic change.

Clinical features

There is a disturbance of memory in which information cannot be stored. In addition the normal temporal sequence of established memories is disrupted, resulting in a semifictionalised account of the circumstances which the patient may find him/herself in (*confabulation*). This memory disturbance can only be tested for when the confusion of Wernicke's disease has cleared.

Treatment

None – no evidence that replacement, at this stage, will help.

B$_{12}$ DEFICIENCY – SUBACUTE COMBINED DEGENERATION OF THE SPINAL CORD

B$_{12}$ deficiency produces the specific neurological syndrome of subacute degeneration of the spinal cord (SADC).

Two cobalamin-dependent enzymatic reactions occur in humans. The first reaction converts methylmalonyl-coenzyme A (CoA) to succinyl-CoA. The second involves the synthesis of methionine from homocysteine. Deficiency in B$_{12}$ therefore results in an accumulation of homocysteine. Despite the importance of methionine to myelin sheath phospholipid methylation, the basis of neurological damage remains uncertain.

Causes

- Inadequate diet
- Increased need – pregnancy
- Defective absorbtion – Pernicious anaemia – decreased intrinsic factor (necessary for absorption)
  – malabsorption (pancreatitis, coeliac disease, gastric surgery, tapeworm infestation etc.)

Pathology

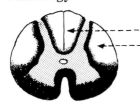

Spinal cord demyelination with eventual axon loss – affects: posterior columns and lateral columns (corticospinal and spinocerebellar tracts). Corticospinal degeneration is most evident in the lower cord, posterior column degeneration in the upper cord. The white matter of the cerebral hemispheres can also be affected. Peripheral nerve large myelinated fibre degeneration also occurs.

B$_{12}$ deficiency resulting in neurological damage is usually associated with a macrocytosis, though a normal peripheral blood film may be found.

Clinical features

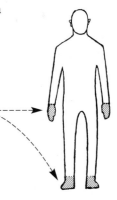

Onset is subacute, though can be acutely precipitated by exposure to nitrous oxide anaesthesia.

Paraesthesia of extremities is the presenting symptom.

Numbness and distal weakness follow.

Walking becomes unsteady and spasticity is evident in the lower limbs with flexor or extensor spasms. More widespread neurological features including optic atrophy, cerebral demyelination with encephalopathy and dementia develop in untreated cases.

Examination

- Gait is ataxic with positive Romberg's test (sensory ataxia).
- Motor power is diminished distally.
- Plantar responses are extensor.
- Sensory loss: loss of vibration and joint position sensation in the lower limbs. Stocking/glove sensory loss is found when peripheral nerves are involved.
- Reflex findings are variable and depend on the predominance of peripheral nerve or corticospinal tract involvement.

Mini mental status examination (MMSE) test may suggest dementia.
Optic pallor and centrocaecal scotoma can be demonstrated.

B$_{12}$ DEFICIENCY – SUBACUTE COMBINED DEGENERATION OF THE SPINAL CORD

Diagnosis
Suspect in paraparesis with combined upper and lower motor neuron signs with 'stocking/glove' sensory loss.

Differentiate from other causes of acute myelopathy, e.g. cord compression, multiple sclerosis.

Investigation
Peripheral blood film – may show a megaloblastic anaemia
Serum B$_{12}$/Folate – low B$_{12}$. (If folate low – investigate causes: diet/drugs/malabsorption)
If serum B$_{12}$ low (normal > 190 ng/l)
  – measure intrinsic factor antibody
  – Schilling test (measure of capacity to absorb) – if normal – dietary
                                                 – if low – repeat with intrinsic factor
                                                   (normal = pernicious anaemia,
                                                   abnormal = malabsorption and
                                                   investigate accordingly)

MRI – may show spinal and cerebral white matter hyperintensity on T2 images
Nerve conduction studies – may show axonal neuropathy

Treatment
Consider treatment for patients who have serum B$_{12}$ level of less than 130 ng/l (neurological dysfunction normally occurs with levels < 100 ng/l).

Initiate treatment with vitamin B$_{12}$, 1000 micrograms intramuscularly given daily for 3 to 7 days, then weekly for 4 weeks.

Continue maintenance therapy for life.

Course and progression
Untreated, the disorder is progressive, the patient eventually becoming bed-bound and comatose. If diagnosed and treated early (within 2 months of onset), complete recovery can be anticipated. In established cases, only progression may be halted.

Caution:
When folic acid is prescribed alone, it will improve the haematological picture of B$_{12}$ deficiency but cause rapid often irreversible neurological deterioration.

Tocopherol (vit. E).
In its active form – D α tocopherol – it acts as a membrane stabilizer and anti-oxidant. Deficiency occurs in chronic fat malabsorption (e.g. coeliac disease or cystic fibrosis) and results in widespread neurological disturbances – ataxia, ophthalmoplegia, seizures and corticospinal tract dysfunction. These are halted and often reversed by i.m. vit. E. It has been speculated that the antioxidant effect might make vitamin E a candidate for cytoprotection and repair within the nervous system. Studies in Parkinson's disease, multiple sclerosis and stroke are disappointing.

Abetalipoproteinaemia (Bassen-Kornzweig syndrome) predisposes to Vit E deficiency (the vitamin is transported by low-density lipoproteins). These patients have acanthocytes in the peripheral blood and a pigmentary retinopathy.

NUTRITIONAL POLYNEUROPATHY

Deficiency of vitamin B complex – B_1 (Thiamine), B_2 (Riboflavin), B_3 (Nicotinic acid), B_5 (Pantathenic acid) or B_6 (Pyridoxine) – results in peripheral nerve damage.

The combination of polyneuropathy and cardiac involvement is referred to as BERI-BERI. When oedema is also present it is termed wet beri-beri and, when absent, dry beri-beri. Beri-beri occurs in rice eating countries.

In Western countries, alcoholism is the major cause of nutritional polyneuropathy with or without cardiac involvement, otherwise world wide famine and starvation is responsible.

Pathology

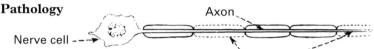

Axon

Nerve cell

Segmental demyelination and axonal degeneration occur simultaneously

The distal portions of nerves are initially affected.

Anterior horn cells and dorsal root ganglion cells undergo chromatolysis.

Vagus nerve and sympathetic trunk involvement occurs in severe cases.

Clinical features
Onset: gradual

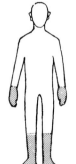

Symptoms: Progressive distal weakness and sensory loss with painful tingling paraesthesia involving initially lower limbs.
Autonomic complaints – impotence, dizziness (orthostatic hypotension) and disordered sweating – are common.

Signs:
- Varying degrees of *areflexia* (only ankle reflexes are lost initially).
- *Weakness* which is more marked distally than proximally and initially involves the lower limbs.
- *Sensory loss* of a 'stocking/glove' type involving all modalities of sensation.
- *Autonomic* involvement results in sweating soles of feet and postural blood pressure drop.
- *Vagus nerve* involvement results in a hoarse voice and disturbance of swallowing.

Associated signs
Shiny skin on legs with poor distal hair growth. 'Hyperpathic' painful soles of feet. Evidence of liver failure.

Diagnosis
Suggested by nutritional/alcohol history.
Supported by investigation such as peripheral blood film (elevated MCV) and disturbed liver function tests.
Nerve conduction studies reveal mildly reduced motor and sensory conduction velocities.

Differential diagnosis
Consider other causes of subacute or chronic sensorimotor neuropathy (see page 435).

Treatment
A high calorie (3000) diet should be supplemented daily with Thiamine (25 mg), Niacin (100 mg), riboflavin (10 mg), Pantathenic acid (10 mg) and Pyridoxin (5 mg).
Burning paraesthesia may respond to carbamazepine or phenytoin.
Recovery may be very slow and incomplete but with the withdrawal of alcohol and adequate vitamin supplementation some improvement should occur.

TOBACCO–ALCOHOL AMBLYOPIA

A large number of toxic substances can produce impaired vision. Methyl alcohol causes sudden and permanent blindness. Chronic painless visual loss from optic neuritis develops in malnourished patients with a high tobacco consumption (Tobacco-alcohol amblyopia). This is caused by exposure to cyanide from tobacco smoking associated with low vitamin levels due to poor nutrition and absorption associated with drinking alcohol. Other potential toxins include methyl alcohol (moonshine) and ethylene glycol (antifreeze).

Pathology
Damage involves the papillomacular bundle within the optic nerves, chiasma and optic tracts. Retinal ganglion cells in the macular region are also affected.

Clinical features
– The condition slowly develops over weeks.
– Vision in each eye becomes hazy and blurred.
– Colour vision (red/green discrimination) is involved early.

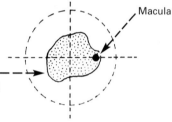

Macula

Examination
– Bilateral involvement.
– Reduced visual acuity.
– Centrocaecal scotoma
  (a central field defect spreading from blind spot to macula and most easily detected with a red target).

Treatment
Vitamin B supplementation, including B_{12}, should be administered. B_{12} possesses the capacity for cyanide detoxification. Recovery is poor if visual loss is well established.

– Fundal examination is normal, though optic atrophy will occur eventually.
– Coexistent Wernicke Korsakoff syndrome or polyneuropathy are common.

ALCOHOL RELATED DISORDERS

ALCOHOL MYOPATHY
Muscle damage (elevated creatine phosphokinase) is not uncommon in alcoholics following acute ingestion. The cause of alcoholic myopathy is uncertain; mitochondrial disturbances, potassium depletion, rhabdomyolysis (due to seizures or local compression) have all been suggested.

There are two forms of alcoholic muscle disease

1. *Acute necrotizing myopathy* occurs after 'binge' drinking.
– Acute muscle necrosis ensues with pain/cramping and muscle tenderness/swelling.
– Myoglobin is excreted in the urine (myoglobinuria) after release from damaged muscles.
– Symptoms of alcohol withdrawal – delirium, etc. – coexist.
– Limb involvement may be markedly asymmetrical.
– Sometimes calf muscles are swollen and tender.
– Improvement occurs over weeks to months.
– Serum creatine phosphokinase (CPK) is elevated. Marked myoglobinuria when present may result in renal failure.
– Elevated serum K^+ may provide cardiac arrhythmias.

2. *Chronic myopathy*
Painless proximal weakness sometimes associated with cardiomyopathy. Muscle biopsy showing type 2 fibre atrophy.

Management is abstinence, vitamin supplementation and IV saline in *acute necrotizing myopathy* with myoglobinuria to prevent renal failure.

ALCOHOL RELATED DISORDERS

ALCOHOLIC DEMENTIA

Experimentally, chronic alcohol consumption results in neuronal loss. CT evidence of atrophy and neuropsychological impairment is common in alcoholics. However, whether or not these result from the direct toxic and dementing effect of alcohol remains uncertain.

ALCOHOLIC CEREBELLAR DEGENERATION

Probably the commonest cause of acquired ataxia, alcoholic patients may develop a chronic cerebellar syndrome either as a sequel of Wernicke's syndrome or as a distinct clinical entity. A long history of alcohol abuse is obtained. Males are predominantly affected. Onset is gradual and symptoms often stabilise. Ataxia of gait with lower limb inco-ordination predominates. The upper limbs are spared. Nystagmus is rarely present. Cerebellar dysarthria is usually mild. Coexistent signs of peripheral neuropathy are often found.

Investigations: – Abnormal liver function tests e.g. elevation of enzymes – γ GT.
– Macrocytosis in peripheral blood film.
– CSF examination normal.
– CT and MRI reveal cerebellar vermal atrophy.

Progression → may evolve rapidly and reverse with improved nutrition and alcohol withdrawal.
→ may evolve subacutely.
→ may evolve chronically and slowly progress over many years.

Pathology: – All the cellular elements of the cerebellar cortex are affected, but particularly Purkinje cells of the anterior and superior vermis and the anterior portion of the anterior lobes.

Pathogenesis: – The disorder may be due to *nutritional deficiency*, especially thiamine, or else result from the direct toxic effect of alcohol or electrolyte disturbance on the cerebellum.

Differential diagnosis: – Distinguish from hereditary and other acquired ataxias, e.g. hypothyroidism.

Treatment: – Alcohol withdrawal, a well balanced diet and adequate vitamin supplementation.

CENTRAL PONTINE MYELINOLYSIS

Alcohol abuse, debilitating disease or rapid correction of hyponatraemia may precipitate presentation.
The lesion is one of demyelination with cavitation. Microscopically, myelin is lost, oligodendrocytes degenerate but neurons and axons are spared.
Clinically, an acute or subacute pontine lesion is suspected, evolving over a few days, with bulbar weakness and tetraparesis (locked-in syndrome).
The limbs are flaccid with extensor plantar responses.
With progression of the lesion, eye signs become evident and conscious level becomes depressed → coma → death.

Investigations:

Electrolytic disturbances (low sodium, low phosphate) are found.
Liver function is normal. CSF examination is normal.
MRI is more sensitive than CT showing an abnormality in the pons.

Recognition of this condition before death is important in view of its reversibility, though prior to CT/MRI availability it was diagnosed at autopsy. Vigorous supportive therapy with correction of metabolic abnormalities and vitamin supplementation is advised. In patients with severe hyponatraemia (< 110 mmol/l), especially alcoholics, slow correction is essential.

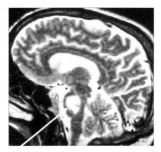

MRI (T2) – increased signal filling the pons

CORPUS CALLOSUM DEMYELINATION

(syn: Marchiafava–Bignami disease)
This is a rare disorder occurring in malnourished alcoholics. Occasionally diagnosed premortem by MRI, progressing to death over some weeks.
The clinical picture is that of personality change with signs of frontal lobe disease. The condition occurs most commonly in persons of Italian origin.

NON-METASTATIC MANIFESTATIONS OF MALIGNANT DISEASE

Disturbance of neurological function can occur in association with malignancy without evidence of metastases (0.1% of all cancer patients). Brain, spinal cord, peripheral nerve and muscle may be affected, either separately or in combination.

Small cell carcinoma of the lung, gynaecological malignancy and lymphoma are the commonest associated disorders. Specific antibodies (anti-neuronal), are responsible for certain syndromes. These are directed towards antigens in the nervous system and the tumour and may explain the trend toward greater life expectancy in those with, rather than those without, such non-metastatic disorders.

The non-metastatic manifestations of malignancy are rare.

These are not discrete, e.g. neuropathy and myopathy may coexist → carcinomatous neuromyopathy; encephalitis and myelopathy → carcinomatous encephalomyelitis.

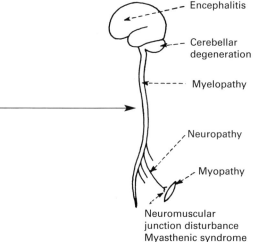

Encephalitis

Cerebellar degeneration

Myelopathy

Neuropathy

Myopathy

Neuromuscular junction disturbance
Myasthenic syndrome

ENCEPHALITIS (anti-Hu syndrome)
Associated commonly with small cell lung cancer (SCLC) usually *before* this becomes clinically manifest.

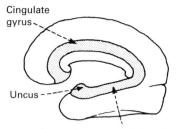

Cingulate gyrus

Uncus

Limbic system   Parahippocampal gyrus

Pathology
The encephalitic process selectively affects the limbic system – with neuronal loss, astrocytic proliferation and perivascular inflammatory changes.

Clinical features
Disturbance in behaviour precedes the development of complex partial (temporal lobe) seizures and memory impairment. Autonomic dysfunction and sensory neuropathy often co-exist. Progression is rapid.

Investigations. Most cases are anti-Hu antibody positive. MRI is normal. ECG may show temporal lobe abnormalities. CSF reveals a mild lymphocytosis with protein elevation.

CEREBELLAR DEGENERATION (anti-Yo syndrome) associated with breast or ovarian carcinoma.

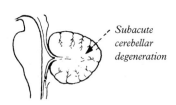

Subacute cerebellar degeneration

Pathology:
Characterised by Purkinje cell loss with some involvement of the dentate muscles. Brain stem changes also occur.

Clinical features:
The patient presents with a rapidly developing ataxia.

Brain stem involvement results in nystagmus, opsoclonus and vertigo.

The course is usually rapid.

Investigations
MRI shows cortical and vermal cerebellar atrophy.

CSF is mild abnormal and anti-Yo antibodies are present in 50% of suspected cases.

NON-METASTATIC MANIFESTATIONS OF MALIGNANT DISEASE

NEUROPATHY (see page 440)

Sensory neuropathy: Destruction of the posterior root ganglion combined with axonal and demyelinative peripheral nerve damage causes progressive sensory symptoms. The neuropathy is subacute or chronic in evolution. Clinically dysaesthesia and numbness starts in extremities and spreads. Associated with SCLC and anti-Hu antibodies.

Sensorimotor neuropathy: A mixed neuropathy with weakness and sensory loss. The syndrome may predate the recognition of the underlying neoplasm. Rate of progression is slow and predominantly motor forms may be mistaken for ALS (page 551) associated with Hodgkin's and other lymphomas.

Rarely an acute neuropathy indistinguishable from postinfectious polyneuropathy occurs.

NECROTISING MYELOPATHY:

Flaccid paraplegia develops subacutely. Spinal MRI may show a swollen cord. Mechanism is uncertain.

MYOPATHY

Muscle weakness in malignancy takes several forms.

Proximal myopathy: A slowly progressive syndrome with weakness of proximal limb muscles.

Inflammatory myopathy (polymyositis/dermatomyositis) (see page 472):

The overall incidence of associated neoplasm in inflammatory myopathy is 15%. The typical patient is in middle age with a proximal weakness, elevated ESR and muscle enzymes with or without the skin features of dermatomyositis.

Myopathy with endocrine disturbance: Ectopic hormone production (by malignant cells) may induce a myopathy characterised by chronic progressive proximal weakness, e.g. ectopic ACTH production from small cell carcinoma of lung.

Cachetic myopathy occurs in terminally ill, wasted patients.

Investigation and treatment of non-metastatic syndromes
Successful treatment of the underlying tumour offers the only hope of improvement. The search must be exhaustive and repeated where first negative. Tumour markers (AFP, CEA, PSA etc), chest and abdominal CT, pelvic ultrasound, mammography are advised with PET (FDG) if available. Treatment with steroids, immunosuppressants (AZT, cyclosporine, etc), IVIG or plasma exchange is of uncertain benefit.

THE MYASTHENIC SYNDROME (Eaton-Lambert syndrome)

An autoimmune disorder of the neuromuscular junction. IgG voltage-gated calcium channel antibodies (VGCCAs) block the cholinergic synapse resulting in reduced acetylcholine release. The autonomic synapses are also affected. In men the association with underlying malignancy warrants detailed investigation (see above).

Clinical features
The patient develops weakness of lower then upper limbs with a tendency to fatigue. Following brief exercise, power may paradoxically suddenly improve – second wind phenomenon. In contrast to myasthenia gravis ocular and bulbar muscles are rarely affected. Examination reveals a proximal pattern of wasting and weakness with diminished tendon reflexes. Up to 50% of patients experience symptoms of autonomic (cholinergic) dysfunction – impotence, dry mouth and visual disturbance.

Diagnosis
Confirmed electrophysiologically; the 'second wind phenomenon' is shown up as an incrementing response to repetitive nerve stimulation (as opposed to the decrementing response in myasthenia gravis, page 482). VGCCAs are detected in serum.

Treatment
Guanidine hydrochloride and 4-aminopyridine enhance acetylcholine release. These treatments are effective but toxic. 3,4-diaminopyridine (less toxic), steroids, anticholinesterases, plasmapheresis or IVIG may help.

This syndrome may respond to the removal of the underlying neoplasm if present.

DEGENERATIVE DISORDERS

Introduction

This heterogeneous group of neurological diseases characterised by selective neuronal loss, is grouped together by the lack of known aetiology. As causes of such disease are identified (e.g. metabolic, viral) they have been reclassified in their appropriate category. Of the remaining conditions many are age related or familial and in some there is an identifiable genetic basis.

Characteristically these disorders:

– are gradually progressive
– are symmetrical (bilateral symptoms and signs)
– may affect one or several specific systems of the nervous system
– may demonstrate a specific pathology or just show neuronal atrophy and eventual loss without other features.

Classification

Degenerative disoders are classified according to the specific part or parts of the central/peripheral nervous system affected and according to the ensuing clinical manifestations. These degenerative disorders may be alternatively termed the system degenerations because of their propensity to affect only part of the nervous system.

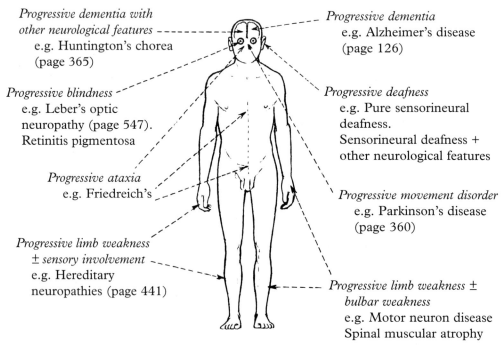

Progressive dementia with other neurological features
e.g. Huntington's chorea (page 365)

Progressive blindness
e.g. Leber's optic neuropathy (page 547).
Retinitis pigmentosa

Progressive ataxia
e.g. Friedreich's

Progressive limb weakness ± sensory involvement
e.g. Hereditary neuropathies (page 441)

Progressive dementia
e.g. Alzheimer's disease (page 126)

Progressive deafness
e.g. Pure sensorineural deafness.
Sensorineural deafness + other neurological features

Progressive movement disorder
e.g. Parkinson's disease (page 360)

Progressive limb weakness ± bulbar weakness
e.g. Motor neuron disease
Spinal muscular atrophy

Most of these conditions are discussed in other chapters.

PROGRESSIVE BLINDNESS

LEBER'S HEREDITARY OPTIC NEUROPATHY (LHON)

Leber's optic neuropathy is a familial disorder of maternal inheritance with a tendency to affect males significantly more than females. It is classified as a mitochondrial disorder due to DNA mutation (page 478). Most individuals have one of three point mutations of mitochondrial DNA (mtDNA).

Pathology

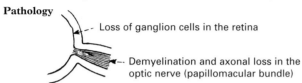

Loss of ganglion cells in the retina

Demyelination and axonal loss in the optic nerve (papillomacular bundle)

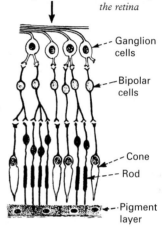

Light source   *The layers of the retina*

Ganglion cells

Bipolar cells

Cone

Rod

Pigment layer

Clinical features

Onset of visual loss in late teens/early twenties.
– Both eyes are simultaneously affected (rarely one eye months before the other).
– Central vision is lost with large bilateral scotomata.
Characteristically, blue/yellow colour discrimination is affected before red/green. The optic disc initially appears pink and swollen with an increase in small vessels, eventually becoming pale and atrophic.
Visual impairment progresses with peripheral construction of the fields.
Complete visual loss seldom occurs.
Associated symptoms and signs of a more generalised nervous system disorder occur in a proportion of cases – dementia, ataxia, progressive spastic paraplegia – and confusion with multiple sclerosis may arise. In contrast to bilateral optic neuritis, 'leakage' occurs with fluorescein angiography. Genetic counselling for LHON is complicated by the sex and age-dependent penetrance. The mother of an affected male has the mitochondrial mutation and may or may not have symptoms. No treatment exists. Quinone analogues (ubiquinone and idebenone) may help during periods of rapid visual worsening.

RETINITIS PIGMENTOSA

A heterogeneous hereditary disorder of the retina which may be inherited as an autosomal dominant, recessive or X-linked disorder. All layers of the retina are affected. Posterior pole cataracts and glaucoma are occasionally associated.

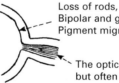

Loss of rods, degeneration of cones. Bipolar and ganglion cells are also affected. Pigment migrates to superficial layers

The optic nerve may show some gliosis, but often is remarkably normal.

Clinical features

Onset of visual loss in childhood. Both eyes are simultaneously affected. Initially there is a failure of twilight vision. The patient has difficulty in making his/her way as darkness falls (nyctalopia). The retina around the macular area is first affected resulting in a characteristic ring scotoma. This gradually spreads outwards; eventually only a small 'tunnel' of central vision is left. Finally, complete blindness occurs. The majority of patients are completely blind by 50 years of age. The fundal appearance is diagnostic as a result of the superficial migration of pigment.
The *electroretinogram* – recording the electrical activity of the retina – is eventually lost.

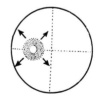

Treatment

None. Vitamins and steroids have been tried unsuccessfully.

Associated conditions in retinitis pigmentosa

Several conditions are associated with retinitis pigmentosa:
– Hypogonadism/obesity/mental deficiency
– Spinocerebellar ataxis
– Laurence Moon syndrome
– Friedreich's ataxia

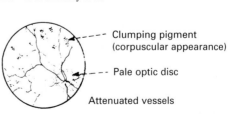

Clumping pigment (corpuscular appearance)

Pale optic disc

Attenuated vessels

The association with neuropathy and ataxia (NARP), or progressive external ophthalmoplegia and heart block (Kearns-Sayre syndrome) are due to mitochondrial disease (page 478).

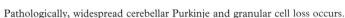

PROGRESSIVE ATAXIA

The degenerative disorders manifested by progressive ataxia are termed *spinocerebellar-ataxias*.

These may be classified by age of onset, presence of associated features, but increasingly by mode of inheritance.

RECESSIVELY INHERITED ATAXIAS

ATAXIA TELANGIECTASIA (Louis-Bar Syndrome)

This multisystem disorder is characterised by progressive cerebellar ataxia, ocular and cutaneous telangiectasia and immunodeficiency.

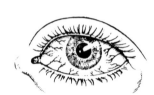

The gene maps to chromosome 11q23 associated with mutations in the ATM gene. The ATM protein is a member of the family of proteins involved in DNA repair.

Pathologically, widespread cerebellar Purkinje and granular cell loss occurs.

A progressive ataxia develops in infancy. Telangiectasia develops later, becoming more obvious after exposure to the sun. Prevalence similar to Freidrich's ataxia.

Patients are eventually confined to a wheelchair and, because of associated low serum immunoglobulin levels are susceptible to repetitive infections.

Malignant neoplasms (lymphoreticular tumours) occur in 10%.

Patients are unusually sensitive to X-rays. Treatment of malignancy with conventional dosages of radiation can prove fatal.

Death occurs in second or third decade from infection or malignancy (often lymphoma).

FRIEDREICH'S ATAXIA

Friedreich's ataxia is the commonest inherited ataxia with an incidence of 1/50000 in European populations and carrier frequency of 1/20.

It is caused by mutations in the FRDA gene located on chromosome 9 which encodes the protein Frataxin. It is the first autosomal recessive disease identified in which a triplet repeat expansion (GAA) is responsible.

Pathology:

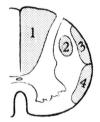

Spinal: The spinal cord is shrunken, especially in the thoracic region.

There is degeneration, demyelination and gliosis of:
  1. – Posterior columns.
  2. – Corticospinal tracts
  3. – Dorsal spinocerebellar tracts
  4. – Ventral spinocerebellar tracts.
Dorsal roots and peripheral nerves are shrunken in advanced cases.

Cerebellar: Changes in the cerebellum are less marked, there is Purkinje cell loss and atrophy of the dentate nucleus.

Peripheral nerves show loss of large myelinated axons and segmental demyelination. The corticobulbar tract and cerebrum are relatively spared.

RECESSIVELY INHERITED ATAXIA

FRIEDREICH'S ATAXIA (*cont'd*)

Clinical features

Friedreich's ataxia is characterised by progressive gait ataxia and limb incordination, hypertrophic cardiomyopathy and increased incidence of diabetes mellitus/impaired glucose tolerance.

Sexes are equally affected. Onset of symptoms is normally around puberty, and always before 25 years of age; most patients become wheelchair bound by their late twenties. Cardio-pulmonary failure is the usual common cause of death.

Disturbance of balance is the initial symptom, often associated with the development of scoliosis. A spastic, ataxic gait develops with inco-ordination of the limbs.

Corticospinal tract involvement results in limb weakness with absent abdominal reflexes and extensor plantar responses.

Posterior column involvement results in loss of vibration and proprioception in the extremities.

Dorsal root and *peripheral nerve* involvement results in absent lower limb reflexes.

Involvement of myocardial muscle (cardiomyopathy) is common and results in cardiac failure or dysrhythmias. *Musculoskeletal abnormalities* occur in 80% of cases.

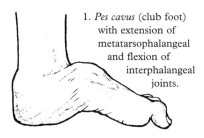

1. *Pes cavus* (club foot) with extension of metatarsophalangeal and flexion of interphalangeal joints.

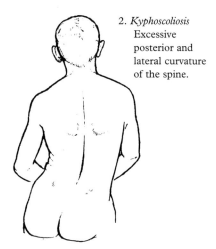

2. *Kyphoscoliosis* Excessive posterior and lateral curvature of the spine.

Optic atrophy and deafness coexist in many cases.

There is a clinical resemblance to mitochondrial encephalopathies as well as reduced respiratory enzyme activities in some patients (Friedreich's has been suspected to involve some degree of disturbance of mitochondrial respiration).

Investigation

Identification of the gene and availability of diagnostic testing has limited the value of other ancillary investigations such as imaging and neurophysiology. Regular cardiac assessment and monitoring of blood glucose is important.

Treatment

Although there is no specific treatment for Friedreich's ataxia, many of its symptoms can be managed. Orthopaedic intervention can alleviate scoliosis, and orthopaedic appliances and physical therapy help maintain ambulation. Cardiac problems can be successfully treated pharmacologically and insulin therapy may be necessary to control diabetes mellitus.

Other causes of areflexic ataxia

Abetalipoproteinaemia (Bassen Kornzweig disease)
- Malabsorption syndrome
- Acanthocytes (thorn-shaped red blood cells)
- Low serum cholesterol, triglycerides and fatty acids
- Low vitamin E.

Hexosaminidase deficiency
- Accumulation of GM_2 gangliosides in brain and skin.

Xeroderma pigmentatosum
- Sensitive to ultraviolet light
- Keratosis and skin cancer.

DOMINANTLY INHERITED AND OTHER ATAXIAS

Classification of the dominantly inherited, late-onset, cerebellar ataxias is complex and controversial. The term 'late-onset' is misleading given that these disorders may present in childhood and adolescence. Commonly other neurological features co-exist: ophthalmoplegia, optic atrophy, retinal pigmentation, deafness, dysarthria, dysphagia, dementia, extra pyramidal and pyramidal signs and peripheral neuropathy. This bewildering condition is classified into 3 different types.

	Autosomal dominant Cerebellar ataxia (ADCA) Type 1	Autosomal dominant Cerebellar ataxia (ADCA) Type 2	Autosomal dominant Cerebellar ataxia (ADCA) Type 3
Clinical features	Ataxia ± Ophthalmoplegia Mild dementia Optic atrophy Spasticity	Ataxia + Retinopathy (progressive visual loss) ± Dementia – extrapyramidal features	Ataxia (alone) – Age of onset > 50 years

At least 13 different gene loci have been reported to be responsible – the spinocerebellar ataxia or SCA mutations. SCA1, SCA2, SCA3 (also known as Machado-Joseph disease), SCA4, SCA5, SCA6, SCA7, SCA8, SCA10, SCA11, SCA12, SCA13, and SCA14. Causative genes have been identified as expansions of trinucleotide CAG repeat for SCA1, SCA2, SCA3, SCA6, SCA7, and SCA12, and the CTG repeat for SCA8. DNA testing is diagnostic though new loci remain to be discovered.

IDIOPATHIC LATE ONSET ATAXIA

Some may be new mutations of ADCA. For diagnosis all other causes of acquired ataxia – inflammatory, infective, nutritional, metabolic, endocrine and non-metastatic – must be excluded by appropriate investigations.

Type 1 – Age of onset 35–55 years – ataxia ± dementia, spasticity
Type 2 – Age of onset > 55 years – mid-line ataxia sparing speech/limbs
Type 3 – Age of onset 50–60 years – ataxia, titubation and tremor

THE HEREDITARY INTERMITTENT ATAXIAS

These disorders are characterized by brief paroxysmal episodes with no neurological impairment between attacks. Two types can be distinguished on the basis of the length of the attacks, the presence of myokymia (facial twitching), precipitating factors, response to acetazolamide and the nature of the genetic defect.

Type 1, attacks are precipitated by sudden movements, emotional stress, fatigue, exercise, or hunger. Stiffness, generalized myokymia, vertigo, nausea, diplopia and tremor also occur. The attacks last 10 minutes or less. This disorder is associated with a variety of point mutations in the voltage-gated potassium channel gene, KCNA1, located on chromosome 12p13.

Type 2, myokymia is absent, the prominent symptoms being ataxia of gait and limbs, dysarthria, and gaze-evoked nystagmus. The attacks begin abruptly and last from 15 minutes to a few hours though sometimes days. Emotional stress, physical exertion, but not movement trigger attacks. The carbonic anhydrase inhibitor acetazolamide is very effective in preventing attacks. This disorder is associated with mutations in CACNL1A4 (subunit of a voltage-gated calcium channel gene) located on chromosome 19p. SCA-6 is also associated with a small expansion of CAG repeats in this gene as is familial hemiplegic migraine, a condition sharing similar features.

MOTOR NEURON DISEASE/AMYOTROPHIC LATERAL SCLEROSIS (ALS)

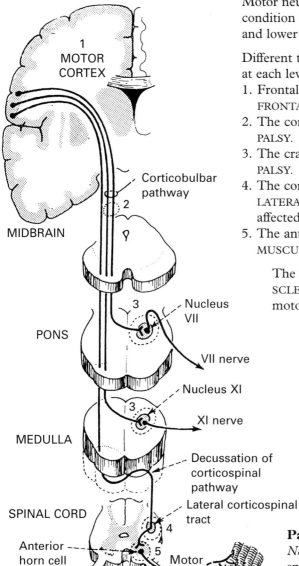

Motor neuron disease (MND) is a progressive condition characterised by degeneration of upper and lower motor neurons.

Different terms are used to describe involvement at each level:
1. Frontal atrophy in the precentral gyrus – FRONTAL DEMENTIA.
2. The corticobulbar pathway: PSEUDOBULBAR PALSY.
3. The cranial nerve nuclei: progressive BULBAR PALSY.
4. The corticospinal tract: (Called PRIMARY LATERAL SCLEROSIS when this tract alone is affected)
5. The anterior horn cell: PROGRESSIVE MUSCULAR ATROPHY.

The term AMYOTROPHIC LATERAL SCLEROSIS (ALS) is used synonymously with motor neuron disease.

Epidemiology
Incidence: 2 per 100 000 per year, with a prevalence of 6 per 100 000. Clusters and conjugal cases have been reported.
Familial ALS accounts for 5% of cases and is usually inherited as a dominant trait.
Sex ratio: male/female – 1.5:1
Mean age of onset – 55 years.
Mean survival – 3 years (50%).

Pathology
Naked eye: Thinning of anterior roots of spinal cord. Most noticeable in cervical and lumbosacral regions.

Microscopic: Loss of neurons in motor cortex.
Loss of neurons in cranial nerve nuclei and anterior horns.
Section of brain stem: reduction of corticobulbar and corticospinal fibres.
No evidence of inflammatory response is seen in involved structures.

551

MOTOR NEURON DISEASE/ALS

AETIOLOGY

The cause of motor neuron disease is unknown. Several possibilities have been suggested:

– **Genetic:** Mutations in the SOD1 gene (responsible for producing the enzyme superoxide dismutase) are found in 20% of familial cases of ALS. Superoxide dismutase is important in removing toxic superoxide radicals and converting them into non-harmful substances. Defects in the enzyme lead to accumulation and anterior horn cell death.

– **Viruses:** Chronic virus infection has been suggested. Polio virus will acutely damage the anterior horn cell and chronic polio infection could theoretically produce motor neuron disease. Some claim that motor neuron disease follows acute poliomyelitis; however, when this occurs the clinical picture is not typical and may resemble more closely Spinal Muscular Atrophy (see later). Polio antibody titres remain normal. Virus-like particles have been reported in some patients with MND, but transmission to non-human primates has been unsuccessful. HIV-associated ALS like syndromes with similar pathological evidence of anterior horn cell loss have raised the possibility that ALS could be due to retroviral infection (retroviruses persist by integration into the host's DNA and would be ideal suspects)

– **Toxins:** Certain metals, lead, selenium, mercury and manganese have been incriminated, but again evidence is inconclusive.

– **Minerals:** Clinical similarities between MND and neurological involvement in hyperparathyroidism and phosphate deficiency suggest a relationship with chronic calcium deficiency.

The final common pathway of anterior horn cell death, irrespective of what actually triggers the process, is a complex interaction of genetic factors, oxidative stress and glutamate excess (excitatory injury). Abnormal clumps of proteins (neurofilaments) can be found in motor neurons that may themselves be toxic or by-products of overwhelming cell injury. Calcium channel antibodies have been isolated and these further accelerate injury by stimulating additional glutamate release and intracellular calcium influx activating enzymes that promote additional cell damage.

CLINICAL FEATURES

At onset:
Asymmetric weakness and wasting of extremities – 75%
Bulbar or pseudobulbar features – 25% – dysphagia or dysarthria

Frontal dementia
This occurs in 3–5% of all patients, but is more prevalent in familial cases.

Pseudobulbar palsy
Features are due to degeneration of corticobulbar pathways to V, VII, X, XI and XII cranial nerve motor nuclei (with sparing of III, IV and VI).

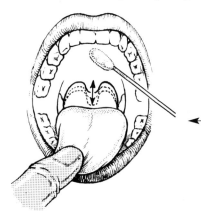

There is an apparent weakness of the muscles of mastication and expression, the patient has difficulty in chewing and the face is expressionless. The jaw jerk (page 15) is exaggerated.

Food and fluid enter nasopharynx when swallowing – palatal weakness (X).
Gag reflex is brisk when soft palate is stimulated.
Speech is drawling and monotonous.
Swallowing for solids is difficult (X).
Tongue is immobile, pointed and cannot protrude (XII).
Emotional lability – unprovoked outbursts of laughing or crying occur.

MOTOR NEURON DISEASE/ALS

Progressive bulbar palsy

The symptoms and signs are due to a disturbance of the motor cranial nuclei rather than corticobulbar tracts. The condition is distinguished from pseudobulbar palsy by the presence of lower motor neuron (nuclear) signs.

Atrophy and *fasciculations* are present in cranial nerve innervated muscles.

Fasciculations are visible muscle twitches which occur spontaneously and represent groups of discharging motor units.

The tongue appears wasted and folded; fibrillations produce a writhing appearance. Jaw jerk and gag reflex are absent.

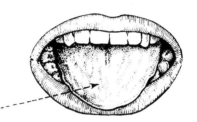

Corticospinal involvement

Signs of corticospinal tract disturbance with:
- Increased tone.
- Brisk reflexes.
- Extensor plantar responses.
- Distinctive distribution of weakness

(extensors in upper limbs; flexors in lower limbs).
Spasticity is rarely severe (intact extrapyramidal inhibition).

(Primary lateral sclerosis is a slowly progressive form of ALS restricted to the cortical spinal tract.)

Progressive muscular atrophy

Signs and symptoms are due to anterior horn cell involvement.
Atrophy, weakness and fasciculations are the cardinal features.

The patient is often aware of fasciculation.
Muscle cramps are common.
Weakness is not as severe as the degree of wasting suggests.

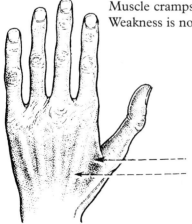

In the hand: wasting is evident.
1st dorsal interosseous muscle and tendons become prominent as hand muscles waste, giving 'guttered' appearance – SKELETON HAND.

As the disease progresses, all levels of the motor system become involved. Respiratory muscle weakness ultimately occurs and is the usual cause of death.

MOTOR NEURON DISEASE/ALS

Differential diagnosis includes disorders which produce combined upper and lower motor neuron signs, e.g.

Cervical spondylosis

Spinal tumours.

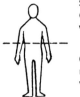

Segmental (LMN signs) weakness

Corticospinal muscle weakness

Hexosaminidase deficiency (autosomal recessive disorder) may mimic ALS.

An ALS like syndrome can occur with *elevated serum paraproteins, lymphoproliferative disease, lead poisoning and HIV infection.*

Hyperthyroidism and *hyperparathyroidism* produce muscle wasting and hyperreflexia.

Pseudobulbar palsy may result also from cerebrovascular disease or multiple sclerosis.

Progressive muscular atrophy may be confused with a spinal muscular atrophy, limb girdle dystrophy, diabetic amyotrophy or lead neuropathy.

N.B. IN MOTOR NEURON DISEASE: – *Sensory signs do not occur*

         – *Bladder is never involved*

         – *Ocular muscles are never affected.*

Investigations

EMG reveals denervation with fibrillation.

Nerve conduction studies shows normal velocities and exclude in all limbs multifocal neuropathy with conduction block.

MRI (or myelography) where appropriate excludes foramen magnum or spinal cord compression.

Thyroid and calcium studies exclude endocrine or metabolic disease.

In selected cases screen for paraproteinaemia, lymphoreticular disease and hexosaminidase deficiency.

MOTOR NEURON DISEASE/ALS

Diagnostic criteria (El Escorial criteria for MND/ALS – World Federation of Neurology)

Presence of –
  LMN signs in at least 2 limbs.
  UMN signs in at least 1 region (bulbar/cervical/lumbosacral)
  Progression of disease.

Absence of –
  Sensory signs.
  Neurogenic sphincter disturbance.
  Other clinically evident CNS/PNS disease.
  Exclusion of ALS-like syndromes

TREATMENT

Treatment is primarily that of managing symptoms and supporting both patient and family as these progress and their needs change.

Counselling is essential to a full understanding of the illness and its natural history. Support from a Nurse Specialist is invaluable to meeting the challenges of each phase of illness and issues of feeding and methods of ventilatory support are best discussed well in advance so that informed decisions can be made. The comprehensive care of patients is challenging with medical, legal and ethical considerations.

Symptomatic treatment:

Anarthria and dysarthria: – Speech assessment and communication aids when indicated.
Dysphagia and aspiration: – Percutaneous endoscopic gastrostomy (PEG).
Nutrition: – Estimate calorific content and supplement diet with vitamins.
Muscle weakness: – Physiotherapy, walking aids. Splints, etc.
Respiratory failure: – As vital capacity drops respiratory failure becomes inevitable. Non-invasive ventilatory assistance should be considered, if requested, when this falls below 70%. Mechanical ventilation should only be provided in those who insist upon it. Rarely ALS can present with early respiratory failure before treatment issues have been discussed. This creates a major management dilemma.

Disease-modifying treatment

Riluzole is a drug with energy buffering and anti-glutamate properties. It is the only approved treatment and in a dose of 100 mg daily is safe with a marginal effect in prolonging survival by 2 months.

Recombinant human insulin-like growth factor requires further evaluation. Anti retroviral treatment (Indinavir) is currently under trial. Recent research suggests that anti-oxidant drugs may be beneficial but a greater understanding of the molecular basis of this illness is required to design more promising treatments.

INHERITED MOTOR NEURON DISORDERS

SPINAL MUSCULAR ATROPHIES (SMAs)

Spinal muscular atrophy is the second most common fatal, autosomal recessive disease in Caucasians (after cystic fibrosis). The disorder is characterised by degeneration of the anterior horn cells and symmetrical muscle weakness and wasting.

Depending on the age of onset, degree of muscular involvement and length of survival, 3 types of recessive SMA are recognised: All map to the gene locus 5q12.2-q13.3.

With an incidence of 1/10 000, the offspring of patients have a disease risk of approximately 1%.

Type I – Werdnig Hoffman disease (Acute Infantile SMA)

This is an autosomal recessive disorder.
Incidence 1:25 000 births

Clinical features:

Reduced fetal movements in late pregnancy with weakness and hypotonia at birth.
Swallowing and sucking are impaired
The child lies with arms and legs abducted
and externally rotated (hypotonic posture) ⎫
Contractures, wasting and fasciculation ⎬ different from other
gradually become evident ⎭ causes of 'floppy' infant.
All motor milestones are delayed; 95% of all patients are dead by 18 months.

Type II – Kugelberg Welander disease (Late infantile or juvenile SMA)

Pathological features similar to Werdnig Hoffman disease.

Clinical features:

Limb girdle muscles affected.

It is slowly progressive with great variability even within the same family. Median age at death 12 years. Survival to adulthood occurs in the dominant form.

Type III (Adult onset SMA)

Onset between 2nd and 5th decade with progressive limb girdle weakness. Distinction from progressive muscular atrophy form of ALS is difficult. A benign course supports the former.

Distal and scapuloperoneal forms

Differentiation from HMSN types I and II (page 441) and scapuloperoneal dystrophy (page 467) is clinically difficult and separation may only be possible on histological and neurophysiological grounds.

Spinal and bulbar muscular atrophy (Kennedy's syndrome)

X-linked adult-onset neurogenic muscular atrophy with late distal and bulbar involvement (Gene Locus: Xq11-q12). Onset of fasciculations followed by muscle weakness and wasting occur at approximately 40 years of age. Bulbar signs and facial fasciculations are characteristic. Babinski sign is negative. The disorder is compatible with long life.

Management of spinal muscular atrophies

There is no specific treatment. Care is supportive. Genetic counselling is essential.

NEUROCUTANEOUS SYNDROMES

Previously called Phakomatoses – Phakos Greek: birthmark
These disorders are hereditary, characterised by multiorgan malformations and tumours. The literature includes many varieties of such conditions; most are extremely rare. Only the more major disorders are described below.

NEUROFIBROMATOSIS
Two distinct types occur:

Type 1 (NF1)
Characterised by café au lait spots and neurofibromas (Von Recklinghausen's disease).
Incidence: 1:4000
Inheritance: Autosomal dominant
Gene localised to 17q22

Type 2 (NF2)
Characterised by tumours (schwannomas) of the eighth cranial nerve (vestibular division).
1:50 000
Autosomal dominant
Gene localised to chromosome 22.

Pathology (type 1):

An embryological disorder in which localised overgrowth of *mesodermal* or *ectodermal* tissue produces tumours of:

| meninges | vascular system | skin, viscera | peripheral and central nervous systems |

Pathology (type 2): See page 395
Clinical features (type 1):
Skin manifestations: – Café au lait spots:
light brown patches on the trunk with well demarcated edges.
Subcutaneous neurofibromata lying along peripheral nerves and enlarging with age.
Mollusca fibrosa:
cutaneous fibromas – large, pedunculated and pink in colour.
Plexiform neuroma:
diffuse neurofibroma associated with skin and subcutaneous overgrowth and occasional underlying bony abnormality.
Skeletal manifestations: – 50% of patients exhibit scoliosis.
Subperiosteal neurofibromas may give rise to bone hypertrophy or rarification with pathological fractures.
Sphenoid wing dysplasia is a rare but diagnostic abnormality.
Ocular: – Lisch nodules are melanocytic hamartomas of the iris and are seen on slit-lamp examination in 90% of patients
Neoplasia: – A high incidence of leukaemia, neuroblastoma, medullary thyroid carcinoma, and multiple endocrine neoplasia occurs.
Neurological manifestations: – Mental retardation and epilepsy occur in 10–15% of patients without intracranial neoplasm.

Cerebrovascular accidents as a consequence of intimal hyperplasia are not uncommon. Three patterns of neurological neoplasia are recognised:

1. *Intracranial neoplasms:*
   Optic nerve glioma
   Multiple meningioma.

2. *Intraspinal neoplasms:*
   Meningioma
   Neurofibroma
   Glioma.

3. *Peripheral nerve neoplasms:*
   Neurofibroma – a proportion of which become sarcomatous.

Clinical features (type 2)
Skeletal manifestations are absent. Café au lait spots rare. Posterior subcapsular cataracts occur in 50% of cases. The condition is defined by bilateral vestibular schwannomas but may present as early unilateral acoustic neuroma plus a family history of NF2. Other intracranial and intraspinal neoplasms occur.

NEUROCUTANEOUS SYNDROMES

NEUROFIBROMATOSIS (cont'd)

Diagnosis

A family history is obtained in over 50% of patients. In type 1, the cutaneous manifestations are characteristic, though they may be extremely mild with only café au lait spots (more than 6 in an individual is diagnostic). As a rule, the more florid the cutaneous manifestations the less likely is there nervous system involvement. CT scanning, MRI and myelography may be necessary when nervous system involvement is suspected. Type 2 is diagnosed when imaging (MRI) confirms bilateral vestibular schwannomas. The recent cloning of the type 2 gene to chromosome 22 may lead to direct gene testing in persons at risk.

Treatment

Plexiform neuromas may be removed for cosmetic reasons. The management of intracranial and intraspinal tumours has already been discussed.

TUBEROUS SCLEROSIS

Incidence: 1:30 000.
Autosomal dominant inheritance with high sporadic mutation rate. Linkage studies suggest loci on chromosome 9 (TSC.1) and 16 (TSC.2).

Characterised by cutaneous, neurologic, renal, skeletal, cardiac and pulmonary abnormalities.

Pathology

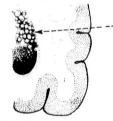

An embryological disorder.
Hard gliotic 'tubers' arise anywhere within the hemisphere but commonly around the ventricles. Projection into the ventricles produces a typical appearance like 'dripping candle wax'.

Tubers in the brain result from ⟶ Transition may occur
astrocytic overgrowth with large from gliosis to a
vacuolated cells and loss of subependymal
surrounding myelin. astrocytoma.

As well as skin lesions, primitive renal tumours and cystic lung hamartomas occur.

Clinical features

Skin manifestations

The cutaneous lesions are characteristic – adenoma sebaceum, a red raised papular-like rash over the nose, cheeks and skin, appears towards the end of the 1st year, though occasionally as late as the 5th year.
Depigmented areas on the trunk resembling vitiligo are common (Shagreen patch).
Fibromas and café au lait spots occur occasionally. Teeth are pitted.

Neurological manifestations: – Mental retardation is present in 60% of patients, though the onset and its recognition may be delayed.
Seizures occur in almost all patients, often as early as the 1st week of life. Attacks are initially focal motor and eventually become generalised. The response to anticonvulsants is variable.
Intracranial neoplasms – astrocytomas – arise from tubers usually close to the ventricles and may result in an obstructive hydrocephalus.
Neoplasia: – Renal carcinoma occurs in 50% of patients. Retinal tumours (hamartomas) and muscle tumours (rhabdomyomas) are common, the latter often involving the heart.

Diagnosis:

The presence of epilepsy and adenoma sebaceum is diagnostic.

CT scan may show subependymal areas of calcium deposition. MRI shows uncalcified subependymal tubers. Other developmental abnormalities may be evident, e.g. microgyria.

Treatment:

Anticonvulsant therapy for epilepsy. Surgical removal of symptomatic lesions. High mutation rate indicates that antenatal diagnosis will not significantly reduce incidence.

NEUROCUTANEOUS SYNDROMES

STURGE-WEBER SYNDROME

This disorder is characterised by a facial angioma associated with a leptomeningeal venous angioma. There is no clear pattern of inheritance. Practically all cases are sporadic.

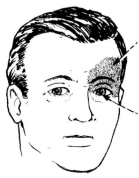

CAPILLARY NAEVUS or 'port wine stain' usually involving forehead and eyelid conforming to the 1st or 1st and 2nd divisions of the trigeminal nerve.

EYE DISORDERS are common -buphthalmos (congenital glaucoma), choroidal angioma.

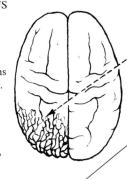

Thickened leptomeninges, commonly ipsilateral to the facial naevus and full of abnormal vessels, overlie an ATROPHIC HEMISPHERE with degenerative changes and vascular calcification usually most marked in the parieto-occipital vessels.

EPILEPSY occurs in 75% usually presenting in infancy.

HEMIPARESIS, HOMONYMOUS HEMIANOPIA occur in 30%.
BEHAVIOURAL DISORDER AND MENTAL RETARDATION occur in 50%.

Skull X-rays show parallel linear calcification (tram-line sign) and CT scan, in addition, shows the associated atrophic change. Angiography demonstrates dilated deep cerebral veins with decreased cortical drainage. Arteriovenous and dural venous sinus malformations are present in 30%.

Treatment

Intractable epilepsy may require lobectomy, or even hemispherectomy. Some recommend early excision of the surface lesion, but the rarity of the condition prevents thorough treatment evaluation.

VON HIPPEL-LINDAU DISEASE

An autosomal dominant disorder in which haemangioblastomas are found in the cerebellum, spinal canal and retina, and are associated with a number of visceral pathologies:
- – Renal angioma
- – Renal cell carcinoma
- – Phaeochromocytoma
- – Pancreatic adenoma/cyst
- – Cysts and haemangiomas in liver and epididymis.

Mutation in a tumour suppressor gene is found in 60% of affected families. Any of the above may produce signs and symptoms.

Retinal haemangioblastoma is seen on fundoscopy 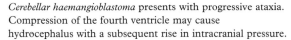 and may produce sudden blindness. These often produce the earliest clinical manifestation of disease. Confirm with fluorescin angiography and treat with cryosurgery or photocoagulation.

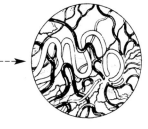

Cerebellar haemangioblastoma presents with progressive ataxia. Compression of the fourth ventricle may cause hydrocephalus with a subsequent rise in intracranial pressure.

Spinal canal haemangioblastoma – intradural or intramedullary lesion presenting with signs and symptoms of cord or root compression.

Diagnosis is established from family history and cranial imaging (MRI or CT). Renal ultrasound, abdominal CT and urinary amine estimations are required to complete the evaluation. In patients at risk, regular screening for renal, adrenal, pancreatic and intracranial tumours is recommended.

ATAXIA TELANGIECTASIA – see page 548.

BRADLEY, W. et al (eds) (2000) Neurology in Clinical Practice, 3rd Edition, Butterworth-Heinemann, Oxford.

GRAHAM, D.I., LANTOS, P. L. (eds) (2002) Greenfield's Neuropathology, 7th Edition, Arnold, London.

KLEIHUES, P., CAVENEE, W.K. (eds) (2000) Pathology and Genetics of Tumours of the Nervous System. WHO Classification of Tumours. IARC Press, Lyon.

PATTEN, J.P. (1995) Neurological Differential Diagnosis, 2nd Edition, Springer, London.

ROWLAND, L. (ed) (2000) Merritt's Neurology, 10th Edition, Lippincott, Williams & Wilkins, Philadelphia.

SAMUELS, M. (ed) (1999) Manual of Neurologic Therapeutics, 6th Edition, Lippincott, Williams & Wilkins, Philadelphia.

WINN, H.R., YOUMANS, J.R. (2003) Youmans Neurological Surgery, 5th Edition, Saunders, London.

INDEX